T0295210

Techniques in Small Animal Wound Management

Techniques in Small Animal Wound Management

Edited by

Nicole J. Buote DVM, DACVS-SA
ACVS Founding Fellow Minimally Invasive Surgery (Soft Tissue)
Associate Professor
Department of Clinical Sciences
Small Animal Surgery Section
Soft Tissue Service
Cornell University School of Veterinary Medicine
Ithaca, NY, USA

WILEY Blackwell

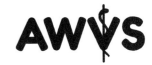

Copyright © 2024 by John Wiley & Sons Inc. All rights reserved.

Published by John Wiley & Sons, Inc., Hoboken, New Jersey.
Published simultaneously in Canada.

No part of this publication may be reproduced, stored in a retrieval system, or transmitted in any form or by any means, electronic, mechanical, photocopying, recording, scanning, or otherwise, except as permitted under Section 107 or 108 of the 1976 United States Copyright Act, without either the prior written permission of the Publisher, or authorization through payment of the appropriate per-copy fee to the Copyright Clearance Center, Inc., 222 Rosewood Drive, Danvers, MA 01923, (978) 750-8400, fax (978) 750-4470, or on the web at www.copyright.com. Requests to the Publisher for permission should be addressed to the Permissions Department, John Wiley & Sons, Inc., 111 River Street, Hoboken, NJ 07030, (201) 748-6011, fax (201) 748-6008, or online at http://www.wiley.com/go/permission.

Trademarks: Wiley and the Wiley logo are trademarks or registered trademarks of John Wiley & Sons, Inc. and/or its affiliates in the United States and other countries and may not be used without written permission. All other trademarks are the property of their respective owners. John Wiley & Sons, Inc. is not associated with any product or vendor mentioned in this book.

Limit of Liability/Disclaimer of Warranty: While the publisher and author have used their best efforts in preparing this book, they make no representations or warranties with respect to the accuracy or completeness of the contents of this book and specifically disclaim any implied warranties of merchantability or fitness for a particular purpose. No warranty may be created or extended by sales representatives or written sales materials. The advice and strategies contained herein may not be suitable for your situation. You should consult with a professional where appropriate. Neither the publisher nor author shall be liable for any loss of profit or any other commercial damages, including but not limited to special, incidental, consequential, or other damages. Further, readers should be aware that websites listed in this work may have changed or disappeared between when this work was written and when it is read. Neither the publisher nor authors shall be liable for any loss of profit or any other commercial damages, including but not limited to special, incidental, consequential, or other damages.

This textbook is dedicated to my family, whom I love the most and the best. Thank you for pushing me, for supporting me, and understanding me.

To my parents, Robert and Sharon, thank you for always urging me to think big and work hard. I have not and will not "settle."

Nathan, thank you for all your support during the creation of this book. I know it has been hard, and I couldn't have done it without you.

To my boys, William and Nicholas, thank you for all the hugs and support and for making me take a break occasionally. I hope you see the value in all this hard work. Love you best.

Contents

List of Contributors

Angela C. Banz, DVM, DACVS
VCA Northwest Veterinary Specialists
Clackamas, OR, USA

Cheryl Braswell, DACVECC, CHT-C, CVPP, CHPV
Spring City, TN, USA

Nicole J. Buote, DVM, DACVS-SA
ACVS Founding Fellow, Minimally Invasive
Surgery (Soft Tissue)
Department of Clinical Sciences
Cornell University
Ithaca, NY, USA

Ryan P. Cavanaugh, DVM, DACVS-SA
ACVS Founding Fellow, Surgical Oncology
Associate Professor of Small Animal Surgery
Ross University School of Veterinary Medicine
St. Kitts, West Indies

Colin Chik, DVM
Department of Clinical Sciences
Cornell University
Ithaca, NY, USA

Kristin A. Coleman, DVM, MS, DACVS-SA
Gulf Coast Veterinary Specialists
Houston, TX, USA

James D. Crowley, BVSc
Small Animal Specialist Hospital
Sydney, Australia

Rebecca M. Harman, PhD
Department of Microbiology and Immunology
Baker Institute for Animal Health
Cornell University
Ithaca, NY, USA

Galina Hayes, BVSc, PhD, DACVECC, DACVS
Department of Clinical Sciences
Cornell University
Ithaca, NY, USA

Celine S. Kermanian, DVM
VCA West Los Angeles Animal Hospital
Los Angeles, CA, USA

M.S. Amarendhra Kumar, BVSc., MVSc., MS, PhD
Department of Medical Education
Tufts University Schools of Medicine
and Dental Medicine
Boston, MA, USA

Daniel J. Lopez, DVM, DACVS-SA
Department of Clinical Sciences
Cornell University
Ithaca, NY, USA

Jill K. Luther, DVM, MS, DACVS-SA
Heartland Veterinary Surgery, LLC
Columbia, MO, USA

Brian Marchione, DVM, DACVO
Ocuvet Inc., Los Angeles, CA, USA

Megan Mickelson, DVM, DACVS-SA
ACVS Fellow of Surgical Oncology
College of Veterinary Medicine
University of Missouri
Columbia, MO, USA

Nathan Peterson, DVM, MS, DACVECC
Department of Clinical Sciences
Cornell University
Ithaca, NY, USA

Kathryn A. Pitt, DVM, MS, DACVS-SA
ACVS Fellow, Surgical Oncology
Wanderlust Veterinary Services
Academic and Private Practice Locum

Aarthi Rajesh, PhD
Department of Microbiology and Immunology
Baker Institute for Animal Health
Cornell University
Ithaca, NY, USA

Desiree D. Rosselli, DVM, DACVS-SA
VCA West Los Angeles Animal Hospital
Los Angeles, CA, USA

Bryden J. Stanley, BVMS, MANZCVS, MVetSc, MRCVS, Diplomate ACVS
Animal Surgical Center of Michigan
Flint, MI, USA

Julia P. Sumner, BVSc, DACVS-SA
Small Animal Specialist Hospital
Sydney, Australia

Gerlinde R. Van de Walle, DVM, PhD
Department of Microbiology and Immunology
Baker Institute for Animal Health
Cornell University
Ithaca, NY, USA

Foreword

It is with great pleasure that I write this foreword for the outstanding textbook, *Techniques in Small Animal Wound Management*, edited by Dr. Nicole J. Buote. I am acutely aware of the impact full-thickness wounding has on our small animal patients as well as how profoundly devastating and overwhelming it is for owners to be faced with the seemingly monumental task of restoring pain-free function to their much-loved family member. Our competence and confidence in effectively managing a challenging open wound play an essential role for the health and well-being of both patients and owners.

Wound management is both science and art, and as veterinarians, we are often faced with many complex issues, commonly requiring a multidisciplinary approach. Appropriate management of the wound and periwound until both are healthy is the first crucial step. Only then can clinicians choose the optimal reconstructive technique which is critical to successful healing. The choices we face at each step can at times appear too numerous and bewildering. The field is constantly evolving, requiring the unwavering commitment of wound care practitioners to maintaining an open mind, and researching newer therapies and modalities. Each wound is different, and each patient presents a unique set of challenges and complications. Every owner is different, and communication becomes a vital part of the journey. This remarkable compendium offers a comprehensive and insightful guide that will undoubtedly become a cornerstone in the education of veterinary students, veterinarians, and specialists alike, instilling knowledge and confidence. Dr. Buote, with her vision and dedication, has brought together a formidable assembly of experts who have collectively amassed and generously shared their knowledge.

"*Techniques in Small Animal Wound Management*" is well-structured, beginning with a solid foundation in anatomical considerations, principles of wound healing, and factors influencing this intricate and fascinating progression. Understanding how a wound heals is essential, as it forms the bedrock upon which successful wound management strategies are built. Wound complications are, unfortunately, a reality, and this textbook equips readers with the knowledge and skills to recognize and address them appropriately – a necessary reminder for us to maintain adaptability and critical thinking. Wound terminology is nuanced, and this textbook clearly outlines how we classify wounds, how we describe wounds, and the language of wound closure. Effective communication among veterinary professionals is indispensable, and understanding the terminology is the bridge that connects us in our pursuit of excellence.

The journey through this book continues with a comprehensive exploration of the initial evaluation of the patient and the wound, emphasizing the all-important basic tenets of initial wound management, which are so critical for laying the groundwork for effective wound care. The book progresses to discussing a plethora of topical treatments, dressings, and bandages, providing insights into the latest advancements in wound care. The chapters on topical treatments and dressings, ranging from traditional to cutting-edge biologic and regenerative therapies, exemplify the evolving nature of wound management in veterinary medicine. These exciting newer therapies hold the promise of not only accelerating healing but also improving the overall quality of the repaired tissues.

The art of reconstructing wounds is an intricate endeavor full of decision-making, and the latter part of the textbook offers a solid guide to mastering variously shaped wounds, tension-relieving techniques, skin flaps, and free grafting. These skills are critical in the pursuit of a robust wound closure with excellent functional outcomes, and becoming familiar with such procedures greatly improves our competence. The inclusion of a chapter covering specific wound types, including several case studies, serves as a valuable tool, guiding readers through real-life scenarios and underscoring the unique nature of every wound and the necessity of individualized care.

Each wound, each patient, each owner, is a journey to be undertaken and a family story waiting to be told. It is our responsibility to guide that journey safely to the best possible outcome so that the story can be told well. Dr. Buote's *Techniques in Small Animal Wound Management* will facilitate veterinarians' ability to be successful in this responsibility. In closing, I extend my heartfelt gratitude to Dr. Nicole Buote and the contributors of this extraordinary textbook. Your dedication to the advancement of small animal wound management is evident on every page, and your commitment to spreading knowledge and improving care is inspiring.

8 October 2023

Bryden J. Stanley, BVMS, MANZCVS, MVetSc, MRCVS, Diplomate ACVS

Preface

Since the origin of medical practice, wound management has been critical to human and animal survival. Beginning with the Barber Surgeons of Henry V through the robotic surgeons of today, the treatment of wounds has captivated students, clinicians, and researchers. Whether you are a general practitioner, an emergency doctor, or a specialist, wounds will likely comprise a consistent part of your practice. The ability to assess and successfully treat wounds is therefore one of the most important skills you as a veterinarian can possess. The treatments available for wounds are as varied as their causes, and the complexity of their management is often challenging, leaving clinicians either elated or frustrated. These cases test a doctor's examination skills, clinical decision-making, and client communication. Clinicians of all experience levels require up-to-date information to ensure the best outcomes for their patients.

Even if wound management is a daily occurrence in your practice, the volume of new information published on a yearly basis can be overwhelming. There are already amazing resources on the biology of wounds and reconstruction techniques. We hope to complement these texts with the most current information in clinically relevant, easy-to-read sections. This textbook offers a depth of anatomy and physiology knowledge that is emphasized with clinical case examples and specific treatment recommendations in an effort to provide "something for everyone." Some information, such as the stages of wound healing, wound terminology, and initial evaluation, is a requirement for any text on wounds and can be found within; but we have added in-depth chapters on the anatomy of tissues most often affected by wounds and common complications that clinicians are likely to encounter to provide important clinical context. Many authors in this book are leaders in the field, publishing ground-breaking research on the treatments they discuss and providing insight from years of experience. On a specific note, this textbook includes 14 chapters on specific wound types, delivering detailed information about unique wound characteristics, treatment recommendations, and prognosis. While some chapters necessarily delve into advanced techniques (e.g. hyperbaric oxygen therapy, negative pressure wound therapy, stem cells, etc.), this text also includes hundreds of photographs and illustrations describing the basics of bandaging, drain placement, and the reconstructive techniques a recent graduate may need.

As wound treatments continue to evolve, so will this book, and we hope the online resources and videos add value for our readers. It is my intent to add updated references and product lists on a yearly basis to supplement the information contained in this textbook in between editions since wound management changes rapidly. I believe that giving back to the veterinary community is important; therefore, a portion of the proceeds from the sale of this book will be donated to the Association of Women Veterinary Surgeons (AWVS, www.awvs.org), an organization intent on supporting female surgeons and house officers to ensure they succeed and thrive. A textbook of this type is not produced solely by the editor, and I want to extend my deepest gratitude to every contributor for their tireless work as well as many of my colleagues at Cornell University who provided chapters, pictures, drawings, and encouragement. The time and energy spent to better prepare students, residents, and our colleagues is well worth it, and we hope this textbook helps you care for your patients and clients for years to come.

Knowing what must be done does away with fear.
—*Rosa Parks*

Nicole J. Buote, DVM, DACVS-SA
ACVS Founding Fellow Minimally Invasive Surgery (Soft Tissue)
Associate Professor
Department of Clinical Sciences,
Small Animal Surgery Section,
Soft Tissue Service,
Cornell University School of Veterinary Medicine,
930 Campus Road,
Ithaca, NY 14853, USA
E-mail address: Njb235@cornell.edu

About the Companion Website

This book is accompanied by a companion website:

www.wiley.com/go/buote/wounds

The website includes:

- Videos that are supplementary to the script.

1

The Skin

M.S. Amarendhra Kumar

Department of Medical Education, Tufts University Schools of Medicine and Dental Medicine, Boston, MA, USA

The **integument** comprises the skin and its appendages (referred to as the **adnexa**), including structures such as hair, glands, digital pads, and claws [1–3]. The adnexal structures are of epidermal origin; they are continuous with the epidermal layer of the skin, supported by the underlying connective tissue.

Skin: The **skin** (**cutis**) is one of the body's largest and most important organs, for it forms a protective layer against the external environment and plays a crucial role in homeostasis. It is composed of three layers [4], the epidermis, dermis, and hypodermis (or subcutis), all firmly attached to each other. Important differences between cats and dogs exist (Table 1.1) and effect the healing properties and treatment options available when managing injuries. Skin transmits various stimuli from the external environment to the central nervous system (CNS). The nerve fibers carrying these stimuli penetrate the tissues (muscles and fascia) underlying the hypodermis and travel to the CNS, often within the fascial planes that ultimately merge with the periosteum of the appendicular and axial skeletal elements (Figure 1.1). Fascial planes form distinct compartments for individual muscles in many regions of the body. The skin's vascular components travel by similar routes and are responsible for maintaining body temperature within physiologic limits and regulating systemic blood pressure.

Epidermis: The epidermis of the skin is avascular and serves as the outermost protective layer of the body (Figure 1.2). It minimizes trans-epidermal water loss, prevents invasion by infectious agents and other harmful substances, absorbs ultraviolet radiation by the melanocytes, and aids in Vitamin D biosynthesis. The basic structure of the epidermis is similar in all domesticated mammals with some minor regional and species differences. The thickness of the epidermis is inversely proportional to the density of the hair coat. In dogs and cats, since most of the skin surface is covered with hair, the epidermis is relatively thin. In the dog, the epidermis consists of two to three layers of living cells increasing to 10 layers [5–7] while in the cat, the epidermis is slightly thinner. The average time for epidermal turnover is 22 days in carnivores regardless of the thickness of the epidermis [8, 9]. Dermal papillae are small fingerlike extensions into the epidermis, surrounded by rete ridges of the epidermis. These two structures interlock with each other, anchoring the epidermis. Epidermal rete ridges are absent in most of the skin in carnivore skin due to the dense haircoat [10, 11]. The hair follicles extend into the dermis, firmly anchoring the epidermis. In sparsely haired regions such as the scrotum, inguinal, and axillary areas, the epidermis is slightly thicker and epidermal rete ridges may be observed. The term **glabrous skin** is applied to areas devoid of hairs, such as the nasal plane, lips, and genitals as well as parts of the limb extremities such as digital pads. These regions may have several layers of living keratinocytes, prominent basement membranes, and form epidermal rete ridges [10].

The epidermal layer rests upon a meshwork of extracellular fibers (**dermal–epidermal junction**) upon which the keratinocytes rest, called the **basement membrane** (or **basal lamina**), which is acellular and avascular (Figure 1.2). If the basement membrane is disrupted, as with a skin wound, other cells (such as activated fibroblasts and neutrophils) will pass through it from beneath to participate in healing processes, forming scars, extending capillary loops, and developing granulation beds. Otherwise, the basal lamina remains impassable. Beneath it is the dermis, the vascularized second layer of the skin.

Nonkeratinocytes: Several cell types are contained in these two major layers of the skin (the epidermis and dermis). The most common cells within the epidermis are **keratinocytes**, making up 85% of all epidermal cells. The nonkeratinocytes account for approximately 15% of the epidermis and include the melanocytes, tactile epithelioid cells (*Merkel cells*), and

Techniques in Small Animal Wound Management, First Edition. Edited by Nicole J. Buote.
© 2024 John Wiley & Sons, Inc. Published 2024 by John Wiley & Sons, Inc.
Companion website: www.wiley.com/go/buote/wounds

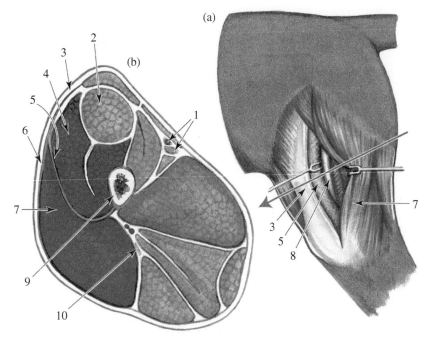

Figure 1.1 (a) Lateral approach to the shaft of the femur is shown. The fascia lata is split along the cranial margin of the biceps femoris m. (b) Cross-sectional view of left thigh. Note the location of nerves and blood vessels between the fascial planes. 1, Femoral artery and vein; 2, Rectus femoris m; 3, Fascia lata; 4, Vastus lateralis m; 5, Deeper lamina of fascia lata which runs between the vastus lateralis and biceps femoris muscles and reaches the shaft of the femur. The biceps femoris and vastus lateralis are therefore separated along this plane to reach the femur shaft; 6, Superficial lamina of fascia lata; 7, Biceps femoris; 8, Lateral shaft of femur; 9, Sciatic nerve.

intraepidermal macrophages (or *Langerhans* cells). **Melanocytes** are derived from neural crest cells. **Dendritic cells** (DCs) are a heterogeneous group of antigen-presenting leukocytes with a common origin that play an important role in the activation of the immune system. These cells have potent antigen-presenting capabilities with characteristic dendritic morphology. Three main cutaneus DC populations have been described: intraepidermal Langerhans cells (LCs), dermal myeloid DCs, and dermal plasmacytoid DCs (pDCs). The **intraepidermal macrophages (*Langerhans cells*)** are interspersed among the much more numerous keratinocytes (Figure 1.3) and act as antigen-presenting cells [13]. The LCs are one type of antigen-presenting DCs involved in cutaneus hypersensitivity reactions. They are capable of inducing

Table 1.1 Summary of skin differences between dogs and cats.

Item	Dog	Cat
Number of living epidermal cell layers	2–3 in most places, up to 10 layers in some places	Fewer layers of living epidermal cells
Merkel cell carcinoma	Relatively benign	Relatively aggressive
Melanocytes	More numerous	Fewer
Angiosomes (cutaneus perforating vessels)	Greater number of cutaneus perforating vessels in dermis/hypodermis	Fewer number of cutaneus perforating vessels in dermis/hypodermis
The density of tertiary and higher-order vessels	Higher density of tertiary and higher-order vessels	A lower density of tertiary and higher-order vessels
Hairs	Fewer secondary hairs (~9)	More secondary hairs (~12)
Wool (secondary) hairs	No medulla	Contains a medulla
Scrotal skin	Usually, sparse hair	Hairy
Facial sebaceous glands	Fewer on the face	More numerous on the face
Tail glands (modified sebaceous glands)	Located caudal to Ca 7 vertebra	Located at the baser of the tail
Dermis/hypodermis collagen production	May have a higher rate of collagen production	May have a lower rate of collagen synthesis ability
Wound repair	Rapid granulation tissue production	Delayed granulation tissue production

antiviral-specific immune responses *in vivo* [14]. The LCs survey the epithelium constantly for pathogens and migrate to the lymph nodes where they present microbial antigens to T-cells. This results in developing tolerance and maintaining tissue homeostasis [15]. Langerhans cells in the skin are continuously replenished from circulating bone marrow precursors [16, 17]. There is steady-state migration of LCs to skin-draining lymph nodes, perhaps to induce and maintain tolerance to cutaneus antigens. Their number in the epidermis is small compared to keratinocytes, and they are largely present in the upper stratum spinosum.

Tactile epithelioid cells (*Merkel* cells) are in the stratum basale of hairless and hairy skin and are numerous in the nasal plane of carnivores. These cells, in association with sensory nerve endings, function as epidermal mechanoreceptors (Figure 1.3) that transmit tactile sensations (touch) through cutaneus nerves [18]. Merkel cells are neurosecretory cells thought to be derived from neural crest cells [19, 20]. However, recent studies in mice and humans indicate they may be derivatives of epidermal cells [21, 22]. They are slowly adapting cutaneus mechanoreceptors located in the basal layer of the epidermis. Merkel cell afferents are gentle touch receptors activated by steady skin indentation [21]. In humans, Merkel cell carcinoma is a rare cutaneus neuroendocrine carcinoma that is a highly malignant skin cancer most often associated with the presence of Merkel cell poliovirus genes (MCPyV) [22–24]. Originally thought to arise from Merkel cells, recent studies indicate in humans, the cancer cell origin is from primitive epidermal stem cells, early B-cells, or dermal fibroblasts [25–27]. In canine and feline Merkel cell carcinoma, MCPyV genes were not detected, indicating a different etiology for cancer [28]. In addition, Merkel cell carcinoma appears to be more benign in dogs but more aggressive in cats [29–31].

Cutaneus Immune Barrier

Skin, as an immunologic organ, is present at the critical junction between the host and the environment. The most important function is to guard against potentially damaging agents such as microbes, toxins, and radiation. This is effectively accomplished by the presence of anatomical, biochemical, and immunologic barriers. The anatomical barrier consists of the tight cell-to-cell junctions and associated skeletal proteins of the stratum corneum. This barrier is enhanced by sebaceous gland secretions. Biochemical barriers include hydrolytic enzymes, acids, lipids, and antimicrobial proteins. The immunologic barrier is composed of cellular and humoral constituents of the immune system. Within this barrier exist cooperative arms of innate and adaptive immunity [32]. The **innate immune system** is a primitive defense mechanism comprised immune cells such as macrophages, neutrophils, and LCs, and their associated inflammatory mediators such as cytokines and chemokines. To mount a defensive reaction against the invading pathogen, the innate immune system must discriminate between "self" and "non-self." Several molecules exist in pathogens absent in the host, collectively known as pathogen-associated molecular patterns (PAMPs). Innate immune cells use pattern recognition receptors (PRRs) such as toll-like receptors (TLRs), and peptidoglycan receptors (PGNs) to identify PAMPs in pathogens. Identification of pathogens triggers a cascade of inflammatory reactions including the secretion of cytokines and chemokines. These mediators further enhance the offensive assault on pathogens. Some of

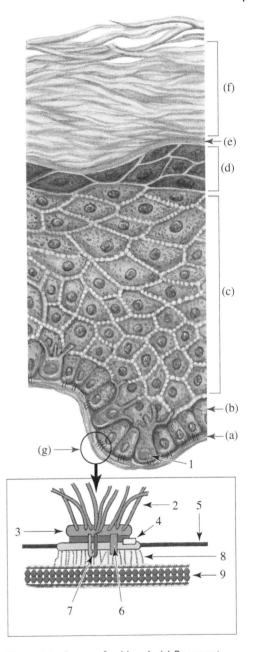

Figure 1.2 Layers of epidermis. (a) Basement membrane. (b) Stratum basale. (c) Stratum spinosum. (d) Stratum granulosum. (e) Stratum lucidum. (f) Stratum corneum. (g) Cells of stratum basale are anchored to the basement membrane by hemidesmosomes. 1, Melanocyte; 2, Keratin filaments (tonofilaments); 3, Plate; 4, Bullous pemphigoid antigen-1; 5, Plasma membrane; 6, Bullous pemphigoid antigen-2; 7, Integrin; 8, Anchoring filaments; 9, Basal lamina.

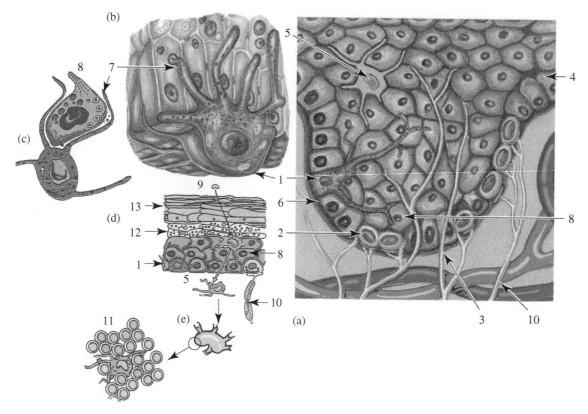

Figure 1.3 Keratinocytes and nonkeratinocytes of the epidermis. (a) Epidermis showing a melanocyte (1), Langerhans cell (5) and keratinocytes (8). (b) A melanocyte shown in-situ with its dendritic processes. (c) An isolated melanocyte shown transferring melanosomes along its cytoplasmic processes to an adjacent keratinocyte. (d) A Langerhans cell ingests an antigen by phagocytosis. It will then migrate from the epidermis to local lymph nodes; (e) Once the Langerhans cells reach a lymph node and transform into dendritic cells, they stimulate T lymphocytes. 1, Melanocyte; 2, Tactile epithelioid (*Merkel*) cells are mechanoreceptors derived from the neural crest. They are shown with their sensory nerve endings exhibiting a broad nerve plate (*Merkel* cell-neurite complex or the tactile hair disc, shown in blue); 3, Unmyelinated nerve fibers that penetrate the epidermis. These nerve endings mainly detect temperature and pain sensations; 4, Stratum basale; 5, A Langerhans cell, which belongs to the immune system. It detects foreign antigens and presents them to T-lymphocytes; 6, Basement membrane; 7, Cytoplasmic processes of a melanocyte; 8, A keratinocyte adjacent to a melanocyte receiving melanosomes; 9, Antigens that penetrate the epidermis are detected by the Langerhans cells; 10, A sensory nerve fiber terminating on a Merkel cell; 11, T-lymphocytes activated by Langerhans cell in the lymph node; 12, Stratum granulosum; 13, Stratum corneum. *Source:* Concept Adapted from Kierszenbaum [12].

the primary players such as lymphocytes and DCs mediate and augment **adaptive immunity** (humoral immunity), which is more evolved and allows immunologic memory.

Melanocytes (Figure 1.3): Melanocytes are derived from the neural crest and are present mainly in the epidermal stratum germinativum and in hair follicles. **Melanophores** (Chromatophores) are found in lower vertebrates (fishes and amphibians) and differ from melanocytes in how they transfer melanin pigment to adjacent areas. Unlike melanocytes which can produce only **eumelanin** (brown/black) or **pheomelanin** (red/yellow), melanophores can synthesize several pigments [33, 34]. Melanophores are also derived from the neural crest and their main function is pigment aggregation in the center of the cell or dispersion throughout the cytoplasm, allowing the animal to effect color changes important for camouflage and social interactions. In mammals, melanocytes transfer **melanosomes** to adjacent keratinocytes of the basal layer via dendritic processes, protecting deeper layers of the skin from ultraviolet radiation (which is particularly damaging to cells during mitosis). Although melanocytes maintain close contact with keratinocytes via dendritic processes, they have a slower turnover rate than keratinocytes. In the dog, on average, one melanocyte exists for every 10–20 keratinocytes, while in the cat, there are fewer melanocytes [35]. The melanocytes, unlike the keratinocytes, are a stable population of cells living many years without undergoing cell division, while keratinocytes divide actively and live only a few days. If melanocytes decide to divide, the consequences are usually serious due to the development of malignant tumors [36].

Melanocyte and melanosome activities are largely regulated by the pituitary hormone, alpha-melanocyte-stimulating hormone [37, 38] (α-**MSH**, also called **intermedin**). In some mammalian species (rat, rabbit, ox, etc.), the pars intermedia of the pituitary is well-defined and contains large amounts of α-MSH, but in other mammals (and birds) it is practically vestigial, and so α-MSH is thought to originate from the adenohypophysis. In the carnivores, the pars intermedia secretes α-MSH. Alpha-MSH shares an amino acid sequence with another pituitary hormone, adrenocorticotrophic hormone (**ACTH**). The adrenocorticotrophic hormone is composed of 39 amino acids, of which the first 13 represent α-MSH. Because of the common amino acid sequence of these two hormones, hyperpigmentation has been described in some animals with pituitary-dependent hyperadrenocorticism [39], and in others with Addison's-like disease where ACTH levels are increased.

Coat Color and Temperature: The color gene, the dominant C gene, codes for the enzyme tyrosinase (TYR), which is involved in the first step of melanin pigment production. Mutations in the TYR gene result in temperature-sensitive pigment production, producing *Burmese* and *Siamese* colors. Mutation of the TYR gene is also associated with the inhibition of fur pigmentation when temperatures rise above a certain level. When Siamese and Himalayan kittens are born, they are uniformly white due to the reasonably constant temperature of the intrauterine environment. Soon after birth, cooler segments of the body, mainly the extremities, begin to develop pigmentation. In older Siamese cats, the fur darkens as the entire body becomes slightly cooler, due to age-related reductions in cutaneus blood flow. Removal of fur in these cats' results in darker pigmentation of exposed growing hair due to a decrease in surface temperature. For this reason, unnecessary clipping of hair should be avoided in show cats of these breeds.

Alpha-MSH (and ACTH) cause melanosome dispersion, and thus skin darkening, while melatonin (from the pineal gland) and catecholamines cause melanosome concentration (and thus skin pallor). The term **melanoderma** is used to refer to increased melanin pigmentation of the skin, whereas the term **leukoderma** (Vitiligo) refers to a loss of this pigmentation [40]. Autoimmune dermatoses affecting melanocytes result in vitiligo in humans. Dogs and cats are also susceptible to this condition [41]. In dogs and cats, depigmentation mainly affects the face, including eyelashes, nasal planum, oral cavity, ears, and muzzle, but also noticed on footpads, scrotum, nails/claws. White coat color in cats is associated with blue (occasionally orange) eyes, and these animals sometimes exhibit a genetic predisposition to deafness. Calico coat color is sex-linked in cats [42] and is associated with females with XX chromosomes, or males with an extra X chromosome (Klinefelter's Syndrome, with XXY).

The **dermal–epidermal junction**: The dermal–epidermal junction is known as the **basement membrane zone** (Figure 1.2) consisting of the **basement membrane**. The basement membrane has a gate-keeping function controlling the bi-directional traffic of cells and bioactive molecules [43]. The basement membrane region is crucial to stabilizing epidermal attachment to the dermis, and it also acts as a barrier and filter zone. However, nutrients and water can freely diffuse through the basement membrane zone from the dermal side of the skin toward the epidermis. Although the terms "**basal lamina**" and "basement membrane" are used interchangeably, the term basal lamina is usually employed with electron microscopic descriptions, while the term "basement membrane" is generally used with light microscopy. The basement membrane zone is continuous along the entirety of the dermal–epidermal junction and the dermal intersection between hair follicles and skin glands. Based upon electron microscopic studies of this junction, two components of the basal lamina have been described, the **lamina lucida** (40 nm electron-lucent zone, mainly containing the glycoprotein laminin) and the **lamina densa** (50 nm electron-dense zone, composed mainly of collagen). The basement membrane core structural components include collagen IV, laminins, nidogens, and heparin sulfate proteoglycans [44]. The mechanical stability of the basement membrane depends largely on collagen IV scaffold [45]. The stratum basale cells of the epidermis are anchored to the basement membrane zone and dermis through specialized attachments called **hemidesmosomes** (so named because of their appearance as half-desmosomes, Figure 1.2). The outer layer of the hemidesmosomes interfaces with the plasma membrane while its inner layer interfaces with intermediate filaments. Anchoring filaments from hemidesmosome span across the lamina lucida to join lamina densa [46]. This junction is also often associated with numerous disease processes. Protein components such **bullous pemphigoid antigen** is a component of hemidesmosomes [47]. Bullous pemphigoid (BP) is an autoimmune disease in both humans and in animals, associated with antibody formation against the bullous pemphigoid antigen [48–50]. Transient cells also pass through the basement membrane, such as neoplastic cells in certain cancers, neutrophils, and other leukocytes during inflammation. Apparently, invading cells secrete proteolytic enzymes to dissolve the basement membrane [51, 52].

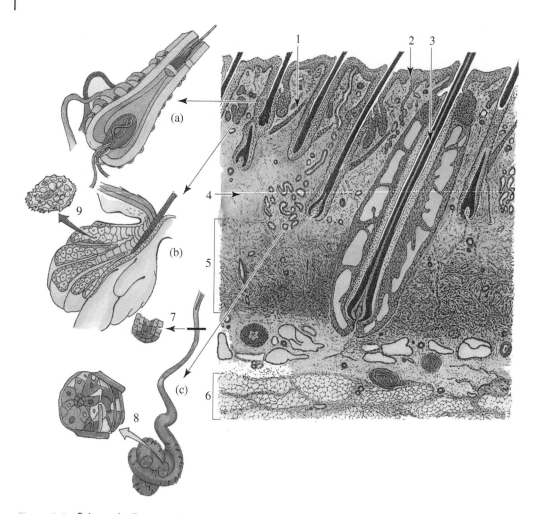

Figure 1.4 Schematic diagram of skin showing hairs and associated structures. (a) Simple hair follicle. (b) Sebaceous gland. (c) An eccrine sweat gland. 1, Arrector pili m; 2, Papillary layer of the dermis; 3, Sinus hair; 4, Dermis; 5, Reticular layer of the dermis; 6, Hypodermis with fat cells; 7, Cross sectional view of a sweat gland excretory duct; 8, Schematic view of the secretory portion of a sweat gland; 9, A sebaceous gland cell. *Source:* Adapted from Konig [53].

Other Structures: Among the epidermal adnexa of the skin are other structures such as hair follicles and sweat and sebaceous glands (Figure 1.4), all of which leave the confines of the epithelial layer and penetrate, some quite deeply, into the dermis [1–3]. Hair follicles are important not only for generating the hairs that insulate the body; but also, for serving as reservoirs for various stem cell populations, including keratinocyte precursors. The follicular bulb regions of the epidermal external root sheaths of some primary hair shafts (Figure 1.9) are associated with smooth muscles (*arrector pili* mm). These structures penetrate the deep dermal region, sometimes even to the hypodermis (Figure 1.5), and are distally attached to fibers in the superficial region of the dermis. These muscles raise the hairs to trap air and insulate the animal when its core body temperature falls.

Skin thickness varies widely in different regions of the body, with mean skin thickness in dogs varying from 0.5 to 5.0 mm and 0.4 to 2 mm in cats [5, 54, 55], depending on a variety of physiological variables including breed, anatomical region of the body, sex, age, and degree of skin hydration [56]. A report indicates a significant negative correlation between age and skin thickness in dogs [55]. The breed of the dog also influences skin thickness, Labrador retrievers exhibited thicker skin than other breeds [55]. The skin is extremely thick in areas prone to abrasions (e.g., footpads), yet thin in other regions (e.g., the flank). The stratum corneum is highly cornified where the skin is subjected to mechanical damage, as in the digital pads. Thick and thin skins are differentiated primarily based on the relative thickness of the stratum corneum, the outermost of the five layers of the epidermis. Hyperadrenocorticism results in thinning of the skin as a physical sign exposed to glucocorticoids [57].

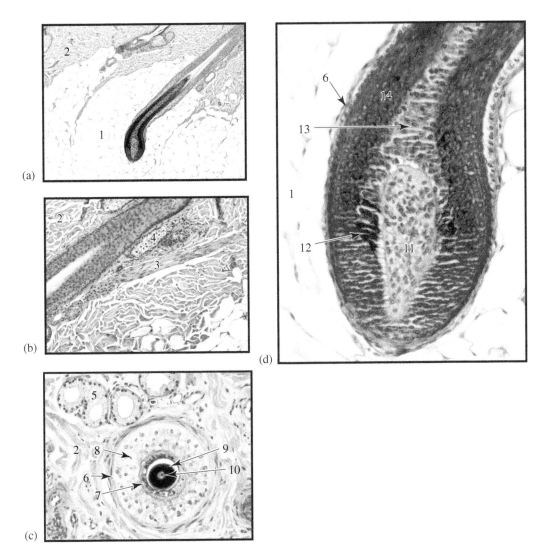

Figure 1.5   Histological features of hair. (a) Hair in the anagen stage (note the characteristic bend; 10×). (b) Arrector pili m. (20×). (c) Cross section of a hair shaft (20×). (d) Hair bulb (40×). 1, Fat cells; 2, Connective tissue of dermis; 3, Arrector pili m.; 4, Sebaceous gland; 5, Sweat gland; 6, Connective tissue around the outer epithelial sheath of the hair shaft; 7, Inner epithelial sheath with cells showing trichohyaline granules; 8, Outer epithelial sheath; 9, Hair cuticle around hair cortex; 10, Medulla of hair; 11, Dermal papilla; 12, Melanin; 13, Cells destined to form the medulla; 14, Cells destined to form the cortex and inner sheath. *Source:* Courtesy of Caceci T, Ph.D., Virginia-Maryland Regional College of Veterinary Medicine.

Epidermal Layers: Thick and thin skins are differentiated primarily based on the relative thickness of the stratum corneum, the outermost of the five layers of the epidermis. These epidermal layers are composed almost entirely of keratinocytes, with some transient cells as well.

The **stratum basale** is the innermost epidermal layer, resting on the basement membrane. The term "stratum germinativum" is sometimes used to describe this layer, referring to this layer's ability to produce daughter cells by mitosis; but as mitosis is also encountered in the next layer (the stratum spinosum), "stratum basale" is the preferred term in this chapter. Cells of the stratum basale contain water-insoluble keratin assembled into cytoplasmic tonofilaments. The stratum basale itself consists of a single layer of cells in continuous mitosis, maintaining the stem cell population while adding new cells that gradually move to the surface (undergoing the keratinization process) and slough off. Intercellular junctions called **desmosomes** bind cells of the stratum basale at their apical and lateral surfaces (Figure 1.6), while hemidesmosomes anchor these cells to the basement membrane (Figure 1.2). The basal cell layer serves as a progenitor cell layer and contributes to basement membrane formation. The structural components of desmosomes include several

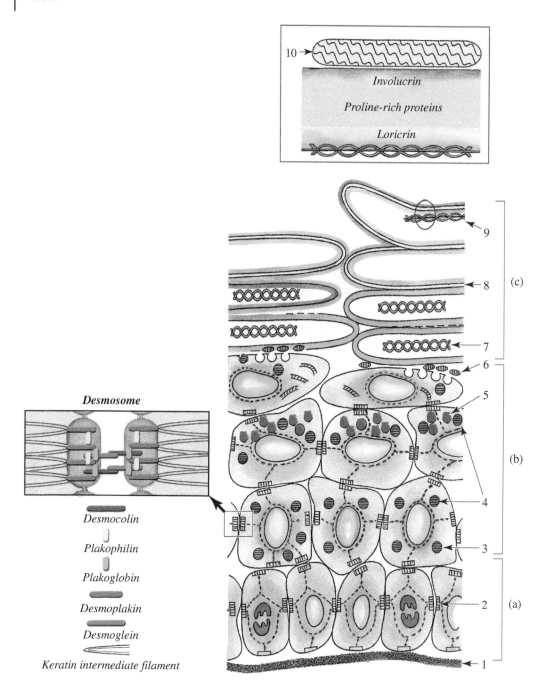

Involucrin

Proline-rich proteins

Loricrin

Desmosome

Desmocolin

Plakophilin

Plakoglobin

Desmoplakin

Desmoglein

Keratin intermediate filament

Figure 1.6 Schematic diagram of the epidermis depicting the differentiation of keratinocytes and the formation of the water barrier. (a) Stratum basale. (b) Stratum spinosum and granulosum. (c) Stratum corneum. The stratum basale cells divide by mitosis, with some of the daughter cells forming the stratum spinosum. These cells mature into stratum granulosum, and the type of keratin molecules manufactured changes from *keratins 5,14* (stratum spinosum) to *keratins 1,10*. The cytoplasm of the stratum spinosum cells exhibits *lamellar bodies* (derived from lipids). The cells of the stratum granulosum are flattened nucleated keratinocytes that manufacture more lamellar bodies and *filaggrin*, a non-filamentous protein that induces aggregation of keratins. The keratohyalin granules lose their limiting membranes and are associated with tonofilaments. The products of the lamellar bodies are released into intercellular spaces, adding waxy coats to the stratum corneum cells. This is the principal water-proofing layer. 1, Basal lamina; 2, Desmosome; 3, Melanosome; 4, Lamellar body; 5, Filaggrin granule; 6, Extruded lipids; 7, Keratin filaments; 8, Cell envelope; 9, Keratin-filaggrin complex lining the inner surface of the cell membrane; 10, Multilayered lipid linked to involucrin. *Source:* Adapted from Kierszenbaum [12].

core glycoproteins (desmoglein and desmocollin) and desmosomal plaque proteins (desmoplakin I and II, plakoglobin, and plakophilin). Cats and dogs apparently do not differ in the distribution of core glycoproteins in the skin [58].

The **stratum spinosum** (or prickle cell layer) is the next layer of the epidermis, and the thickest layer, often consisting of two to four tiers of cells. Extremely thick skin may exhibit more than 40 cell layers. Cells of stratum spinosum display characteristic "spines" under light microscopy. These spines are fixation artifacts at the locations where **desmosomes** hold adjacent keratinocytes together [59, 60] (Figure 1.2). In most resources, they are referred to as "intercellular bridges," but in fact, there is no continuity of cytoplasm; the adjacent plasma membranes remain intact. The desmosomes are anchored to the cells themselves via **intermediate filaments**. Intermediate filaments are a very broad class of fibrous proteins that play an important role as both structural and functional elements of the cytoskeleton of epithelial cells. For example, epidermal cells contain **keratins**, a diverse family of intermediate filaments, one purpose of which is to connect adjacent cells through desmosomes. Keratin filaments (tonofilaments) are more organized in these cells, forming **tonofibrils**. Currently, the term "keratin" covers all intermediate filament-forming proteins with specific physicochemical properties. The best-known function of keratins and keratin filaments is to provide a scaffold (through self-bundling and by forming thicker strands) with which epithelial cells and tissues can sustain mechanical stress, maintain their structural integrity, and ensure mechanical resilience [61].

The **stratum granulosum** is the next layer, often consisting of two to three layers of flattened epithelial cells with cytoplasm rich in keratohyalin granules. **Keratohyalin granules** are non-membrane-bound aggregates containing highly phosphorylated proteins, which cause the granules to stain with basic dyes (Figure 1.7). Keratohyalin granules are formed and deposited on intermediate filaments during the maturation of keratinocytes. **Profilaggrin** is the main component of these abundant, basophilic keratohyalin granules from which the granular layer of the epidermis derives its name. Profilaggrin is a phosphorylated polymer of high molecular weight (>400 kDa), composed of tandem repeats of filaggrin monomers joined by small linker peptides. During the transition from stratum granulosum to stratum corneum, the conversion of profilaggrin to monomeric **filaggrin** (filament aggregating protein) occurs by site-specific proteolysis and dephosphorylation. Filaggrin is an intermediate filament-associated protein that aids in the packing of keratin filaments during the terminal differentiation of keratinocytes. Filaggrin gene mutation or altered Filaggrin expression disrupts its normal function and may result in skin diseases and accelerated pathogen penetration [62]. Keratohyalin material may not be visible in some types of skin and is often lacking in thin regions. The stratum granulosum usually consists of one to three layers of granular cells that are transcriptionally active and deposit a cornified envelope of cross-linked proteins beneath the plasma membrane. The more distally located cells gradually lose their nuclei and become metabolically inert as they transition into the stratum corneum.

The **stratum lucidum** is a layer present only on the nose and footpads and as such, generally not recognized as a distinct layer by most histologists. This is an extremely thin and translucent layer, being apparent only in a thick and hairless epidermis. The stratum lucidum contains a thin layer of flattened cells continuing to undergo keratinization. The nuclei and most of the organelles of the cells are undergoing degeneration. The stratum lucidum may not be visible histologically (depending on the type of skin being studied) but the changes that occur in the stratum lucidum must occur in all keratinocytes for them to become fully keratinized. This layer has no apparent cytological features that distinguish it from stratum corneum and is generally considered absent in carnivores [5, 6, 10, 63].

The **stratum corneum is t**he outermost epidermal layer (Figure 1.7), consisting of several layers of flat, cornified usually a nuclear cells filled with arrays of tonofibrils embedded in a keratohyalin matrix, surrounded by a water-insoluble "cell envelope" [12, 64]. The stratum corneum may be compared with a brick wall, the flattened protein-rich corneocytes representing the bricks, and mortar, and represented by intercellular lipid-rich matrix [65, 66]. The layer provides the barrier against the entry of noxious chemicals and pathogens and against the desiccating effects of the environment [67]. The thickness of this layer of cells depends on the body region where it is found. In general, the stratum corneum is 3–35 μm in cats and 5–150 μm microns in dogs [68]. The stratum corneum in the dog was reported to have 47 cell layers in thickness [6]. The outermost laminae of cornified cells slough off (a process called **desquamation**), being continually replaced by keratinocytes of the inner layer. The rate of desquamation in normal skin normally matches the rate of cell proliferation in the stratum basale (and perhaps in the lower regions of stratum spinosum). The stratum corneum is maintained in perfect equilibrium, with renewal and replacement of desquamated cell layers by well-balanced epidermal proliferation, and progressive differentiation consisting of the synthesis of the lipid-enriched **lamellar bodies** and secretory organelles. The secretion of lamellar bodies before the cornification process promotes lipid accumulation around each corneocyte. Lamellar bodies begin at the suprabasilar epidermal layer and accumulate in significant amounts in the uppermost cells of stratum granulosum, accounting for 20% of the cell volume. The thick corneocyte

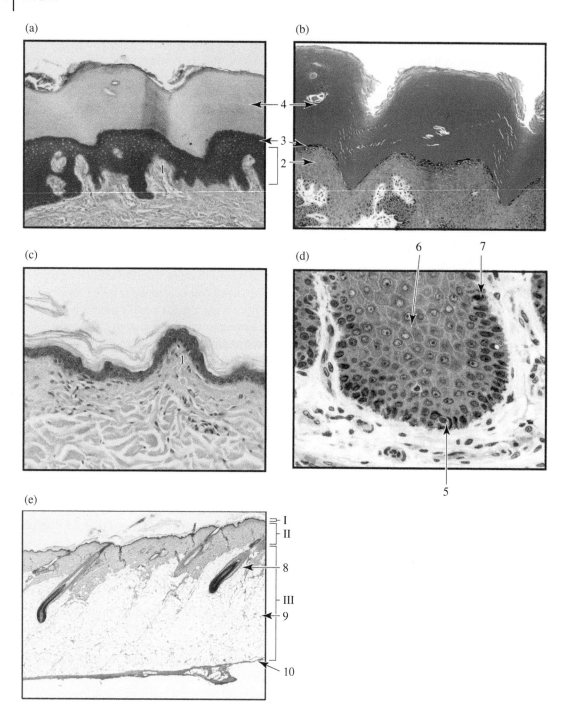

Figure 1.7 Examples of thick and thin skin. (a,b) Thick epidermis, palmar skin (10×). (c) Thin epidermis (20×). (d) Stratum germinativum and stratum spinosum (40×). 1, Dermal projections; 2, Stratum spinosum; 3, Stratum granulosum; 4, Stratum corneum; 5, Melanocyte; 6, "Intercellular bridges" of stratum spinosum; 7, Stratum basale; (e) Low magnification view of the skin showing 3 layers; I, Epidermis; II, Dermis; III, Hypodermis; 8, Hair follicle; 9, Fat cells; 10, Cutaneus muscle. *Source:* Courtesy of Caceci, T Ph.D., Virginia-Maryland College of Veterinary Medicine.

membrane forms from the synthesis and sequestration of keratin protein intracellularly. The entire **cycle of epidermal renewal** takes approximately 15–30 days. The mechanisms responsible for well-regulated desquamation are complex and involve the elimination of corneocyte cohesion by proteolytic degradation of desmosomes. Stratum **corneum chymotryptic enzyme** (SCCE) is a serine protease enzyme [69] that has been identified and characterized as having a specific function in corneocyte desquamation. This enzyme may be responsible for the degradation of the desmosomes that bind the keratinocytes together. Corneocyte desquamation occurs in a biphasic manner, with an initial phase that begins early after the formation of stratum corneum with already exhibiting extensive corneodesmosomal degradation. This is continued by a second phase of desquamation at the peripheral region of the stratum corneum resulting in the shedding of surface corneocytes [70].

The Normal Keratinization Process

The keratinization (or cornification) process starts with mitotic activity in the stratum basale and terminates with the formation of the stratum corneum (Figure 1.6). These cells contain keratohyalin granules, which stain basophilic with hematoxylin and eosin (H & E) stains. Cell division alters cell mechanics in neighboring cells from overcrowding, resulting in compressive stress, altering cell adhesion, and increasing the probability of delamination (a division of single-layered epidermis into complex stratified epithelia) at the site [71–73]. Mitotic inhibition has been shown to reduce delamination [71]. The proliferating basal layer of cells is tightly packed, attached to both the basement membrane as well as the terminally differentiated postmitotic suprabasal layer which moves outwards by delamination, filling the many layers of the epidermis. During their upward migration, the keratinocytes maintain tight cell–cell junctions. Within the epithelial tissue, desmosomes provide a robust linkage of cytoskeletal elements, with actin cytoskeleton playing a major role in desmosome assembly [74]. Epithelial cell migration in the skin requires tightly regulated desmosome assembly and disassembly [74]. The process of desmosomal disassembly and reassembly also occurs in events such as wound healing or tumor cell migration. Upon reaching the most superficial layer, the keratinocytes lose their nuclei and die, forming the cornified layer [71].

Keratinocytes (a term reserved for epidermal cells destined to form a stratum corneum) produce an intermediate filament protein called **keratin**, which makes the skin and hair pliable and insoluble, thus helping to form an unreactive barrier against the external environment. The dense meshwork of intracellular keratin filaments interconnected between cells by desmosomes provides the basis for the mechanical strength within the epidermis. **Keratohyalin granules** are matrix proteins that increase in concentration within cells of the stratum granulosum layer [75], promoting the assembly of keratin filaments into larger bundles. The complex mixture of fibrous structural proteins in the epidermis is collectively referred to as **keratin proteins** [76]. Historically, keratin proteins stood for all the proteins extracted from horns, hairs, claws, hooves, and skin.

Calcineurin is a serine/threonine protein phosphatase that is widespread in many tissues, especially in the immune system and neural tissues. In the immune system, inhibition of calcineurin by cyclosporine leads to disruption of T-cell function [77]. Inhibition of calcineurin has been shown to inhibit the proliferation of cultured keratinocytes [78], probably due to inhibition of p21 expression resulting in downregulation of keratinocyte differentiation [79] and survival [80]. Wound healing depends on keratinocyte proliferation, differentiation, and migration. Cell motility/migration depends on calcineurin/nuclear factor of activated T cell (NFAT) signaling pathway [81, 82], induced by calcium–calmodulin complex. Calcium influx into keratinocytes induces their motility, driven by T-plastic (an action-bundling protein) through crosslinking to actin filaments and their synthesis regulated by calcineurin/NFAT pathway [83].

Cells of the stratum spinosum begin forming intermediate filaments into organized bundles (**tonofibrils**), which extend into the cytoplasm, attaching to desmosomes. Keratin is packaged into membrane-bound organelles within the stratum spinosum cells, which are referred to as **lamellar bodies** (also membrane-coating granules or *Odland* bodies) in the more distally located cells of the epidermis. These lamellar bodies are rich in glycosphingolipids, phospholipids, cholesterol, and numerous hydrolases. Keratinocytes become flattened as they continue to migrate toward the surface, forming the next layer, the stratum granulosum. These cells contain numerous keratohyalin granules without a limiting membrane. In addition to the keratohyalin granules, these cells also continue to accumulate more lamellar bodies and begin to release the lamellar glycolipid acylglucosylceramide (a glucocerebroside) into intercellular spaces. This waxy glycolipid forms wide sheets in the intercellular spaces of the stratum granulosum, coating keratinocytes of the upper layers, but principally the stratum corneum, and providing a water barrier for the epidermis. The stratum granulosum and stratum corneum also show nuclear fragmentation (karyorrhexis) and modification of cytoplasmic organelles. Cells of the stratum corneum lack nuclei and other intracellular organelles in normal circumstances, and their cytoplasm contains keratin cross-linked with another matrix protein, filaggrin. The keratin-filaggrin complex lines the inside of the cell membrane, forming the "cell envelope," which is cross-linked with the waxy acylglucosylceramide across the cell membrane. The cell envelope is a complex array of proteins such as periplakin, envoplakin, involucrin, and loricrin, which are cross-linked by transglutaminase-1, providing structural and mechanical integrity to the cells forming a water barrier [84]. The stratum corneum keratinocytes are rich in sphingolipids (ceramides), which are a major component of the liquid barrier. Thus, an important role of the keratinization process is to produce a stratum corneum, the main barrier system of the epidermis. In addition to aiding the assembly of keratin bundles, hydrolysis of filaggrin is regulated in such a manner as to yield free amino acids in extracellular spaces of the stratum corneum, promoting its water-holding properties.

The Abnormal Keratinization Process

The importance of the stratum corneum is highlighted in burn victims, where large areas of this barrier may be lost, resulting in life-threatening infections. Additionally, repeated application of detergents to the skin, or dietary essential fatty acid deficiencies (e.g., linoleic acid), may result in lipid depletion of the stratum corneum; breakdown of the liquid barrier; and frequently epidermal hyperplasia, producing scaling, roughness, and alopecia. Cytokines released by the epidermis may also initiate acute dermal inflammation. In certain conditions (such as **primary seborrhea** in the cocker spaniel [85]), there is a proliferation abnormality in which the total cell cycle time and the active proliferative pool of basal keratinocytes are increased, resulting in an accumulation of scale, excessively dry or greasy skin [86]. The final step in keratinization is desquamation, and failure to exfoliate dead cells in cats and dogs may result in scaly skin (primary/secondary exfoliative dermatoses).

Pemphigus and **Bullous Pemphigoid** (BP) are chronic autoimmune skin diseases that lead to mucosal and/or epidermal blisters and ulcers [87]. They do so by disrupting either the intraepidermal intercellular attachments of the keratinocytes and mucosal epithelial cells (pemphigus) or the epidermal and mucosal attachments to the basement membrane. Clinically, pemphigus and BP are often indistinguishable. Their lesions are usually apparent on the face (most strikingly so on the planum nasale) and there are accompanying lesions of the feet and/or mouth. Pemphigus and BP have characteristic microscopic lesions that, together with clinical findings, serve as the basis for diagnosis.

Hairs: Hairs (*pili*) (Figures 1.4, 1.5, and 1.8), which are important for thermoregulation, are epidermal derivatives. Small bundles of arrector pili muscles serve to raise hairs from the skin, trapping air between them; as air makes a good insulator, this conserves body temperature. The arrector pili are innervated by postganglionic sympathetic nerve endings, which are sometimes referred to as **pilomotor nerve** endings. Arrector pili are best developed along the dorsal line of the neck, back, and tail [2, 3, 68, 88]. The hair coat consists of **outer hair** (*capilli*, cover hair, primary hair, or guard hair), and **wool hair** (*pili lanei* or secondary hair; Figure 1.8d) situated below the outer coat. The outer hair is thick, consisting of an outer cuticle and cortex, and a central medulla. The primary hair is surrounded by several secondary hairs. Wool hairs are finer and may (in the cat) or may not (in the dog) contain a medulla. Relative proportions of pigment, air bubbles, and the extent of pigment distribution in the cortical/medullary layers of outer hairs determine various hues of coat color, ranging from white (no pigment) to yellow (small amount of pigment), red (more pigment), and black (abundant pigment). Coat color does not necessarily reflect skin color, as a white-coated animal may have dark skin beneath the hair coat. The term **melanotrichia** refers to increased melanin hair pigmentation, whereas the terms **leukotrichia** and **poliosis** refer to a loss of hair pigmentation (graying of hair).

Each hair has two components, the hair follicle, and the hair shaft. The **hair follicle** is a tubular invagination of the epidermis, consisting of a **hair bulb** (i.e., the proximal end of the invaginated hair follicle) resting on a vascularized dermal core called the **dermal papilla** (from which it is separated by a thin basement membrane). Each hair shaft has an inner medulla and an outer cortex [68]. The cortex is sheathed in a cuticle, and each hair follicle is sheathed in a connective tissue coat. The cuticle is formed by a single layer of flat keratinized cells whose free edges overlap like shingles on a roof, all directed toward the distal end of the shaft. The cuticle of the internal root sheath is formed by overlapping keratinized cells like those of the cuticle of the hair, except that the free edges are oriented in the opposite direction toward the hair bulb. This arrangement results in solid implantation of the hair root in the hair follicle and helps to explain why hairs are not easily pulled out as well as why catagen and telogen hairs do not simply fall out.

The arrector pili are attached to the shaft of the hair follicle at a region called the **follicular bulb** (or the **bulge region**, Figure 1.9), which contains stem cells (**clonogenic keratinocytes**). These stem cells can migrate to regenerate hair shafts, form new sebaceous glands, or even contribute to the regeneration of the surface epithelium [89–93] (Figure 1.9). Thus, stem cells are clinically relevant in repairing skin wounds [12, 94, 95], and regenerating interfollicular epidermis [93, 96]. These stem cells may also contribute to tumorigenesis on canine tumors of skin origin, such as trichoblastomas, trichoepitheliomas, and tricholemmomas [97].

Hairs are generally arranged in clusters (hair beds), and these beds in dogs and cats may contain hair follicles opening either independently or through a common opening at the epidermal surface (compound hairs, Figure 1.8). Dorsal and

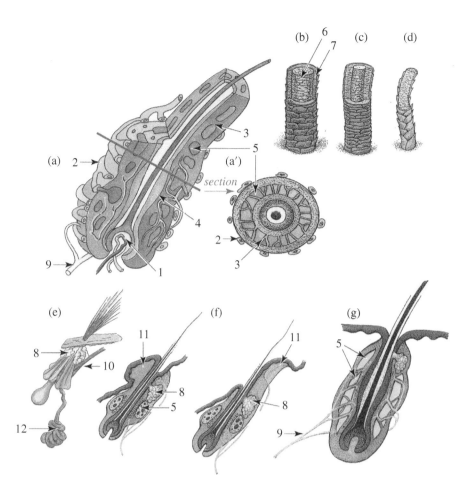

Figure 1.8 Different types of hairs in animals. (a,f,g) Tactile (or sinus) hairs are found on the face. They are deeply rooted into the subcutis or even in the superficial muscles on the face. A few sinus hairs are also found on the medial aspect of the carpus of the cat (**carpal organ**). The hairs are surrounded by venous sinuses. (b,c) Guard hairs with different thicknesses of cortex and medulla; (d) A wool hair. In carnivores, wool hairs are medullated, while in ungulates, they lack a medulla. (e) A complex hair follicle with a single primary hair surrounded by several secondary hairs. (a′) Cross-sectional view of a sinus hair shaft. 1, Dermal papilla with blood vessels and nerve endings; 2, Veins draining blood sinuses; 3, Connective tissue trabeculae surrounding the venous sinuses; 4, Epidermal wall of hair follicle; 5, Blood sinus; 6, Medulla of hair shaft; 7, Cortex of hair shaft; 8, Sebaceous gland; 9. Sensory nerve ending; 10, Arrector pili m; 11, Tactile elevation; 12, An apocrine sweat gland.

lateral aspects of the body exhibit a denser hair coat than ventral aspects of the thorax and abdomen, medial aspects of the thigh, and ventral aspects of the tail. Hairs are sparse on the canine scrotum, but cats exhibit a hairy scrotum. Cats and dogs exhibit compound hair follicles that possess numerous hairs emerging from a common pore [98]. Compound hairs generally consist of one guard hair surrounded by up to nine wool hairs (up to 12 in the cat). The arrector pili muscle bundles from individual hairs join to form a single muscle bundle that inserts into the dermis, while secondary hairs may be associated with sebaceous glands. In addition to these more common hairs, specialized hairs are found in certain regions of the body. For example, **tactile hairs** (or sinus hairs, also called vibrissae, Figure 1.8) are found over the face. These hairs exhibit blood sinuses around the base of the hair follicles designed to amplify the wave motion of the hair and stimulate nerve endings. Walls and trabeculae within the blood sinuses are richly supplied by sensory nerve endings. Scattered over the body surface are specialized sinus guard hairs (**tylotrich hair**) associated with small but visible elevations of the skin called **tactile elevations** [88] (*torus tactiles,* Figure 1.8f). The term is taken from the Greek *tylos*, "a knot or callus." These tylotrich hairs are extremely touch-sensitive. The tactile elevations (or integumentary papules) are small, knob-like structures (0.16–0.42 mm in diameter). The tactile elevations are also touch-sensitive. The tylotrich guard hairs are modified sinus hairs and as such exhibit small venous sinuses.

Hair Replacement: Hairs, except for tactile hairs, are periodically replaced in animals [1, 99]. Outdoor cats and dogs living in colder regions shed hair during the spring and fall, while indoor cats and dogs (especially short-haired breeds) shed throughout the year. Grooming habits of cats serve to remove loose hairs and ectoparasites, stimulate oil glands of the

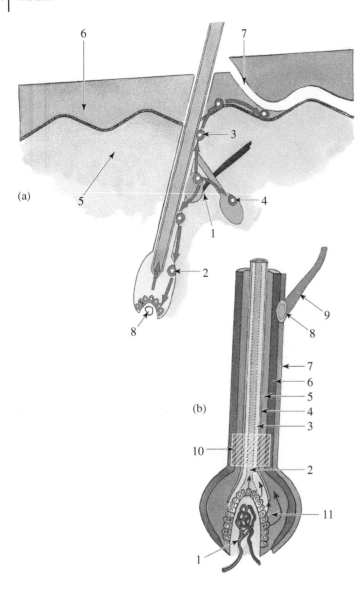

(a)

(b)

Figure 1.9 Structure of skin, schematic. (a) Keratinocyte stem cells are present in the follicular bulb (1), a part of the external root sheath of the hair follicle where the arrector pili m. attaches; 2, Stem cells can migrate to populate the apex of the dermal papilla to the form the internal root sheath, the cortex and medulla; 3, Stem cells can migrate into the epidermis along the basal lamina and reform the epidermal layer; 4, Stem cells can also differentiate to form sebaceous glands; 5, Dermis; 6, Epidermis; 7, Damaged epidermal layer. Stem cells from hair follicles may eventually restore damaged epidermis; 8, Dermal papilla. (b) Structure of a hair follicle. 1, Dermal papilla; 2, Medulla; 3, Cortex; 4, Cuticle; 5, Internal root sheath; 6, External root sheath; 7, Connective tissue sheath; 8, Follicular bulb region; 9, Arrector pili m.; 10, Cross-hatched region is the keratogenous zone where hard keratin accumulates; 11, Arrows indicate hair bulb cells forming internal and external root sheaths. *Source:* Adapted from Kierszenbaum [12].

skin to waterproof the hair coat, and aid in thermoregulation through the evaporative cooling of saliva. The shedding pattern of hairs depends on several factors, including external temperature and humidity, nutritional status, and health of the animal. The hair cycle can be summarized as follows [98, 100, 101]:

- Anagen, a long period of growth.
- Catagen, the transitional period from growing to resting
- Telogen, a long period of inactivity.

Glands of the Skin: **Sebaceous glands** are associated with hair follicles (Figure 1.4). Their oily secretions help keep the hair coat soft and water-resistant, and contraction of the arrector pili may help to express sebaceous gland secretions. Cats have more sebaceous glands in the face than dogs [65]. **Sweat glands** are classified into two types based on the nature of their secretion. True sweat glands (**merocrine** or **eccrine** glands) are independent of hair follicles (Figure 1.4), and, in carnivores, are predominantly confined to the footpads [1–3] (which are devoid of sebaceous glands). **Apocrine** sweat glands are diffusely distributed over the entire body of the carnivore and are associated with hair follicles [68]. Apocrine glands may release pheromones. Several contractile elements (i.e., myoepithelial cells) surround the sweat glands, which contract to empty the contents of the sweat glands to the body exterior. Sweat glands are supplied by **secretomotor** sympathetic nerve fibers. Circumscribed **tail glands** are modified sebaceous glands found on the dorsal aspect of the tail in an area measuring up to 5 cm in length, caudal to the level of the seventh caudal vertebra of the dog [88] (but located at the base of the feline tail). The tail gland region appears slightly yellowish and waxy due to secretions of glands in this region. The hairs over this region are coarser than the surrounding region and emerge from single follicular shafts. Tail glands may function to promote sexual behavior through pheromone secretion and conspecific (i.e., belonging to the same species) recognition.

Dermis

The **dermis** (or **corium**) is the layer of the skin below the epidermis (Figure 1.10). It is highly vascular and supports the epidermis. It is separated from the epidermis by a thin basement membrane. The dermis is a connective tissue structure derived from embryonic mesoderm (mesenchyme), while the epidermis is of ectodermal origin. Since the epidermis is avascular, the dermis provides for the needs of the epidermis with several vascular complexes located at different levels.

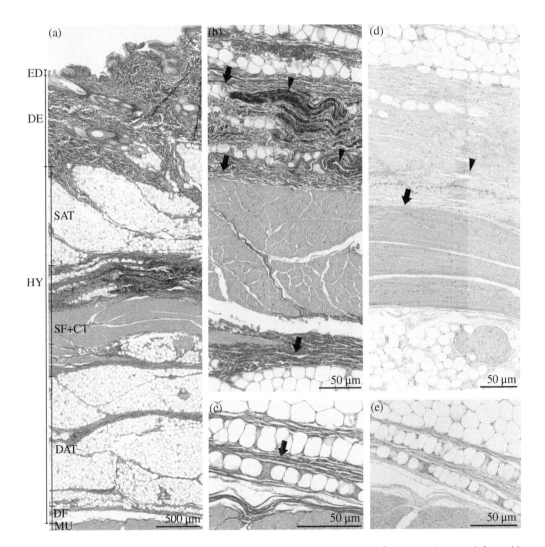

Figure 1.10 Transverse sections of *regio abdominis lateralis* of the dog. (a) Overview micrograph from skin to muscle representing the fascia layers in the dog section. DAT, deep adipose tissue; DE, dermis; DF, deep fascia; ED, epidermis; HY, hypodermis; MU, muscle; SAT, superficial adipose tissue; SF, superficial fascia; SF+CT, superficial fascia inclusive *m. cutaneus trunci*. (b) Elastic fibers are present along the regular collagen fibers in SF (arrows) and along the blood vessels (arrowheads). (c) The DF is loosely attached to the underlying *m. obliquus externus abdominis*. Elastic fibers (arrow) are present in the layers of DF. (d) Alcian blue staining, indicating the presence of hyaluronan, is intense in the layers of SF in relation to muscle (arrow) and blood vessels (arrowhead). (e) Hyaluronan is present within the layers of DF. (a–c) Weigert's Resorcin Fuchsin stain; (d,e) Alcian blue stain. *Source:* Ahmed et al. [102]/Reproduced with permission from John Wiley & Sons, INC.

Dermal thickness varies in different regions of the body [103], being quite thick in the nose and footpads. It is thicker on the dorsal surface than it is on the ventral surface of the body, and the lateral versus the medial surfaces of the limbs. The mean dermal thickness in the dog reported was 0.77 mm (ranging from 0.55 to 1.25 mm). The dermis is thick dorsally (0.95 mm), intermediate laterally on the flank (0.17 mm), and thin ventrally (0.62 mm) [103]. The papillary layer of the cat is relatively low, exhibiting only shallow undulations [1]. The dermis is composed of cellular and extracellular fibrous components of connective tissue (such as fibroblasts, macrophages, plasma cells, and mast cells) and collagenous (most abundant), reticular, and elastic fibers. The extracellular matrix of the dermis is composed of type I, III, and type V collagen fibrils, with type I collagen fibers being the most predominant, microfibrils, and elastic fibers supported by a mucopolysaccharide matrix that is hydrated by an ultrafiltrate of plasma (the source of interstitial fluid and the liquid fraction of lymph) provides the tensile strength and elasticity. Other components of, or found extending within, the dermis include blood and lymph vessels, nerves, glands, hair follicles, and smooth muscle fibers. The hair follicles and glands are epidermal derivatives located at various levels of the dermis but are physically and physiologically separated from it by a basement membrane. Where there are hairs, discrete bundles of smooth muscle called **arrectores pilorum** (arrector pili, *pl.*) extend from near the base of each hair follicle to the superficial papillary layer of the dermis [1–3] (Figure 1.7). The arrector pili insert onto the external basement membrane of the hair follicle and originate in fibers of the superficial dermis.

The dermis has both a superficial and a deeper layer. Where hairs are sparse (as in the digital pads), the superficial layer is called the **papillary layer**, as it forms finger-like projections below the epidermis (Figure 1.7c). Dermal papillae may be wavy and indistinct in regions of the body less prone to friction (for example, heavily-haired skin such as the dorsal aspect of the neck). In regions prone to high friction (such as the footpads), dermal papillae are rather pronounced and interlock with corresponding indentations of the epidermis (epidermal rete ridges) to prevent epidermal sloughing. The papillary layer consists of loose collagenous tissue containing numerous vascular plexuses and nerve endings. The papillary projections are relatively low in cats [1]. The deeper dermis is called the **reticular layer**, based on the lattice-like appearance of collagen fibers in the matrix (Figure 1.10). However, in dogs and cats, the dermis is classically divided into superficial and deep layers rather than papillary and reticular layers [10, 104]. Where the skin has cutaneus muscle (e.g., cutaneus trunci, Figure 1.10), the skeletal muscle fibers are tightly anchored to the superficial layer of the dermis to facilitate movements of the skin.

Cells of the dermis (Figure 1.11): Many cell types populate the dermis, including fibroblasts, myofibroblasts, macrophages (*histiocytes*), and mast cells, with the latter involved in immediate hypersensitivity reactions. Cats have been reported to have more numerous mast cells in the dermis (up to 20/high-power field) than dogs (4–12/high-power field) [10, 54].

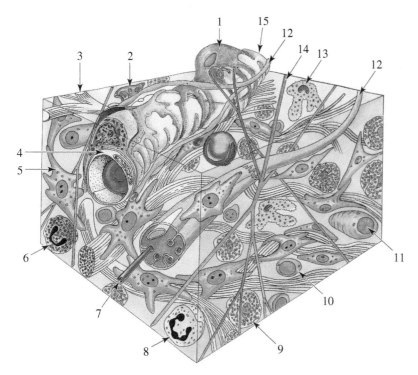

Figure 1.11 Cells and other components of loose connective tissue (superficial fascia). 1, Pericyte; 2, Adipocyte; 3, Collagen fibrils; 4, Capillary endothelium; 5, Fibroblast; 6, Eosinophil; 7, Nonmyelinated axon; 8, Neutrophil; 9, Mast cell; 10, Lymphocyte; 11, Plasma cell; 12, Nonmyelinated axons enclosed by a neurilemmal cell; 13, Macrophage; 14, Elastin fiber; 15, Capillary. Adapted from Williams and Warwick [105].

Fibroblasts and myofibroblasts are important sources of extracellular collagen that is important during wound healing [106]. In cats, activation of fibroblasts and myofibroblasts seems to be slower than in the dog, which may play a role in delayed/or altered open wound contracture [107, 108], perhaps also contributing to a higher risk of wound dehiscence due to pseudo-wound healing [109]. Mast cells of the dermis release vasoactive amines (e.g., serotonin and histamine) as well as pro-inflammatory mediators that can induce immediate hypersensitivity reactions. DCs migrate from the epidermis and are often found in the dermis en route to local lymph nodes.

The Hypodermis (Subdermis or Subcutis or Superficial Fascia)

Beneath the dermis, mesenchymal cells (see fascia) form a layer of loose (or areolar) connective tissue, the hypodermis, consisting of irregular bundles of collagen and elastic fibers and various types of connective tissue cells. The hypodermis is referred to as **subcutaneous connective tissue** by histologists, and as **superficial fascia** by gross anatomists. The hypodermis is relatively thin in carnivores and contains more abundant elastic fibers than that of other domesticated mammals. The hypodermis serves to bind the skin to deeper structures. In some regions, the superficial fascia is directly continuous with the deep fascia (a more organized connective tissue structure, Figures 1.12 and 1.13) or with the periosteum, as on the dorsum of the nose.

The hypodermis is responsible for the following functions: It stores fat as an energy source and serves as a shock absorber, it attaches the dermis to bones and cartilage, it provides support for nerves and blood vessels, and it helps to regulate body temperature. Diseases affecting the dermis can easily spread into the hypodermis and sometimes may also involve muscle bundles as in the case of burns and scars [111]. The adipose tissue in the hypodermis is important for energy homeostasis, and actively secretes adipokines, including adiponectin, interleukin 6, and tumor necrosis factor-alpha (TNFα). Adiponectin has anti-inflammatory and anti-atherosclerotic properties [112, 113] as well as insulin-sensitizing and lipid-lowering effects [114]. Adipocytes of hypodermis appear to secrete higher concentrations of adiponectin and lower concentrations of interleukin 6 and TNFα compared with visceral adipocytes [115].

(a) (b)

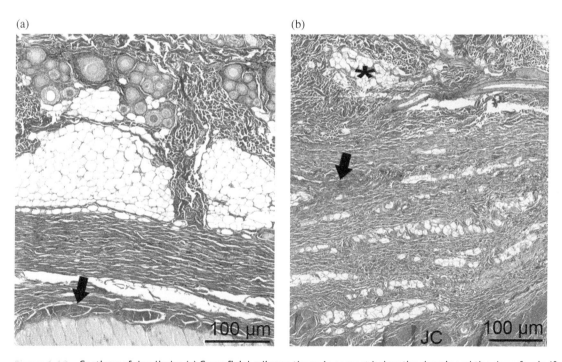

Figure 1.12 Sections of dog limbs. (a) Superficial adipose tissue is present below the dermis and the deep fascia (*fascia lata*; arrow) in this region, which is thick and composed of dense collagen fibers and tightly attached to the epimysium of *m. biceps femoris*. The superficial fascia and deep fascia are fused. (b) Fat deposits (asterisk) are present in the hypodermis of the carpus. Elastic fibers (arrow) are present in the loose areolar tissue in relation to blood vessels. The articular capsule (JC) of the intercarpal joint is present in the section. (a,b) Weigert's Resorcin Fuchsin stain. *Source:* Ahmed et al. [102]/Reproduced with permission from John Wiley & Sons, INC.

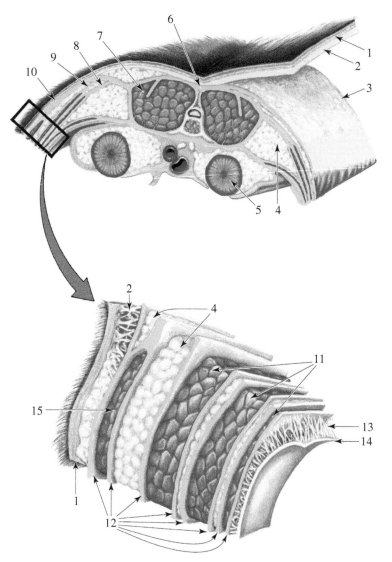

Figure 1.13 Organization of superficial and deep fascia. 1, Skin; 2, Superficial fascia; 3, Fat cells in the superficial fascia, reflected along with deep fascia; 4, Fat; 5, Kidney; 6, Median fibrous raphe (deep fascia attaching to spinous processes of vertebrae); 7, Epaxial muscle; 8–10, 12, Layers of deep fascial laminae; 11, Abdominal muscles; 13, Subserous fascia; 14, Parietal layer of serous membrane; 15, Latissimus dorsi m. *Source:* Adapted from Adams [110].

The hypodermis is a composite of fibrous collagenous tissue (Figure 1.12) in a viscoelastic ground substance of fibroblast origin composed of glycosaminoglycans. It forms an envelope layer beneath the skin. Loss of large amounts of subcutaneus tissue during surgery may impede wound healing [116–118]. This is due to the cellular (e.g., fibroblast that produces collagen fibers required for wound repair) and vascular components of the subcutis that are important for forming granulation tissue. Based on clinical observations of wound healing, cats may have a lower ability to synthesize collagen in the dermis and subdermis [116] than dogs.

The hypodermis connects the skin to underlying structures and permits some degree of skin movement, designed to transmit and dissipate tensional force [119–121]. In certain regions of the body, the hypodermis is characteristically infiltrated by numerous fat cells, thus forming a thick layer of adipose tissue (**panniculus adiposus**). It is divided into superficial adipose tissue exhibiting large fat globules surrounded by perpendicularly oriented fibrous septa (*retinacula cutis superficialis*), and deep adipose tissue with well-defined obliquely oriented fibrous septa (*retinacula cutis profunda*, Figure 1.12) [122]. These adipocytes function as energy stores as well as cushions against concussive forces applied against the skin. Panniculus adiposus is well-defined over the gluteal region. In other regions of the body, a thin layer of striated muscle develops within the hypodermis, giving rise to **panniculus carnosus**. The cutaneus trunk muscle (Figure 1.10) is an example.

Nerve Supply to the Skin: Skin is generously innervated by nerve endings (Figure 1.14). Sensory nerve endings may terminate in the skin as free nerve endings in the epidermis (nonencapsulated receptors), or they may be encapsulated

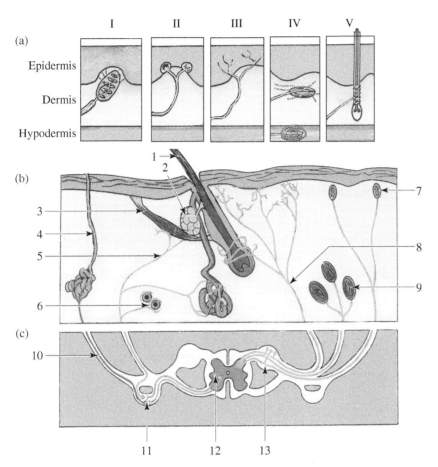

Figure 1.14 (a) Sensory structures of the skin. Various types of receptors are located in the skin. Some are encapsulated; I, *Meissner* corpuscles are in the dermal papillae and detect touch; II, Tactile epithelioid cells (*Merkel* cells) are mechanoreceptors; III, Free nerve endings penetrate the epidermis and respond to pain and temperature differences; IV, *Ruffini* end organs are located in the dermis, and are anchored to the surrounding tissue by fine collagen fibrils and respond to stretch; V, Peritrichial nerve endings wrap around the base and shaft of hair follicles and are responsive to hair movement. (b) Schematic structure of the skin and associated structures. 1, Hair; 2, Sebaceous gland; 3, Arrector pili m.; 4, True (eccrine) sweat gland; 5, Pilomotor (postganglionic sympathetic) nerve to arrector pili m.; 6, Vasomotor (postganglionic sympathetic) nerve to the smooth muscles of blood vessels; 7, *Meissner* corpuscle; 8, Naked sensory nerve endings to hair follicle (peritrichial nerve ending) and to the superficial layers of the dermis and deep layers of the epidermis; 9, *Pacinian* corpuscle and its nerve endings. *Pacinian* corpuscles located in the hypodermis and deep fascial layers respond to pressure. (c) Schematic of the spinal cord level showing nerves to the skin. On the left side of the spinal cord, sympathetic components to the skin are shown, while the right side depicts sensory input from skin structures; 10, Secretomotor (postganglionic sympathetic nerve) fibers to sweat glands; 11, Postganglionic sympathetic neurons located in sympathetic trunk ganglia; 12, Preganglionic sympathetic neurons in the lateral horn; 13, Dorsal root ganglion containing sensory nerve cell bodies. *Source:* Adapted from Kierszenbaum [12] and McGavin and Zachary [123].

by specialized structures within the dermis (encapsulated receptors). **Encapsulated receptors** vary in shape, structure, and function, and are found in the dermis as well as other parts of the body [2]. The simplest is the bulb corpuscle, which is touch-sensitive. Other encapsulated terminals such as the tactile and lamellated corpuscles are mainly pressure-sensitive. **Nonencapsulated nerve endings** are nonmyelinated axons distributed widely in epithelia, hair follicles, connective tissues, periosteum of bones, tendons, joints, and muscles. Cutaneus nerve endings extend into the epidermis from the dermis as nonmyelinated fibers. They are usually confined to the stratum basale and stratum spinosum and perceive pain and temperature variations and are dispersed among keratinocytes, and in the dermis in association with blood vessels and fibroblasts [124]. Other free nerve endings terminate within the epidermis as leaf-like expansions (**nerve plates**, also called the Merkel cell-neurite complexes or the tactile hair discs) in association with specialized epidermal cells called **tactile epithelioid cells**. The cytoplasm of these cells contains abundant granules, presumably neurotransmitters. These cells are thought to serve as mechanoreceptors (or mechanoceptors). Nonencapsulated nerve endings in the dermis that surround hair follicles form peritrichial nerve endings at the base of these follicles (Figure 1.8) and are sensitive to hair movement.

Sensory and autonomic cutaneus nerve endings in the skin can release several neuropeptides when stimulated. These neuropeptides act as neurotransmitters, paracrine factors, or hormones [125]. Keratinocytes, Merkel cells, and fibroblasts among other cells of the skin have been shown to release neuropeptides [126, 127]. This, in concert with neuropeptides released from nerve endings, may play a role in wound healing. Several of these neuropeptides can act on G protein-coupled receptors [128]. These peptides include Substance P, neurokinin A, calcitonin gene-related peptide (CGRP), and vasoactive intestinal peptide [129]. These molecules, along with the neuropeptides released from the other skin cells may play a crucial role in wound healing [124, 130]. For example, Substance P stimulates vasodilatation [131], upregulates adhesion molecule expression on endothelial cells, monocyte chemotaxis, inflammatory cell activity [132, 133], and synthesis and release of pro-inflammatory cytokines during the inflammatory phase of wound healing [134]. Denervated skin delays wound healing [135, 136]. Diabetic neuropathies have been shown delay wound healing [137, 138].

Blood Supply to the Skin: The epidermis has no direct blood supply of its own; therefore, passive diffusion of fluids from the underlying dermis must provide metabolic support to the deeper, metabolically active epidermal cell layers. The skin is nourished by numerous **cutaneus arteries** (their terminal branches are seen in Figure 1.15). These arteries supply blood to the vascular plexuses that nourish the skin and its appendages [56]. These direct cutaneus vessels can be incorporated into large skin flaps (vascular pedicle grafts), forming **axial pattern flaps** for closing large skin wounds secondary to trauma or resection of diseased skin (Figure 1.16). These are called axial pattern flaps because they include a direct specific artery within the longitudinal axis. A significant amount of blood can be stored in cutaneus vascular plexuses, depending on whether the blood vessels are dilated or not. Dilation or constriction of cutaneus blood vessels (i.e., vasomotion) is controlled by the sympathetic nervous system, whose postganglionic fibers to these vessels form **vasomotor nerve** endings. Increased blood flow to the skin facilitates heat loss by various mechanisms [140], including sweating, and is mediated by

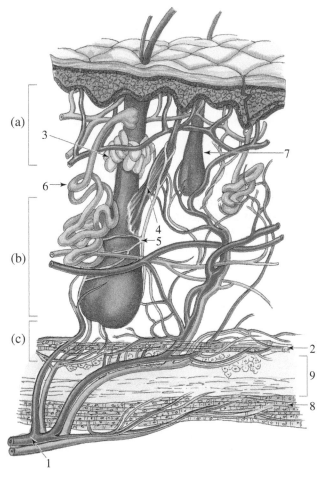

Figure 1.15 Cutaneus circulation in the dog and cat (schematic from neck region). (a) Superficial (papillary) vascular plexus. (b) Middle (or cutaneus) vascular plexus. (c) Deep (or subdermal) vascular plexus. 1, Terminal branches of the direct cutaneus vessels at the level of the cutaneus muscle which supply the subdermal plexus; 2, Subdermal plexus (surrounding a superficial cutaneus muscle); 3, Sebaceous gland; 4. Arrector pili m; 5, Postganglionic sympathetic nerve fibers supplying the arrector pili m; 6, Apocrine sweat gland; 7, Hair follicle; 8, Deeper cutaneus muscle; 9, Panniculus adiposus.

Figure 1.16 Cutaneus blood vessels are important for surgical repositioning of skin flaps. (a) Main cutaneus arteries and the extent of their vascularization: The arrows indicate the direction and the extent to which the skin flap may be moved. (b) The right side of the dog shows the flap extending from the opposite side. (c) Shows the caudal superficial epigastric axial pattern flap. 1, Prescapular branch of superficial cervical artery; 2, Thoracodorsal artery; 3, Caudal superficial epigastric artery; 4, Deep circumflex iliac artery; 5, Moving the skin from the left to right side retaining the deep circumflex iliac arterial supply; 6, Moving the skin supplied by the left thoracodorsal artery to the right side; 7, Caudal superficial epigastric axial pattern flap can be rotated into a variety of positions as indicated by the arrows. *Source:* Adapted from Pavletic [139].

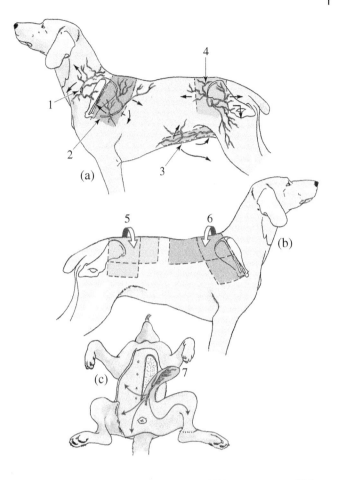

arteriovenous anastomoses (AVAs) under smooth muscle control. Peripheral blood vessels exhibit numerous AVAs between arterioles and venules, which are thus located proximal to terminal capillary plexuses. The AVAs are controlled by sympathetically innervated smooth muscle sphincters. Relaxation of the AVA results in the shunting of large volumes of blood into superficial veins, resulting in radiation heat loss from the skin surface. Thus, the major function of AVAs is to aid in thermoregulation.

Footpad Differences Between the Dog and Cat: Dog footpad exhibits well-defined elongated cornified conical papillae. The epithelium is quite thin underneath these papillae, consisting of three to five cell layers. The dermis exhibits prominent dermal papillae with microvasculature units consisting of several capillaries immediately below the basement membrane, intermeshed with a few venules in the core of the papillae. The Venules form a venous plexus around footpad dermal arteries in the dog, while in the cat, the periarterial venous plexus is not observed in the core of the dermal papillae [141]. AVAs are frequently found in the dermal papillary core. In the cat, the footpad surface is smooth lacking conical papillae. The dermal papillae of the cat are also smaller than those of the dog. The cat also has fewer AVAs in the dermis, with a less complex periarterial network of veins [141]. The periarterial venous network around AVAs serves as countercurrent heat exchangers. The footpads of the cat may be more susceptible to cold injuries such as frostbite.

The cutaneus vasculature is described in terms of arteriosomes and venosomes, each arteriosome consisting of arterial network from a major artery. Similarly, venosomes are described on the venous network draining into a major vein. A three-dimensional block of tissue, consisting of the integument and underlying deep structures, supplied, and drained by specific and dominant named vessels (i.e., matched artriosome and venosome, for example, the thoracodorsal vessels over the lateral flank region) is termed an **angiosome** [142, 143]. Dogs have been shown to have a higher density of tertiary and higher branching of vessels than cats, especially in the trunk region [56, 116, 144]. This may be a reason why the granulation tissue during wound healing appears dark red in dogs while it is of a lighter pink hue in cats [145].

Blood vessels in the skin are organized into three intercommunicating vascular plexuses [88, 104, 146, 147] (Figure 1.15). Some variations in the cutaneus blood supply described herein are encountered in the ears and footpads and at mucocutaneus junctions. The general description given applies as well to the hairy parts of the skin in dogs and cats.

- The deepest **subcutaneus** (or **subdermal**) **plexus** is directly derived from numerous small cutaneus arteries encountered during dissection when the skin is reflected. This is an important vascular plexus of the subcutis that not only provides blood to overlying vascular plexuses, but also to hair bulbs and follicles, sweat glands, and their ducts, and arrector pili. Blood vessels of the subdermal plexus generally run in subcutaneus fatty tissue (panniculus adiposus) and/or the cutaneus muscles (panniculus carnosus), which are associated with the superficial fascia. Where a cutaneus muscle is present, the subdermal plexus is present on either side of the cutaneus muscle. To help preserve skin circulation during surgical manipulation, it is important to undermine the skin along the fascial plane beneath the cutaneus muscle to maintain the integrity of the subdermal plexus and any associated direct cutaneus vessels. In areas lacking a cutaneus muscle layer, undermining is directed to the hypodermal layer below the dermis to ensure the integrity of the subdermal plexus.
- The middle **(or cutaneus) plexus** is derived from secondary arteries running off the subdermal plexus, and it supplies blood to sebaceous glands and hair follicles.
- The most superficial **papillary** (or subpapillary) **plexus** is formed by blood vessels derived from the cutaneus plexus, and it supplies the dermal papillary region. Unlike humans and pigs, carnivores do not exhibit well-defined vascular loops in their dermal papillae, thereby explaining why dog skin does not usually blister in response to superficial burns.

The deep venous plexus of the dermis is located at the interface of the dermis and hypodermis, and the deep subpapillary venous plexus is located between the superficial and deep layers of the dermis. The superficial papillary venous plexus is located beneath the basement membrane [68, 144, 146, 147].

Cutaneus arteries are important for **pedicle flaps**, which are patches of epidermis and dermis that are partially detached from one site, and then grafted to an adjacent site to cover surface defects (Figure 1.16). The pedicle flaps require an intact blood supply for survival. The cutaneus anatomy and its relationship to the blood supply must be considered for safely manipulating skin as in undermining skin to facilitate wound closure or in creating skin flaps [99, 148–151]. The primary course of circulation to the skin is through the deep or subdermal plexus; direct cutaneus arteries, traveling parallel to the overlying skin, supply this vascular network.

The surgical assessment of the skin's laxity or inherent elasticity is important in determining how best to close the wound. Although the skin is elastic, fibrous components (collagen and elastic fibers) within the skin and underlying attachment of the dermis to the hypodermis contribute to pulling the skin in predetermined directions over the body. Cleavage lines of skin tension lines [152–155] (Figure 1.17) represent areas where the skin is pulled in preset tracks over

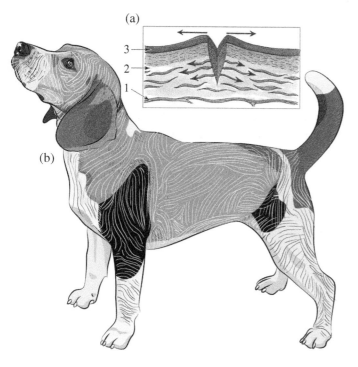

(a)

3
2
1

(b)

Figure 1.17 Skin tension lines in the dog. (a) Skin has a natural tendency to gape when cut due to the elastic fibers found in the dermis. (b) Tension lines indicate the orientation of the elastic fibers in the skin. 1, an intact elastic fiber; 2, severed and contracted dermal elastic fibers; 3, gaped epidermis. *Source:* Adapted from Oiki et al. [152].

the body surface and can be used as general guides to minimize tension during wound closing. As minimizing skin tension is an important consideration in proper wound closure, it is better to close wounds parallel to tension lines whenever possible. Excessive tension perpendicular to the incision can result in suture failure and wound reopening (dehiscence). Too much tension can also compromise circulation to regional skin and adjacent tissues. Furthermore, this tautness can contribute to the progressive widening of a postoperative surgical scar, thereby minimizing optimal cosmetic results.

Cutaneus Pharmacology: Intramuscular and subcutaneus injections are common means of parenteral drug administration. Subcutaneusly administered drugs may cause pain, tenderness, and local tissue necrosis, especially if the solution is alkaline. The topical application of drugs is also routinely employed in veterinary medicine. Drugs suspended in organic solvents (such as alcohol) or in an oil base tend to be absorbed through the skin, with the drugs exerting both local and systemic effects. The diffusion rate of a drug through the skin is largely determined by the compound's lipid solubility (lipophilicity). The stratum corneum possesses an increased lipid content with densely packed cells, thus creating a formidable barrier against rapid drug penetration. Therefore, the relative thickness of the stratum corneum determines the rate of penetration of even highly lipid-soluble compounds through the skin. Lipid-soluble drugs more readily penetrate the skin by diffusion through hair follicular shafts, sebaceous glands, and sweat glands. The skin of the scrotum and ventral abdomen, for example, is more permeable to lipid-soluble drugs than the skin on the back, thus requiring lesser amounts of a given drug for an equivalent effect.

Transdermal modality of drug delivery: "Transdermal" means across the skin. This method of drug delivery is achieved by the slow release of a drug from a compounded emulsion or from a patch applied on the skin. The drug diffuses across the epidermis to reach the blood vessels of the underlying dermis. The patch mode of drug delivery is popular in human medicine and is gaining acceptance among veterinarians as a preferred route of administration for certain drugs. Fentanyl, for example, is administered transdermally to both humans and animals before and after surgery to reduce pain. The fentanyl patch is applied to the skin, usually on the underside of the earflap. Transdermal drug delivery should be considered only if oral or other means of drug delivery are unavailable. In addition, since a transdermally administered drug requires a longer period to work, it may not be the desired route for drugs that are required immediately. For certain drugs, the effective endpoint may not be quantifiable to determine, whether it is delivered transdermally or not. Other disadvantages of transdermal patches include the patch falling off, getting stuck to another pet or human, or the risk of a pet swallowing it. To prevent these, a transdermal patch should usually be secured by a bandage. The stratum corneum is an excellent barrier to the passage of charged molecules and large molecules. **Iontophoresis** is a technique to facilitate the transport of charged (ionic) molecules into a tissue by passage of a direct electric charge through the electrolyte solution containing the charged therapeutic molecules [156–158]. The epidermis Despite these drawbacks, there are still several advantages to transdermal administration, including the elimination of gastrointestinal side effects, the elimination of daily pill administration, and an effective route for pain control.

Connective Tissue and Fascia

Fascia: Fascia (pl. fasciae) is an important structural component of tissues and organs found beneath the skin [159] (Figures 1.1, 1.10, and 1.12), and this term generally refers to the sheets or layers of predominantly fibrous connective tissue, of varying tensile strength, elasticity, and density, covering those structures. Fascia is the adult remnant of the leftover fetal mesenchyme after the other mesodermal structures were formed during fetal development. It quite literally holds the body together, connecting the dermis and skeletal muscles to the structural core of the skeleton [160], and investing the body cavities and internally suspended visceral organs with a continuous connective tissue covering. The fascial compartments of the skeletal muscles are estimated to account for 10–15% of myofascial force transmission on the skeleton [161]. Thus, nerves, blood vessels, muscles, and internal organs are all covered by fascia. Fascia spans from the dermis toward the skeletal muscles and deeper structures of the body and can be described separately as consisting of superficial fascia, deep fascia, skeletal muscle fascia consisting of epimysium, perimysium, and endomysium, and finally periosteum or visceral fascia covering internal organs [162]. Where the fusion between the superficial and deep fascia is extensive, as in the areas distal to the carpal region, the skin is less mobile and may be more prone to abrasions. Toward the extremities, the superficial fascia is tightly bound to the skin, with similar results, for example, at the tip of the nose. Conversely, where the skin is supple and extensively mobile, the superficial fascia is abundant and without close connections to the deep fascia. For example, in the antebrachium, the cephalic vein is loosely enveloped by superficial fascia with minimal connection to the deep fascia. Conversely, where the superficial fa the skin is supple and extensively mobile when the superficial fascia is abundant and without close connections to the antebrachium, where the superficial fascia loosely envelops the cephalic vein. In such regions, one must take extra care to avoid hematomas following a venipuncture.

Superficial fascia (*tela subcutanea* or subcutaneus tissue or the hypodermis) is located immediately beneath the skin. It is loose, containing numerous cellular and fibrous components, and accumulates edematous fluid under certain pathophysiologic states. The fascia consists of abundant collagenous and elastic fibers. Within the fibrous interstices of the hypodermis (Figure 1.11) are found, besides the fibroblasts/fibrocytes and other cells of the hypodermis, migrant white blood cells, mast cells, variable numbers of adipocytes [163] which, in some regions of the body (e.g., over gluteal and flank regions), organize into consistently located structural fat pads. Mast cells are of bone marrow derivation, they respond to allergies and inflammation, by releasing a cascade of biomolecules including histamine, serotonin, heparin, prostaglandins, proteolytic enzymes, and other pro-inflammatory molecules. Mast cell tumors account for 16–21% of skin tumors in dogs; and approximately 20% of skin tumors in cats [164]. The fascia is also an active pool of various progenitor stem cells that possess fibroblastic, chondrogenic [165], osteogenic, and adipogenic differentiation potential [165–168]. Fibroblasts derived from fascia play a major role in wound healing, helping to seal large open wounds [169].

A fat-filled region of superficial fascia is usually referred to as **panniculus adiposus** when it forms a continuous layer of grossly visible fat. These areas are also commonly called fat depots. They perform both a mechanical function as well as serve as nutritional reserves [122, 170]. During starvation, fat is mobilized from all subcutaneus regions, and visceral fat depots (around the heart, kidneys, intestines, and in bone marrow) simultaneously, but subcutaneus fat is depleted first. Thus, one only sees sunken eyes and bony haunches in animals experiencing the extremes of starvation.

Striated muscle fibers (**panniculus carnosus)** develop within superficial fascia in certain regions of the body. These cutaneus skeletal muscles (Figure 1.18) are well-defined, and those present in the trunk region are referred to as cutaneus trunci muscles. The cutaneus trunci muscles are quite extensive in the cat, covering the entire gluteal and femoral

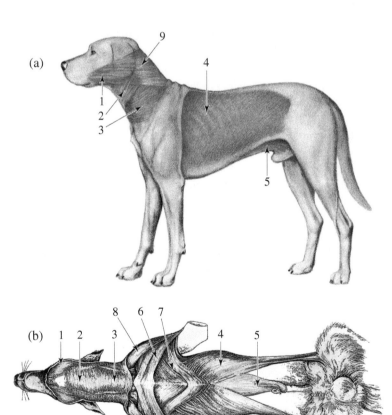

Figure 1.18 Cutaneus muscles of the dog.
(a) Lateral view of a dog showing various cutaneus muscles in relation to surface landmarks.
(b) Ventral view of a dog with skin removed to show cutaneus as well as some superficial skeletal muscles. 1, Facial part of platysma (cutaneus faciei m.); 2, 3, Sphincter colli superficialis m. (this muscle may not be well defined in some dogs, but better defined in the cat); 4, Cutaneus trunci m.; 5, Cranial preputial m. (in the female this muscle is the supramammarius derived from cutaneus trunci m); 6, Superficial pectoral m.; 7, Deep pectoral m.; 8, Brachiocephalicus m; 9, Platysma. *Source:* Adapted from Nickel et al. [159].

regions [159]. In both the male dog and cat, a muscular slip from the cutaneus trunci continues into the prepuce as the cranial preputial muscle (Figure 1.18). The equivalent muscle in females is the supramammary muscle, located deep within the mammary glands. Other cutaneus muscles include the platysma, and the superficial and deep sphincters of the neck (sphincter colli; not always well-defined). Cutaneus muscles play an important role in ridding the skin of irritants, such as insects, by twitching the skin (e.g., the **panniculus reflex**) [171, 172]. The cutaneus trunci muscle is innervated by the lateral thoracic nerve.

Superficial fascia, which in addition to its cellular components is made up mainly of loose areolar tissue allows the skin to move freely; its bulk, along with its adipocyte content, allows it to act as a thermal insulator. Picking up a fold of skin over the nape is normally an easy task in animals, and when the skin is released, it should readjust to its original location immediately. The skin of dehydrated dogs may take longer to fall back into place due to loss of skin elasticity.

Superficial fascia contains several cell types, and it is usually rich in lymphatics, blood vessels, and nerves (Figure 1.11). The nerves and vessels, which course within the areolar tissue of the hypodermis, can stretch without breaking due to their histologic architectures (the vessels are tortuous). Subcutaneously injected agents are easily absorbed into the systemic circulation due to the abundant vasculature of superficial fascia. Because there are no compartments in the superficial fascia the initial "buffalo hump" noted when animals are given a large volume of subcutaneus fluid eventually dissipates and the fluid migrates to the most dependent position on the animal's body. Large veins such as the cephalic, saphenous, and external jugular are enclosed by a layer of this superficial fascia. The superficial fascia with its loosely knit fibrous structure is also continuous with the deep fascia. The loosely arrayed fibers of the elastic and mobile superficial fascia blend imperceptibly with the denser and more oriented fibers of the deep fascia. Where two leaves of deep fascia lie side by side (as can be found when one considers the **epimysia** [*pl.*], or the deep fascial envelopes, that surround two neighboring skeletal muscles) there is a transitional zone of loose areolar tissue, which permits gliding movements as muscles contract independently. These planes of areolar tissue constitute the "planes of dissection" one finds during anatomical laboratory dissections or during blunt dissection maneuvers made by a surgeon.

Superficial fascia underlying the dermis of the skin on the trunk of carnivores is not rigidly attached to the **linea alba** (the ventral median fibrous band of the abdominal wall to which the bilaterally symmetrical abdominal muscles attach) nor is it rigidly attached to the mid-dorsal periosteum and ligaments of the spinous processes of the thoracic and lumbar vertebrae, therefore allowing for greater movement of skin from one side to the other. Superficial fascia is scarce over the ears, where the skin is tightly attached to underlying cartilage, and over the muzzle, where the superficial fascia fuses the epimysium of facial muscles to the overlying skin. It is also sparse toward the extremities, yet abundant over ventral regions of the body where the skin is more movable [88].

Deep fascia is composed of densely arranged collagenous fibers that form distinct sheets (Figure 1.13). It is well-developed over the thoracolumbar (also referred to as thoracodorsal), gluteal, femoral, crural, and antebrachial regions; it surrounds all muscles, and it also extends as intermuscular septa between certain essentially fused muscles [159] (e.g., the lumbar portions of the iliocostalis and longissimus muscles). Some of the extrinsic muscles of the limbs (e.g., latissimus dorsi), trunk (e.g., abdominal muscles), and back (e.g., epaxial muscles) arise from the internal aspects of the deep fascial envelopes surrounding them (Figure 1.13). The deep fascial layers between the trunk and limb muscles continue inward, fusing with the fibrous layer of the periosteum, thus providing additional resistance to the pull of attached muscles. The deep fascial envelopes of the limb muscles, loosely connected by fibers of the intervening areolar tissue, which blends from one deep fascial leaf to the next, provide for individual muscle separation, which assists in reducing friction when adjacent muscles are contracting/relaxing. These fascial envelopes also increase the surface area available for muscle attachment. In some regions of the body (e.g., thoracolumbar region), the deep fascia is directly continuous with flat tendinous attachments of trunk muscles, such as the latissimus dorsi and the oblique abdominal muscles.

Since deep fascia is often layered into multiple laminae, for ease of description it can, itself, be further subdivided into **superficial** and **deep** layers. Adipose tissue, within the bridging areolar tissue, is usually present between layers of deep fascia [173] (Figure 1.13). For example, the thoracolumbar deep fascia is attached to the supraspinous ligament and the spinous processes of the thoracic and lumbar vertebrae. It divides into a superficial layer that is practically the aponeurosis of the latissimus dorsi muscle and deeper layers that provide attachments to the serratus dorsalis cranialis, serratus dorsalis caudalis and the external and internal abdominal oblique muscles. An even deeper lamina, which is continuous with the fascia covering the epaxial muscles, arises from the transverse processes of the lumbar vertebrae and serves as the origin of the transverse abdominis muscle. In addition to providing attachments to these muscles, a thin layer of areolar tissue is found between layers of trunk muscles where it provides a gliding surface for muscle contraction.

Skeletal Muscle

Organization of Skeletal Muscle: Skeletal muscle normally accounts for about 50% of body weight (57% in greyhounds and 44% in other dogs [174]). These muscle fibers can be considered specialized organs, containing not only muscle tissue, but also nerve endings, blood vessels, and connective tissue. The basic functional unit of skeletal muscle is the muscle fiber (or cell). Each muscle fiber is loosely invested with a random arrangement of collagen fibrils (**endomysium**) to allow for movement during contraction.

Groups of muscle fibers form a **muscle fascicle**, with a thin connective tissue layer, the **perimysium**, surrounding each muscle fascicle [2]. The multisheet-layered perimysium runs transversely to fibers and holds groups of fibers in place. Several muscle fascicles are bundled together by a connective tissue capsule known as the **epimysium**. The epimysium extends inside each muscle and is continuous with the perimysium and endomysium. It is also continuous with the intermuscular connective tissue septa formed by deep fascia. Orthopedic surgeons often make use of intermuscular connective tissue planes to separate adjacent muscles, thus gaining access to bone (Figure 1.1).

Intramuscular connective tissue components account for 1–10% of skeletal muscle, of which the endomysial content can vary between 0.5% and 1.2% of muscle dry weight, and the perimysium can account for between 0.4% and 4.8%. This relatively small variation between muscles in endomysial versus perimysial connective tissue content has been taken to indicate that these differences may dictate their functional differences. Intermuscular connective tissue may play a role in force transmission [175].

Some muscle fibers run the entire length of the muscle fascicle, and these can be up to 20 cm in length. However, most are much shorter with tapered ends that overlap adjacent fibers and are bound together by connective tissue fibers of the endomysium. Tendons extend the endomysium at the ends of individual muscle fibers, forming bundles of parallel fibers, which are composed mainly of collagen, the most abundant protein in the body.

Each skeletal muscle fiber has several nuclei located immediately beneath the cell membrane (**sarcolemma**). Approximately 80% of the cytoplasm (**sarcoplasm**) is occupied by myofibrils and mitochondria. Each myofibril, in turn, is composed of numerous myofilaments [176]. Myofilaments are contractile proteins organized parallel to the long axis of the muscle fiber, and each is made up of numerous actin (thin) and myosin (thick) filaments [1–3].

Nerve Supply to Muscle: Skeletal muscles are associated with both afferent/sensory and efferent/motor nerves. Any nerve terminating inside a muscle cell may carry α and γ motor fibers, which innervate extrafusal and intrafusal fibers, respectively. Postganglionic sympathetic nerve fibers supply unitary smooth muscles of blood vessels, particularly arterioles [177, 178]. Visceral afferent nerves carry sensory information from blood vessels while general somatic afferent nerve fibers provide sensory information from neuromuscular spindles and tendons. Encapsulated and sensory receptors associated with muscle tendons may constitute up to 40–50% of nerve fibers supplying skeletal muscle [179]. These sensory fibers are proprioceptive, and they are concerned with muscle reflex control (such as maintaining muscle tone and coordinated contraction of different muscle groups). Visceral sensory fibers arise from larger blood vessels within skeletal muscles, which travel with the larger nerves that innervate the skeletal muscles. These fibers play a role in local vascular reflexes and pain perception.

The distribution of nerve branches within a muscle follows a fixed pattern, and in general, nerves enter a muscle where it is least mobile. Such an arrangement protects against accidental stretching of nerves when the muscle contracts. Once a nerve enters a muscle, it repeatedly branches along connective tissue planes within. In a fusiform muscle (such as the extensor carpi radialis), major nerve fibers run along the length of the muscle to reach individual muscle fibers. Nerves may run transverse to fibers in a wide muscle [180] (such as the serratus ventralis).

Blood Supply to Muscle: In general, blood vessels and lymphatics accompany the nerve supply to a muscle. The blood supply to a particular muscle may not be as specific as its nerve supply. In addition, the branching pattern of blood vessels varies between muscles; therefore, injury to a given blood vessel may damage one muscle more seriously than the other muscle fibers of the same group. Because of their high oxygen and nutrient demands, muscles depend on a rich blood supply to function properly [181].

Collateral blood supply is a common muscle feature, but due to heavy metabolic demands, major arterial vascular supplies should not be interrupted during surgical procedures since collateral blood supplies will be insufficient in preventing muscle damage. In general, blood and nerve branches are bundled together in **neurovascular pedicles** as they enter a muscle at or close to its attachments. This makes it easy to preserve them during surgical procedures, especially during orthopedic or muscle flap procedures. Complete interruption of blood supply to a muscle will result in **gangrene** (death) of the muscle. Partial blockage of blood supply (**ischemia**) may result in extreme muscle pain due to metabolite build-up (namely H^+ ions) [182].

Each muscle has a characteristic blood supply pattern; the most common is a single set of vessels entering the upper end, with another set at the middle. An additional set of blood vessels is usually seen supplying the muscle at the musculotendinous intersection. Trunk muscles are generally supplied by a series of minor blood vessels, in addition to one or two major vessels. Vascular supplies to these muscles usually tend to be segmental in origin from major blood vessels. Once blood vessels enter a muscle, their branches spread parallel to the long axis of muscle fascicles. These branches pierce the perimysium, forming a capillary network surrounding each muscle fiber that is supported by endomysial fibers (Figure 1.19).

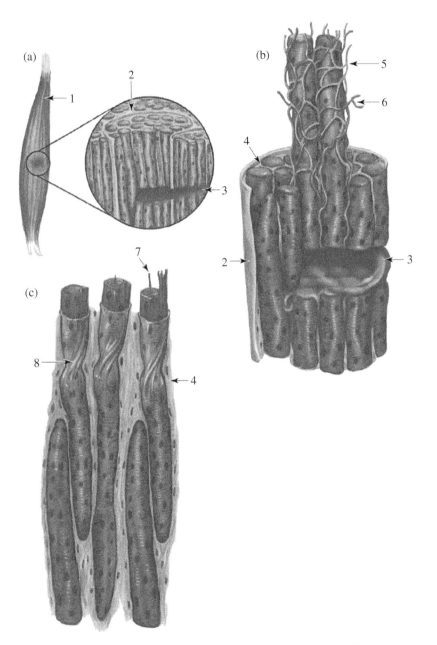

Figure 1.19   Muscle damage and repair. (a) Injury resulting in muscle fiber disruption and interstitial hemorrhage between disrupted muscle fibers. (b) Higher magnification of injury to a muscle. Note the rich blood and lymph capillary plexus surrounding each muscle fiber. The capillaries are sufficiently tortuous to permit their accommodation to changes in length of the fibers. Blood clot formation disrupts blood flow within the muscle fascicle bundled by the perimysium. Resulting inflammation within the fiber bundle contributes to congestion within the perimysium. The fascial compartment overlying the bruised region may appear tight and painful. (c) Muscle may also suffer from crush injuries. In this case, the sarcolemma is not disrupted, and local repair may occur by synthesis of contractile proteins. If the injury disrupts the sarcolemma, regeneration does not occur and the area is invaded by fibroblasts and fibrous scar tissue is formed; 1, Muscle; 2, Perimysium; 3, Hemorrhage; 4, Endomysium; 5, Lymph capillaries; 6, Blood capillaries; 7, Muscle fibril; 8, Crush injury to muscle fibers showing sarcolemma.

Lymphatics originate from lymphatic capillaries surrounding muscle fibers, and they carry away fluid and substances (e.g., proteins) that are too large to enter blood capillary beds. Due to high muscle vascularity, most drugs administered intramuscularly are absorbed more rapidly into the circulation than following subcutaneus injection.

Denervation: When a skeletal muscle loses its motor nerve supply, it also loses its contractile stimulus and fibers gradually degenerate and are replaced by connective tissue. However, for a short period following the loss of motor innervation, muscle exhibits heightened sensitivity to Acetylcholine (**denervation hypersensitivity**), and a period of slight twitching (**fibrillation**) ensues that eventually dissipates. Fibrillation is thought to be due to spontaneous rhythmic discharge within the muscle a few days following denervation. Muscle degeneration can be reversed over a period of months if nerve fibers succeed in reinnervating. Electrical stimulation and muscle massage have been shown to increase blood supply and slow degenerative muscle changes. Once reinnervated, the muscle can gradually regain strength. It is also believed that satellite cells found among muscle fibers can form new muscle cells.

Skeletal Muscle Trauma and Regeneration

Muscle injuries often occur due to over-stretching (**strain**), resulting in the rupture of muscle fibers, and external trauma may also result in the rupture of muscle fibers (**contusion**). These injuries may also result in localized bleeding and edema, due to the rich network of capillaries around individual muscle fibers (Figure 1.19). If the endomysial sheathing and sarcolemma are intact, the muscle fiber regenerates by replenishing myofibrils (Figure 1.19). Bleeding inside muscle is also of clinical importance since blood clots and fluid accumulation may disrupt blood flow (Figure 1.19). Due to the nature of connective tissue sheathing around groups of muscle fibers (perimysial compartments), increased interstitial fluid accumulation may cause pressure occlusion of the incoming blood supply leading to muscle necrosis (compartmental syndrome). If damage to muscle fibers is extensive, dead cells are replaced by connective tissue (**scarring**).

Replacement of muscle tissue with fibrous tissue following injury may result in **muscle contracture**. This type of condition most frequently involves the infraspinatus and quadriceps muscles. Severe strain and irreversible damage of the infraspinatus can occur in hunting dogs, resulting in infraspinatus contracture. Quadriceps muscle injuries following distal femoral fractures or extended limb immobilization following surgery may result in quadriceps contracture, or tie-down, in young dogs. Muscle contracture lesions also occur less commonly in the gracilis and semitendinosus of German shepherd dogs and Belgian shepherds.

Skeletal Muscle Stem Cells: Skeletal muscle fibers are prone to the constant stresses of exercise, weight-bearing, and trauma. Because they are generally considered to be irreversibly post-mitotic, skeletal myofibers require an everlasting source of cells for muscle repair and regeneration (Figure 1.20). Damaged, dysfunctional muscle cells are removed by apoptosis, and new muscle cells may form from satellite cells. Skeletal muscle stem cells, or **satellite cells**, are a pool of undifferentiated reserve cells considered to be the primary source for replacing damaged muscle fibers following injury [184–186]. These satellite cells are set aside underneath the basal lamina of each muscle fiber during fetal development, and function as a major source of myogenic cells crucial to postnatal muscle repair. Only a small population of satellite cells seems to serve as myogenic stem cells [187, 188]. Undifferentiated satellite cells are normally dormant; however, following muscle injury, some satellite cells be stimulated to proliferate, by reentering the cell cycle, then differentiate into myoblasts, and finally join with each other to form multinucleated myotubes. These newly formed myotubes can then fuse with a part of an injured myofiber that survived the initial trauma. Although signals triggering activation and proliferation of satellite cells have not been fully identified, many growth factors and cytokines have been shown to influence the proliferation, differentiation, and fusion of myogenic precursor cells *in vitro*. A variable number of satellite cells are observed within each muscle throughout life, as their number as well as their ability to renew muscle fibers, decreases with age. The number of divisions that satellite cells are capable of appears to be limited [184, 187, 188].

There are believed to be at least two major populations of satellite cells in mature skeletal muscle: (i) committed satellite cells, which differentiate immediately to myoblasts after muscle injury, and (ii) stem satellite cells, which undergo cell division before differentiation [168]. Muscle stem cells remain in a homeostatic or regenerative status regulated by secreted factors and by direct cell–cell contact between stem cells and muscle fibers [189]. Stem satellite cells are capable of replenishing new satellite cells for possible future needs. Additionally, under appropriate conditions, some of these cells are multipotent, exhibiting abilities to differentiate not only into myogenic lineages, but also different mesenchymal cell lineages, and even neural or endothelial cells. Denervation results in muscle atrophy. Satellite cells proliferate within three months

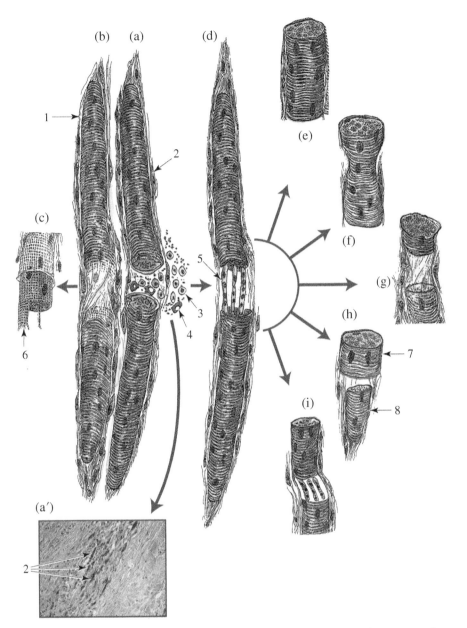

Figure 1.20   Schematic illustration of skeletal muscle fiber regeneration after segmental necrosis and its possible sequelae. (a) Injury to a muscle fiber – during the early phase of regeneration macrophages invade to clean up tissue debris (a′). Satellite cells transform into myoblasts; (b) If the sarcolemma is intact the muscle fiber may regenerate by internal repair – which includes synthesis of myofibrils (c). (d). Later stage of regeneration – myoblasts align themselves end-to-end and fuse to form myotubes. The myotubes now occupy the necrotic segment of the muscle fiber, and a number of possible paths from this stage are schematically indicated; (e) Completely successful restoration of normal fiber caliber. (f) The Regenerated segment is of a smaller caliber than the rest of the fiber. (g) Failure of regeneration results in an empty basement membrane sleeve, which may subsequently scar. (h) Multiple independent fibers due to lack of fusion of the myotubes with the surviving fiber stump. (i) Forked fibers due to incomplete lateral fusion of myotubes. 1, Basal lamina (endomysium); 2, Satellite cell; 3, Macrophage; 4, Myoblast; 5, Myotube; 6, Myofibrils; 7, Surviving stump; 8, Independent regenerated fiber. *Source:* Adapted from Schematically illustrated based on data from Carpenter and Karpati [183].

after denervation [190]. Immune cells infiltrate muscle injury sites and release several cytokines, which play a crucial role in facilitating muscle repair and regeneration [191, 192]. In addition, recent research indicates that injured muscles can release several cytokines that are important in myogenic differentiation [193]. However, muscle stem cell therapy for muscle or tissue repair (to date) is still in its infancy [194].

References

1 Nickel, R., Schummer, A., and Seiferle, E. (1981). The anatomy of domestic animals. In: *The Circulatory System, Skin, and the Cutaneous Organs of the Domestic Animals*, vol. 3. New York, NY: Springer Verlag.

2 Banks, W.J. (1993). *Applied Veterinary Histology*. St Louis, MO: Mosby.

3 Dellmann, H.D. and Brown, E.M. (1981). *Textbook of Veterinary Histology*, 2e. Philadelphia, PA: Lea & Febiger.

4 Sajid, A., Maryam, S., and Nabeel, S. (2015). The structure of skin and transdermal drug delivery system- a review. *Res. J. Pharm. Tech.* 8: 103–109.

5 Strickland, J.H. and Calhoun, M.L. (1963). The integument system of the cat. *Am. J. Vet. Res.* 24: 1018–1029.

6 Lloyd, D.H. and Garthwaite, G. (1982). Epidermal structure, and surface topography of canine skin. *Res. Vet. Sci.* 33: 593–603.

7 Webb, A.J. and Calhoun, M.L. (1954). The microscopic anatomy of the skin of mongrel dogs. *Am. J. Vet. Res.* 15: 274–280.

8 Lever, W.F. and Schaumberg-Lever, G. (1990). *Histopathology of the Skin*, 7e, 1–43. Philadelphia, PA: JB Lippincott.

9 Dover, R. and Wright, N.A. (1993). Epidermal cell kinetics. In: *Dermatology in General Medicine*, 4e (ed. T.B. Fitzpatrick, A.Z. Eisen, K.F. Wolff, et al.), 79–145. New York, NY: McGraw-Hill.

10 Muller, G.H., Kirk, R.W., and Scott, D.W. (1989). *Small Animal Dermatology*, 4e, 1–48. Philadelphia, PA: WB Saunders.

11 Al-Bagdadi, F. (1993). Integument. In: *Miller's Anatomy of Dog*, 3e (ed. H.E. Evans), 98–121. Philadelphia, PA: WB Saunders.

12 Kierszenbaum, A.L. (2002). *Histology and Cell Biology, an Introduction to Pathology*. St Louis, MO: Mosby.

13 Epaulard, O., Adam, L., Poux, C. et al. (2014). Macrophage- and neutrophil-derived TNF-alpha instructs skin Langerhans cells to prime antiviral immune responses. *J. Immunol.* 193: 2416–2426.

14 Hovav, A.-H. (2018). Mucosal and skin Langerhans cell- nurture calls. *Trends Immunol.* 39: 788–800.

15 Doebel, T., Voisin, B., and Nagao, K. (2017). Langerhans cells- the macrophage in dendrite cell clothing. *Trends Immunol.* 38: 817–828.

16 Collin, M. and Milne, P. (2016). Langerhans cell origin and regulation. *Curr. Opin. Hematol.* 23: 28–35.

17 Merad, M., Ginhoux, F., and Collin, M. (2008). Origin, homeostasis, and function of Langerhans cells and other langerin-expressing dendritic cells. *Nat. Rev. Immunol.* 8: 935–947.

18 Marshall, K.L., Clary, R.C., Baba, Y. et al. (2016). Touch receptors undergo rapid remodeling in healthy skin. *Cell Rep.* 17: 1719–1727.

19 Szeder, V., Grim, M., Halata, Z., and Sieber-Blum, M. (2003). Neural crest origin of mammalian Merkel cells. *Dev. Biol.* 253: 258–263.

20 Grim, M. and Halata, Z. (2000). Developmental origin of avian Merkel cells. *Anat. Embryol.* 202: 401–410.

21 Iggo, A. and Muir, A.R. (1969). The structure and function of a slowly adapting touch corpuscles in hairy skin. *J. Physiol.* 200: 763–796.

22 Tilling, T., Wladykowski, E., Failla, A.V. et al. (2014). Immunohistochemical analyses point to epidermal origin of human Merkel cells. *Histochem. Cell Biol.* 141: 407–421.

23 Woo, S.H., Stumpfova, M., Jensen, U.B. et al. (2010). Identification of epidermal progenitors for the Merkel cell lineage. *Development* 137: 3965–3971.

24 Feng, H., Shuda, M., Chang, Y., and Moore, P.S. (2008). Clonal integration of a poliovirus in human in Merkel cell carcinoma. *Science* 319: 1096–1100.

25 Zur Hausen, A., Rennspiess, D., Winnepenninckx, V. et al. (2013). Early B-cell differentiation in Merkel cell carcinoma: clues to cellular ancestry. *Cancer Res.* 73: 4982–4987.

26 Tilling, T. and Moll, I. (2012). Which are the cells of origin in Merkel cell carcinoma? *J. Skin Cancer* 2012: 680410.

27 Sauer, C.M., Haugg, A.M., Rennspiess, C.E. et al. (2017). Reviewing the current evidence supporting early B-cells as their cellular origin or Merkel cell carcinoma. *Crit. Rev. Oncol. Hematol.* 116: 99–105.

28 Van der Steen, F.E.M.M.M., Grinwis, G.C.M., Weerts Erk, A.W.S., and Teske, E. (2021). Feline and canine Merkel cell carcinoma: a case series and discussion on cellular origin. *Vet. Comp. Oncol.* 19: 393–398.

29 Dohata, A., Chambers, J.K., Uchida, K. et al. (2015). Clinical and pathological study of feline Merkel cell carcinoma with immunohistochemical characterization of normal and neoplastic Merkel cells. *Vet. Pathol.* 52: 1012–1018.

30 Sumi, A., Chambers, J.K., Doi, M. et al. (2018). Clinical features, and outcomes of Merkel cell carcinoma in 20 cats. *Vet. Comp. Oncol.* 16: 554–561.

31 Nickoloff, B.J., Hill, J., and Weiss, L.M. (1985). Canine neuroendocrine carcinoma. A tumor resembling histiocytoma. *Am. J. Dermatopathol.* 7: 579–586.

32 Antonio, Q.J. and Simoes. (2019). Organization of the skin immune system and compartmentalized immune responses in infectious diseases. *Clin. Microbiol. Rev.* 32 (32): e00034-18. https://doi.org/10.1128/CMR.00034-18.

33 Reedy, M.V., Parichy, D.M., Erickson, C.A. et al. (1998). Chapter 5. The regulation of melanoblast migration and differentiation. In: *The Pigmentary System: Physiology and Pathophysiology* (ed. J.J. Nordland, R.E. Boissy, V.J. Hearing, et al.), 75–95. Oxford University Press.

34 Kelsh, R.N. (2004). Genetics and evolution of pigment patterns in fish. *Pigment Cell Res.* 17: 326–336.

35 Affolter, V.K. and Moore, K. (1994). Histologic features of normal canine and feline skin. *Clin. Dermatol.* 12: 491–497.

36 Smedley, R.C., Sebastian, K., and Kiupel, M. (2022). Diagnosis and prognosis of canine melanocyte neoplasms. *Vet. Sci.* 9: 175. https://doi.org/10.3390/vetsci9040175.

37 Shi, Y. (2004). Beyond skin color: emergence of melanin-concentrating hormone in energy homeostasis and other physiological functions. *Peptides* 25: 1605–1611.

38 Sulaimon, S.S. and Kitchell, B.E. (2003). The biology of melanocytes. *Vet. Dermatol.* 14: 57–65.

39 Stratakis, C.A. (2016). Skin manifestations of Cushing's syndrome. *Endocr. Metab. Disord.* 17: 283–286.

40 Tham, H.L., Linder, K.E., and Olivry, T. (2019). Autoimmune diseases affecting skin melanocytes in dogs, cats and horses vitiligo and the uveodermatological syndrome: a comprehensive review. *BMC Vet. Res.* 15: 1–17.

41 Kibar, M., Aslan, O., and Arslan, K. (2014). Uveodermatological syndrome (Vogt-Koyanagi-Harada-like syndrome) with depigmentation in a Siberian husky. *Revue Méd. Vét.* 165: 57–60.

42 Stelow, E.A., Bain, M.J., and Kass, P.H. (2016). The relationship between coat color and aggressive behaviors in the domestic cat. *J. Appl. Anim. Welfare Sci.* 19: 1–15.

43 Breitkreutz, D., Mirancea, N., and Nischt, R. (2009). Basement membranes in skin: unique matrix structures with diverse functions? *Histochem. Cell Biol.* 132: 1–10.

44 Pozzi, A., Yurchenco, P.D., and Iozzo, R.V. (2017). The nature and biology of basement membranes. *Matrix Biol.* 57-58: 1–11.

45 Pöschl, E., Schlötzer-Schrehardt, U., Brachvogel, B. et al. (2004). Collagen IV is essential for basement stability but dispensable for initiation of its assembly during early development. *Development* 131: 1619–1621.

46 Keene, D.R., Marinkovich, M.P., and Sakai, L.Y. (1997). Immunodissection of the connective tissue matrix in human skin. *Microsc. Res. Tech.* 38: 394–406.

47 Dalegrave, S., Francisco, D., Fiorin, T. et al. (2021). Penfigoide bolhoseo em cao. *Acta Sci. Vet.* 49 (Suppl 1): 609–613.

48 Ross, F.P. and Christiano, A.M. (2006). Nothing but skin and bone. *J. Clin. Invest.* 116: 1140–1149.

49 Ackerman, L.J. (1985). Pemphigus and pemphigoid in domestic animals: an overview. *Can. Vet. J.* 26: 185–189.

50 Olivry, T., Bizikova, P., Dunston, S.M. et al. (2010). Clinical and immunological heterogeneity of canine subepidermal blistering dermatoses with anti-laminin-332 (laminin-5) autoantibodies. *Vet. Dermatol.* 21: 345–357.

51 Cavallo-Medved, D., Rudy, D., Blum, G. et al. (2009). Live-cell imaging demonstrates extracellular matrix degradation in association with active cathepsin B in caveolae of endothelial cells during tube formation. *Exp. Cell Res.* 315: 1234–1246.

52 Valastyan, S. and Weinberg, R.A. (2011). Tumor metastasis: molecular insights and evolving paradigms. *Cell* 147: 275–292.

53 Konig, H.E. and Liebich, H.G. (2004). *Veterinary Anatomy of Domestic Animals*. Blackwell.

54 Scott, D.W. (1980). Feline dermatology 1900-1978: a monograph. *J. Am. Anim. Hosp. Assoc.* 16: 349–364.

55 Young, L.A., Dodge, J.C., Guest, K.J. et al. (2002). Age, breed, sex and period effects on skin biophysical parameters for dogs fed canned dog food. *J. Nutr.* 132: 1695S–1697S.

56 Miller, W.H., Griffin, C.E., Campbell, K.L., and Muller, G.H. (2013). *Muller & Kirk's Small Animal Dermatology*, 7e, 1–70. Philadelphia, PA: WB Saunders.

57 Peterson, M.E. (2007). Diagnosis of hyperadrenocorticism in dogs. *Clin. Tech. Small Anim. Pract.* 22: 2–11.

58 Miragliotta, V., Coli, A., Ricciardi, M.P. et al. (2005). Immunohistochemical analysis of the distribution of desmoglein 1 and 2 in the skin of dogs and cats. *Am. J. Vet. Res.* 66: 1931–1935.

59 Denning, M.F., Guy, S.G., Ellerbroek, S.M. et al. (1998). The expression of desmoglein isoforms in cultured human keratinocytes is regulated by calcium, serum and protein kinase C. *Exp. Cell Res.* 239: 50–59.

60 Scott, D.W., Miller, W.H., and Griffin, C.E. (2001). Structure and function of the skin. In: *Small Animal Dermatology*, 6e, 1–70. Philadelphia, PA: WB Saunders.

61 Garrod, D. and Chidgrey, M. (2008). Desmosome structure, composition, and function. *Biochim. Biophys. Acta* 1778: 572–587.

62 Gunnaporn, S., Sirin, T., and Prapat, S. (2004). Filaggrin in canine skin. In: *Filaggrin* (ed. J.P. Thyssen and H.I. Maibach), 209–219. Berlin, Heidelberg: Springer-Verlag.

63 Thomsett, L.R. (1986). Structure of canine skin. *Br. Vet. J.* 112: 116–123.

64 Jackson, S.M., Williams, M.L., and Feingold, K.R. (1993). Pathobiology of stratum corneum. *West. J. Med.* 158: 279–285.

65 Neilsen, S.W. (1953). Glands of the canine skin. *Am. J. Vet.* 14: 448–454.

66 Nishifuji, K. and Yoon, J.S. (2013). The stratum corneum: the rampart of the mammalian body. *Vet. Dermatol.* 24: 60. -e16.

67 Elias, P.M. (2005). Stratum corneum defensive functions: an integrated views. *J. Invest. Dermatol.* 125: 183–200.

68 Banks, W.J. (1992). *Histologia Veterinária Aplicada*, 2e, 629. São Paulo: Manole.

69 Egelrud, T. (1993). Purification and preliminary characterization of stratum corneum chymotryptic enzyme: a proteinase that may be involved in desquamation. *J. Invest. Dermatol.* 101: 200–204.

70 Chapman, S.J. and Walsh, A. (1990). Desmosomes, corneosomes and desquamation – an ultrastructural study of adult-pig epidermis. *Arch. Dermatol. Res.* 282: 304–310.

71 Miroshnikova, Y.A., Le, H.Q., Schneider, D. et al. (2017). Adhesion forces and cortical tension couple cell proliferation and differentiation to drive epidermal stratification. *Nat. Cell Biol.* 20: 69–80.

72 Youssef, J., Nurse, A.K., Freund, L.B., and Morgan, J.R. (2011). Quantification of the forces driving self-assembly of three-dimensional microtissues. *Proc. Natl. Acad. Sci. USA* 108: 6993–6998.

73 Maitre, J.L., Berthoumieux, H., Gabriel Krens, S.F. et al. (2012). Adhesion functions in cell sorting by mechanically coupling the cortices of adhering cells. *Science* 338: 253–256.

74 Roberts, B.J., Pashaj, A., Johnson, K.R., and Wahl, J.K. (2011). Desmosome dynamics in migrating epithelial cells requires the actin cytoskeleton. *Exp. Cell Res.* 317: 2814–2822.

75 Freeman, S.C. and Sonthalia, S. (2022). *Histology, Keratohyalin Granules*. StatPearls.

76 Bragulla, H.H. and Homberger, D.G. (2009). Structure and functions of keratin proteins in simple, stratified, keratinized and cornified epithelia. *J. Anat.* 214: 516–559.

77 Rusnak, F. and Mertz, P. (2000). Calcineurin: form and function. *Physiol. Rev.* 80: 1483–1521.

78 Fisher, G.J., Duell, E.A., Nickoloff, B.J. et al. (1988). Levels of cyclosporin in epidermis of treated psoriasis patients differentially inhibit growth of keratinocytes cultured in serum-free versus serum-containing media. *J. Invest. Dermatol.* 91: 142–146.

79 Santini, M.P., Talora, C., Seki, T. et al. (2001). Cross talk among calcineurin, Sp1/Sp3, and NFAT in control of p21(WAF1/CIP1) expression in keratinocyte differentiation. *Proc. Natl. Acad. Sci. USA* 98 (17): 9575–9580.

80 Pena, J.A., Jacqueline, L., Losi-Sasaki, L., and Gooch, J.L. (2010). Loss of calcineurin Aα alters keratinocyte survival and differentiation. *J. Investig. Dermatol.* 130: 135–140.

81 Jauliac, S., López-Rodriguez, C., Shaw, L.M. et al. (2002). The role of NFAT transcription factors in integrin-mediated carcinoma invasion. *Nat. Cell Biol.* 4: 540–544.

82 O'Connor, R.S., Mills, S.T., Jones, K.A. et al. (2007). A combinatorial role for NFAT5 in both myoblast migration and differentiation during skeletal muscle myogenesis. *J. Cell Sci.* 120: 149–159.

83 Brun, C., Demeauxc, A., Guaddachi, F. et al. T-Plastin expression downstream to the calcineurin/NFAT pathway is involved in keratinocyte migration. *PLoS One* 9 (9): e104700. https://doi.org/10.1371/journal.pone.0104700.

84 Sevilla, L.M., Nachat, R., Groot, K.R. et al. (2007). Mice deficient in involucrin, envoplakin, and periplakin have a defective epidermal barrier. *J. Cell Biol.* 179: 1599–1612.

85 Scott, D.W. and Miller, W.H. (1996). Primary seborrhoea in English Springer spaniels: a retrospective study of 14 cases. *J. Small Anim. Pract.* 37: 173–178.

86 Englar, R.E. (2019). *Scale and Crusts. Common Clinical Presentations in Dogs and Cats*, 209–219. Wiley.

87 Pamela, E., Ginn, J.E., Mansell, K.L., and Pauline, M.R. (2007). Skin and appendages, chapter 5. In: *Jubb, Kennedy & Palmer's Pathology of Domestic Animals*, 5e, vol. 1 (ed. M.G. Maxie). New York, NY: Elsevier.

88 Hermanson, J.W., de Lahunta, A., and Evans, H.E. (2019). *Miller and Evan's Anatomy of the Dog*, 5e, vol. 2019, 61–77. Elsevier; Saunders.

89 Kobayashi, T., Shimizu, A., Nishifuji, K. et al. (2009). Canine hair-follicle keratinocytes enriched with bulge cells have the highly proliferative characteristic of stem cells. *Vet. Dermatol.* 20: 338–346. https://doi.org/10.1111/j.1365-3164.2009.00815.x.

90 Cotsarelis, G., Sun, T.T., and Lavker, R.M. (1990). Label retaining cells reside in the bulge area of pilosebaceaous unit: implications for follicular stem cells, hair cycle, and skin carcinogenesis. *Cell* 61: 1329–1337.

91 Kobayashi, T., Iwasaki, T., Amagai, M., and Ohyama, M. (2010). Canine follicle stem cell candidates reside in the bulge and share characteristic features with human bulge cells. *J. Invest. Dermatol.* 130: 1988–1995.

92 Gerhards, N.M., Sayar, B.S., Origgi, F.C. et al. (2016). Stem cell-associated marker expression in canine hair follicles. *J. Histochem. Cytochem.* 64: 190–204.

93 Kobayashi, T., Enomoto, K., Wang, Y.H. et al. (2013). Epidermal structure created by canine hair follicle keratinocytes enriched with bulge cells in a three-dimensional skin equivalent model in vitro implications for regenerative therapy of canine epidermis. *Vet. Dermatol.* 24: 77–83.

94 Ito, M., Liu, Y., Yang, Z. et al. (2005). Stem cells in the hair follicle bulge contribute to wound repair but not to homeostasis of the epidermis. *Nt. Med.* 11: 1351–1354.

95 Wiener DJ, Dohen MG, Muller EJ, Welle MM. Spatial distribution of stem cell-like keratinocytes in dissected compound hair follicles of the dog. *PLoS One* 11 (1): e0146937. 10.1371/journal.pone.0146937.2013):

96 Levy, V., Lindon, C., Harte, B.D., and Morgan, B.A. (2005). Distinct stem cell populations regenerate the f ollicle and interfollicular epidermis. *Dev. Cell* 9: 855–861.

97 Brachelente, C., Porcellato, I., Storna, M. et al. (2013). The contribution of stem cells to epidermal and hair follicle tumours in the dog. *Vet. Dermatol.* 24: 188–194.

98 Baker, K.P. (1974). Hair growth and replacement in the cat. *Br. Vet. J.* 130: 327–335.

99 Pavletic, M.M. (2010). *Atlas of Small Animal Wound Management and Reconstructive Surgery*. Wiley-Blackwell Publishing.

100 Ackerman, L. (2008). *Atlas of Small Animal Dermatology*. Buenos Aires: Inter-Medica.

101 Müntener, T., Doherr, M.G., Guscetti, F. et al. (2011). The canine hair cycle- a guide for the assessment of morphological and immunological and immunohistochemical criteria. *Vet. Dermatol.* 22: 383–395.

102 Ahmed, W., Kulikpowska, M., Ahlmann, T. et al. (2019). A comparative multi-site and whole-body assessment of fascia in the horse and dog: a detailed histological investigation. *J. Anat.* 235: 1065–1077.

103 Rojko, J.L., Hoover, E.A., and Martin, S.L. (1978). Histologic interpretation of cutaneous biopsies from dogs with dermatologic disorders. *Vet. Pathol.* 15: 579–589.

104 Scott, D.W., Miller, D.H., and Griffin, C.E. (2001). *Muller and Kirk's Small Animal Dermatology*, 6e, 1528. Philadelphia, PA: Saunders.

105 Williams, P.L. and Warwick, R. (1980). *Gray's Anatomy*, 36ee. London: WB Saunders.

106 Pakshir, P., Noskovicova, N., Lodyga, M. et al. (2020). The myofibroblast at a glance. *J. Cell Sci.* 133: jcs227900. https://doi.org/10.1242/jcs.227900.

107 Bohling, M.W., Henderson, R.A., Swaim, S.F. et al. (2004). Cutaneous wound healing in the cat: a macroscopic description and comparison with cutaneous wound healing in the dog. *Vet. Surg.* 33: 579–587.

108 Rudolph, R., Vande Berg, J., and Ehrlich, H.P. (1992). Wound contraction and scar contracture. In: *Wound Healing: Biochemical and Clinical Aspects* (ed. I.K. Cohen, R.F. Diegelmann, and W.J. Lindblad), 96–114. Philadelphia, PA: WB Saunders.

109 Pavletic, M.M. (2018). Basic principles of wound healing. In: *Atlas of Small Animal Wound Management and Reconstructive Surgery*, 4e (ed. M.M. Pavletic), 17–31. Ames, IA: Wiley-Blackwell.

110 Adams, D.R. (1986). *Canine Anatomy*. Ames: The Iowa State University Press.

111 Hellström, M., Hellström, S., Engström-Laurent, A., and Bertheim, U. (2014). The structure of the basement membrane zone differs between keloids, hypertrophic scars and normal skin: a possible back-ground to an impaired function. *J. Plast. Reconstr. Aesthet. Surg.* 67: 1564–1572.

112 Ouchi, N., Kihara, S., Arita, Y. et al. (2000). Adiponectin, an adiposite-derived plasma protein, inhibits endothelial NF-kappaB signaling through a cAMP-dependent pathway. *Circulation* 102: 1296–1301.

113 Kadowaki, T. and Yamauchi, T. (2005). Adiponectin and adiponectin receptors. *Endocr. Rev.* 26: 439–451.

114 Karbowska, J. and Kochan, Z. (2006). Role of adiponectin in the regulation of carbohydrate and lipid metabolism. *J. Physiol. Pharmacol.* 57: 103–113.

115 Mazaki-Tovi, M., Bolin, S.R., and Schenck, P.A. (2016). Differential secretion of adipokines from subcutaneous and visceral adipose tissue in healthy dogs: association with body condition and response to troglitazone. *Vet. J.* 216: 136–141.

116 Bohling, M.W. and Henderson, R.A. (2006). Differences in cutaneous wound healing between dogs and cats. *Vet. Clin. Small Anim. Prac.* 36: 687–692.

117 Lascelles, B.D.X. and White, R.A.S. (2001). Combined omental pedicle grafts and thoracodorsal axial pattern flaps for the reconstruction of chronic, nonhealing axillary wounds in cats. *Vet. Surg.* 30: 380–385.

118 Brockman, D.J., Pardo, A.C., Conzemius, M.G. et al. (1996). Omentum-enhanced reconstruction of chronic nonhealing wounds in cats: techniques and clinical use. *Vet. Surg.* 25: 99–104.

119 Schleip, R., Klingler, W., and Zorn, A. (2010). Biomechanical properties of fascial tissues and their role as pain generators. *J. Musculoskelet. Pain* 18 (4): 393–395.

120 Schleip, R., Jäger, H., and Klingler, W. (2012). What is 'fascia'? A review of different nomenclatures. *J. Bodyworks Mov. Ther.* 16: 496–502.

121 Schleip, R., Duerselen, L., Vleeming, A. et al. (2012). Strain hardening of fascia: static stretching of dense fibrous connective tissues can induce a temporary stiffness increase accompanied by enhanced matrix hydration. *J. Bodyworks Mov. Ther.* 16: 94–100.

122 Stecco, C., Macchi, V., Porzionato, A. et al. (2011). The fascia: the forgotten structure. *Ital. J. Anat. Embryol.* 116: 127–138.

123 McGavin, M. and Zachary, J. (2007). *Pathologic Basis of Veterinary Disease*. Elsevier.

124 Ashraft, M., Baguneid, M., and Bayat, A. (2016). The role of neuromediators and innervation in cutaneous wound healing. *Acta Dermatol. Venereol.* 96: 587–594.

125 Schaffer, M., Beiter, T., Becker, H.D., and Hunt, T.K. (1998). Neuropeptides: mediators of inflammation and tissue repair? *Arch. Surg.* 133: 1107–1116.

126 Leung, M.S. and Wong, C.C. (2000). Expressions of putative neurotransmitters and neuronal growth-related genes in Merkel cell-neurite complexes of the rats. *Life Sci.* 66: 1481–1490.

127 Wang, H., Xing, L., Li, W. et al. (2002). Production and secretion of calcitonin gene-related peptide from human lymphocytes. *J. Neuroimmunol.* 130: 155–162.

128 Roosterman, D., Goerge, T., Schneider, S.W. et al. (2006). Neuronal control of skin function: the skin as a neuroimmunoendocrine organ. *Physiol. Rev.* 86: 1309–1379.

129 Sternini, C. (1997). Organization of the peripheral nervous system: autonomic and sensory ganglia. *J. Investig. Dermatol. Symp. Proc.* 2: 1–7.

130 Ansel, J.C., Kaynard, A.H., Armstrong, C.A. et al. (1996). Skin-nervous system interactions. *J. Invest. Dermatol.* 106: 198–204.

131 Baraniuk, J.N., Kowalski, M.L., and Kaliner, M.A. (1990). Relationships between permeable vessels, nerves, and mast cells in rat cutaneous neurogenic inflammation. *J. Appl. Physiol.* 68: 2305–2311.

132 Lindsey, K.Q., Caughman, S.W., Olerud, J.E. et al. (2000). Neural regulation of endothelial cell-mediated inflammation. *J. Investig. Dermatol. Symp. Proc.* 5: 74–78.

133 Helme, R.D., Eglezos, A., and Hosking, C.S. (1987). Substance P induces chemotaxis of neutrophils in normal and capsaicin-treated rats. *Immunol. Cell Biol.* 65: 267–269.

134 Luger, T.A. and Lotti, T. (1998). Neuropeptides: role in inflammatory skin diseases. *J. Eur. Acad. Dermatol. Venereol.* 10: 207–211.

135 Smith, P.G. and Liu, M. (2002). Impaired cutaneous wound healing after sensor denervation in developing rats: effects on cell proliferation and apoptosis. *Cell Tissue Res.* 307: 281–291.

136 Souza, B.R., Cardoso, J.F., Amadeu, T.P. et al. (2005). Sympathetic denervation accelerates wound contraction but delays reepithelialization in rats. *Wound Repair. Regen.* 13: 498–505.

137 Fahey, T.J., Sadaty, A., Jones, W.G. 2nd et al. (1991). Diabetes impairs the late inflammatory response to wound healing. *J. Surg. Res.* 50: 308–313.

138 Cheng, C., Singh, V., Krishnan, A. et al. (2013). Loss of innervation and axon plasticity accompanies impaired diabetic wound healing. *PLoS One* 8: e75877.

139 Pavletic, M. (1999). *Atlas of Small Animal Surgery*. Elsevier.

140 Ninomiya, H., Akiyama, E., Simazaki, K. et al. (2011). Functional anatomy of the footpad vasculature of dogs: scanning electron microscopy of vascular corrosion casts. *Vet. Dermatol.* 22: 475–481.

141 Ninomiya, Y., Yamazaki, K., and Inomata, T. (2013). Comparative anatomy of the vasculature of the dog (Canis familiaris) and domestic cat (Felis catus) paw pad. *J. Vet. Med.* 3: 11–15.

142 Taylor, G.I. and Minabe, T. (1992). The angiosomes of the mammals and other vertebrates. *Plast. Reconstr. Surg.* 89: 181–215.

143 Fujii, M. and Terashi, H. (2019). Angiosome and tissue healing. *Ann. Vasc. Dis.* 12: 147–150.

144 Perc, B. and Erjavec, V. (2022). Overview of wound healing differences between dogs and cats. *Proc. Socratic Lectures* 7: 167–172.

145 Bohling, M.W. (2014). Wound healing. In: *Feline Soft Tissue and General Surgery* (ed. S.J. Langey-Hobbs, J.L. Demetriou, and J.F. Ladlow), 171–175. Velika Britanija: Elsevier Ltd.

146 Bragulla, H., Budras, K.D., Mülling, C. et al. (2004). Tegumento comum. In: *Anatomia dos Animais Domésticos: texto e atlas colorido*, vol. 2 (ed. H.E. König and H.G. Liebick), 325–380. Porto Alegre: Artmed.

147 Hargis, A.M. and Ginn, P.E. (2007). The integument. In: *Pathologic Basis of Veterinary Disease*, 4e (ed. M.D. McGavin and J.F. Zachary), 1107–1261. St Louis: Mosby Elsevier.

148 Pavletic, M.M. (2000). Use of an external skin-stretching device for wound closure in dogs and cats. *J. Am. Vet. Med. Assoc.* 7: 350–354.

149 Pavletic, M.M. (1980). Caudal superficial epigastric arterial pedicle grafts in the dog. *Vet. Surg.* 9: 103–107.

150 Pavletic, M.M. (1981). Canine axial pattern flaps, using omocervical, thoracodorsal, and deep circumflex iliac direct cutaneous arteries. *Am. J. Vet. Res.* 42: 391–406.

151 Pavletic, M.M. (1989). Thoracodorsal and caudal superficial epigastric axial pattern skin flaps in cats. *Vet. Surg.* 18: 380–385.

152 Oiki, N., Nishida, T., Ichihara, N. et al. (2003). Cleavage line patterns in beagle dogs: as a guideline for use in dermatoplasty. *Ant. Histol. Embryol.* 32: 65–69.

153 Gardner, J.H. and Raybuck, H.E. (1951). Cleavage line patterns of the cat. *Anat. Rec.* 110: 549–555.

154 Irwin, D.H.G. (1966). Tension lines in the skin of the dog. *J. Small Anim. Pract.* 7: 593–598.

155 Deroy, C., Destrade, M., McAlinden, A., and Ni, A.A. (2017). Non-invasive evaluation of skin tension lines with elastic waves. *Skin Res. Technol.* 23: 326–335.

156 Vranic, E. (2003). Iontophoresis: fundamentals, developments, and application. *Bosnian J. Basic Med. Sci.* 3: 54–58.

157 Kalia, Y.N., Naik, A., Garrison, J., and Guy, R.H. (2004). Iontophoretic drug delivery. *Adv. Drug Deliv. Rev.* 56: 619–658.

158 Rawat, S., Vengurlekar, S., Rakesh, B. et al. (2008). Transdermal delivery by iontophoresis. *Indian J. Pharm. Sci.* 70: 5 10.

159 Nickel, R., Schbummer, A., Seiferle, E. et al. (1986). The anatomy of the domestic animals. In: *The Locomotor System of the Domestic Mammals*, vol. 1. Berlin-Hamburg: Verlag Paul Parey, Springer Verlag.

160 Blottner, D., Huang, Y., Trautmann, G., and Sun, I. (2019). The fascia: continuum linking bone and myofascial bag for global and local body movement control on earth and space. A scoping review. *Rev. Human Space Explor.* https://doi.org/10.1016/j.reach.2019.100030.

161 Huijing, P.A., Maas, H., and Baan, G.C. (2003). Compartmental fasciotomy and isolating a muscle from neighboring muscles interfere with myofascial force transmission within the rat anterior crural compartment. *J. Morphol.* 256: 306–321.

162 Paoletti, S. (2006). *The Fasciae: Anatomy, Dysfunction and Treatment*. Seattle: Eastland Press.

163 Zhang, D., Dong, Y., Zhang, Y. et al. (2019). Spatial distribution and correlation of adipocytes and mast cells in the superficial fascia of rats. *Histochem. Cell Biol.* 152: 439–451.

164 Blackwood, L., Murphy, S., Buracco, P. et al. (2012). European consensus document on mast cell tumours in dogs and cats. *Vet. Comp. Oncol.* 10: el–e29.

165 Li, G., Zheng, B., Meszaros, L.B. et al. (2011). Identification and characterization of chondrogenic progenitor cells in the fascia of postnatal skeletal muscle. *J. Mol. Cell Biol.* 3: 369–377.

166 Choi, M.Y., Kim, H.I., Yang, Y.I. et al. (2012). The isolation and in situ identification of MSCs residing in loose connective tissues using a niche-preserving organ culture system. *Biomaterials* 33: 4469–4479.

167 Wong, H.L., Siu, W.S., Fung, C.H. et al. (2015). Characteristics of stem cells derived from rat fascia: in vitro proliferative and multilineage potential assessment. *Mol. Med. Rep.* 11: 1982–1990.

168 Phinney, D.G. and Prockop, D.J. (2007). Concise review: mesenchymal stem/multipotent stromal cells: the state of transdifferentiation and modes of tissue repair. *Curr. Views Stem Cell* 25: 2896–2902.

169 Correa-Gallegos, J.D., Christ, S., Ramesh, P. et al. (2019). Patch repair of deep wounds by mobilized fascia. *Nature* 576: 287–305.

170 Nakajima, H., Imanishi, N., Minabe, T. et al. (2004). Anatomical study of subcutaneous adipofascial tissue: a concept of the protective adipofascial system (PAFS) and lubricant adipofascial system (LAFS). *Scand. J. Plast. Reconstr. Surg. Hand Surg.* 38: 261–266.

171 Fox, M.W. (1963). Clinical observations on the panniculus reflex in the dog. *J. Am. Vet. Med. Assoc.* 142: 1296–1299.

172 Foss, K.D., Hague, D.W., and Selmic, L. (2021). Assessment of the cutaneus trunci reflex in neurologically healthy cats. *J. Feline Med. Surg.* 23: 287–292.

173 Adams, D.R. (2003). *Canine Anatomy: A Systemic Study*. Iowa State Press.

174 Gunn, H.M. (1978). The proportions of muscle, bone and fat in two different types of dogs. *Res. Vet. Sci.* 24: 277–282.

175 Huijing, P.A. and Baan, G.C. (2001). Myofascial force transmission causes interaction between adjacent muscles and connective tissue: effects of blunt dissection and compartmental fasciotomy on length force characteristics of rat extensor digitorum longus muscle. *Arch. Physiol. Biochem.* 109: 97–109.

176 Peckham, M. (2008). Engineering a multi-nucleated myotube, the role of the actin cytoskeleton. *J. Microsc.* 231: 486–493.

177 Saltin, B. and Mortensen, S.P. (2012). Inefficient functional sympatholysis is an overlooked cause of malperfusion in contracting skeletal muscle. *J. Physiol.* 590: 6269–6275.

178 Khan, M.M., Lustrino, D., Silveira, W.A. et al. (2016). Sympathetic innervation controls homeostasis of neuromuscular junctions in health and disease. *Proc. Natl. Acad. Sci. USA* 113: 746–750.

179 Banks, R.W., Hullinger, M., Saed, H.H., and Stacey, M.J. (2009). A comparative analysis of the encapsulated end-organs of mammalian skeletal muscles and of their sensory nerve endings. *J. Anat.* 214: 859–887.

180 Kumar, M.S.A. (2015). *Clinically Oriented Anatomy of the Dog and Cat*, 2e, Chapter 4. Ronkonkoma, NY: Linus Learning.

181 Joyner, M.J. and Casey, D.P. (2015). Regulation of increased blood flow (hyperemia) to muscles during exercise: a hierarchy of competing physiological needs. *Physiol. Rev.* 95: 549–601.

182 Queme, L.F., Ross, J.L., and Jankowski, M.P. (2017). Peripheral mechanisms of ischemic myalgia. *Front. Cell. Neurosci.* 11: 419. https://doi.org/10.3389/fncel.2017.00419.

183 Carpenter, S. and Karpati, G. (2001). *Pathology of Skeletal Muscle*. Oxford University Press.

184 Hardy, D., Besnard, A., Latil, M. et al. (2015). Comparative study of injury models for studying muscle regeneration in mice. *PLoS One* 11 (1): e0147198. https://doi.org/10.1371/journal.pone.0147198.

185 Wang, Y.X., Dumont, N.A., and Rudnicki, M.A. (2014). Muscle stem cells at a glance. *J. Cell Sci.* 127: 4543–4548.

186 Chen, J.C.J. and Goldhamer, D.J. (2003). Skeletal muscle stem cells. *Reprod. Biol. Endocrinol.* 1: 101–107.

187 Chargé, S.B.P. and Rudnicki, M.A. (2003). Cellular and molecular regulation of muscle regeneration. *Physiol. Rev.* 84: 209–238.

188 Ono, Y., Masuda, S., Nam, H.-S.W. et al. (2012). Slow-dividing satellite cells retain long-term self-renewal ability in adult muscle. *J. Cell Sci.* 125: 1309–1317.

189 Kann, A.P., Hung, M., and Krauss, R.S. (2021). Cell-cell contact and signaling in the muscle stem cell niche. *Curr. Opin. Cell Biol.* 73: 78–83.

190 Wu, J., Sun, X., Zhu, M. et al. (2012). Muscles and myoblast stem cells. *Int. J. Morphol.* 30: 1532–1537.

191 Tidball, J.G. (2017). Regulation of muscle growth and regeneration by the immune system. *Nat. Rev. Immunol.* 17: 165–178.

192 Tidball, J.G. and Villalta, S.A. (2010). Regulatory interactions between muscle and the immune system during muscle regeneration. *Am. J. Physiol. Regul. Integr. Comp. Physiol.* 298: R1173–R1187.

193 Waldemer-Streyer, R.J., Kim, D., and Chen, J. (2022). Muscle cell-derived cytokines in skeletal muscle regeneration. *FEBS J.* 289: 6463–6483.

194 Narayanan, N., Lengemann, P., Kim, K.H. et al. (2021). Harnessing nerve-muscle cell interactions for biomaterials- based skeletal muscle regeneration. *J. Biomed. Mater. Res.* 109: 289–299.

2

Physiology of Wound Healing and Clinical Considerations

Daniel J. Lopez

Department of Clinical Sciences, Cornell University, Ithaca, NY, USA

Stages of Wound Healing

The physiology of wound healing can be classified into three stages: inflammation, proliferation, and maturation [1–6]. The following stages, and their substages, are discussed below and this organizational scheme is highlighted in Table 2.1. While these stages are discussed distinctly, there is often significant commingling of the physiological processes between stages. In addition, varying regions of large wounds may progress through the stages at different rates. Finally, while proposed timelines of each stage are frequently present throughout the literature, each wound will follow its own unique timeline. Therefore, it is more important to determine the stage of a wound through observation as compared to tracking the days since injury. While the discussion below will primarily pertain to traumatic wounds of the epidermis and dermis, this classification can be applied to any biological wound, including surgical spay incisions, intestinal resection anastomosis, traumatic open wounds, and bony fractures.

From a clinical standpoint, the veterinarian's ultimate goal is to restore organ function. With regards to the skin, this is accomplished by successfully restoring the epidermal integrity of a wound, whether through primary intention or second intention healing. To achieve this goal, the veterinarian's initial focus should be to promote the transition of the wound from the inflammatory stage to the proliferative stage. This focus is crucial toward restoring and maintaining epithelial integrity, as the success of this transition marks the shift from response to repair.

Inflammatory Stage

The inflammatory phase of wound healing begins immediately following the disruption of the epithelium (such as the epidermis), whether purposefully or traumatically. It encompasses the periods of hemostasis and debridement and concludes as repair commences (characterized clinically by the appearance of granulation tissue). Overall, the inflammatory phase is highlighted by the body's innate reaction to epidermal disruption and its attempts to prevent infection.

Substages

Hemostasis
Key Cellular Regulator   The Platelet.

Timeframe   The hemostatic process begins immediately after epithelial disruption. While clot formation occurs quickly, the cytokines and growth factors released by platelet degranulation direct wound healing for several days after (e.g., PDGF, TGF β, FGF, EGF) [7–9].

Techniques in Small Animal Wound Management, First Edition. Edited by Nicole J. Buote.
© 2024 John Wiley & Sons, Inc. Published 2024 by John Wiley & Sons, Inc.
Companion website: www.wiley.com/go/buote/wounds

Table 2.1 Summary of stages of wound healing.

Stage	Substage	Key cellular regulator	Purpose	Clinical appearance
Inflammatory stage	Hemostasis	Platelet	Halting hemorrhage	Presence of clot or thrombosed vessels (Figure 2.1)
	Early inflammation/ debridement	Neutrophil	Removal of non-viable and foreign material. Provision of innate immune system	Presence of exudate, non-viable tissue, and possibly foreign material (Figure 2.2)
	Late inflammation/ wound programming	Macrophage	Coordinating the transition from response to repair	A noted decrease in the amount of exudate from early inflammation, with minimal nonviable tissue remaining (Figure 2.3)
Proliferative stage	Angiogenesis	Endothelial cell	Development of new vasculature	Progressive increase in bright red-to-pink "fleshy" cobblestone tissue within the wound (Figure 2.5)
	Granulation tissue	Fibroblast	Deposition of collagen into the feedback	
	Epithelialization	Keratinocyte	Restore function through epithelial continuity	Characterized as the colloquial "scar," which appears as a white, shiny, hairless, and glandless tissue covering (Figure 2.6)
	Contraction	Myofibroblast	Restore function through epithelial continuity	Best observed via wound size reduction across serial bandage changes (Figure 2.7)
Maturation stage		Fibroblast	Improve overall wound strength	Decrease in scar size and appearance, with less palpable thickening of the "wound ridge" as the collagen remodels (Figure 2.8)

Clinical Appearance   Presentation during the hemostatic phase is rather uncommon in veterinary medicine, as in most cases hemostasis has already occurred prior to presentation. It is not uncommon for owners to communicate with the veterinarian that "severe" hemorrhage was noted following the occurrence of the wound (hence prompting the emergent presentation), only for the hemorrhage to have "magically" ceased by the time of presentation. This is the hemostatic phase in action and may sometimes be evident by large blood clots within the wound that has stabilized the hemorrhage (Figure 2.1a). In addition, closer evaluation of local vasculature may reveal traumatized and thrombosed blood vessels, characterized by purple vessels that contract upon their length (Figure 2.1b). However, in some cases, the wound may demonstrate active hemorrhage from large vessels that have not been stabilized by a clot.

(a)

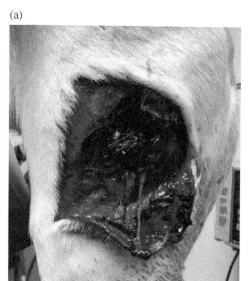

(b)

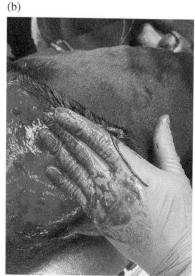

Figure 2.1 Hemostasis. (a) A sharp traumatic laceration presenting within approximately 5–10 minutes of the initial trauma. Note the dark fibrin clots present within the wound providing hemorrhage control. (b) A thrombosed and vasoconstricted vessel apparent within an acutely presenting wound. *Source:* Courtesy of Daniel Lopez, DVM DACVS-SA.

Summary Wound healing starts immediately after epithelial and endothelial injury, with IL-1 released secondary to keratinocyte injury and platelet aggregation/activation developing secondary to subendothelial tissue factor and collagen exposure [9]. This leads to the formation of a platelet plug via primary hemostasis [10]. Local vasoconstriction aids in hemostasis via the release of catecholamines, prostaglandin 2-α, and thromboxane-A2 from the site of injury and from the platelet plug [11]. Following the initial platelet plug, secondary hemostasis results in the formation of a fibrin clot. The fibrin clot is noted to be a crucial component of wound healing as it provides a mechanical environment that facilitates cellular infiltration and migration [3, 7, 12]. It also provides a biological environment rich in growth factors and cytokines (previously mentioned) secondary to platelet degranulation that aid in wound healing [12]. These growth factors and cytokines promote recruitment and differentiation of cells necessary for wound healing, such as neutrophils, macrophages, fibroblasts, keratinocytes, or endothelial cells [7, 8].

Clinical Considerations While hemostasis often occurs naturally secondary to vasoconstriction and clot formation, larger vessels continuing to hemorrhage at presentation may require surgical ligation or the application of electrosurgery. While hematomas are often retained within internal wounds (e.g., long bone fracture), these larger clots are frequently lost either in environment or during flushing/debridement of more superficial wounds. Therefore, while clearly beneficial to wound healing, there does not appear to be a necessity for hematoma retention for successful integumentary wound healing [12].

Early Inflammation
Key Cellular Regulator The Neutrophil.

Timeframe While inflammation and innate immune response begin almost immediately, neutrophil migration peaks at 24–48 hours [2, 13].

Clinical Appearance In most cases, traumatic wounds present to the veterinarian during the early inflammatory phase. Depending on the cause of trauma, wounds may appear clean (e.g., sharp laceration), may be contaminated with significant foreign material, or may have areas of significant trauma and devitalization (see Chapter 4 for in-depth discussion of wound classification). Over the course of the next 24–48 hours, continued declaration of previously traumatized tissues may become apparent characterized by color changes within tissue. Typically, the amount of exudate, either septic or non-septic, increases during this stage secondary to the suppurative response [3]. The wound will demonstrate the cardinal signs of inflammation, including warmth [calor], redness [rubor], swelling [tumor], and pain [dolor]. An example of a wound in the early inflammatory phase is provided in Figure 2.2.

Summary Exhaustion of the vasoconstrictor mechanisms, in conjunction with the local release of serotonin from platelet granules and histamine from mast cells, results in subsequent vasodilation. This vasodilation gives rise to the cardinal signs of inflammation described above [3, 11]. Neutrophils undergo chemotaxis and migrate into the wound under the influence of cytokines/growth factors including IL-1, PDGF, and TGA-β as well as by bacteria byproducts [3, 11]. Neutrophils function to aid in autolytic debridement, removal of foreign material, and to provide the initial innate immune defense against bacteria [12]. As neutrophils complete their job, they are either shed into the environment, which we identify as suppurative inflammation, or phagocytized via macrophages [11, 12].

Clinical Considerations The early inflammatory phase is ripe with opportunity for the veterinarian to provide a positive intervention for wound healing. Although previously thought that inflammation would "burn out" with time, it is now recognized that complex bioactive mechanisms must occur to facilitate

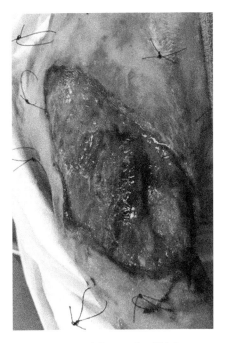

Figure 2.2 Early inflammation. This image depicts a wound localized on the caudal aspect of the left stifle following a traumatic injury one day post-initial injury. The wound demonstrates an exudate effusion, with varying areas of darkened color of the underlying musculature and skin edges with questionable viability. Both surgical and autolytic debridement were initiated to minimize the inflammatory burden of the wound. *Source:* Courtesy of Daniel Lopez, DVM DACVS-SA.

the transition from response to repair [3, 14, 15]. Therefore, minimizing continued inflammation is crucial for this complex transition. Examples of minimizing niduses of inflammation include serial removal of inflammatory debris and foreign material via flushing and sharp surgical debridement (see Chapter 5) [16, 17]. Autolytic debridement can be supported through hyperosmotic debridement dressings (see Chapters 7 and 8) [18, 19]. While the application of negative pressure wound therapy (Chapter 10) may be beneficial for continued removal of debris and suppurative exudate, a balance between the positives of this therapy versus the positives of daily macroscopic debridement should be weighed [20, 21].

Late Inflammation
Key Cellular Regulator   The Macrophage.

Timeframe   Macrophage migration peaks at 48–96 hours after the initial injury [5, 22, 23]. However, wound macrophages persist long into the healing process and provide continued direction via cytokine release [2, 22, 23].

Clinical Appearance   During the late inflammatory phase, the wound generally takes a "static" appearance during serial wound evaluations. No further tissue declaration is noted during sequential wound evaluations, and the need for sharp surgical debridement is reduced or absent. In addition, a gradual decrease in the amount of exudate may be noted. However, granulation tissue has yet to appear. Care should be taken not to confuse underlying musculature, if exposed, with granulation tissue, as the appearance can be similar (Figure 2.3).

Summary   As the veterinarian continues to work to minimize the niduses of inflammation, the cellular domination begins to shift from the neutrophil to the wound macrophage [2, 3, 5, 12]. The wound macrophage is the central cell that aids in the transition from the inflammatory phase to the proliferative phase; the experimental exclusion of macrophages has been demonstrated to be detrimental to healing [22–24]. This is accomplished through the release of growth factors and bioactive substances that promote the proliferative phase, as well as transformation of the macrophage from an inflammatory phenotype (M1) to the anti-inflammatory phenotype (M2) [23]. For example, macrophages influence the release of cytokines that differentiate local mesenchymal stem cells into fibroblasts (FGF-2) or promote angiogenesis (VEGF-A) [2]. In addition, macrophages both release and direct the production of matrix-metalloproteinases (MMPs), which facilitate the movement of cells, such as fibroblasts and endothelial cells, throughout the wound [3].

Clinical Considerations   The late inflammatory phase also provides opportunity for positive interventions by the veterinarian. Continued removal of inflammatory debris via flushing and debridement should occur as necessary. However, often during this phase, the need for surgical debridement has decreased and autolytic debridement can be supported through hyperosmotic debridement dressings (see Chapters 7 and 8). In addition, as the inflammation continues to subside,

(a)

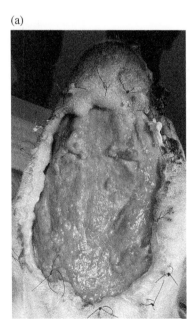

(b)

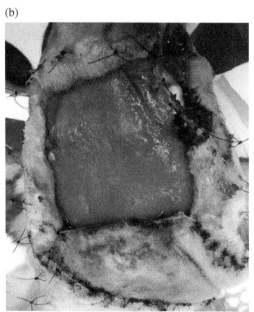

Figure 2.3   Late inflammation. These images are of the same patient, with the image (a) being taken approximately seven days prior to the image (b). Image (a) represents the period of late inflammation, which is characterized by a progressively decreasing amount of exudate and the lack of any necrotic tissue. Although the tissue appears pink to red, note that this is mainly exposed to underlying musculature and should not be confused with a robust granulation bed (as observed in image b). Note: a flap was instituted between images (a,b) to recruit epithelial tissue. *Source:* Courtesy of Daniel Lopez, DVM DACVS-SA.

dressings targeting debridement may slowly be transitioned to dressings targeting moist wound healing to aid in the progression to the proliferative phase and minimize trauma to early granulation tissue [18, 19]. Finally, a strong consideration can be given to negative pressure wound therapy during the late inflammatory phase to promote the transition to the proliferative phase through supporting angiogenesis and collagen production [20, 21].

Proliferative Stage

The transition to the proliferative phase represents a major milestone in wound healing, as the body's response shifts from reacting to the wound to repairing the wound. There are four hallmarks to the proliferative stage of wound healing; angiogenesis, granulation tissue formation, epithelialization, and wound contraction. The process of each step is illustrated in Figure 2.4a–d. These hallmarks aim to develop a robust and sustainable blood supply to the wound, to fill the wound defect with a rugged collagen bed, and finally provide an epithelial covering to restore function.

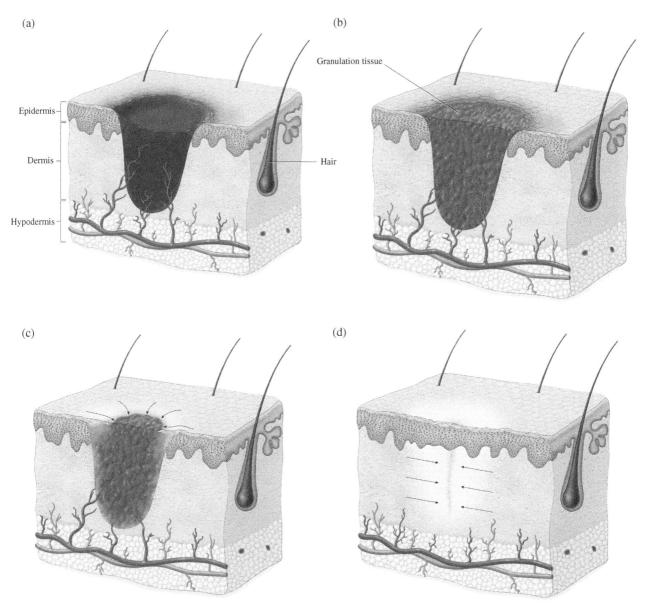

Figure 2.4 **Hallmarks of the proliferative stage**. These illustrations depict the hallmarks of the proliferative stage, including angiogenesis (a), granulation tissue formation (b), epithelialization (c), and contraction (d). *Source:* Courtesy of Daniel Lopez, DVM DACVS-SA.

With regards to large open wounds, advanced reconstructive techniques can be considered to hasten epidermal continuity. Their indications and considerations are discussed in Chapter 16 as well as other references. The success of these techniques is often improved through the development of a healthy wound bed via a robust proliferative response.

Although many previous reports provide a guideline regarding the time frame of the proliferative phase, with reviews noting this phase beginning as early as three to four days, the true onset of the proliferative phase can be highly variable [3, 5]. This variability is dependent on the success of minimizing inflammatory niduses, as persistent inflammation can stall or dampen a robust proliferative response [3, 5, 15]. If a veterinarian expects a wound to have a robust proliferative phase yet the wound appears stagnant, additional diagnostics and interventions may be necessary (see inherent detriments to wound healing below).

Substages

Angiogenesis
Key Cellular Regulator   The Endothelial Cell.

Clinical Appearance   See description of granulation tissue below.

Summary   While the process of angiogenesis begins immediately following injury via platelet degranulation, the cumulative and clinical impact of this angiogenesis is not observed until several days later [2, 5]. Endothelial cell proliferation and subsequent neovascularization are stimulated by both local hypoxia and cytokines [2, 5]. The primary cytokines influencing angiogenesis are FGF and VEG-F, which are released by both platelets, macrophages, and keratinocytes [5, 25, 26]. This endothelial proliferation leads to the development of new blood vessels that support collagen deposition and aid in immune function through improved tissue perfusion [15, 27].

Clinical Considerations   While clinically apparent angiogenesis takes time, it can likely be accelerated using negative pressure wound therapy [20, 21]. Given the high prevalence of multidrug-resistant bacteria within hospitals, the clinical importance of angiogenesis cannot be understated. Improving wound perfusion improves the delivery of oxygen and innate immune cells to the wound, thereby allowing a natural response to fight the infection [15, 27]. In addition, improved wound perfusion maximizes the delivery of systemic antibiotics to the desired target [28].

Granulation Tissue Formation
Key Cellular Regulator   The Fibroblast.

Clinical Appearance   The clinical appearance of granulation tissue demarks the transition into the proliferative stage, and its recognition is key to determining that the wound is progressing appropriately. Early granulation tissue is characterized in appearance by a bright red-to-pink "fleshy" cobblestone tissue that is easily traumatized. The red color of granulation tissue and its granular appearance is a result of angiogenesis and the formation of new capillary buds throughout the collagen stroma [26]. As time progresses, the bright red color of granulation tissue shifts to be paler in color as the ratio of blood vessels to collagen decreases with maturation (Figure 2.5) [2, 6].

(a)

(b)

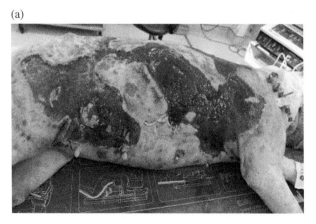 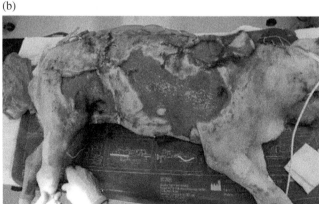

Figure 2.5   (a,b) **Granulation tissue**. These images are from a patient who suffered severe burn injuries. The image on the left (a) is representative of early granulation tissue, which is redder in color secondary to the newly developing blood vessels during angiogenesis. The image on the right (b) represents a more mature granulation bed, which has greater collagen dominance and vascular maturation resulting in an overall paler color. *Source:* Courtesy of Daniel Lopez, DVM DACVS-SA.

Summary Granulation tissue consists of collagen and associated fibroblasts, capillaries, and macrophages [2]. Quiescent mesenchymal cells residing in local tissues differentiate into fibroblasts under the influence of wound cytokines produced by the macrophage and migrate throughout the wound with the aid of matrix-metalloproteinases [2]. Fibroblasts produce collagen (initially thinner type 3 collagen as compared to stronger residual type 1), which in combination with angiogenesis gives rise to the characteristic appearance of granulation tissue [2, 3]. The deposition of collagen eventually exceeds angiogenesis as time progresses, resulting in a paler color change with collagen dominance [6]. Granulation tissue synthesis continues and aims to fill the dead space of the wound, thereby aiding in contraction and providing a surface for epithelization to occur.

Clinical Considerations Moist wound environments have been documented to be beneficial for the production and support of granulation tissue [18, 19]. Wound dressings can differ in both their absorptive capacity and their antibacterial properties, such as silver versus honey; therefore, dressing choice should be determined based on wound assessment, clinical experience, and response to previous treatment. Dressings are discussed in further detail in Chapter 8. Exuberant granulation tissue is defined as the production of granulation tissue that exceeds the height of the surrounding epidermis. Exuberant granulation tissue is rather uncommon in small animals, and generally only occurs mildly when present. More severe cases may benefit from judicious reduction of exuberant granulation tissue by sharp dissection to support contraction and epithelialization. Finally, a significant species differences is noted with regards to the production of granulation tissue; cats are noted to produce both less granulation tissue with a more peripheral distribution compared to dogs [29].

Epithelialization
Primary Cellular Regulator Keratinocyte.

Clinical Appearance Epithelization produces the colloquial "scar," which is characterized by a white, shiny, hairless, and glandless tissue covering. This process is demonstrated in Figure 2.6. The lack of hair covering is secondary to the lack of dermal layer, which normally supports the epidermis but is replaced by granulation tissue during second intention healing.

Figure 2.6 (a,b) **Epithelialization**. These images are from a severe degloving/shearing wound over the antebrachium of a dog. The image on the left (a) was taken during the proliferative phase, where a robust granulation bed covered the previously exposed bone. The image on the right (b) was taken several weeks later, which demonstrates epithelial continuity achieved primarily through epithelialization which is observed as the white, shiny, hairless covering of the granulation bed. Secondary to the extent of epithelialization due to the lack of contraction capability given the wound location, this epidermal covering was fragile and frequently traumatized. *Source:* Courtesy of Daniel Lopez, DVM DACVS-SA.

(a)

(b)

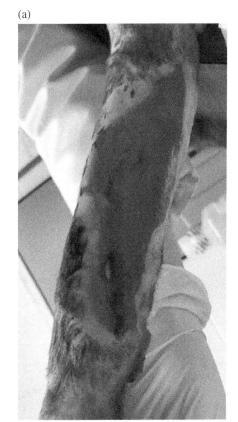
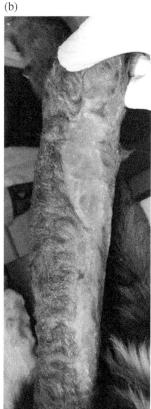

Summary Relatively quickly after initial wounding, epithelial cells begin migrating from the wound edges in an attempt to restore epithelial continuity [2, 12]. In the wake of migration, epithelial cells proliferate to restore epidermal thickness [2]. This process is influenced by wound cytokines such as EGF, FGF, or TGF-β, and is accelerated as the underlying wound matrix matures during the proliferative process [2, 3, 7]. The capability of proliferation and migration is not limitless however and is therefore synergistic with wound contraction to restore epidermal coverage for larger wounds.

Clinical Considerations Epithelization is encouraged in a moist wound environment [18, 19]. In cases where epithelization stalls, epidermal recruitment techniques can be employed. For example, island skin grafts can be inserted into a healthy wound bed, providing additional epithelial cells for radial proliferation and migration. Skin grafts are further discussed in Chapter 16. While epithelialization is beneficial for restoring epithelial continuity, this layer can be relatively fragile and prone to injury. This fragility is clinically apparent by continual splitting/breaking and resealing with relatively benign trauma. Therefore, considerations for advanced reconstructions may be necessary to provide a more robust epidermal covering.

Wound Contraction

Primary Cellular Regulator Myofibroblast.

Clinical Appearance It is often difficult to observe contraction at a single time point; therefore, it is best observed serially over multiple bandage changes. The surface area of the wound gradually decreases in size with each subsequent evaluation (Figure 2.7). An important step for monitoring wound healing includes objective measurement of the wound's surface area. Keeping detailed records of the largest dimension in two axes allows for accurate assessment of progress. This reduction in size is more than what is observed via concurrent epithelialization. On occasion, with profound contraction, the skin may carry a "shrinking" appearance.

Summary Fibroblasts within the wound undergo a phenotypic transition to myofibroblasts under the influence of mechanical tension and cytokines/growth factors, primary PDGF, and TGF-β [12, 30]. A hallmark characteristic of the myofibroblast is the development of smooth muscle actin fibers [30]. Myofibroblasts reorient themselves along the tension lines of the wound, anchor themselves both to the extracellular matrix and to each other, and trigger wound contraction through shortening of the smooth muscle actin [6, 30]. Contraction can occur at a rate of 0.75 mm per day in humans [2, 5].

(a) (b)

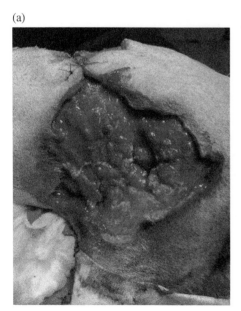 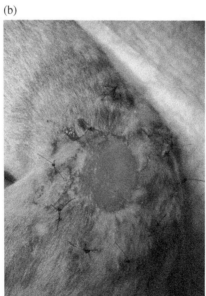

Figure 2.7 (a,b) **Contraction**. These images are from a patient who suffered a severe bite wound overlying the left and right dorsal flank with subsequent necrosis. The image on the left (a) was taken immediately after initial debridement and is representative of the early inflammatory phase of wound healing. The degree of defect raised concern for the potential need for advanced reconstructive pictures. However, the wound was allowed to heal initially by second intention and the image on the right (b) was taken approximately one month later. The degree of contraction noted over this time was profound. Notice in comparison to the previous epithelialization images (a,b), the wound's closure is minimally due to the white, shiny, hairless tissue (observed at the wound edge). This emphasizes that the majority of this wound closure has occurred by contraction, which maintains a dermal component, as compared to epithelialization. *Source:* Courtesy of Daniel Lopez, DVM DACVS-SA.

Clinical Considerations   As with the previous substages, a moist wound environment supports wound contraction [18, 19]. Given the relatively loosely adherent skin in small animals, contraction can provide a significant reduction in wound size. The shape of the wound likely influences the success of wound contraction as well, with linear wounds contracting faster in comparison to circular wounds in humans [5]. Providing radial traction on the wound edges, toward the center of the wound, may support contraction through aiding in local stress relaxation of elastin fibers. This radial traction can be generated from the radial pull of a tie over bandages, or a vacuum-assisted closured device. Caution should be had relying on contracture over certain areas, such as joints or near orifices, as the resulting contracture may alter the function of the adjacent structures.

Primary Intention Considerations   While we often cannot visualize the proliferative phase in wounds undergoing primary closure, this phase is still a crucial process for primary intention wound healing. Epithelialization is often the primary component of restoring epidermal continuity in wounds closed by primary intention. Wounds healing through primary intention can form an epidermal seal within 24 hours [5]. Therefore, when suturing wounds primarily, the promotion of dermal (and epidermal) apposition is crucial to minimize the distance necessary for epithelial cell migration and limit the need for wound contraction. This is exceptionally important when creating permanent stomas (e.g., perineal urethrostomy, tracheostomy, etc.), as contraction and excessive granulation tissue formation due to poor tissue layer apposition contributes to stoma stricture. Collagen production, or granulation tissue, still occurs within wounds closed primarily, thereby filling the dead space and bridging the incision to increase wound strength. This "wound ridge" is readily palpable within the incision, and its absence may suggest a failure in wound remodeling and raises a concern for overall wound strength [5].

Maturation Phase

Primary Cellular Regulator
Fibroblasts.

Peak Timeframe
While starting in combination with the late proliferative phase, it continues over the next 12–18 months [2]. The net production of collagen peaks by approximately day 21, and the rate of wound strength gain tapers off by six weeks post-wounding [2].

Clinical Appearance
Over time, the scar becomes less apparent and the wound ridge becomes less palpable secondary to remodeling and maturation of the deeper tissue layers and the epithelial surface (Figure 2.8).

(a)   (b)   (c)

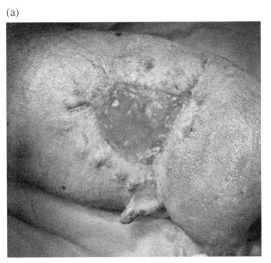 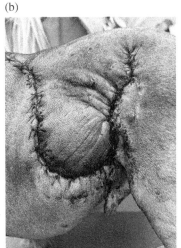 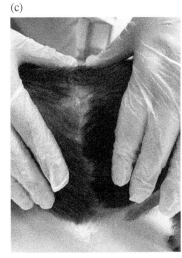

Figure 2.8   (a–c) **Wound maturation**. These pictures are serially taken from a patient with a severe flank wound (a) that was augmented with a rotational subdermal plexus flap to achieve epidermal continuity (b). The image in the middle (b) was taken approximately three days postoperatively. Note the moderate swelling of the tissues and the prominence of the incision. The image on the right (c) was taken approximately two months later, emphasizing complete remodeling of both the incision and the underlying granulation tissue resulting in a smooth, relatively unnoticeable scar. *Source:* Courtesy of Daniel Lopez, DVM DACVS-SA.

Summary

The maturation phase is often a second thought after the complexities of the inflammatory and the proliferative phase. However, the continued reorganization, cross-linkage, and replacement of haphazardly produced type 3 collagen fibers to type 1 collagen fibers result in progressive increase in wound strength that is necessary to maintain organ function [2, 6]. This wound strength reaches approximately 50% of the wound strength at three months in the skin, but peaks at 70–80% of non-wounded tissues long-term [6].

Clinical Considerations

Luckily, maturation often occurs without significant support from the veterinarian. However, given the lack of return to normal skin strength, the scar remains a weak point. Failures in maturation may lead to reopening of previously closed scars, which can be a source of frustration to both the owner and the veterinarian. Indolent pocket wounds, whether developing during primary or second intention healing, provide a clinical example of maturation failure [31–33]. While the focus of skin healing is often aimed at healing tissues "side-to-side," catastrophic complications can occur if "superficial-to-deep" (or dermal to granulation bed) is not emphasized. Indolent pocket wounds occur secondary to this failure of "superficial-to-deep" healing, whereas the dermal/epidermal surface and the granulation surfaces fail to adhere and subsequently progress through the healing process separately [33].

The formation of an indolent pocket wound during primary closure may result in a phenomenon termed "pseudohealing" [32]. Failure of the "superficial-to-deep" healing during primary closures results in both excessive dead space and failure of collagen deposition to bridge across the wound (the aforementioned wound ridge), thereby decreasing overall wound strength [5, 32]. Normal daily activities, such as grooming, overwhelm the strength of the maturing epidermal seal resulting in complete dehiscence [32].

Indolent pocket wounds also occur during second intention wound healing, where indolent ulcers develop characterized by failure of adherence of the epidermal/dermal layer to the underlying granulation tissue. Attempts at wound contraction result in inward rolling of the epidermal edge as opposed to along the granulation bed. Attempts at epithelialization result in migration of the keratinocytes between the granulation and dermal bed instead of across the surface of the granulation bed. As time progresses, the epithelialized edges of the wound become fibrotic and wound healing stalls completely. In both instances, restoring fresh epithelial edges and ensuring appropriate contact between the dermal and granulation bed/minimizing dead space are crucial for success.

Inherent Detriments to Wound Healing

In conjunction with targeting wound therapy based on the underlying pathophysiology, the veterinarian should also consider if patient comorbidities may influence the normal progression of wound healing (Table 2.2). Inherent physiological changes within a patient often alter the patterns of inflammation and cytokine distribution, which ultimately can derail the normal processes of wound healing [15, 32–34].

Table 2.2 Summary of factors acting as inherent detriments to wound healing.

Local wound factors	Systemic patient factors
Poor tissue oxygenation	Older age
Infection	Species variation (dog versus cat)
Residual foreign material	Poor nutritional status
	Metabolic diseases
	Medications
	Radiation therapy

Tissue Oxygenation

Appropriate oxygen supply to a wound is crucial for progressive healing [27, 35]. Angiogenesis, collagen deposition and fibroplasia, epithelialization, contraction, and immune function are all dependent on the relative supply of oxygen within a wound [27, 34]. Therefore, ensuring appropriate oxygen delivery is crucial to support all stages of wound healing. The wound initially is relatively hypoxic secondary to the high oxygen consumption via metabolically active cells and poor perfusion [35]. Local hypoxia is overcome through angiogenesis to improve oxygen delivery [26]. However, the clinician should aim to maximize both oxygen availability and delivery prior to robust angiogenesis.

Interventions to improve oxygen delivery can be as simple as ensuring patients are hemodynamically resuscitated to maintain cardiac output or providing supplementary oxygen to patients with concurrent respiratory comorbidities. More complex treatments include maximizing oxygen delivery through hyperbaric oxygen therapy (see Chapter 13). While hyperbaric oxygen therapy has been utilized in humans to improve local oxygen delivery, the efficacy in veterinary medicine remains unclear and the availability uncommon [36].

Infection

With disruption of the epithelial barrier, microorganisms are provided easy access to the normally protected deeper tissues. While the innate immune system aims to limit the consequences of these microorganisms, this system can become overwhelmed resulting in the progression from contamination to colonization to infection (see Chapters 4 and 5).

Complications with wound healing occur because of the presence of bacteria and the body's response to those bacteria. In the presence of infection, the body remains in a pro-inflammatory phase via the production of proinflammatory cytokines, including IL-1 and TNF-α, which stalls the transition into the proliferative phase [34, 37]. In addition, unregulated bacterial byproducts, such as collagenases and matrix metalloproteinases, counter attempts at a robust repair [34, 37]. This is often best characterized in the environment of anastomotic healing in patients with concurrent septic peritonitis. Unfortunately, infections in wounds can be extremely challenging to overcome, given the initial reduction in perfusion (hampering the efficacy of antibiotics) and the formation of wound biofilms. Management of wound infections is discussed in further detail in Chapters 4 and 5.

Residual Foreign Material

Similar to infection, retained foreign material potentiates a chronic inflammatory response. This proinflammatory environment continues to stagnate the progression of the proliferative stage, negatively impacting wound healing [5, 16].

Age

While age is not a disease, it has been associated with alterations in wound healing both in humans and veterinary species. In humans, it is generally thought that it is the rate of progression of healing, rather than the overall quality, that is impacted via changes in both the inflammatory and proliferative phases [34, 38, 39]. These changes may also be attributed to reductions in dermal thickness and microcirculation as the patient ages [6, 40]. Age has been implicated as a risk factor in wound healing in veterinary patients undergoing gastrointestinal surgery as well [41].

Species

Species differences in both primary intention and second intention healing have been documented (Table 2.3). These changes may be related to their dermal blood supply, with dogs demonstrating a greater density of collateral subcutaneous trunk vessels than cats [42]. For patients undergoing primary intention healing, wounds in cats were documented to only be 50% as strong as wounds in dogs at day 7 [29]. During this first week, cats are also demonstrated to have decreased cutaneous perfusion in comparison to dogs; however, these differences appear to disappear after seven days [29]. Finally, while subcutaneous tissues play an important role in supporting wound healing, their function appears to be more important in cats than dogs [43]. While wound healing is often successful in feline patients, these differences support the clinical perception of cats taking longer to heal open wounds than dogs.

Nutritional Status

The nutritional and metabolic status of patients, both acutely and chronic, warrants evaluation to optimize wound healing. In an acute wound setting, the metabolic need of the patient significantly increases as the patient enters a catabolic state.

Table 2.3 Species differences.

Anatomical differences	Dogs have a higher density of collateral subcutaneous trunk vessels
	Cats have decreased skin perfusion during first week of healing
Primary closure incisions	Dogs have a 2× breaking strength compared to cats at seven days
Secondary intention healing	
Granulation	Cats: less granulation tissue; takes mean of 6.3 days first observation and a mean of 19 d to cover the wound
	Dogs: more granulation tissue; takes a mean of 4.5 days to first observation and a mean of 7.5 days to cover the wound
Epithelialization	Cats: 13% of wound area reepithelialized by day 14
	Dogs: 44% of wound area reepithelialized by day 14

This is especially apparent in burn patients. These increased metabolic demands can be difficult to overcome given the concurrent inflammatory cascade which may contribute to an overall feeling of malaise and patient inappetence. Therefore, supplementary feeding techniques to aid in matching patient demands (which likely exceed resting energy requirement) may be necessary. Early enteral nutrition has been documented to have a positive effect in human and veterinary patients; however, further research is needed in veterinary species [41, 44–54]. Chronic malnutrition may impede wound healing ability secondary to the chronic negative energy balance and lack of appropriate reserves to combat the catabolic wound healing state [15, 34]. Obesity in the veterinary field is becoming increasingly more common and may have a greater impact on wound healing than is currently comprehended. Obese human patients have been documented to have impaired wound healing, likely secondary to either adipokines or increased tension on wounds [15, 34].

While intricacies of nutrition are highly complex, with many factors coming into play, the most important nutritional component pertaining to wound healing is likely protein availability. Amino acids are crucial for collagen production and immune function [34]. Therefore, deficiencies in proteins can impair capillary formation, decrease collagen production, increase the risk of wound infection, and negatively impact wound healing [34]. In veterinary patients, diets deficient in proteins have been demonstrated to delay wound healing and decrease wound strength, with a recommendation of maintaining serum proteins higher than 2.0 g/dL to minimize these consequences [1, 4, 15, 55]. The consequences of decreased serum proteins have also been observed in some patients undergoing gastrointestinal anastomotic healing, as hypoalbuminemia has been identified as a risk factor for intestinal dehiscence [56, 57].

Metabolic Diseases

While the relationship between metabolic diseases and wound healing is extensively investigated in human medicine, these investigations in veterinary medicine are rather incomplete. Metabolic diseases implicated to negatively impact wound healing in veterinary patients include hyperadrenocorticism and hypothyroidism [58]. Excessive endogenous glucocorticoids negatively impact wound healing through the atrophy of epidermal and granulation tissue and impaired macrophage activity, limited fibroblast proliferation, decreased collagen synthesis, and decreased synthesis of matrix metalloproteinases (MMP) [4, 6, 59, 60]. Chronic stress in veterinary patients may be an underrecognized source of endogenous glucocorticoids, as stress is implicated in impaired wound healing in humans by reducing the number of pro-inflammatory cytokines, including IL-1 and TNF-α [34]. Wound complications and immunosuppression secondary to diabetes is a well-documented association in humans, with hyperglycemia affecting leukocyte function, MMP expression and function, and altering vascular supply [15, 34]. While this relationship is fully established in humans, a connection between impaired wound healing has yet to be made in veterinary patients. Regardless, continued glycemic control should be recommended to minimize any potential risk [15]. Other encountered metabolic diseases, such as renal disease, liver disease, immunosuppressive diseases (IMHA, ITP, etc.), and cancer may all dysregulate the inflammatory process leading to alterations in wound healing or altering the metabolic demands of cells [4, 15, 34]. Regardless of the metabolic disease, attempting to regulate the disease prior to wound creation may result in improved wound healing. However, in many cases, this is not possible, such as with unplanned traumatic wounds, and the veterinarian should inform the owner of the potential for increased complications and longer time to healing.

Medications

The administration of medications can alter the natural inflammatory pathway and change cytokine profiles. The administration of glucocorticoids has been documented to lead to reductions in granulation tissue, decreased wound contraction, delayed wound healing, and reduced tensile strength in human and animal models [34]. These associations are likely both time and dose-dependent. In addition, secondary immunosuppression from higher doses may lead to an increased likelihood of local infection. Therefore, veterinarians should identify the lowest tolerated steroid dose, if necessary, to minimize the risk of wound complications. While the short-term administration of non-steroidal anti-inflammatory drugs has not been shown to impact wound healing, the long-term administration of this class of drug has been documented to have an anti-proliferative effect through impairing wound contraction, epithelization, angiogenesis, and collagen strength [34, 61]. While this association has not been identified in skin healing in the veterinary species, it has been identified with delayed bone healing [62]. Finally, chemotherapeutic agents target rapidly dividing cells, inhibit cellular metabolism, and inhibit angiogenesis. These targets are unfortunately all major participants in normal wound healing. Therefore, the use of these medications decreases wound matrix production, collagen production, fibroblast proliferation, and leads to immunosuppression, all negatively affecting wound healing [4, 34, 63]. In most cases, chemotherapeutic agents are not recommended until after epidermal continuity (aka incisional healing and suture remove) is complete.

Radiation Therapy

Radiation therapy has long been documented to impair normal wound healing, although the pathogenesis is complex and remains poorly understood [64]. Several pathological mechanisms likely occur in concert, including cellular depletion (reduction in proliferating cells secondary to ionizing radiation damage), fibroblast dysfunction (decreased growth rates, replicative capacity, and contractility), alterations in the extracellular matrix (dysregulation of collagen production and maturation), microvascular impairment (development of a fibrotic microangiopathy leading to decreased perfusion/delivery of oxygen and reduced neovascularization) and cytokine/growth factor derangements (increased production of proinflammatory cytokines including IL-1 and TNF-α) [4, 64, 65]. Clinically, flaps occurring in a previously irradiated fields of veterinary patients have been demonstrated to have increased risk for wound complications [66].

Conclusion

The body has an amazing healing capability, and the phrase "wounds heal in spite of the veterinarian, not because of" does carry some truth. To support this healing process, the veterinarian's initial focus should be to aid the wound in its transition from the inflammatory phase to the proliferative phase. If this transition stalls, the veterinarian should evaluate both the wound and the patient for factors that may be deterring this transition. Finally, once the wound shifts from response to repair, the veterinarian's focus should aim to restoring epithelial continuity, whether through delayed primary closure, secondary closure, or second intention healing.

References

1 Balsa, I.M. and Culp, W.T.N. (2015). Wound care. *Vet. Clin. Small Anim.* 45: 1049–1065.
2 Baum, C.L. and Arpey, C.J. (2005). Normal cutaneous wound healing: clinical correlation with cellular and molecular events. *Dermatol. Surg.* 31: 674–686.
3 Broughton, G. 2nd, Janis, J.E., and Attinger, C.E. (2006). The basic science of wound healing. *Plast. Reconstr. Surg.* 117: 12S–34S.
4 Buote, N. (2021). Updates in wound management and dressings. *Vet. Clin. Small Anim.* 52 (2): 289–315.
5 Singh, S., Young, A., and McNaught, C. (2017). The physiology of wound healing. *J. Surg.* 35 (9): 473–477.
6 Stanley, B.J. and Cornell, K. (2018). Wound healing. In: *Veterinary Surgery: Small Animal*, 2e (ed. S.A. Johnston and K.M. Tobias), 132–148. St. Louis: Elsevier Health Sciences.
7 Barrientos, S., Stojadinovic, O., Golinko, M.S. et al. (2008). Growth factors and cytokines in wound healing. *Wound Repair Regener.* 16: 585–601.
8 Vaidyanathan, L. (2021). Growth factors in wound healing- a review. *Biomed. Pharmacol. J.* 14: 1469–1480.
9 Henry, G. and Garner, W.L. (2003). Inflammatory mediators in wound healing. *Surg. Clin. North Am.* 83: 483–507.

10 Furie, B. and Furie, B.C. (2008). Mechanism of thrombus formation. *N. Engl. J. Med.* 359: 938–949.

11 Broughton, G. 2nd, Janis, J.E., and Attinger, C.E. (2006). Wound healing: an overview. *Plast. Reconstr. Surg.* 117: 1e-S–32e-S.

12 Singer, A.J. and Clark, R.A.F. (1999). Cutaneous wound healing. *N. Engl. J. Med.* 341: 738–746.

13 Kim, M.H., Liu, W., Borjesson, D.L. et al. (2008). Dynamics of neutrophil infiltration during cutaneous wound healing and infection using fluorescence imaging. *J. Invest. Dermatol.* 128: 1812–1820.

14 Dovi, J.V., Szpaderska, A.M., and DiPietro, L.A. (2004). Neutrophil function in the healing wound: adding insult to injury? *Thromb. Haemost.* 92: 275–280.

15 Franz, M.G., Robson, M.C., Steed, D.L. et al. (2008). Guidelines to aid healing of acute wounds by decreasing impediments of healing. *Wound Repair Regener.* 16: 723–748.

16 Ayello, E.A. and Cuddigan, J.E. (2004). Debridement: controlling the necrotic/cellular burden. *Adv. Skin Wound Care* 17: 66–75.

17 Kirshen, C., Woo, K., Ayello, E.A. et al. (2006). Debridement: a vital component of wound bed preparation. *Adv. Skin Wound Care* 19: 506–517.

18 Junker, J.P.E., Kamel, R.A., Caterson, E.J., and Eriksson, E. (2013). Clinical impact upon wound healing and inflammation in moist, wet, and dry environments. *Adv. Wound Care* 2: 348–356.

19 Nuutila, K. and Eriksson, E. (2021). Moist wound healing with commonly available dressings. *Adv. Wound Care* 10: 685–698.

20 Demaria, M., Stanley, B.J., Hauptman, J.G. et al. (2011). Effects of negative pressure wound therapy on healing of open wounds in dogs. *Vet. Surg.* 40: 658–669.

21 Pitt, K.A. and Stanley, B.J. (2014). Negative pressure wound therapy: experience in 45 dogs. *Vet. Surg.* 43: 380–387.

22 Koh, T.J. and DiPietro, L.A. (2013). Inflammation and wound healing: the role of the macrophage. *Expert Rev. Mol. Med.* 13: 1–14.

23 Snyder, R.J., Lantis, J., Kirsner, R.S. et al. (2016). Macrophages: a review of their role in wound healing and their therapeutic use. *Wound Rep. Reg.* 24: 613–629.

24 Leibovich, S.J. and Ross, R. (1975). The role of the macrophage in wound repair: a study with hydrocortisone and antimacrophage serum. *Am. J. Pathol.* 78: 71–100.

25 Ferrara, N. (2000). Vascular endothelial growth factor and the regulation of angiogenesis. *Recent Prog. Horm. Res.* 55: 15–35.

26 Tonnesen, M.G., Feng, X., and Clark, R.A.F. (2000). Angiogenesis in wound healing. *J. Investig. Dermatol. Symp. Proc.* 5: 40–46.

27 Castilla, D.M., Liu, Z., and Velazquez, O.C. (2012). Oxygen: implications for wound healing. *Adv. Wound Care* 1: 225–230.

28 Magnum, L.C., Gacia, G.R., Akers, K.S., and Wenke, J.C. (2019). Duration of extremity tourniquet application profoundly impacts soft-tissue antibiotic exposure in a rat model of ischemia-reperfusion injury. *Injury* 50: 2203–2214.

29 Bohling, M.W., Henderson, R.A., Swaim, S.F. et al. (2004). Cutaneous wound healing in the cat: a macroscopic description and comparison with cutaneous wound healing in the dog. *Vet. Surg.* 33: 579–587.

30 Chitturi, R.T., Balasubramaniam, A.M., Parameswar, R.A. et al. (2015). The role of myofibroblasts in wound healing, contraction, and its clinical implications in cleft palate repair. *J. Int. Oral Health* 7: 75–80.

31 Demetriou, J. and Stein, S. (2011). Causes and management of complications in wound healing. *In Prac.* 33: 392–400.

32 Pavletic, M.M. (2018). Basic principles of wound healing. In: *Atlas of Small Animal Wound Management and Reconstructive Surgery*, 4ee (ed. M.M. Pavletic), 17–32. Hoboken, NJ: Wiley.

33 Pavletic, M.M. (2018). Common complication in wound healing. In: *Atlas of Small Animal Wound Management and Reconstructive Surgery*, 4ee (ed. M.M. Pavletic), 143–172. Hoboken, NJ: Wiley.

34 Guo, S. and DiPietro, L.A. (2010). Factors affecting wound healing. *J. Dent. Res.* 89: 219–229.

35 Sen, C.K. (2009). Wound healing essentials: let there be oxygen. *Wound Repair Regener.* 17: 1–18.

36 Latimer, C.R., Lux, C.N., Roberts, S. et al. (2018). Effects of hyerbaric oxygen therapy on uncomplicated incisional and open wound healing in dogs. *Vet. Surg.* 47: 827–836.

37 Jones, S.G., Edwards, R., and Thomas, D.W. (2004). Inflammation and wound healing: the role of bacteria in the immuno-regulation of wound healing. *Int. J. Low Extrem. Wounds* 3: 201–208.

38 Ashcroft, G.S., Mills, S.J., and Ashworth, J.J. (2002). Ageing and wound healing. *Biogerontology* 3: 337–345.

39 Gosain, A. and DiPietro, L.A. (2004). Aging and wound healing. *World J. Surg.* 28: 321–326.

40 Norman, D. (2004). The effects of age-related skin changes on wound healing rates. *Rev. J. Wound Care* 13: 199–201.

41 Lopez, D.J., McCalla, S., Korten, B. et al. (2021). Comparison of patient outcome in dogs following enterotomy versus intestinal resection and anastomosis for treatment of intestinal foreign bodies. *J. Am. Vet. Med. Assoc.* 258: 1378–1385.

42 Bohling, M.W. and Henderson, R.A. (2006). Differences in cutaneous wound healing between dogs and cats. *Vet. Clin. North Am. Small Anim. Prac.* 36: 687–692.

43 Bohling, M.W., Henderson, R.A., Swaim, S.F. et al. (2006). Comparison of the role of the subcutaneous tissues in cutaneous wound healing in the dog and cat. *Vet. Surg.* 35: 3–14.

44 Doig, G.S., Heighes, P.T., Simpson, F. et al. (2009). Early enteral nutrition, provided within 24 h of injury or intensive care unit admission, significantly reduces mortality in critically ill patients: a meta-analysis of randomised controlled trials. *Intens. Care Med.* 35: 2018–2027.

45 Hoffberg, J.E. and Koenigshof, A. (2017). Evaluation of the safety of early compared to late enteral nutrition in canine septic peritonitis. *J. Am. Anim. Hosp. Assoc.* 53: 90–95.

46 Kawasaki, N., Suzuki, Y., Nakayoshi, T. et al. (2009). Early postoperative enteral nutrition is useful for recovering gastrointestinal motility and maintaining the nutritional status. *Surg. Today* 39: 225–230.

47 Levine, G.M., Deren, J.J., Steiger, E. et al. (1974). Role of oral intake in maintenance of gut mass and disaccharide activity. *Gastroenterology* 67: 975–982.

48 Lewis, S.J., Andersen, H.K., and Thomas, S. (2009). Early enteral nutrition within 24 h of intestinal surgery versus later commencement of feeding: a systematic review and meta-analysis. *J. Gastrointest. Surg.* 13: 569–575.

49 Liu, D.T., Brown, D.C., and Silverstein, D.C. (2012). Early nutritional support is associated with decreased length of hospitalization in dogs with septic peritonitis: a retrospective study of 45 cases (2000– 2009). *J. Vet. Emerg. Crit. Care* 22: 453–459.

50 Marks, S.L. (1998). The principles and practical application of enteral nutrition. *Vet. Clin. North Am. Small Anim. Prac.* 28: 677–708.

51 Marik, P.E. and Zaloga, G.P. (2001). Early enteral nutrition in acutely ill patients: a systematic review. *Crit. Care Med.* 29: 2264–2270.

52 Martos-Benítez, F.D., Gutiérrez-Noyola, A., Soto-García, A. et al. (2018). Program of gastrointestinal rehabilitation and early postoperative enteral nutrition: a prospective study. *Updates Surg.* 70: 105–112.

53 Moss, G., Greenstein, A., Levy, S. et al. (1980). Maintenance of GI function after bowel surgery and immediate enteral full nutrition. I. Doubling the canine colorectal anastomotic bursting pressure and intestinal wound mature collagen content. *J. Parenter Enter. Nutr.* 4: 535–538.

54 O'Keefe, G.E., Shelton, M., Cuschieri, J. et al. (2008). Inflammation and the host response to injury, a large-scale collaborative project: patient-oriented research core—standard operating procedures for clinical care VIII—nutritional support of the trauma patient. *J. Trauma* 65: 1520–1528.

55 Perez-Tamayo, R. and Ihnen, M. (1953). The effect of methionine in experimental wound healing; a morphologic study. *Am. J. Pathol.* 29: 233–249.

56 Grimes, J.A., Schmiedt, C.W., Cornell, K.K., and Radlinski, M.A. (2011). Identification of risk factors for septic peritonitis and failure to survive following gastrointestinal surgery in dogs. *J. Am. Vet. Med. Assoc.* 238 (4): 486–494.

57 Ralphs, S.C., Jessen, C.R., and Lipowitz, A.J. (2003). Risk factors for leakage following intestinal anastamosis in dogs and cats: 115 cases (1991–2000). *J. Am. Vet. Med. Assoc.* 223: 73–77.

58 Nicholson, M., Beal, M., Shofer, F. et al. (2002). Epidemiologic evaluation of postoperative wound infection in clean-contaminated wounds: a retrospective study of 239 dogs and cats. *Vet. Surg.* 31: 577–581.

59 de Almeida, T.F., de Castro, P.T., and Monte-Alto-Costa, A. (2016). Blockade of glucocorticoid receptors improves cutaneous wound healing in stressed mice. *Exp. Biol. Med.* 241: 353–358.

60 Stephens, F.O., Hunt, T.K., Jawetz, E. et al. (1971). Effect of cortisone and vitamin a on wound infection. *Am. J. Surg.* 121: 569–571.

61 Fairweather, M., Heit, Y.I., Buie, J. et al. (2015). Celecoxib inhibits early cutaneous wound healing. *J. Surg. Res.* 194: 717–724.

62 Gallaher, H.M., Butler, J.R., Wills, R.W. et al. (2019). Effects of short- and long-term administration of nonsteroidal anti-inflammatory drugs on osteotomy healing in dogs. *Vet. Surg.* 48: 1318–1329.

63 Laing, E.J. (1990). Problems in wound healing associated with chemotherapy and radiation therapy. *Probl. Vet. Med.* 2: 433–441.

64 Jacobson, L.K., Johnson, M.B., Dedhia, R.D. et al. Impaired wound healing after radiation therapy: a systematic review of pathogenesis and treatment. *Jpras Open* 13: 92–105.

65 Lux, C. (2022). Wound healing in animals: a review of physiology and clinical evaluation. *Vet. Dermatol.* 33: 91–e27.

66 Seguin, B., McDonald, D.E., Kent, M.S. et al. (2005). Tolerance of cutaneous or mucosal flaps placed into a radiation therapy field in dogs. *Vet. Surg.* 34: 214–222.

3

Postoperative Complications

Ryan P. Cavanaugh

Ross University School of Veterinary Medicine, St. Kitts, West Indies

Introduction

Despite continued improvements in the understanding of the physiologic complexities associated with wound healing and expanded access to sophisticated surgical technology, postoperative complications are still routinely encountered in companion animals receiving surgical therapy. Veterinary studies conducting active surveillance of peri- and postoperative complications reported incidences ranging from 17% and 41% with surgical site infection (SSI) representing one of the most encountered complications [3, 4]. The introduction of institutional surgical safety checklists (SSCs) to facilitate the unification of the surgical and anesthetic teams and to highlight patient-specific needs and concerns prior to the initiation of the procedure resulted in a reduction in the incidence of complications to 10% and 29%, respectively [3, 4]. Human studies evaluating the utility of SSCs have documented even more significant impacts on postoperative complication rates with reported rate reductions ranging from 36% to 66% [5–7]. This validates the importance of an active institutional surveillance program so that complications can be detected and mitigated in a timely fashion. Stickney and colleagues demonstrated that without active postoperative surveillance, SSIs would have been missed in 28% of the cohort evaluated, further emphasizing the utility of an active surveillance program [8].

Contributing causes of postoperative complications in companion animals are well-described and multifactorial. The provision of a sanitary operating room environment and observation of strict aseptic technique integrated with the utilization of contemporary patient preparation protocols are all variables that the surgeon has direct control over to help limit complications such as SSI (Table 3.1) [9–15].

Systemic patient factors such as nutritional deficiencies precipitating hypoproteinemia, the presence of comorbidities such as hyperadrenocorticism, and the administration of immunosuppressive medications can all deleteriously impact healing and should be mitigated prior to elective surgical intervention whenever possible. Species differences in wound healing should also be respected as felids have reduced collateral vascular perfusion of the subcutaneous tissue compared to dogs which translates into slower healing of surgically reconstructed wounds (see Chapter 1). Likewise, open wound management in cats progresses at a slower rate compared to dogs which is suspected to be secondary to blunted capacity to develop granulation tissue and secondary to deposition of this tissue laterally within a wound compared to centrally as in canids. The anatomic location of the surgical site can also be assessed as a potential trigger for heightened complication risk with wounds centered over articular and peri-articular locations being the most problematic. Postoperative rigid or semirigid coaptation of high-motion surgical sites may serve to strategically diminish complication risk. Wounds reconstructed under excessive tension are also prone to complications such as surgical dehiscence and wounds adjacent to or within mucosal-laden orifices carry a higher risk for SSI based on increased bacterial demographics.

Based on the multitude of variables that impact wound healing and to decrease the potential for preventable postoperative complications, it is suggested that a structured, systematic, evidence-based approach be deployed for the provision of individual wound care in clinical practice. One such tool used in the human healthcare sector is called the TIME clinical decision support tool (CDST).

3

Postoperative Complications

Ryan P. Cavanaugh

Ross University School of Veterinary Medicine, St. Kitts, West Indies

Introduction

Despite continued improvements in the understanding of the physiologic complexities associated with wound healing and expanded access to sophisticated surgical technology, postoperative complications are still routinely encountered in companion animals receiving surgical therapy. Veterinary studies conducting active surveillance of peri- and postoperative complications reported incidences ranging from 17% and 41% with surgical site infection (SSI) representing one of the most encountered complications [3, 4]. The introduction of institutional surgical safety checklists (SSCs) to facilitate the unification of the surgical and anesthetic teams and to highlight patient-specific needs and concerns prior to the initiation of the procedure resulted in a reduction in the incidence of complications to 10% and 29%, respectively [3, 4]. Human studies evaluating the utility of SSCs have documented even more significant impacts on postoperative complication rates with reported rate reductions ranging from 36% to 66% [5–7]. This validates the importance of an active institutional surveillance program so that complications can be detected and mitigated in a timely fashion. Stickney and colleagues demonstrated that without active postoperative surveillance, SSIs would have been missed in 28% of the cohort evaluated, further emphasizing the utility of an active surveillance program [8].

Contributing causes of postoperative complications in companion animals are well-described and multifactorial. The provision of a sanitary operating room environment and observation of strict aseptic technique integrated with the utilization of contemporary patient preparation protocols are all variables that the surgeon has direct control over to help limit complications such as SSI (Table 3.1) [9–15].

Systemic patient factors such as nutritional deficiencies precipitating hypoproteinemia, the presence of comorbidities such as hyperadrenocorticism, and the administration of immunosuppressive medications can all deleteriously impact healing and should be mitigated prior to elective surgical intervention whenever possible. Species differences in wound healing should also be respected as felids have reduced collateral vascular perfusion of the subcutaneous tissue compared to dogs which translates into slower healing of surgically reconstructed wounds (see Chapter 1). Likewise, open wound management in cats progresses at a slower rate compared to dogs which is suspected to be secondary to blunted capacity to develop granulation tissue and secondary to deposition of this tissue laterally within a wound compared to centrally as in canids. The anatomic location of the surgical site can also be assessed as a potential trigger for heightened complication risk with wounds centered over articular and peri-articular locations being the most problematic. Postoperative rigid or semirigid coaptation of high-motion surgical sites may serve to strategically diminish complication risk. Wounds reconstructed under excessive tension are also prone to complications such as surgical dehiscence and wounds adjacent to or within mucosal-laden orifices carry a higher risk for SSI based on increased bacterial demographics.

Based on the multitude of variables that impact wound healing and to decrease the potential for preventable postoperative complications, it is suggested that a structured, systematic, evidence-based approach be deployed for the provision of individual wound care in clinical practice. One such tool used in the human healthcare sector is called the TIME clinical decision support tool (CDST).

Techniques in Small Animal Wound Management, First Edition. Edited by Nicole J. Buote.
© 2024 John Wiley & Sons, Inc. Published 2024 by John Wiley & Sons, Inc.
Companion website: www.wiley.com/go/buote/wounds

Table 3.1 Surgical hand preparation methods.

Protocols	Time to scrub (s)	Traumatic to skin	Water usage	Residual antimicrobial effect	Risk of recontamination during hand rinsing
Aqueous scrub containing povidone-iodine	180–300	Yes	20 l/surgeon (10–15 l w/ motion-activated water tap)	Limited	Yes
Aqueous scrub containing 4% chlorhexidine gluconate	180–300	Yes	20 l/surgeon (10–15 l w/ motion-activated water tap)	Yes	Yes
[a]Alcohol-based rubs	90–180	No	0	Limited	No
[a]Alcohol-based rubs containing additional active ingredients (i.e., Chlorhexidine)	90–180	No	0	Yes	No

[a] The World Health Organization currently recommends the usage of an alcohol-based hand rub for surgical hand preparation over an aqueous scrub solution. Utilization of an alcohol-based hand rub with additional additives such as chlorhexidine contributes to a long-lasting residual antimicrobial effect that can protect the patient in instances of breaks in aseptic technique secondary to accidental glove puncture.

The TIME principle was first described by Schultz and colleagues and concentrated on optimization of the local wound bed in preparation for application of advanced wound healing therapies or to allow for the augmentation of endogenous healing mechanisms [16]. The four components of the TIME system include: (i) **T**ISSUE – Debridement of necrotic or nonviable tissue, (ii) **I**NFECTION/INFLAMMATION – Achieving bacterial balance by inhibiting the critical colonization of the wound, (iii) **M**OISTURE IMBALANCE – Utilization of appropriate moisture retentive dressings to prevent desiccation and control volume of exudate to prevent spillover and subsequent maceration of peri-wound tissue, (iv) **E**DGE – Lack of advancement at the epidermal margin prompts investigation into inhibitors of epithelialization and wound contraction. Since its inception, the TIME principle has been heralded as an effective tool for guiding practitioners in the identification of causative variable(s) impeding the successful progression of hard-to-heal wounds and is now recognized as the most commonly used wound assessment tool in Europe [17, 18]. Critics of the system purport that it is too narrowly focused with over-emphasis on the wound but insufficient focus on the global status of the patient [18, 19]. Objective assessment and refinement of the TIME paradigm by wound practitioners has led to its current evolution, TIME CDST.

The CDST incorporates five components that facilitate a holistic patient assessment in conjunction with treating the elements of TIME, followed by an objective evaluation of the efficacy of the treatment and appropriateness of the wound management [18]. The CDST elements include: (i) **A**ssess – The accuracy of the diagnosis of the patient and their wound, (ii) **B**ring – A multidisciplinary team to promote holistic care, (iii) **C**ontrol – and treat systemic contributions to the wound, (iv) **D**ecide – Appropriate treatment, (iv) **E**valuate – the treatment and wound management goals (Figure 3.1) [18].

Objective assessment of the impact of TIME CDST supports that usage of the tool enhances clinical care, especially for chronic poor healing wounds predisposed to biofilm accumulation such as those seen with diabetic foot ulcers in people [18, 20]. Although usage of the tool is not commonplace in veterinary medicine, the industry would likely benefit from the introduction of a standardized algorithm that facilitates comprehensive assessment and management of the wounded patient. Recent veterinary publications have introduced the TIME CDST concepts; however, widespread integration will be the next logical step as wound practitioners strive to enhance their clinical practice [21, 22].

Seromas

Disruption of connective tissue planes or the creation of large tissue deficits, whether a result of accidental wounding or purposeful manipulation during reconstruction allows an avenue for the accumulation of extracellular fluid in these areas of so-called "dead space." Physical disruption of the normal lymphatic pathways in combination with the typical inflammatory exudates produced during surgical manipulation further compound the issue [23]. This phenomenon, known as seroma development, is one of the most common complications associated with surgical wound management in companion animals.

Assess patient, wellbeing and wound

Bring in multidisciplinary colleagues

Control or treat underlying causes of wound

Decide appropriate treatment

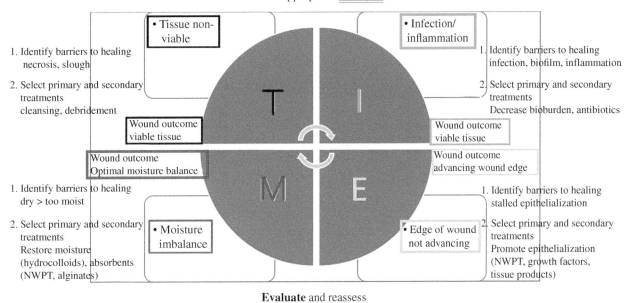

1. Identify barriers to healing
   necrosis, slough

2. Select primary and secondary
   treatments
   cleansing, debridement

Wound outcome
viable tissue

Wound outcome
Optimal moisture balance

1. Identify barriers to healing
   dry > too moist

2. Select primary and secondary
   treatments
   Restore moisture
   (hydrocolloids), absorbents
   (NWPT, alginates)

• Tissue non-
  viable

• Infection/
  inflammation

1. Identify barriers to healing
   infection, biofilm, inflammation

2. Select primary and secondary
   treatments
   Decrease bioburden, antibiotics

Wound outcome
viable tissue

Wound outcome
advancing wound edge

1. Identify barriers to healing
   stalled epithelialization

2. Select primary and secondary
   treatments
   Promote epithelialization
   (NWPT, growth factors,
   tissue products)

• Moisture
  imbalance

• Edge of wound
  not advancing

Evaluate and reassess

Figure 3.1   Visual depiction of the components of the TIME assessment system. *Source:* Courtesy of Nicole Buote, DVM, DACVS.

Established risk factors for seroma development in human surgery include the type of surgical procedure being performed, excessive mobility in the postoperative period, administration of preoperative chemotherapy or radiation, and whether dead space is closed during reconstruction [24]. Interestingly, usage of electrocautery to facilitate skin flap development for reconstruction has also been shown to predispose to a seroma; however, in certain instances, the beneficial contributions of the utilization of this surgical tool to facilitate hemostasis may outweigh the theoretical risk of seroma development [24, 25].

The reported incidence of seroma development will vary depending on the invasiveness and location of the surgical procedure but in certain commonly performed reconstructive procedures in human medicine such as abdominoplasty, rates of occurrence have been reported to be as high as 43% (range, 5–43) [26]. In veterinary surgery, even routine wound closures associated with the most commonly performed surgical interventions such as ovariohysterectomy (OVH) produce high rates of seroma development. In two single-center, randomized, blinded, controlled trials at a veterinary teaching hospital, the reported rate of seroma occurrence within 30 days after OVH in dogs was 17.7% and in cats was 32.3%, respectively [27, 28]. More advanced reconstructive interventions such as those requiring integration of an axial pattern flap have also yielded high rates of seroma formation (22%) even when active mitigation strategies such as drain placement and postoperative coaptation are utilized [29].

Although commonly self-limiting, veterinary surgeons should proactively integrate techniques to facilitate a reduction in seroma occurrence as their development has been associated with complications such as infection and wound dehiscence/flap necrosis because of increased pressure on the reconstructed tissue [26]. Seromas may elicit discomfort in the treated patient and can also be unsightly, prompting concerns from the client and potentially tarnishing trust in the attending veterinarian. In rare instances, chronic seromas left untreated have been reported to develop into pseudocysts [30].

The clinical diagnosis of a seroma is generally straightforward, rarely requiring invasive testing to confirm a diagnosis. A non-painful, fluid-filled, fluctuant swelling at the site of recent surgery without any systemic signs in the patient would generally be sufficient to establish a working diagnosis of a seroma (Figure 3.2a,b). Indiscriminate drainage with a needle during out-patient evaluation is discouraged as this could introduce bacteria and elicit infection at the surgical site that otherwise contains a sterile accumulation of extracellular fluid. When a seroma develops after surgery in the cervical

(a) (b)

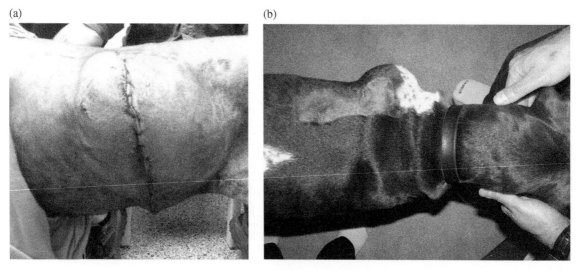

Figure 3.2 (a,b) Typical appearance of incisional seromas affecting the lateral thorax of a dog after wound reconstruction. Note the lack of incisional erythema and inflammation which is typical for this presentation. *Source:* Courtesy of Julius M. Liptak, BVSc, MVetClinStud, FANZCVSc, DACVS-SA, DECVS, ACVS Founding Fellow, Surgical Oncology and Oral and Maxillofacial Surgery, RCVS Specialist in Surgical Oncology.

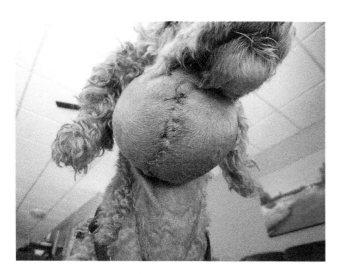

Figure 3.3 Incisional seroma affecting the ventral cervical region in a dog after wound reconstruction. Prophylactic drainage may be indicated in wounds such as this when progressive swelling is documented or if the patient demonstrates evolving signs of respiratory difficulty. *Source:* Courtesy of Julius M. Liptak, BVSc, MVetClinStud, FANZCVSc, DACVS-SA, DECVS, ACVS Founding Fellow, Surgical Oncology and Oral and Maxillofacial Surgery, RCVS Specialist in Surgical Oncology.

region, proactive surveillance is important to ensure that the swelling does not enlarge to a point where it could compress oropharyngeal structures and compromise breathing (Figure 3.3). Intentional drainage of these seromas would be considered appropriate if the seroma is trending toward progressive and extensive enlargement or if the patient is demonstrating early signs of respiratory impairment. In rare instances when a presumptive diagnosis cannot be established, cytology of the fluid can be performed which would reveal a paucity of white blood cells and variable amounts of red blood cells [31]. Supportive treatment with heat application to the site to facilitate dilation of local lymphatic vessels which imbibe the extracellular fluid and redistribute it, in conjunction with reinforcing exercise restrictions will result in seroma resolution within one to two weeks in most instances. If the anatomic location of the surgical site is amenable to placement of a compressive bandage, this may also facilitate more rapid resolution of the seroma.

Wounds with large amounts of dead space should be preferentially reconstructed over a drain to facilitate the prevention of seroma development (Figure 3.4a,b). Surgical drains not only control the accumulation of free fluid within a wound bed but also contribute to the removal of residual organic material, bacteria, necrotic debris, and inflammatory mediators [32, 33]. Both open (passive) Penrose and closed (active) suction drainage systems have been validated for use in

(a)

(b)

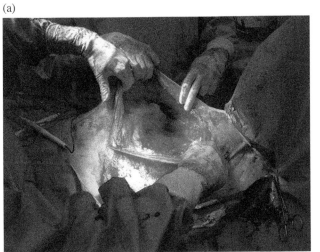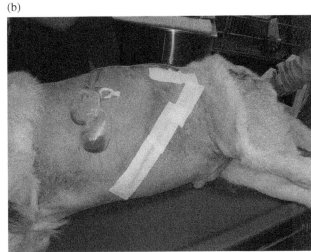

Figure 3.4   (a,b) Extensive dead space in the left lateral flank area of a Siberian Husky dog after removal of a 26 pound lipoma. To avoid seroma development, the wound was reconstructed over the top of a close suction Jackson Pratt drain. *Source:* Courtesy of Ryan P. Cavanaugh, DVM, DACVS-SA, ACVS Founding Fellow, Surgical Oncology.

wound management for companion animals (see Chapter 9). When reconstructing surgically induced wounds (i.e., tumor excision site undergoing single-stage reconstruction) or in instances of delayed primary or secondary closure of a wound that was previously managed openly, closed suction drainage systems are preferentially utilized since Penrose drains have been associated with a higher risk of allowing for opportunistic nosocomial infections [32, 33].

Several commercially available closed suction drainage systems (Wound Evac®, Redovac®, Jackson Pratt®, Mini Redovac®) are available to veterinary practitioners; however, Bristow and colleagues showed that no single system demonstrates superiority with regard to functionality and complication abatement [34]. The author prefers to use the Jackson Pratt drainage system based on its predictable handling characteristics and widespread commercial availability in North America. The placement of any drain within a wound will elicit an inflammatory response and alter the characterization of the wound classification (i.e., convert a clean procedure into a clean-contaminated procedure). Shaver and colleagues demonstrated that closed suction drain removal should be targeted when the wound fluid production rate decreases below 4.8 ml/kg/d [32].

Negative pressure wound therapy (NPWT) is effective at controlling exudates from open wounds and has been explored as a modality for positively supporting reconstructed tissue (see Chapter 10) [35, 36]. When used after wound reconstruction, the technique is termed closed-incision NPWT or ciNPWT. Instrumentation for ciNPWT is slightly different than the classic NPWT setup as the foam dressing is soft and fully integrated into the adhesive drape and suction network. ciNPWT has been shown to reduce incisional drainage and decrease surgical wound dehiscence (SWD) in people [37]. Vallarino and colleagues prospectively evaluated a cohort of 12 dogs that were randomly assigned to receive ciNPWT of their incision after forequarter amputation with 6/12 dogs receiving only a soft-padded bandage, thereby serving as controls [37]. No difference in seroma development was noted between the two groups but additional larger-scale investigations are warranted.

Wound Dehiscence (Indolent Pockets, Pseudo Healing)

SWD, defined as a splitting open or rupture of a previously closed incision site has been correlated with significant increases in morbidity and mortality in addition to imposing additional unexpected healthcare costs on the animal caretakers and workload on the attending surgical team. Objective analysis of data generated from the human healthcare sector helps put in perspective the potential impact that SWD can impose on the patient. Shanmugam and colleagues reported on data extracted from the Nationwide Inpatient Sample Registry evaluating SWD in patients undergoing abdominopelvic surgery and identified a 9.6% increase in mortality and a $40,323 increase in healthcare costs largely attributed to a requisite 9.4 days of additional hospitalization that would not have been required if SWD did not occur. Controlling for variables

Table 3.2 Variables associated with surgical wound dehiscence and factors attributed to the cause.

Related variables	Surgeon	Patient	Wound
Improper suture selection (i.e., size, pattern, resorptive, or tensile properties)	✓		
Excessive tension on the wound	✓		
Sutures placed too close to wound edge (<5 mm)	✓		
Closure of poor-quality tissue or working with scar tissue	✓		
Uncontrolled endocrinopathies		✓	
Uremia		✓	
Malnutrition (hypoalbuminemia)		✓	
Active treatment for Immune-mediated disease or neoplasia		✓	
Irradiated tissue in the wound bed		✓	
Paucity of redundant tissue at surgical site (oral cavity, peri-anal, distal extremities)			✓
Tissue infection	✓		✓
Excessive organic debris in wound	✓		✓
Non-compliance with aftercare instructions	✓	✓	

such as age, gender, and comorbidities, the relative risk of inpatient death and readmission to the hospital within one month was 1.57 and 1.24, respectively [38, 39]. Large-scale studies availing these types of data are lacking in veterinary medicine and should be an area of emphasis in future work evaluating wound complications.

The causes of SWD are multifactorial and generally can be attributed to either surgeon, patient, or wound-related variables (Table 3.2). Common surgeon-related factors include utilization of improper suture materials (size, pattern, or tensile/resorptive properties) or technique (reconstructing the wound without accounting for tension on wound edges, placing suture too tightly or too close to the wound edge (i.e., <5 mm) and operating on poor quality/compromised skin or in scar tissue (Figure 3.5) [40]. Reconstruction of incisions in a nonlinear fashion may also predispose to SWD as the junction of the various components of the incision, particularly at T or Y junctions, are likely under greater tension than the remainder of the incision (Figure 3.5). Utilization of a half-buried horizontal mattress pattern (i.e., "corner stitch") to suture incisional junctions can be an effective tool to offset tension and mitigate the risk of avascular necrosis of the skin edges at these sites [41]. Utilization of objective clinical decision-making tools such as the TIME CDST may facilitate a reduction in technical surgical errors, especially when wound management is being carried out by an inexperienced practitioner.

Patient-related factors include the presence of comorbidities that are known to compromise normal healing pathways such as uncontrolled endocrinopathies (hyperadrenocorticism and diabetes mellitus), uremia, nutritional deficiencies, and

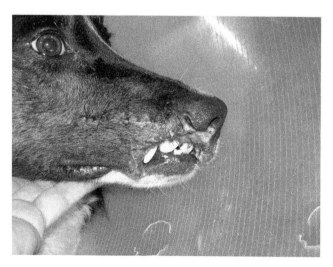

Figure 3.5 SWD of a single pedicle advancement flap used for reconstruction of the rostral lip after full thickness tumor excision. Excessive tension coupled by an inability to restrict lip movement likely contributed to SWD is this dog.
Source: Courtesy of Julius M. Liptak, BVSc, MVetClinStud, FANZCVSc, DACVS-SA, DECVS, ACVS Founding Fellow, Surgical Oncology and Oral and Maxillofacial Surgery, RCVS Specialist in Surgical Oncology.

conditions requiring immunosuppressive therapy such as immune-mediated diseases and neoplasia requiring cytotoxic chemotherapy or radiation therapy treatment [31, 42]. Noncompliance with required postsurgical instructions such as failure to utilize devices (i.e., Elizabethan or BiteNot collar) designed to inhibit self-traumatization of the wound or failure to comply with follow-up scheduling/protocols (allowing for wound dressings to become oversaturated thereby causing maceration of peri-incisional tissue) could also be categorized as patient-related factors [40].

Wound-related factors predisposing to SWD include retained foreign material within the wound bed, abnormal tissue such as a tumor associated with the wound bed, wound location (extremities/digits, perianal and oral, Figures 3.6, 3.7, 3.8, 3.9, 3.10, and 3.11), and infections (Figures 3.12, 3.13, 3.14, and 3.15) – [40]. Certain tumor types such as mast cell tumors (MCTs) have been speculated to be more likely to contribute to postsurgical wound healing complications based on their propensity to secrete proteolytic enzymes and other vasoactive substances that dampen the rate of fibroplasia within a wound bed [31]. Recently, the literature has refuted this proposed theory as a large-scale retrospective study published by Cockburn and colleagues found no observed increase in postoperative complication rate or prolongation of wound healing in marginally excised MCTs when compared to a control population of dogs undergoing surgical removal of soft-tissue sarcomas, a tumor type not previously shown to have associations with wound healing complications after excision [43, 44] (Table 3.2).

A comprehensive literature review by Sandy-Hodgetts and colleagues revealed a prevalence of SWD ranging between 1.3% and 9.3% in people undergoing all types of surgical interventions with obesity and SSI identified as the most common predisposing factors [45]. Although the precise contribution of each variable to SWD in veterinary surgical patients is unknown, SSI is one of the more commonly implicated variables.

The true incidence of SSI in companion animals is unknown with reports ranging from 0.8% to 21.3% [46–50]. Based on wound classification, Garcia-Stickney and colleagues reported rates of SSI for clean procedures at 2.7%, clean-contaminated at 3.2%, contaminated at 4.3%, and dirty at 12.5% [8]. When considered on the whole, the incidence of SSI for clean, soft-tissue procedures has recently been reported to be 5.7% [51].

Established risk factors for the development of SSI include the following: Surgical classification of procedure type (clean versus clean contaminated versus contaminated), increasing length of anesthesia time (>90 minutes and >240 minutes) [52, 53], anesthetic induction using propofol, placement of indwelling implants, concurrent endocrinopathy, increasing

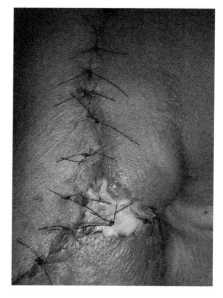

Figure 3.6 SWD of a ventral midline abdominal skin incision at the "T" junction of the incisional arms. When an incision is reconstructed non-linearly, the "T or Y" portion of the incision is most susceptible to SWD as a result of excessive tension and suture placement that can compromise incisional blood supply since sutures must traverse across three sides of the incision. *Source:* Courtesy of Julius M. Liptak, BVSc, MVetClinStud, FANZCVSc, DACVS-SA, DECVS, ACVS Founding Fellow, Surgical Oncology and Oral and Maxillofacial Surgery, RCVS Specialist in Surgical Oncology.

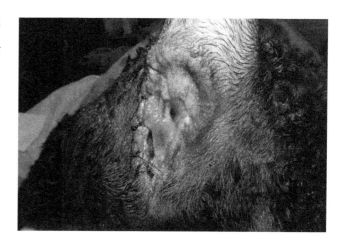

Figure 3.7 Left-sided perianal incision with SWD after removal of an anal sac adenocarcinoma. Based on the anatomic location of the reconstruction immediately adjacent to the anus, a higher incidence of SWD is expected. *Source:* Courtesy of Julius M. Liptak, BVSc, MVetClinStud, FANZCVSc, DACVS-SA, DECVS, ACVS Founding Fellow, Surgical Oncology and Oral and Maxillofacial Surgery, RCVS Specialist in Surgical Oncology.

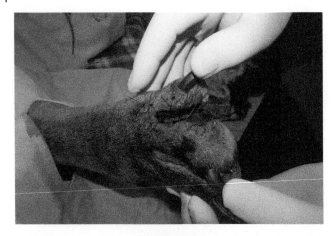

Figure 3.8 Postoperative SWD in a dog after digit amputation was performed to remove a tumor affecting the digit. Foot wounds are more prone to SWD since the incision is exposed to more forces during patient ambulation and since there are higher bacterial loads within the interdigital spaces. Rigid immobilization during the early postsurgical period with a bandage and splint may inhibit splaying of the reconstructed digits, thereby decreasing the incidence of incisional dehiscence in these cases. *Source:* Courtesy of Julius M. Liptak, BVSc, MVetClinStud, FANZCVSc, DACVS-SA, DECVS, ACVS Founding Fellow, Surgical Oncology and Oral and Maxillofacial Surgery, RCVS Specialist in Surgical Oncology.

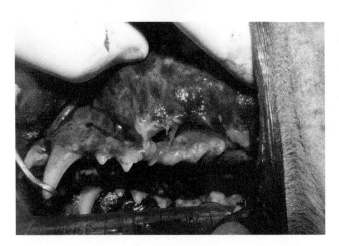

Figure 3.9 SWD of a left-sided maxillectomy reconstruction after wide excision of an oral tumor. Unrestricted motion of the mouth and tongue with potential mastication of food on the affected side, in addition to higher bacterial loads in the oral cavity may predispose intraoral incisions to SWD.
Source: Courtesy of Julius M. Liptak, BVSc, MVetClinStud, FANZCVSc, DACVS-SA, DECVS, ACVS Founding Fellow, Surgical Oncology and Oral and Maxillofacial Surgery, RCVS Specialist in Surgical Oncology.

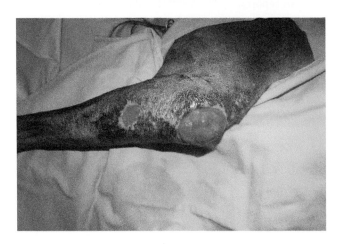

Figure 3.10 SWD of a wound centered over the olecranon of the left thoracic limb. Wounds located over joint surfaces and other high motion regions may be more prone to SWD. Additionally, wounds located over a bony prominence may be higher risk for SWD and therefore provision of rigid immobilization and/or incisional padding may be advantageous to help decrease rates of SWD. *Source:* Courtesy of Julius M. Liptak, BVSc, MVetClinStud, FANZCVSc, DACVS-SA, DECVS, ACVS Founding Fellow, Surgical Oncology and Oral and Maxillofacial Surgery, RCVS Specialist in Surgical Oncology.

body weight, clipping of hair at the surgical site ≥4 hours prior to surgery, increasing length of the surgical incision (>10 cm), and intraoperative hypotension [46, 47, 50, 52–56] (Table 3.3). Although evolution of the veterinary surgical field has resulted in the integration of technical modalities, such as minimally invasive surgery using laparoscopy and thoracoscopy, that has translated into a reduction in the incidence of SSI, other attempts to accomplish this such as through the usage of antimicrobial impregnated suture has not resulted in an observable difference [53, 55].

Reduction in SSI may be best accomplished through the prudent integration of timely and appropriate antimicrobial therapy. Booth and colleagues recommend the application of a "3-D approach" to antimicrobial therapy for the surgical

Figure 3.11 Postoperative image of a dog with a large wound centered over the dorsolateral aspect of the left thigh/perianal region. The wound was reconstructed using a coccygeal axial pattern flap. SWD of the distal tip of the flap is relatively commonly encountered due to chocking of vasculature perfusing the terminal sections of the flap. *Source:* Courtesy of Julius M. Liptak, BVSc, MVetClinStud, FANZCVSc, DACVS-SA, DECVS, ACVS Founding Fellow, Surgical Oncology and Oral and Maxillofacial Surgery, RCVS Specialist in Surgical Oncology.

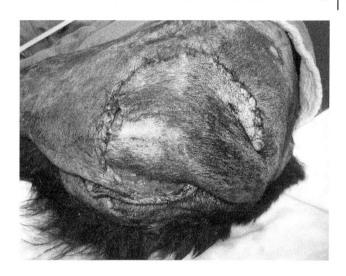

Figure 3.12 Postoperative image of a dog suffering SWD after surgical reconstruction of a proximal antebrachial defect utilizing an axillary flank fold transposition flap. *Source:* Courtesy of Julius M. Liptak, BVSc, MVetClinStud, FANZCVSc, DACVS-SA, DECVS, ACVS Founding Fellow, Surgical Oncology and Oral and Maxillofacial Surgery, RCVS Specialist in Surgical Oncology.

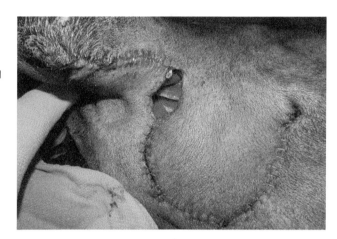

Figure 3.13 SWD of an extremity wound located over the tarsus of a dog. The wound appears grossly infected which was likely the inciting cause of the dehiscence. *Source:* Courtesy of Julius M. Liptak, BVSc, MVetClinStud, FANZCVSc, DACVS-SA, DECVS, ACVS Founding Fellow, Surgical Oncology and Oral and Maxillofacial Surgery, RCVS Specialist in Surgical Oncology.

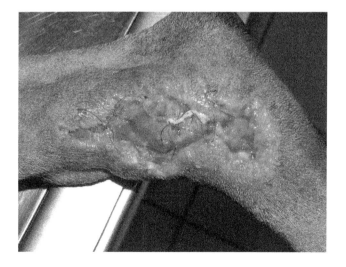

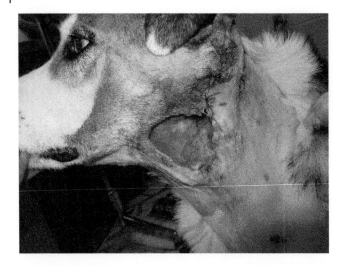

Figure 3.14 Postoperative SWD in a dog with a multidrug resistant *Staphylococcus Pseudintermedius* infection. *Source:* Courtesy of Julius M. Liptak, BVSc, MVetClinStud, FANZCVSc, DACVS-SA, DECVS, ACVS Founding Fellow, Surgical Oncology and Oral and Maxillofacial Surgery, RCVS Specialist in Surgical Oncology.

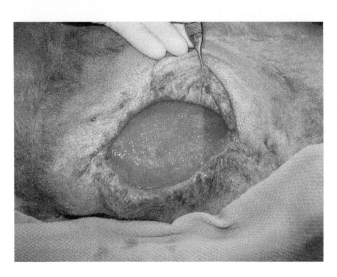

Figure 3.15 Image of an infected wound that has stalled out as it attempts to progress through the normal phases of wound healing. Although discharge from the wound is minimal, the wound edges are unhealthy and fixed to the underlying tissue associated with the lateral border of the wound. This can inhibit wound contraction and epithelialization. *Source:* Courtesy of Julius M. Liptak, BVSc, MVetClinStud, FANZCVSc, DACVS-SA, DECVS, ACVS Founding Fellow, Surgical Oncology and Oral and Maxillofacial Surgery, RCVS Specialist in Surgical Oncology.

Table 3.3   Risk factors for surgical site infection.

Surgical classification of procedure type (clean versus clean contaminated versus contaminated)

Increasing duration of anesthesia (>90 and >240 min both established as variables)

Placement of indwelling implants

Anesthetic induction with propofol

Presence of patient comorbidities (endocrinopathies)

Increasing body weight (i.e., obesity)

Clipping fur from the surgical site >4 h prior to surgery

Increasing length of the surgical incision (>10 cm)

Intraoperative anesthetic complications (hypotension)

patient using the following principles: (i) De-escalation of antimicrobial usage, (ii) development of a regimen that uses doses adequate to kill the entire infecting inoculum and through appropriate, (iii) decontamination of both the surgeon, patient, and operating environment [46]. A list of antimicrobials appropriate for prophylactic usage based on the anatomic location of the surgical intervention is included for review (Table 3.4) [54].

Table 3.4 Recommended antibiotics for antimicrobial prophylaxis based on surgical location.

Location	Common bacteria	IV Antibiotic of choice (class of drug or example)	Oral antibiotic options
Skin	*Staphylococcus* spp. (*S. aureus, S. intermedius*)	Cefazolin (first generation cephalosporin)	Cephalexin (first generation cephalosporin) Cefpodoxime (third generation cephalosporin)
Respiratory tract	*Staphylococcus* spp. *Streptococcus* spp. *Pseudomonas* spp. *Escherichia coli* *Klebsiella* spp. *Pasteurella* spp. *Enterobacter* spp. *Actinomyces pyogenes*	Cefazolin	Cephalexin Clavamox (potentiated penicillin) Baytril (fluoroquinolone)
Hepatobiliary	Gram-negative bacilli *Clostridium* spp. Anaerobes	Cefoxitin (second generation cephalosporin) Ampicillin-sublactam	Clavamox Baytril Metronidazole (nitroimidazole)
Urogenital	*Staphylococcus* spp. *Streptococcus* spp. *Pseudomonas* spp. *Escherichia coli* *Proteus mirabilis* Anaerobes	Cefazolin Ampicillin (penicillin) Ampicillin-sublactam (e.g., Unasyn)	Baytril Clavamox
Oral cavity	*Staphylococcus* spp. *Streptococcus* spp. *Proteus* spp. *Escherichia coli* *Actinomyces pyogenes* *Pasteurella* spp. Anaerobes	Cefazolin Ampicillin-sublactam Clindamycin (lincosamide)	Clavamox Clindamycin
Upper GI tract (stomach, duodenum, proximal jejunum)	Gram-positive cocci Enteric gram-negative bacilli	Cefazolin	Not recommended unless septic Clavamox Baytril
Lower GI tract (distal jejunum, ileum, colon)	Enteric gram-negative bacilli *Pseudomonas* spp. *Escherichia coli* *Klebsiella* spp. *Salmonella* spp. *Enterococcus* spp. Anaerobes	Cefoxitin Ampicillin-sublactam	Not recommended unless septic Clavamox Baytril Metronidazole

Pseudohealing/Indolent Pockets

Puncture wounds and more specifically traumatic bite wounds in companion animals have been associated with the phenomenon called pseudohealing. Deep-seated tissue damage from the initial bite is not evident to the attending clinician as the surface of the skin deceptively appears to be a relatively innocuous puncture wound [57]. The skin associated with the puncture tends to heal rapidly and uneventfully but damage to the underlying tissue continues to evolve until the wound "declares" itself, resulting in a large open and contaminated wound. Based on the mechanism of injury from bites, it is suspected that pseudohealing tends to occur more commonly in cat-to-cat bite wounds since there is typically just focal puncturing of the skin without the tearing and avulsion-type trauma which is frequently observed in dog bite wounds (especially big dog/little dog [BDLD] bite wounds) [57]. One method utilized by practitioners to help minimize complications from pseudohealing is to perform circumferential skin debridement of each puncture wound during the early stages of wound care. This facilitates direct observation of the extent of injury to the underlying tissue and if present, allows the clinician to perform appropriate therapy such as surgical debridement and closure over a drain (Figure 3.16a–d and Video 3.1 🔵).

Predisposition to pseudohealing may occur when extensive damage (from trauma) or loss (due to resection for a tumor or wound debridement) of the subcutis associated with a wound has occurred. Bohling and colleagues showed that widespread loss of the subcutis results in a blunted rate of granulation tissue production, especially in cats. Impaired wound contraction, epithelialization, and a significant reduction in cutaneous perfusion was also observed with the impact lasting for at least two weeks after wounding [58, 59]. For surgically reconstructed wounds, Bohling and colleagues also showed that the breaking strength of a sutured (linear-shaped) incision at the seven-day postoperative time point was only half of the measured strength in dogs. It is speculated that the difference in species is related to significantly greater collagen production in the wounds of dogs compared to cats [60].

(a) (b)

(c) (d)

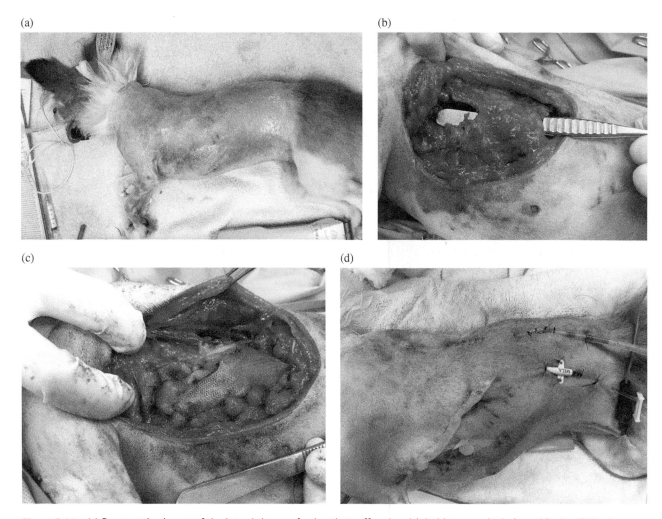

Figure 3.16   (a) Preoperative image of the lateral thorax of a dog that suffered multiple bite wounds during a big dog-little dog (BDLD) attack. (b) Surgical exploration of the wounds reveals extensive damage to the deeper underlying tissue despite minimal damage to the skin. There is full thickness tissue loss of the chest wall with multiple adjacent rib fractures. (c) Intraoperative image showing the chest wall reconstruction using prolene mesh incorporated into the defect by suturing it to surrounding intact rib. (d) Postoperative image showing wound closure over a closed suction Jackson Pratt drain in addition to a thoracostomy tube to facilitate the maintenance of negative intrathoracic pressure during the early postsurgical period. *Source:* Courtesy of Ryan P. Cavanaugh, DVM, DACVS-SA, ACVS Founding Fellow, Surgical Oncology.

Another phenomenon observed in wounds that predispose to complications is that of an indolent pocket. A surgically reconstructed wound may appear healed on the surface, however, within the subcutis or deeper underlying tissue, a granulation tissue-lined pocket develops which fails to contract or fill completely with ancillary mesenchymal tissue [61]. This allows for a wound with inferior strength which may precipitate a pseudohealing event resulting in SWD despite allowing appropriate time for incisional healing and having a wound that grossly appears well healed. To minimize the potential for this clinical scenario to manifest, it is important to ensure adequate skin-subcutis contact during reconstruction. Tacking of the skin and subcutis to deeper tissue layers can also facilitate optimal and sustained skin-subcutis contact. A quilting pattern is commonly used when underlying fascia is present and this technique has been shown to reduce incisional complications (seroma) in dogs and cats and does not predispose to steatitis [27, 28]. In instances where large amounts of the subcutis have been sacrificed, it is imperative that wound reconstruction be completed such that an extended duration of mechanical support be achieved at the wound edges. Tension-relieving techniques such as "walking" sutures, multiple layer closure (subcutis, intradermal, and skin suturing), and interspersed tension-relieving (horizontal/vertical mattress, far-far-near-near, fear-near-near-far) skin sutures between appositional sutures may be of benefit [59].

The risk of pseudohealing increases in wounds located in anatomic locations that undergo excessive motion such as the axilla or the groin. A unique phenomenon in cats occurs with wounds in the axillary region that develop secondary to entrapment of the area (forelimb, head/neck) within a circumferential band, such as a collar, chain, or wire loop. Classically, this situation will manifest in outdoor or feral cats that do not receive daily human observation/care, allowing the wound to become chronic in nature. These so-called "collar wounds" typically present with large regions of chronic, poor-quality granulation tissue which tend to be markedly exudative. This coupled with the fact that the skin in the region is very thin, and the area is under constant motion because of ambulation, predisposes to poor healing by second intention. Likewise, attempts at simple primary reconstruction are often futile, even when localized tissue flaps are harvested to offset tension [61, 62]. Lascelles and colleagues demonstrated that the provision of a vascularized pedicle graft using omentum, which is tunneled through the subcutis from an ipsilateral (to the wound) paracostal incision, resulted in augmentation of the cats healing capacity; however, 30% (7/10) of the wounds did not heal within 24 days and 71% (5/7) of the wounds that healed, ultimately suffered from pseudohealing complications with dehiscence within six weeks of the original reconstruction [61] In another cohort of cats with chronic axillary wounds, Lascelles and colleagues were able to achieve complete healing of the wounds by integrating a thoracodorsal axial pattern flap in conjunction with the previously described omental pedicle graft resulting in complete healing of all wounds within 14 days of surgery, despite suffering minor incisional complications in the acute postoperative period [62]. Subsequent reports have demonstrated that usage of an omocervical axial pattern skin flap in conjunction with omentalization can be an acceptable alternative to the usage of the thoracodorsal axial pattern flap and single-stage closure using the elbow skin fold without omentalization was successful in five cats with chronic axillary wounds [63, 64].

Morel-Lavallée lesions are reported in people and are described as closed degloving injuries that typically occur in the proximal thigh because of blunt force trauma. Shearing forces in conjunction with high-energy impact to the thigh result in the separation of the deeper fascial layers from the more superficial hypodermis thereby disrupting vascular and lymphatic supply to the tissue, resulting in avascular necrosis of the subcutis and surrounding tissue. A chronic inflammatory response is elicited producing a non-resolving, serosanguinous lymphocyte-rich effusion that accumulates within a fibrous capsule in the region of the [65]. McGhie and colleagues recently reported on this syndrome in a young cat that was hit by a car and developed sacrococcygeal luxation in addition to severe soft-tissue trauma in the region. A non-resolving effusion was documented, and multiple procedures were required to achieve resolution of the lesion, including en bloc debridement of the fibrous capsule followed by omentalization of the area [65]. There appears to be an overlap between characteristics of this phenomenon and those observed with collar wounds in cats and collaboration with human surgeons may lead to improved care for feline patients suffering from this syndrome.

Biofilms

What are they – Bacteria are ubiquitous in nature and are identified as having two distinct phenotypic growth patterns. Free-floating bacteria within the environment are noted to be in the planktonic state, whereas when bacteria congregate and adhere to one another and become sessile, they develop into the biofilm-embedded state [54, 66–69]. Biofilm development is complex with multiple colonies of bacterial populations amalgamated beneath a protective extracellular polymeric substance (EPS) which aids in adherence to an acceptable substrate and avails protection against antimicrobial

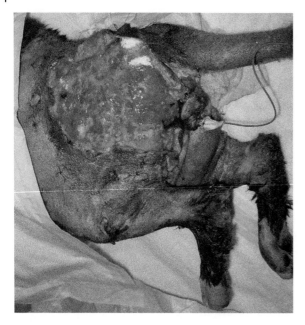

Figure 3.17 Chronic, left caudal thigh and perianal wound in a cat undergoing open wound management. The slimy film covering the surface of the wound is consistent with a biofilm and culture of the wound bed confirmed a multi-drug resistant bacterial infection. *Source:* Courtesy of Ryan P. Cavanaugh, DVM, DACVS-SA, ACVS Founding Fellow, Surgical Oncology.

penetration [66]. Although biofilms are recognized for their propensity to bind to inert substances such as suture, polypropylene catheters, and metallic implants, it is important to understand that not all biofilms are pathogenic as noninert substances such as the gastrointestinal tract, urethra, common bile duct, and oral cavity normally carry biofilms which contribute to the commensal flora in these anatomic regions [54, 69]. The most common bacterial agents associated with pathogenic biofilms in people include *Staphylococcus aureus, Enterococcus faecalis*, and *Pseudomonas aeruginosa* [66, 70].

Any wound may be susceptible to biofilm development but chronic wounds, defined as those that fail to heal after four to six weeks duration, tend to be the most susceptible [66, 71]. Malone and colleagues conducted a meta-analysis exploring the prevalence of biofilms in chronic wounds in people and identified that 78.2% of chronic wounds are likely infected with biofilms [72]. Although the prevalence of biofilms in companion animal wounds has yet to be elucidated, it seems reasonable to assume that prevalence is similarly high, and any nonhealing or chronic wound should be investigated for potential biofilm involvement.

Clinically, the diagnosis of a wound with biofilm should be suspected in a chronic wound with poor quality, friable granulation tissue covered with a slimy film that produces copious (typically non-purulent) exudate which does not diminish after repeated debridement (Figures 3.17 and 3.18a,b) [54, 66, 73]. Recrudescence of infection despite appropriate culture and susceptibility-directed antimicrobial therapy would also be supportive of biofilm infection, especially if the same organism is chronically re-cultured. Additionally, any wound with an indwelling implant should be considered at high risk for biofilm involvement if healing is not progressing appropriately [69]. *In vitro* studies have demonstrated a blunted response by host polymorphonuclear cells and persistence of high levels of interleukins (IL-1B, IL-6) and matrix metalloproteases (MMP-10) within the wound bed after four weeks of

(a)

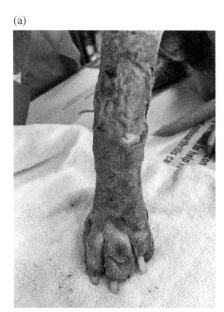

(b)

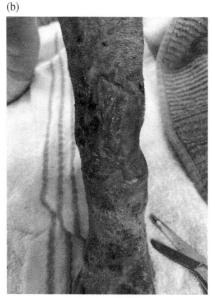

Figure 3.18 (a) Full thickness thoracic limb extremity wound in a dog after being attacked by another dog. The wound was several days old prior to care and in this image the wound is three days post initial surgical debridement. The wound contains poor quality granulation tissue and is covered with a slimy film consistent with that seen in a biofilm-infected wound. (b) Close-up image of the extremity wound seven days post initial surgical debridement. Despite open wound management with a moisture retentive dressing, the wound is not progressing through the normal repair phase of healing which was deemed secondary to biofilm development. *Source:* Courtesy of Ryan P. Cavanaugh, DVM, DACVS-SA, ACVS Founding Fellow, Surgical Oncology.

management, supporting that biofilms are able to effectively stall a wound in the inflammatory phase of healing [66, 74]. This stresses the importance of frequent wound assessment and intellectual interrogation of the healing quality through assessment of clinical characteristics associated with normal progression through the phases of healing.

Effective treatment of biofilm-infected wounds is predicated on accurate bacterial identification and antimicrobial susceptibility testing. Unfortunately, conventional wound swab culture techniques (i.e., Levine technique) predominately isolate the planktonic bacteria and not the biofilm-embedded organisms [69]. Molecular diagnostic techniques such as pyrosequencing and PCR combined with denaturing gradient gel electrophoresis have been shown to result in consistently better bacterial yield when compared to conventional culture and sensitivity and therefore a combination of isolation techniques should be utilized when biofilm involvement is suspected [54]. Even when effective bacterial isolation has been achieved, eradication of bacterial biofilms proves challenging due to innate resistance among the population (quiescent "persister" cells exhibiting high levels of antimicrobial tolerance), in conjunction with the inhibitory effects of the EPS. Additionally, cohorts of bacteria deep within the biofilm become dormant thereby precluding active kill from antimicrobials [75]. For certain antimicrobials, the minimum inhibitory concentration can be 100–1000 times greater than what would be required to neutralize planktonic bacteria of the same strain [54, 69]. Therefore, intentional methodologies must be employed to decimate the EPS and or to penetrate through the layers of the biofilm. Utilization of dual antimicrobial therapy to exploit different mechanisms of EPS penetration or degradation can be achieved through combination antimicrobial therapy using drugs that affect the biofilm through different mechanisms. A comprehensive list of antimicrobial agents that are typically effective against biofilms is included for review (Table 3.5) from [54].

Despite extensive research, a consistently reliable approach to therapy has not been elucidated. Current research is focused on the utilization of combination or co-therapies with biofilm dispersal agents and antibiotics from various classes. Several classes of dispersal agents are available based on their mechanism of action and include (i) Quorum sensing inhibitors (QSIs) that inhibit bacterial communication systems, (ii) free radicals (Nitric oxide and Nitroxides), (iii) Antimicrobial peptides (AMPs) that disrupt bacterial membranes, and (iv) repurposed drugs like mucous inhibitors (i.e., N-acetyl cysteine

Table 3.5 Antibiotics effective against biofilms.

Antibiotic	Type of biofilm	Mechanism of action	Tips for use
Fluoroquinolone	*Staphylococcus* spp. Gram-negative organisms (sessile organisms)	Disrupts extracellular polymeric substance (EPS)	Bacteria develop resistance rapidly so must be used in combination with a second drug
Rifampicin	*Staphylococcus* spp. Medical-device infections Multiple species	Bactericidal to *Staph* spp. even on foreign material Disrupts extracellular polymeric substance (EPS)	Most commonly used as the first antibiotic in a series of two antibiotics
Linezolid	Staphylococcus spp.	Inhibits protein synthesis	Commonly used with rifampicin for joint replacement infections Shunt-related meningitis
Macrolides	*Pseudomonas aeruginosa*	Inhibits quorum sensing	
Clarithromycin	*Staphylococcus epidermis*	Inhibits hexose-containing polysaccharides, decreases hexose synthesis (EPS disruption)	
Others: Colistin Fosfomycin Daptomycin Tigecycline	Sessile *P. aeruginosa* Sessile *P. aeruginosa* Multiple spp. *Staph* spp., *Enterococcus faecalis*	Disrupts EPS Disrupts outer membrane to allow second antibiotic work better Disrupts EPS *In vitro* testing illustrated obstruction of biofilm formation (sub-MIC concentrations)	Rapid development of resistance; use with second antibiotic Use with Fluoroquinolone (synergistic effect) Used for orthopedic implant biofilms, lock solution for IV catheters

and ambroxol) and gold-containing compounds (auranofin) [75]. Although research into co-treatment is mainly limited to *in vitro* studies, a review article by Hawas and colleagues produced objective documentation that combination therapy is more effective than single-agent therapy and purports that this should be a pathway forward as additional therapeutics are studied and developed [75].

Alternative therapies for biofilm-infected wounds that appear promising include cold atmospheric plasma (CAP). The application of CAP to infected wounds has been extensively studied in people and has been validated as an effective modality for controlling wounds containing both mono- and multispecies biofilms. *In vitro* studies support that CAP is not cyto- or genotoxic to host cells and although CAP generators are expensive, potentially limiting their utility in veterinary medicine, the treatment is rapid, environment friendly, and essentially painless which would be attractive for veterinary applications [75].

The current mainstay of localized therapy for biofilm management in veterinary medicine revolves around the combination of aggressive and repetitive, layered or en bloc (when feasible) surgical debridement followed by open-wound management with medicated primary layer and/or negative-pressure dressings [2]. Natural products compatible with open wound management like manuka honey and acetic acid have been evaluated for use in biofilm mitigation and were proven to disrupt their EPS [54]. Novel primary layer dressings termed electroceuticals are capable of generating electric fields within the wound bed which disrupt the bacterium's ability to maintain adhesion to surrounding surfaces. Commercially available electroceutical products are approved by the FDA and available through Arthrex® and Procellera®; however, a recent study by Heald and colleagues introduced a novel product with a battery-powered direct current to the dressing. Proof of concept was confirmed through the successful treatment of a dog and cat wound with multidrug resistant infections, paving way for further development of the product for commercial application [2].

References

1 Sen, C.K., Gordillo, G.M., Roy, S. et al. (2009). Human skin wounds: a major and snowballing threat to public health and the economy. *Wound Repair Regener.* 17 (6): 763–771.

2 Heald, R., Salyer, S., Ham, K. et al. (2022). Electroceutical treatment of infected chronic wounds in a dog and a cat. *Vet. Surg.* 51 (3): 520–527.

3 Cray, M.T., Selmic, L.E., McConnell, B.M. et al. (2018). Effect of implementation of a surgical safety checklist on perioperative and postoperative complications at an academic institution in North America. *Vet. Surg.* 47 (8): 1052–1065.

4 Bergstrom, A., Dimopoulou, M., and Eldh, M. (2016). Reduction of surgical complications in dogs and cats by the use of a surgical safety checklist. *Vet. Surg.* 45 (5): 571–576.

5 Haynes, A.B., Weiser, T.G., Berry, W.R. et al. (2009). A surgical safety checklist to reduce morbidity and mortality in a global population. *N. Engl. J. Med.* 360 (5): 491–499.

6 Weiser, T.G., Haynes, A.B., Dziekan, G. et al. (2010). Effect of a 19-item surgical safety checklist during urgent operations in a global patient population. *Ann. Surg.* 251 (5): 976–980.

7 Bliss, L.A., Ross-Richardson, C.B., Sanzari, L.J. et al. (2012). Thirty-day outcomes support implementation of a surgical safety checklist. *J. Am. Coll. Surg.* 215 (6): 766–776.

8 Garcia Stickney, D.N. and Thieman Mankin, K.M. (2018). The impact of postdischarge surveillance on surgical site infection diagnosis. *Vet. Surg.* 47 (1): 66–73.

9 WHO. (2009). WHO Guidelines Approved by the Guidelines Review Committee. WHO Guidelines on Hand Hygiene in Health Care: First Global Patient Safety Challenge Clean Care Is Safer Care. Geneva: World Health Organization.

10 da Silveira, E.A., Bubeck, K.A., Batista, E.R. et al. (2016). Comparison of an alcohol-based hand rub and water-based chlorhexidine gluconate scrub technique for hand antisepsis prior to elective surgery in horses. *Can. Vet. J.* 57 (2): 164–168.

11 Pittet, D., Allegranzi, B., and Boyce, J. (2009). The World Health Organization guidelines on hand hygiene in health care and their consensus recommendations. *Infect. Control Hosp. Epidemiol.* 30 (7): 611–622.

12 Viljoen, H., Schoeman, J.P., Fosgate, G.T., and Boucher, C. (2022). Comparative antimicrobial efficacy of 4 surgical hand-preparation procedures prior to application of an alcohol-based hand rub in veterinary students. *Vet. Surg.* 51 (3): 447–454.

13 Verwilghen, D.R., Mainil, J., Mastrocicco, E. et al. (2011). Surgical hand antisepsis in veterinary practice: evaluation of soap scrubs and alcohol based rub techniques. *Vet. J.* 190 (3): 372–377.

14 Burgess, B.A. (2019). Prevention and surveillance of surgical infections: a review. *Vet. Surg.* 48 (3): 284–290.

15 Chou, P.Y., Doyle, A.J., Arai, S. et al. (2016). Antibacterial efficacy of several surgical hand preparation products used by veterinary students. *Vet. Surg.* 45 (4): 515–522.

16 Schultz, G.S., Sibbald, R.G., Falanga, V. et al. (2003). Wound bed preparation: a systematic approach to wound management. *Wound Repair Regener.* 11 (s1): S1–S28.

17 Ousey, K., Gilchrist, B., and James, H. (2018). Understanding clinical practice challenges: a survey performed with wound care clinicians to explore wound assessment frameworks. *Wounds Int.* 9 (4): 58–62.

18 Moore, Z., Dowsett, C., Smith, G. et al. (2019). TIME CDST: an updated tool to address the current challenges in wound care. *J. Wound Care* 28 (3): 154–161.

19 Dowsett, C. and Newton, H. (2005). Wound bed preparation: TIME in practice. *Wounds UK* 1 (3): 58.

20 Patton, D., Avsar, P., Wilson, P. et al. (2022). Treatment of diabetic foot ulcers: review of the literature with regard to the TIME clinical decision support tool. *J. Wound Care* 31 (9): 771–779.

21 Aisa, J. and Parlier, M. (2022). Local wound management: a review of modern techniques and products. *Vet. Dermatol.* 33 (5): 463–478.

22 Lux, C.N. (2022). Wound healing in animals: a review of physiology and clinical evaluation. *Vet. Dermatol.* 33 (1): 91. -e27.

23 Janis, J.E., Khansa, L., and Khansa, I. (2016). Strategies for postoperative seroma prevention: a systematic review. *Plastic Reconstruct. Surg.* 138 (1): 240–252.

24 Kottayasamy Seenivasagam, R., Gupta, V., and Singh, G. (2013). Prevention of seroma formation after axillary dissection--a comparative randomized clinical trial of three methods. *Breast J.* 19 (5): 478–484.

25 Porter, K., O'Connor, S., Rimm, E., and Lopez, M. (1998). Electrocautery as a factor in seroma formation following mastectomy. *Am. J. Surg.* 176 (1): 8–11.

26 Seretis, K., Goulis, D., Demiri, E.C., and Lykoudis, E.G. (2017). Prevention of seroma formation following abdominoplasty: a systematic review and meta-analysis. *Aesthet. Surg. J.* 37 (3): 316–323.

27 Travis, B.M., Hayes, G.M., Vissio, K. et al. (2018). A quilting subcutaneous suture pattern to reduce seroma formation and pain 24 hours after midline celiotomy in dogs: a randomized controlled trial. *Vet. Surg.* 47 (2): 204–211.

28 Lopez, D.J., Hayes, G.M., Fefer, G. et al. (2020). Effect of subcutaneous closure technique on incisional complications and postoperative pain in cats undergoing midline celiotomy: a randomized, blinded, controlled trial. *Vet. Surg.* 49 (2): 321–328.

29 Field, E.J., Kelly, G., Pleuvry, D. et al. (2015). Indications, outcome and complications with axial pattern skin flaps in dogs and cats: 73 cases. *J. Small Anim. Pract.* 56 (12): 698–706.

30 Zecha, P. and Missotten, F. (1999). Pseudocyst formation after abdominoplasty–extravasations of Morel-Lavallée. *Br. J. Plastic Surg.* 52 (6): 500–502.

31 Amsellem, P. (2011). Complications of reconstructive surgery in companion animals. *Vet. Clin. North Am. Small Anim. Pract.* 41 (5): 995–1006. vii.

32 Shaver, S.L., Hunt, G.B., and Kidd, S.W. (2014). Evaluation of fluid production and seroma formation after placement of closed suction drains in clean subcutaneous surgical wounds of dogs: 77 cases (2005–2012). *J. Am. Vet. Med. Assoc.* 245 (2): 211–215.

33 Dougherty, S.H. and Simmons, R.L. (1992). The biology and practice of surgical drains part II. *Curr. Probl. Surg.* 29 (9): 643–730.

34 Bristow, P.C., Halfacree, Z.J., and Baines, S.J. (2015). A retrospective study of the use of active suction wound drains in dogs and cats. *J. Small Anim. Pract.* 56 (5): 325–330.

35 Or, M., Van Goethem, B., Kitshoff, A. et al. (2017). Negative pressure wound therapy using polyvinyl alcohol foam to bolster full-thickness mesh skin grafts in dogs. *Vet. Surg.* 46 (3): 389–395.

36 Stanley, B.J., Pitt, K.A., Weder, C.D. et al. (2013). Effects of negative pressure wound therapy on healing of free full-thickness skin grafts in dogs. *Vet. Surg.* 42 (5): 511–522.

37 Vallarino, N., Devriendt, N., Koenraadt, A. et al. (2020). The effect of closed-incision negative pressure wound therapy on clinical and ultrasonographic seroma formation and wound healing following forequarter amputation in large dogs: a randomized pilot trial. *Vlaams Diergeneeskundig Tijdschrift* 89 (4): 198–208.

38 Shanmugam, V.K., Fernandez, S.J., Evans, K.K. et al. (2015). Postoperative wound dehiscence: predictors and associations. *Wound Repair Regener.* 23 (2): 184–190.

39 AHRQ. (2015). Postoperative Wound Dehiscence Rate - Technical Specifications. https://qualityindicators.ahrq.gov/Downloads/Modules/PDI/V50/TechSpecs/PDI_11_Postoperative_Wound_Dehiscence_Rate.pdf.

40 Pavletic, M.M. (ed.) (2012). *Atlas of Small Animal Wound Management and Reconstructive Surgery*, 3e, 5. Ames, IA: Wiley-Blackwell.

41 Meng, F., Andrea, S., Cheng, S. et al. (2017). Modified subcutaneous buried horizontal mattress suture compared with vertical buried mattress suture. *Ann. Plastic Surg.* 79 (2).

42 Balsa, I.M. and Culp, W.T. (2015). Wound care. *Vet. Clin. North Am. Small Anim. Pract.* 45 (5): 1049–1065.

43 Cockburn, E., Janovec, J., Solano, M.A., and L'Eplattenier, H. (2022). Marginal excision of cutaneous mast cell tumors in dogs was not associated with a higher rate of complications or prolonged wound healing than marginal excision of soft tissue sarcomas. *J. Am. Vet. Med. Assoc.* 260 (7): 741–746.

44 Killick, D.R., Rowlands, A.M., Burrow, R.D. et al. (2011). Mast cell tumour and cutaneous histiocytoma excision wound healing in general practice. *J. Small Anim. Pract.* 52 (9): 469–475.

45 Sandy-Hodgetts, K., Carville, K., and Leslie, G.D. (2015). Determining risk factors for surgical wound dehiscence: a literature review. *Int. Wound J.* 12 (3): 265–275.

46 Boothe, D.M. and Boothe, H.W. Jr. (2015). Antimicrobial considerations in the perioperative patient. *Vet. Clin. North Am. Small Anim. Pract.* 45 (3): 585–608.

47 Turk, R., Singh, A., and Weese, J.S. (2015). Prospective surgical site infection surveillance in dogs. *Vet. Surg.* 44 (1): 2–8.

48 Nicoll, C., Singh, A., and Weese, J.S. (2014). Economic impact of tibial plateau leveling osteotomy surgical site infection in dogs. *Vet. Surg.* 43 (8): 899–902.

49 Stevens, D.L. (2009). Treatments for skin and soft-tissue and surgical site infections due to MDR gram-positive bacteria. *J. Inf.* 59 (Suppl 1): S32–S39.

50 Singh, A., Walker, M., Rousseau, J., and Weese, J.S. (2013). Characterization of the biofilm forming ability of staphylococcus pseudintermedius from dogs. *BMC Vet. Res.* 9: 93.

51 Stetter, J., Boge, G.S., Grönlund, U., and Bergström, A. (2021). Risk factors for surgical site infection associated with clean surgical procedures in dogs. *Res. Vet. Sci.* 136: 616–621.

52 Vasseur, P.B., Levy, J., Dowd, E., and Eliot, J. (1988). Surgical wound infection rates in dogs and cats. Data from a teaching hospital. *Vet. Surg.* 17 (2): 60–64.

53 Thieman Mankin, K.M. and Cohen, N.D. (2020). Randomized, controlled clinical trial to assess the effect of antimicrobial-impregnated suture on the incidence of surgical site infections in dogs and cats. *J. Am. Vet. Med. Assoc.* 257 (1): 62–69.

54 Swanson, E.A. (2022). Updates in the use of antibiotics, biofilms. *Vet. Clin. North Am. Small Anim. Pract.* 52 (2S): e1–e19.

55 Mayhew, P.D., Freeman, L., Kwan, T., and Brown, D.C. (2012). Comparison of surgical site infection rates in clean and clean-contaminated wounds in dogs and cats after minimally invasive versus open surgery: 179 cases (2007-2008). *J. Am. Vet. Med. Assoc.* 240 (2): 193–198.

56 Nazarali, A., Singh, A., and Weese, J.S. (2014). Perioperative administration of antimicrobials during tibial plateau leveling osteotomy. *Vet. Surg.* 43 (8): 966–971.

57 Amalsadvala, T. and Swaim, S.F. (2006). Management of hard-to-heal wounds. *Vet. Clin. North Am. Small Anim. Pract.* 36 (4): 693–711.

58 Bohling, M.W., Henderson, R.A., Swaim, S.F. et al. (2006). Comparison of the role of the subcutaneous tissues in cutaneous wound healing in the dog and cat. *Vet. Surg.* 35 (1): 3–14.

59 Bohling, M.W. and Henderson, R.A. (2006). Differences in cutaneous wound healing between dogs and cats. *Vet. Clin. North Am. Small Anim. Pract.* 36 (4): 687–692.

60 Bohling, M.W., Henderson, R.A., Swaim, S.F. et al. (2004). Cutaneous wound healing in the cat: a macroscopic description and comparison with cutaneous wound healing in the dog. *Vet. Surg.* 33 (6): 579–587.

61 Lascelles, B.D., Davison, L., Dunning, M. et al. (1998). Use of omental pedicle grafts in the management of non-healing axillary wounds in 10 cats. *J. Small Anim. Pract.* 39 (10): 475–480.

62 Lascelles, B.D. and White, R.A. (2001). Combined omental pedicle grafts and thoracodorsal axial pattern flaps for the reconstruction of chronic, nonhealing axillary wounds in cats. *Vet. Surg.* 30 (4): 380–385.

63 Brinkley, C.H. (2007). Successful closure of feline axillary wounds by reconstruction of the elbow skin fold. *J. Small Anim. Pract.* 48 (2): 111–115.

64 Gray, M.J. (2005). Chronic axillary wound repair in a cat with omentalisation and omocervical skin flap. *J. Small Anim. Pract.* 46 (10): 499–503.

65 McGhie, J.A., Gibson, I.D., and Herndon, A.M. (2018). Morel-Lavallee lesions: a phenomenon in cats? Case report and review of the literature. *JFMS Open Rep.* 4 (1): 2055116918774469.

66 Gajula, B., Munnamgi, S., and Basu, S. (2020). How bacterial biofilms affect chronic wound healing: a narrative review. *Int. J. Surg. Global Health* 3 (2): e16.

67 Clutterbuck, A.L., Woods, E.J., Knottenbelt, D.C. et al. (2007). Biofilms and their relevance to veterinary medicine. *Vet. Microbiol.* 121 (1–2): 1–17.

68 Swanson, E.A., Freeman, L.J., Seleem, M.N., and Snyder, P.W. (2014). Biofilm-infected wounds in a dog. *J. Am. Vet. Med. Assoc.* 244 (6): 699–707.

69 Walker, M., Singh, A., and S.J. W. (2017). Bacterial biofilms. *Clin. Brief* 103–108.

70 Oliveira, M.A.C., Lima, G.M.G., Nishime, T.M.C. et al. (2021). Inhibitory effect of cold atmospheric plasma on chronic wound-related multispecies biofilms. *Appl. Sci.* 11 (12): 5441.

71 Martin, P. and Nunan, R. (2015). Cellular and molecular mechanisms of repair in acute and chronic wound healing. *Br. J. Dermatol.* 173 (2): 370–378.

72 Malone, M., Bjarnsholt, T., McBain, A.J. et al. (2017). The prevalence of biofilms in chronic wounds: a systematic review and meta-analysis of published data. *J. Wound Care* 26 (1): 20–25.

73 Lenselink, E. and Andriessen, A. (2011). A cohort study on the efficacy of a polyhexanide-containing biocellulose dressing in the treatment of biofilms in wounds. *J. Wound Care* 20 (11): 534. 536–539.

74 Zhao, G., Usui, M.L., Underwood, R.A. et al. (2012). Time course study of delayed wound healing in a biofilm-challenged diabetic mouse model. *Wound Repair Regener.* 20 (3): 342–352.

75 Hawas, S., Verderosa, A.D., and Totsika, M. (2022). Combination therapies for biofilm inhibition and eradication: a comparative review of laboratory and preclinical studies. *Front. Cell. Infect. Microbiol.* 12: 850030.

4

Wound Types and Terminology

Desiree D. Rosselli

VCA West Los Angeles Animal Hospital, Los Angeles, CA, USA

Living tissue sustains a wound when an injury causes a break in the continuity of the skin.

Humans have been describing and treating wounds since ancient times. The Smith Papyrus is one of the earliest known written pieces of evidence of the examination, diagnosis, and treatment of wounds; the Smith Papyrus was written around 1600 BCE, and likely authored several centuries earlier [1].

Today, the classification of wounds can aid in the management of injuries and in assessing or predicting outcomes for healing. The ideal classification system should provide a reliable and valid description of the injury as well as help with treatment options and to allow for prognostication of wound healing [2]. In human medicine, a number of classification schemes for soft tissue injury have been used, which help provide a wound severity scale, as well as assist with surgical decision-making. For example, the Mangled Extremity Severity Score (MESS) [3] assigns a severity score to different variables of wounding such as the velocity of energy that created the wound (low-energy versus high-energy injuries) and the degree of limb ischemia. This system was designed for severe distal limb injuries and used to help predict candidates for salvage or amputation [2]. Another example is the Red Cross wound classification [4] which assigns a score to wounds based on the extent of tissue damage, and the types of structures involved (soft tissue, bone, vital organs). Application of the score has both a clinical decision phase, to determine the need and priority for surgery, as well as a more formal analysis of the wound [2].

The degree of soft tissue injury associated with boney trauma is important to categorize, due to the increased infection rates associated with open fractures [5]. In a veterinary study evaluating 659 traumatic fractures in dogs and cats, 14.1% of cats had open fractures, and 29.2% of dogs had open fractures [6]. The most widely used classification scheme for describing open wounds over a fracture, in both human and veterinary patients, was initially outlined by Gustilo and Anderson in 1976, and later modified as outlined here [7].

Type I: Wound less than 1 cm in length
Type II: Wound more than 1 cm in length, with no extensive soft tissue injury, flap, or avulsion
Type III: Extensive damage to soft tissue; divided into three types:
Type IIIA: The soft tissue coverage over the fracture is adequate, despite extensive laceration, flaps, or high-energy trauma
Type IIIB: Extensive injury and loss of soft tissue, periosteal stripping, bone exposure, and massive contamination
Type IIIC: Any arterial injury that must be repaired, regardless of the degree of soft tissue injury

Classifications of Veterinary Wounds

Below we define specific wound terminology and classifications, based on three different descriptors:

1) Type of wound
2) Age of wound
3) Degree of bacterial contamination

Techniques in Small Animal Wound Management, First Edition. Edited by Nicole J. Buote.
© 2024 John Wiley & Sons, Inc. Published 2024 by John Wiley & Sons, Inc.
Companion website: www.wiley.com/go/buote/wounds

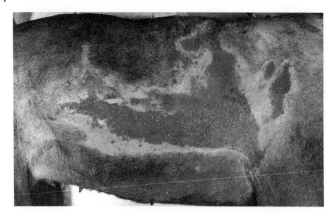

Figure 4.1   An abrasion injury to the right flank of a dog, caused by being dragged by a vehicle. Cranial is to the right of the photograph. *Source:* Courtesy of Desiree D. Rosselli, DVM, DACVS-SA.

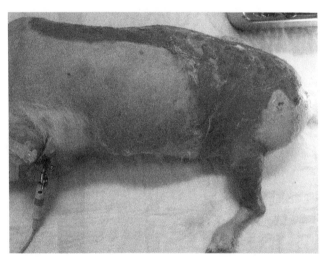

Figure 4.2   A burn wound to the dorsum of a small breed dog, with extension of the wounding down the flank and extremity. Cranial is to the left of the photograph. *Source:* Courtesy of Desiree D. Rosselli, DVM, DACVS-SA.

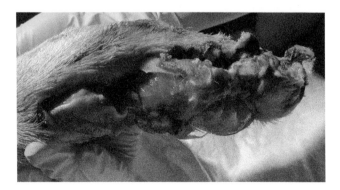

Figure 4.3   A degloving injury to the manus of a dog. Note the exposure of ligaments and bone. The carpus is on the left of the image, and the distal aspect of the paw is on the right of the image. *Source:* Courtesy of Desiree D. Rosselli, DVM, DACVS-SA.

Type of Wound

Broadly, tissue can sustain trauma which causes either closed injury or open injury. Closed injuries such as contusion/bruise, blister, hematoma/seroma, and crush wounds, are often caused by blunt force trauma.

Open wounds are the focus of this chapter and can further be classified based on wound type. Specific wound examples are also discussed in Chapter 17.

Abrasion

An abrasion is a superficial injury to the skin, where the superficial layer of epithelium is rubbed or scraped off, but does not create full-thickness wounding. This type of wound is typically due to friction injuries (Figure 4.1).

Burn

A burn wound is an injury that causes coagulative necrosis of tissues (Figure 4.2). Burn wounds have traditionally been classified by the depth of burn, and/or by the cause of burn [8]. Burns wounds can be caused by the following mechanisms:

Chemical
Electrical
Friction
Frostbite
Radiation
Thermal

Burn wounds are also classified by the total body surface area (TBSA) involved in wounding, and patients with more than 20–30% of TBSA involved are expected to need significant medical and surgical management due to systemic derangements [9].

Degloving/Avulsion/Shearing Wounds

Degloving injuries occur when the skin and/or superficial soft tissues are completely detached or torn from the underlying tissues. These injuries are also termed shearing injuries and often occur to the distal extremities as a result of vehicular trauma (Figure 4.3). Management of degloving injuries can be challenging, particularly if there are large areas of skin loss, instability from joint or ligamentous damage, or bone exposure [10]. Shearing wounds of the limbs were evaluated in 98 dogs and approximately three-fourths of the patients had exposed bone or joint surfaces [11].

Exposed bone and denuded periosteum in a wound cause delays in healing. Exposed bone reduces vascularity, causes reduced formation of healthy granulation tissue, and can inhibit wound epithelization and contraction; desiccated bone presents a risk for infectious osteitis or sequestrum formation [12].

(a)

(b)

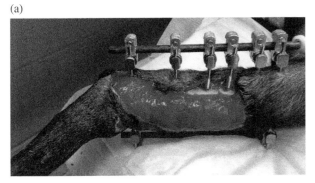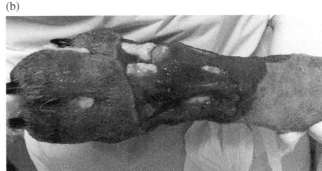

Figure 4.4   (a) Depicts bone exposure of a tibial fracture treated with external skeletal fixation, and the difficulty of epithelization and contraction of the wound over the surface of exposed bone. (b) Shows a degloving injury to the hind limb of a dog; note the bone exposure, and the evidence of bone perforation (forage) created on the metacarpal bones used to help promote granulation tissue formation. *Source:* Courtesy of Desiree D. Rosselli, DVM, DACVS-SA.

One technique to promote the development of granulation tissue over exposed bone is called forage or osteostixis, which is the creation of multiple spaced-out bone perforations by drilling into the medullary canal along the length of the exposed cortex with Kirschner wires or small diameter drill bits [13] (Figure 4.4). The islands of granulation tissue that develop at the perforation sites will subsequently merge with granulation tissue at the periphery of the wound [13]. Free skin grafts or vascularized flaps may also be used to cover areas of bone exposure [10].

Incisions or Surgical Wounds

An incision is a sharp surgical cut created in skin and can extend to deeper tissues. Closure of intentional surgical incisions, with adequate tissue apposition, should enable tissues to proceed through the normal phases of wound healing.

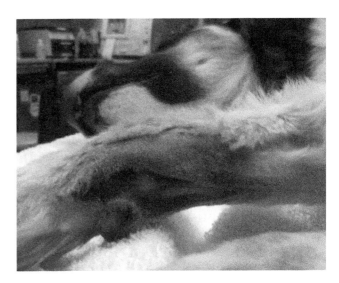

Figure 4.5   A laceration sustained to the caudal aspect of the carpus of a shepherd dog, after jumping over a fence. *Source:* Courtesy of Desiree D. Rosselli, DVM, DACVS-SA.

Laceration/Skin Tear

A laceration is an unintentional cut or tear to the skin and can extend to the deeper tissues (Figure 4.5). These can be linear, or irregular, depending on the mechanism of wounding.

Pressure Ulcers/Sores/Decubitus Ulcers

Pressure sores or decubitus ulcers typically develop in the skin and soft tissues which overlie boney prominences. These types of wounds develop due to sustained or repetitive pressure, usually due to prolonged periods of recumbency (Figure 4.6).

Impairment of vascularity, and likely the presence of infection, are major clinical challenges associated with effective treatment of pressure sores [14, 15]. A chronic wound is often associated with older animals, who have decreased healing potential and often also have concurrent illnesses that may impair wound healing (such as endocrine and metabolic diseases), or in animals with significant neurologic or orthopedic disfunction, where limited mobility and recumbency continually exacerbate wounded areas and do not allow for healing.

Puncture or Penetration Wounds

A penetration can be any wound that extends from the outside of the skin to the inside. Bite wounds and gunshot wounds are the most common penetrating injuries in dogs and cats [16].

(a)   (b)   (c)

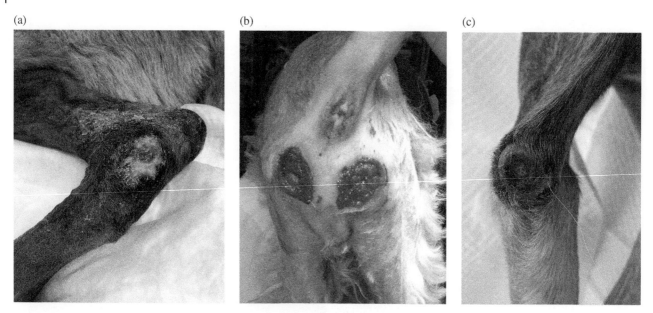

Figure 4.6   (a) Is a pressure sore on the lateral aspect of the hock of a dog; the dog had significant osteoarthritis and difficulty rising. (b) Shows pressure wounds on the caudal aspect of the ischium of a dog; the dog was recovering from paraplegia caused by a myelopathy and was constantly scooting his hind end along when trying to rise. (c) Depicts a pressure sore caused on the caudal aspect of the olecranon of a greyhound due to prolonged bandage management. *Source:* Courtesy of Desiree D. Rosselli, DVM, DACVS-SA.

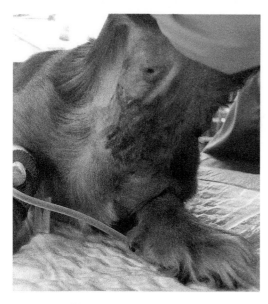

Figure 4.7   Bite wounds to the ventral cervical region of a Dachshund, sustained from a large breed dog. Note that the puncture wounds are very small, compared to the degree of bruising. *Source:* Courtesy of Desiree D. Rosselli, DVM, DACVS-SA.

Bite Wounds   Bite wounds are often sustained during fights between big dogs and small dogs. Tissue damage can occur not only via shearing which causes sharp laceration, but also tensile force that causes skin avulsion, and compression resulting in crush injury to tissues [17]. There can be significant injury to deeper structures, even if there is only minor skin damage [18]. This "tip of the iceberg" phenomena is extremely important to explain to owners as the injuries they see may not accurately indicate the full extent of damage to the skin and underlying tissues microcirculation (Figure 4.7). The thorax, extremities, and head are frequently involved in fights between dogs, and wounds sustained over the thoracic or abdominal cavity are associated with a higher mortality rate [19]. Bite wounds to the abdomen can create intestinal perforations, mesenteric avulsions and urogenital damage therefore an abdominal exploration is always justified in these cases regardless of the visible skin damage.

Gunshot or High Velocity Projectile Wounds   The degree of soft tissue injury sustained by a projectile is related to the characteristics of the object itself, the energy absorbed on impact, and the tissues sustaining the injury [20]. In one retrospective case series of 29 dogs and 8 cats evaluated for gunshot wounds, the limbs were the most common site of wounding (32.4%), followed by thorax (21.6%) and abdomen (13.5%) [21]. The animal triage trauma (ATT) score calculated at admission, was higher for patients who required blood products, those who required surgery, and those who did not survive [21]. The degree of soft tissue wounding is extremely important: in a veterinary study of 97 patients who sustained bone fracture due to gunshot injury, 54% of cases had a poor fracture outcome, and a greater degree of soft tissue trauma at the fracture site was associated with increased likelihood of a poor outcome [22].

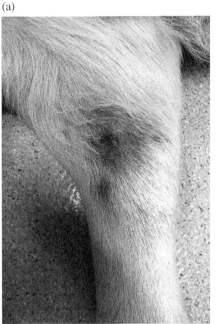 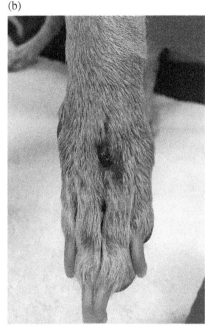

(a) (b)

Figure 4.8 (a) Depicts a draining tract on the medial tibia, overlying a metallic implant. (b) Depicts a draining tract on the manus of a dog, due to a migrating foreign object (foxtail). *Source:* Courtesy of Desiree D. Rosselli, DVM, DACVS-SA.

Impalement Injuries Impalement injuries are sustained due to piercing with a sharp instrument. As with bite wounds, impalement injuries can appear externally as a simple wound, with significant injury to deeper structures. Prognosis after treatment is generally good, even in cases of thoracic impalement requiring thoracotomy, a 93% survival rate is reported [23].

Draining Tracts
A fistulous tract or draining tract connects a focal area of inflammation to the surface of the skin, usually via a small break in the epithelium (Figure 4.8). There are a range of differential diagnoses for draining tracts, which include infectious, non-infectious, and neoplastic etiologies, and a step-wise approach to diagnosis and treatment is usually necessary [24].

Age of Wound

An acute wound, or a fresh wound, is one that has recently occurred. These wounds typically progress through the normal stages of wound healing in an orderly fashion, provided appropriate treatment.

Chronic Wounds
A chronic wound is a wound that fails to progress through the normal stages of healing in a timely manner, meaning that the wound does not heal in the amount of time that should normally be sufficient for wound healing [25]. Failure to heal over a four to six-week period is likely consistent with a chronic wound, although there is not a defined time frame; human patients can have wounds that are present for longer than one year [26, 27]. Some chronic wounds may not progress beyond the inflammatory phase. Chronic wounds may have blunted epithelial edges, epithelium that fails to adhere to the wound bed, or may have uneven, mottled, or friable granulation tissue [15]. Some chronic wounds may not progress to final epithelial closure or functional outcome (Figure 4.9). Chronic wounds represent a very important clinical problem: human and veterinary patients with chronic wounds have poor quality of life as well as substantial economic costs associated with wound care [26]. Many factors can contribute to delayed wound healing and persistence of chronic wounds [14, 25, 28], and these factors can be grouped based on local wound factors and systemic factors:

Local factors that negatively affect wound healing are:

- Impairment to the blood supply
- The presence of infection
- Foreign material in the wound

(a) (b) (c)

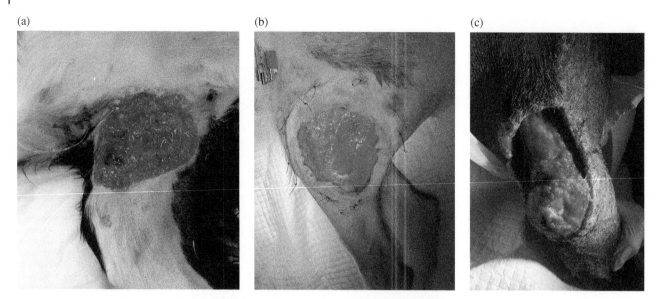

Figure 4.9   (a) Is a chronic wound on the inguinal region of a dog, in an area of high tension and high motion. (b) Is a chronic wound on the lateral pelvic limb of a dog treated with long-term immune suppressive medications. Note the lack of granulation tissue formation, even after weeks of open wound management. (c) Is a chronic wound over the olecranon region of a dog, previously treated with surgical removal of elbow hygromas and subsequent wound healing complications. *Source:* Courtesy of Desiree D. Rosselli, DVM, DACVS-SA.

- Mechanical factors such as excessive tension, motion, or sustained pressure on the wound
- Excessive wound fluid exudate or prolonged tissue desiccation
- Previous local tissue injury such as radiation therapy

Systemic factors that negatively affecting wound healing are:

- Malnourishment
- Older patient age
- Obesity
- Systemic disease such as anemia, vasculitis, hepatic disease, clotting deficiencies, hypoproteinemia, cancer, uremia, shock, or sepsis
- Immune deficiencies or metabolic diseases such as diabetes mellitus, hyperadrenocorticism, FIV; administration of corticosteroids or some chemotherapies

Management of chronic wounds is a significant clinical challenge. Initial management strategies are aimed at amelioration as many of those factors negatively affecting wound healing as possible. Identifying and eliminating the presence of infection is extremely important. Consider obtaining a bacterial culture from a superficial swab which will provide a general picture of wound bacteria affecting the surface of a chronic wound, and comparing this to a deep tissue biopsy which will reflect deeper penetrating organisms [29]. Molecular diagnostic techniques such as PCR assay and pyrosequencing have also been described; these techniques identify bacterial DNA, which can diagnose the presence of organisms that may not grow on a standard bacterial culture such as anaerobic bacteria, slow-growing bacterial species, or fungal organisms [15, 30].

Wound management techniques for chronic wounds may include: aggressive surgical debridement to improve vascularity, use of drains, use of specific dressings (see Chapter 8), use of platelet-rich plasma/stem cells (see Chapter 15), pressure relieving techniques, tension relieving techniques, hyperbaric oxygen therapy (see Chapter 13), and closure with subdermal plexus flaps or axial pattern flaps [16, 31–34].

Negative pressure wound therapy (NPWT) has been used in the management of chronic wounds in humans; in addition to promoting more superficial development of granulation tissue, NPWT leads to clearance of chronic inflammation and edema within the deeper tissue layers [27]. In dogs with complicated wounds, NPWT leads to faster closure and less local signs of infection [35] and has even been reported to help achieve wound healing over an exposed metal implant [36]. NPWT is discussed in depth in Chapter 10.

Recently investigated techniques in veterinary chronic wound treatment include, a printed electroceutical dressing [37], photobiomodulation therapy [38], and allogeneic adipose-derived mesenchymal stem cells [39] have been investigated to assist with promoting healing in chronic wounds.

Degree of Bacterial Contamination of a Wound

The ancient Romans used the following descriptors of "calor, dolor, rubor, tumor" to describe inflammation in terms of heat, pain, redness, and swelling [40]. Although modern wound care has certainly progressed since ancient times, the importance of accurate classification and description of inflammation and infection remains just as important today. Today, the average health care cost for a patient with a surgical site infection is approximately double that compared to a patient without infection [41].

The classification system for surgical wounds was developed by the National Academy of Sciences in 1964 and later modified in the mid-1980s for use by the Centers for Disease Control and Prevention (CDC) [42, 43]. This wound classification system is based on the likelihood and degree of bacterial contamination of a wound as well as structures entered during an operation.

- Clean wounds (Class I): Uninfected wounds without inflammation. The following systems are not entered: respiratory, alimentary, genital, or urinary tracts. Clean wounds are closed primarily, and if necessary, drained with closed drainage. Operative incisional wounds that follow no penetrating trauma are included in this category.
- Clean-contaminated wounds (Class II): Operative wounds or elective entry in the respiratory, alimentary, genital, or uninfected urinary tracts; without unusual contamination.
- Contaminated (Class III): Open, fresh, accidental wounds, or operations with major breaks in sterile technique or gross spillage from the gastrointestinal tract. Also, incisions in which acute, non-purulent inflammation is encountered (Figure 4.10).
- Dirty/Infected wounds (Class IV): Old traumatic wounds with retained devitalized tissue or those that involve existing clinical infection or perforated viscera. Drainage of purulent material is present in the wound. Organisms causing infection were present in the wound prior to the operation (Figure 4.11).

Wound classification is important because it helps with improved assessment of the risk of infection, assists in development of perioperative protocols, and guides decision-making for clinical treatment [44]. Today, the American College of Surgeons – National Surgical Quality Improvement Program (ACS-NSQIP) database can be used to evaluate infection in human wounds based on classifications. Traditionally, wounds classified as clean-contaminated, contaminated, and dirty were at increased risk for infection [43]. Patients with contaminated and dirty wounds had higher odds of complication and need for reoperation as well as increased mortality [44]. Interestingly, over the last 40 years in human medicine, reduced rates of infection are reported regardless of initial wound classification [43, 45, 46], likely due to continued efforts to improve the quality of patient care.

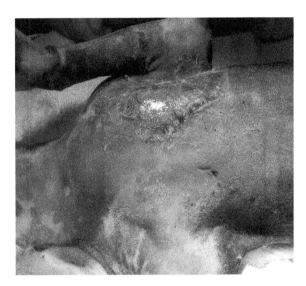

Figure 4.10 A contaminated wound on the ventral thorax of a dog, sustained by a bite wound from a larger dog. The head is located toward the left of the image. *Source:* Courtesy of Desiree D. Rosselli, DVM, DACVS-SA.

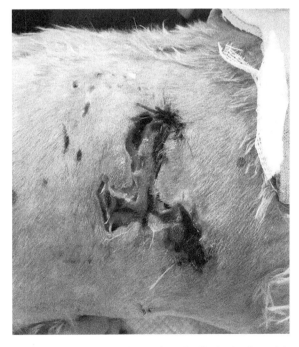

Figure 4.11 An infected wound on the flank of a dog, with evidence of the presence of purulent material from the wound. Cranial is oriented to the right of the image. *Source:* Courtesy of Desiree D. Rosselli, DVM, DACVS-SA.

In veterinary medicine, wound infection rates based on wound classification have been described as follows: clean: 2.5–4.7%, clean contaminated: 4.5–5.0%, contaminated: 5.8–12%, and dirty: 10–18.1% [47, 48]. Research on the effects of wound classification on outcome has not been as extensively studied in veterinary medicine as in human medicine. One veterinary study concluded that wound contamination categories had too much variation to make them useful for predicting animals that would develop surgical site infection [48], and one study showed a wound classification of dirty to be a major risk factor for development of infection [49]. Recently, an association between wound classification and risk of surgical site infection was found following canine limb amputation. Dogs with a wound classification other than clean were more likely to develop surgical site infection compared to dogs with clean wounds [50].

Wound Closure

The first archeological evidence of surgical suturing on a human is from ancient Egypt, around 1100 BCE [1]. Physicians in ancient India even developed special needles for suturing wounds following wound treatment [51]. Toward the end of World War I, tetanus rates were noted to be significantly lower when battlefield injuries were treated initially as open wounds, compared to those treated with immediate and tight closure [52].

Modern wound closure can be classified into the following main categories. A summary is listed in Table 4.1.

- Primary closure
- Delayed primary closure
- Second intention healing
- Secondary closure

Following wounding, tissues should progress through the normal phases of wound healing, going through inflammation, proliferation, and remodeling, as detailed in Chapter 2. Given enough time, many open wounds will likely fill in and heal on their own, which is termed second intention healing (Figure 4.12). Second intention healing is generally elected for wounds that are dirty or contaminated, have significant tissue loss where closure is not possible, or where closure is expected to have excessive tension. Promoting second intention healing of a wound requires time and financial resources, therefore, for many larger wounds, the planned surgical closure of the wound will speed the process of recovery. Surgical closure may become required for some wounds, for example: if an open wound fails to completely epithelialize. Another example is where a surgical closure will result in a more functional outcome compared to a

Table 4.1 Wound closure classifications.

Type of closure	Timing of closure	Candidates	Wound examples
Primary closure	Immediately after wounding to within 6-h of wounding	Clean or clean contaminated wounds	• A surgically created incision • Lacerations without significantly devitalized tissue
Delayed primary closure	3–5 d following open wound management	Initially contaminated or dirty wounds	• Lacerations with devitalized tissue or peri-wound inflammation • An abscess or bite wound • A pressure wound or chronic wounds
Second intention healing	Closure is not performed	Initially contaminated or dirty wounds	• Puncture wounds from a dog bite • Abrasion wounds • Burn wounds • Degloving wounds where wound contraction and epithelialization are progressing

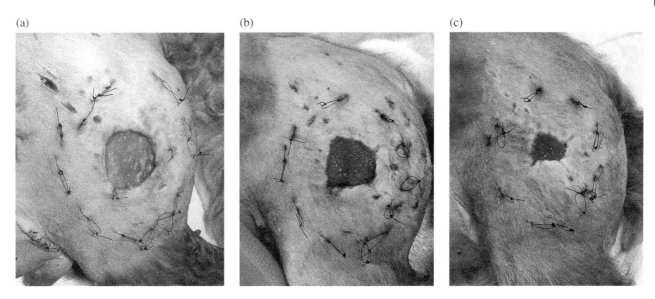

Figure 4.12 These images depict second intention healing of a dog bite wound. (a,b) are taken four days apart, (b,c) are taken seven days apart. Cranial is oriented to the left of the images. *Source:* Courtesy of Desiree D. Rosselli, DVM, DACVS-SA.

wound that had healed with contracture, which is excessive contraction that causes scar tissue formation or constriction of the epithelium (Figure 4.13).

In primary closure, or primary intention, the skin is completely closed following the completion of surgery or initial wound management, regardless of the presence of drains, wicks, or other devices [53]. This is typically employed for wounds that are classified as clean, or clean-contaminated, and wounds without significant tissue loss so that they are not under tension after closure. Traditionally, a clean or clean-contaminated wound was a candidate for primary closure since bacterial colonization was expected to be fewer than the 100,000 colony-forming units of bacteria per gram of tissue necessary to cause infection [54]. An incision or acute wound treated/operated within six-hours of wounding are candidates for primary closure, as there is likely insufficient time for the development of infection [43].

Delayed primary closure allows for a few days of open wound management, prior to a planned closure (Figure 4.14). The goal of the initial period of wound management is to convert the wound into a surgically clean wound that can be closed. Closure may involve excision of part or all of the granulation bed. Closure may be performed over a drain, as discussed in Chapter 9. The duration of open wound management prior to surgical closure varies for individual cases, depending on the size of the wound and the degree of bacterial contamination of the wound. The period of open wound management will typically occur during inflammatory phase of wound healing, usually for days 3–5 after injury.

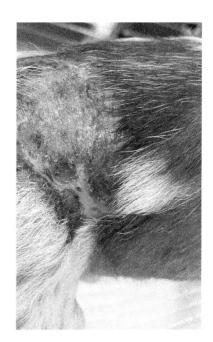

Figure 4.13 A wound healed with contracture on the right flank of a terrier. Cranial is to the right of the photograph. *Source:* Courtesy of Desiree D. Rosselli, DVM, DACVS-SA.

Secondary closure is called third intention healing by some texts, and refers to a longer period of open wound management prior to closure, typically reserved for severely contaminated wounds.

Where direct closure is not possible, other reconstructive techniques may be employed, such as skin grafts, local advancement flaps, or rotational flaps. In depth discussion of reconstructive techniques is found in Chapter 16.

(a)

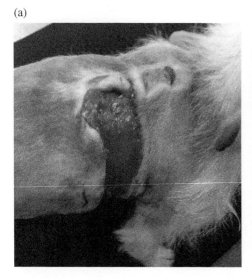

(b)

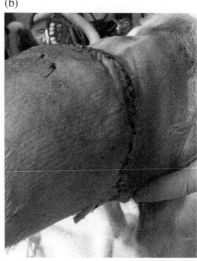

Figure 4.14 An example of delayed primary closure where a bite wound of the right thorax (a) was treated for two weeks prior to debriding and closing the wound (b). *Source:* Courtesy of Desiree D. Rosselli, DVM, DACVS-SA.

References

1 Gabriel, R.A. (2012). *Man and Wound in the Ancient World: A History of Military Medicine from Sumer to the Fall of Constantinople*. Potomac Books Inc.; Chapter 4.

2 Bowyer, G.W. (1999; Chapter 1). General classifications. In: *Classification of Musculoskeletal Trauma* (ed. P.B. Pynsent, J.C.T. Fairbank, and A.J. Carr), 1–12. Butterworth-Heinemann.

3 Johansen, K., Daines, M., Howey, T. et al. (1990). Objective criteria accurately predict amputation following lower extremity trauma. *J. Trauma* 30 (5): 568–572. discussion: 572–573. https://doi.org/10.1097/00005373-199005000-00007.

4 Coupland, R.M. (1992). The red cross classification of war wounds: the E.X.C.F.V.M. scoring system. *World J. Surg.* 16 (5): 910–917. https://doi.org/10.1007/BF02066991.

5 Gustilo, R.B. and Anderson, J.T. (1976). Prevention of infection in the treatment of one thousand and twenty-five open fractures of long bones: retrospective and prospective analyses. *J. Bone Joint Surg. Am.* 58 (4): 453–458.

6 Millard, R.P. and Weng, H.Y. (2014). Proportion of and risk factors for open fractures of the appendicular skeleton in dogs and cats. *J. Am. Vet. Med. Assoc.* 245 (6): 663–668. https://doi.org/10.2460/javma.245.6.663.

7 Gustilo, R.B., Merkow, R.L., and Templeman, D. (1990). The management of open fractures. *J. Bone Joint Surg. Am.* 72 (2): 299–304.

8 Scerri, G.V. (1999. Chapter 3). General classifications of soft tissue injuries. In: *Classification of Musculoskeletal Trauma* (ed. P.B. Pynsent, J.C.T. Fairbank, and A.J. Carr), 26–28. Butterworth-Heinemann.

9 Vaughn, L. and Beckel, N. (2012). Severe burn injury, burn shock, and smoke inhalation injury in small animals. Part 1: burn classification and pathophysiology. *J. Vet. Emerg. Crit. Care* 22 (2): 179–186. https://doi.org/10.1111/j.1476-4431.2012.00727.x.

10 Harris, J.E. and Dhupa, S. (2008). Treatment of degloving injuries with autogenous full thickness mesh scrotal free grafts. *Vet. Comp. Orthop. Traumatol.* 21 (4): 378–381. https://doi.org/10.3415/vcot-07-04-0029.

11 Beardsley, S.L. and Schrader, S.C. (1995). Treatment of dogs with wounds of the limbs caused by shearing forces: 98 cases (1975-1993). *J. Am. Vet. Med. Assoc.* 207 (8): 1071–1075.

12 Hanson, R.R. (2004). Management of avulsion wounds with exposed bone. *Clin. Tech. Equine Prac.* 3 (2): 188–203.

13 Clark, G.N. (2001). Bone perforation to enhance wound healing over exposed bone in dogs with shearing injuries. *J. Am. Anim. Hosp. Assoc.* 37 (3): 215–217. https://doi.org/10.5326/15473317-37-3-215.

14 Bjarnsholt, T., Kirketerp-Møller, K., Jensen, P.Ø. et al. (2008). Why chronic wounds will not heal: a novel hypothesis. *Wound Repair Regener.* 16 (1): 2–10. https://doi.org/10.1111/j.1524-475X.2007.00283.x.

15 Swanson, E.A., Freeman, L.J., Seleem, M.N., and Snyder, P.W. (2014). Biofilm-infected wounds in a dog. *J. Am. Vet. Med. Assoc.* 244 (6): 699–707. https://doi.org/10.2460/javma.244.6.699.

16 Risselada, M., de Rooster, H., Taeymans, O., and van Bree, H. (2008). Penetrating injuries in dogs and cats. A study of 16 cases. *Vet. Comp. Orthop. Traumatol.* 21 (5): 434–439.

17 Holt, D.E. and Griffin, G. (2000). Bite wounds in dogs and cats. *Vet. Clin. North Am. Small Anim. Prac.* 30 (3): 669–679, viii. https://doi.org/10.1016/s0195-5616(00)50045-x.

18 Shahar, R., Shamir, M., and Johnston, D.E. (1997). A technique for management of bite wounds of the thoracic wall in small dogs. *Vet. Surg.* 26 (1): 45–50. https://doi.org/10.1111/j.1532-950x.1997.tb01461.x.

19 Shamir, M.H., Leisner, S., Klement, E. et al. (2002). Dog bite wounds in dogs and cats: a retrospective study of 196 cases. *J. Vet. Med. A Physiol. Pathol. Clin. Med.* 49 (2): 107–112. https://doi.org/10.1046/j.1439-0442.2002.jv416.x.

20 Pavletic, M.M. and Trout, N.J. (2006). Bullet, bite, and burn wounds in dogs and cats. *Vet. Clin. North Am. Small Anim. Prac.* 36 (4): 873–893. https://doi.org/10.1016/j.cvsm.2006.02.005.

21 Olsen, L.E., Streeter, E.M., and DeCook, R.R. (2014). Review of gunshot injuries in cats and dogs and utility of a triage scoring system to predict short-term outcome: 37 cases (2003-2008). *J. Am. Vet. Med. Assoc.* 245 (8): 923–929. https://doi.org/10.2460/javma.245.8.923.

22 Schrock, K., Kerwin, S.C., and Jeffery, N. (2022). Outcomes and complications associated with acute gunshot fractures in cats and dogs. *Vet. Comp. Orthop. Traumatol.* 35 (3): 205–212. https://doi.org/10.1055/s-0041-1739238.

23 Matiasovic, M., Halfacree, Z.J., Moores, A. et al. (2018). Surgical management of impalement injuries to the trunk of dogs: a multicentre retrospective study. *J. Small Anim. Prac.* 59 (3): 139–146. https://doi.org/10.1111/jsap.12767.

24 Daigle, J.C., Kerwin, S., Foil, C.S., and Merchant, S.R. (2001). Draining tracts and nodules in dogs and cats. *Clin. Tech. Small Anim. Prac.* 16 (4): 214–218. https://doi.org/10.1053/svms.2001.26997.

25 Han, G. and Ceilley, R. (2017). Chronic wound healing: a review of current management and treatments. *Adv. Ther.* 34 (3): 599–610. https://doi.org/10.1007/s12325-017-0478-y.

26 Olsson, M., Järbrink, K., Divakar, U. et al. (2019). The humanistic and economic burden of chronic wounds: a systematic review. *Wound Repair Regener.* 27 (1): 114–125. https://doi.org/10.1111/wrr.12683.

27 Bassetto, F., Lancerotto, L., Salmaso, R. et al. (2012). Histological evolution of chronic wounds under negative pressure therapy. *J. Plast. Reconstr. Aesthet. Surg.* 65 (1): 91–99. https://doi.org/10.1016/j.bjps.2011.08.016.

28 Davidson, J.R. (2015). Current concepts in wound management and wound healing products. *Vet. Clin. North Am. Small Anim. Prac.* 45 (3): 537–564. https://doi.org/10.1016/j.cvsm.2015.01.009.

29 Bowler, P.G. (2003). The 10(5) bacterial growth guideline: reassessing its clinical relevance in wound healing. *Ostomy Wound Manage.* 49 (1): 44–53.

30 Cummings, P.J., Ahmed, R., Durocher, J.A. et al. (2013). Pyrosequencing for microbial identification and characterization. *J. Visual. Exp.* 78: e50405. https://doi.org/10.3791/50405.

31 Pavletic, M.M. (2011). Use of commercially available foam pipe insulation as a protective device for wounds over the elbow joint area in five dogs. *J. Am. Vet. Med. Assoc.* 239 (9): 1225–1231. https://doi.org/10.2460/javma.239.9.1225.

32 Jones, C.A. and Lipscomb, V.J. (2019). Indications, complications, and outcomes associated with subdermal plexus skin flap procedures in dogs and cats: 92 cases (2000-2017). *J. Am. Vet. Med. Assoc.* 255 (8): 933–938. https://doi.org/10.2460/javma.255.8.933.

33 Field, E.J., Kelly, G., Pleuvry, D. et al. (2015). Indications, outcome and complications with axial pattern skin flaps in dogs and cats: 73 cases. *J. Small Anim. Prac.* 56 (12): 698–706. https://doi.org/10.1111/jsap.12400.

34 Gouveia, D., Bimbarra, S., Carvalho, C. et al. (2021). Effects of hyperbaric oxygen therapy on wound healing in veterinary medicine: a pilot study. *Open Vet. J.* 11 (4): 544–554. https://doi.org/10.5455/OVJ.2021.v11.i4.4.

35 Nolff, M.C., Albert, R., Reese, S., and Meyer-Lindenberg, A. (2018). Comparison of negative pressure wound therapy and silver-coated foam dressings in open wound treatment in dogs: a prospective controlled clinical trial. *Vet. Comp. Orthop. Traumatol.* 31 (4): 229–238. https://doi.org/10.1055/s-0038-1639579.

36 Bertran, J., Farrell, M., and Fitzpatrick, N. (2013). Successful wound healing over exposed metal implants using vacuum-assisted wound closure in a dog. *J. Small Anim. Prac.* 54 (7): 381–385. https://doi.org/10.1111/jsap.12055.

37 Heald, R., Salyer, S., Ham, K. et al. (2022). Electroceutical treatment of infected chronic wounds in a dog and a cat. *Vet. Surg.* 51 (3): 520–527. https://doi.org/10.1111/vsu.13758.

38 Hoisang, S., Kampa, N., Seesupa, S., and Jitpean, S. (2021). Assessment of wound area reduction on chronic wounds in dogs with photobiomodulation therapy: a randomized controlled clinical trial. *Vet. World.* 14 (8): 2251–2259. https://doi.org/10.14202/vetworld.2021.2251-2259.

39 Enciso, N., Avedillo, L., Fermín, M.L. et al. (2020). Cutaneous wound healing: canine allogeneic ASC therapy. *Stem Cell Res. Ther.* 11 (1): 261. https://doi.org/10.1186/s13287-020-01778-5.

40 Rutgow, I.M. (2022). *Empire of the Scalpel: The History of Surgery*. New York, NY: Schribner; Chapter 2.

41 Broex, E.C., van Asselt, A.D., Bruggeman, C.A., and van Tiel, F.H. (2009). Surgical site infections: how high are the costs? *J. Hosp. Infect.* 72 (3): 193–201. https://doi.org/10.1016/j.jhin.2009.03.020.

42 Simmons, B.P. (1983). Guideline for prevention of surgical wound infections. *Am. J. Infect. Control* 11 (4): 133–143. https://doi.org/10.1016/0196-6553(83)90030-5.

43 Weigelt, J.A. (1985). Risk of wound infections in trauma patients. *Am. J. Surg.* 150 (6): 782–784. https://doi.org/10.1016/0002-9610(85)90429-5.

44 Mioton, L.M., Jordan, S.W., Hanwright, P.J. et al. (2013). The relationship between preoperative wound classification and postoperative infection: a multi-institutional analysis of 15,289 patients. *Arch. Plast. Surg.* 40 (5): 522–529.

45 Ortega, G., Rhee, D.S., Papandria, D.J. et al. (2012). An evaluation of surgical site infections by wound classification system using the ACS-NSQIP. *J. Surg. Res.* 174 (1): 33–38. https://doi.org/10.1016/j.jss.2011.05.056.

46 Onyekwelu, I., Yakkanti, R., Protzer, L. et al. (2017). Surgical Wound classification and surgical site infections in the orthopaedic patient. *J. Am. Acad. Orthop. Surg. Glob. Res. Rev.* 1 (3): e022. https://doi.org/10.5435/JAAOSGlobal-D-17-00022.

47 Vasseur, P.B., Levy, J., Dowd, E., and Eliot, J. (1988). Surgical wound infection rates in dogs and cats. Data from a teaching hospital. *Vet. Surg.* 17 (2): 60–64. https://doi.org/10.1111/j.1532-950x.1988.tb00278.x.

48 Brown, D.C., Conzemius, M.G., Shofer, F., and Swann, H. (1997). Epidemiologic evaluation of postoperative wound infections in dogs and cats. *J. Am. Vet. Med. Assoc.* 210 (9): 1302–1306.

49 Eugster, S., Schawalder, P., Gaschen, F., and Boerlin, P. (2004). A prospective study of postoperative surgical site infections in dogs and cats. *Vet. Surg.* 33 (5): 542–550. https://doi.org/10.1111/j.1532-950X.2004.04076.x.

50 Billas, A.R., Grimes, J.A., Hollenbeck, D.L. et al. (2022). Incidence of and risk factors for surgical site infection following canine limb amputation. *Vet. Surg.* 51 (3): 418–425. http://dx.doi.org.10.1111/vsu.13762.

51 Gabriel, R.A. (2012). *Man and Wound in the Ancient World: A History of Military Medicine from Sumer to the Fall of Constantinople.* Potomac Books Inc.; Chapter 7.

52 Gabriel, R.A. (2012). *Man and Wound in the Ancient World: A History of Military Medicine from Sumer to the Fall of Constantinople.* Potomac Books Inc.; Chapter 2.

53 Center for Disease Control. (2022). Surgical site infection (SSI) event. https://www.cdc.gov/nhsn/pdfs/pscmanual/9pscssicurrent.pdf (accessed 22 August 2022).

54 Robson, M.C. (1997). Wound infection. A failure of wound healing caused by an imbalance of bacteria. *Surg. Clin. North Am.* 77 (3): 637–650. https://doi.org/10.1016/s0039-6109(05)70572-7.

5

Patient Presentation and Evaluation of Wound

Colin Chik

Department of Clinical Sciences, Cornell University, Ithaca, NY, USA

Initial Stabilization of the Wound Patient

All patients with wounds should be initially triaged with a cursory targeted physical examination predominantly assessing the ABC's (airway, breathing, circulation) and overall neurologic status to identify unstable patients that require more immediate attention. These are patients who have typically sustained moderate to severe traumatic injury that result in overall systemic cardiovascular compromise with secondary wounds. In the acute setting, patient stabilization always takes precedence over wound management (Chart 5.1).

Acute Critical Wound Patients

Patients requiring more emergent attention after initial triage assessment should have a detailed targeted physical examination with initial stabilization performed concurrently. Any life-threatening issues should be addressed as they are identified. Flow-by oxygen administration should be provided for any patient presenting with moderate to severe trauma regardless if respiratory compromise is evident (Figure 5.1a–c). Initial full physical examination should further elucidate any cardiorespiratory abnormalities that may rapidly result in cardiopulmonary arrest (e.g., severe hemorrhage, pneumothorax) and be treated promptly. Concurrent intravenous catheter access should be obtained. At time of catheter placement, if hemodynamic status permits, blood for point-of-care analyzers and quick assessment tests should be obtained to guide clinical therapy. Analgesics such as a full-μ agonist opioid and resuscitative fluid boluses (typically 10–20 mL/kg of an isotonic crystalloids over 15–30 minutes) are administered as indicated. Fluid boluses can be repeated pending patient response or have the type of fluid switched pending individual patient needs in order to improve cardiorespiratory and blood pressure parameters. With the increasing availability of point-of-care bedside ultrasound, significant information can be gained on the presence of pneumothorax, cavitary effusion, and/or significant hemorrhage (Figure 5.2). The goals of initial stabilization should focus on improving cardiorespiratory function to restore hemodynamic function, ultimately promoting adequate delivery of oxygen to tissues and preventing cardiopulmonary arrest. Animals sustaining head trauma with depressed mentation should have full neurological examinations and characterized via routinely used scoring systems (e.g., modified Glasgow coma scale). Identification of a Cushing's reflex (a baroreceptor reflex secondary to increased intracranial pressures resulting in systemic hypertension and subsequent bradycardia) can signify traumatic brain injury with concurrent increased intracranial pressure that requires prompt treatment. In-depth discussion about cardiovascular and neurological stabilization of the critical patient is beyond the scope of this chapter but should be the focus of initial care prior to full wound evaluation.

Open wounds on animals presenting in critical states should be flushed briefly by an available irrigant (e.g., sterile saline or tap water) and subsequently covered with sterile lubricant followed by sterile gauze and/or a small bandage during resuscitation to prevent contamination of the wound with nosocomial infections. In some instances, the wounds themselves may be the primary source of patient instability. Hemorrhage from open wounds is often able to be controlled with direct pressure

Techniques in Small Animal Wound Management, First Edition. Edited by Nicole J. Buote.
© 2024 John Wiley & Sons, Inc. Published 2024 by John Wiley & Sons, Inc.
Companion website: www.wiley.com/go/buote/wounds

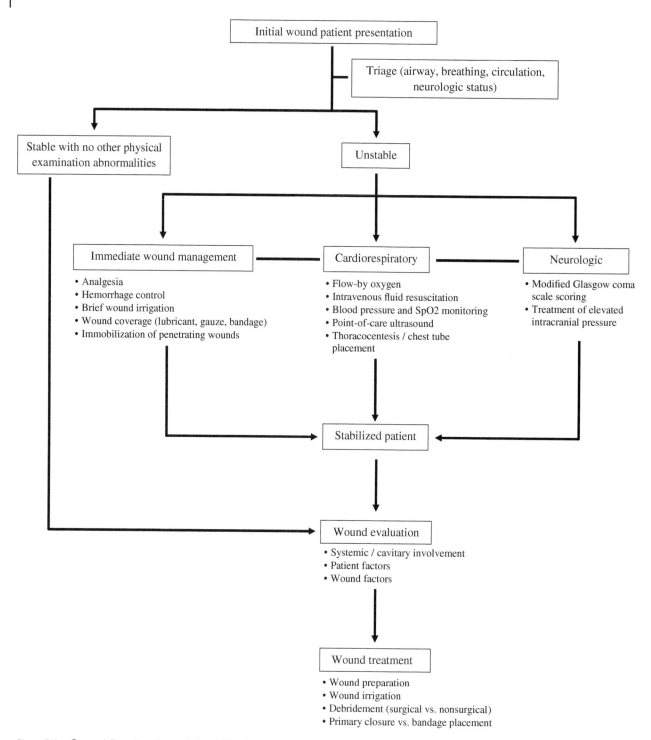

Chart 5.1   General flowchart for initial stabilization of the wound patient.

using sterile gauze, though if hemorrhage is severe and persistent, ligation or cauterization of the bleeding vessel may be required. Other potential therapies for control of hemorrhage include the application of calcium alginate dressings, epinephrine/phenylephrine-soaked gauze, or hemostasis-promoting products (Gelfoam, Surgicel). Visible penetrating foreign bodies should be left in place during stabilization and should be immobilized with the patient as best as possible to prevent movement from causing additional trauma to underlying tissues or organs (Figure 5.3). Penetrating foreign bodies can be trimmed shorter, if possible, with a small portion remaining out of the patient. Broad-spectrum antimicrobial coverage should be

Figure 5.1 Photographs of patients being provided supplemental oxygen. (a) Patient with flow-by oxygen mask. (b and c) Patient with nasal prong oxygen supplementation. *Source:* Courtesy of Nicole Buote, DVM, DACVS.

(a)

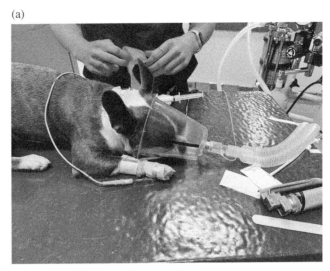

(b)   (c)

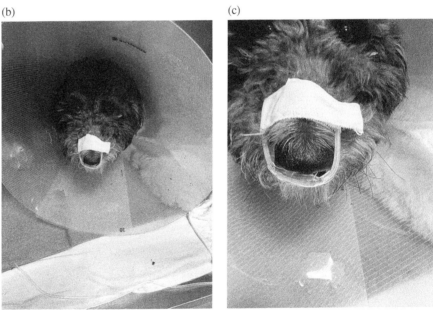

instituted promptly, especially if intracavitary communication of the penetrating foreign body is identified (see Chapter 17 for more specific recommendations). Any wounds on the chest should be promptly evaluated to identify potential intrathoracic involvement that may lead to the development of a pneumothorax or tension pneumothorax. Presence of air-sucking or whistling sounds may indicate communication with the thoracic cavity, and the wound should be covered with a non-porous wrap such as plastic wrap to prevent further air accumulation and development of a tension pneumothorax. Lung auscultation, use of point-of-care ultrasound, patient respiratory status, and pulse oximetry may assist in the diagnosis and assessment of stability. Diagnostic and therapeutic thoracocenteses and/or chest tube placement should be performed as indicated pending patient response to stabilization and recurrence of pneumothorax (Figure 5.4a–c, Videos 5.1 ☺, 5.2 ☺, and 5.3 ☺). Caution should also be exercised during clipping of thoracic wounds to prevent inadvertent entrance into the thoracic cavity, resulting in rapid clinical decline. Thus, it may be more prudent to fully evaluate thoracic wounds when a surgical team is ready and prepared for potential thoracic cavity exploration (Figure 5.5). Following patient stabilization, further characterization of wounds can be performed through both additional diagnostic imaging and wound exploration as indicated. Intracavitary penetration of wounds (traumatic penetrating foreign bodies, severe or extensive bite wounds) may warrant emergent surgical exploration following appropriate resuscitation. Appropriate characterization of the severity of wounds and severity of patient illness are paramount in the acute wound patient.

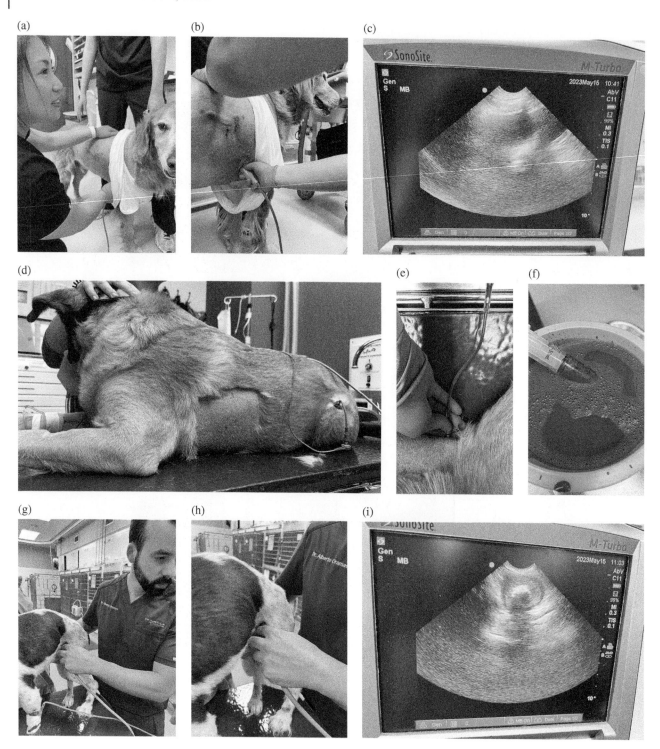

Figure 5.2   Photographs of point-of-care ultrasounds. (a,b) Photographs of a TFAST being performed for a patient with thoracic effusion. (c) Photograph of a TFAST image showing fluid around the lungs. *Source:* Courtesy of Nicole Buote, DVM, DACVS. (d–f) Photographs of a patient presenting with hemothorax. *Source:* Courtesy of Jessica Sands, DVM. (d) Lateral thorax clipped and prepped for thoracocentesis. (e) 1.5 in long 18g needle attached to an extension line removing hemorrhagic effusion. (f) Bowl of non-clotting hemorrhagic effusion. (g–i) Photographs of an AFAST being performed to check for intestinal motility and presence of peritoneal effusion in a postoperative patient. (i) Photograph of an AFAST image showing mild peritoneal effusion surrounding an intestinal loop. *Source:* Courtesy of Nicole Buote, DVM, DACVS.

(a)

(b)

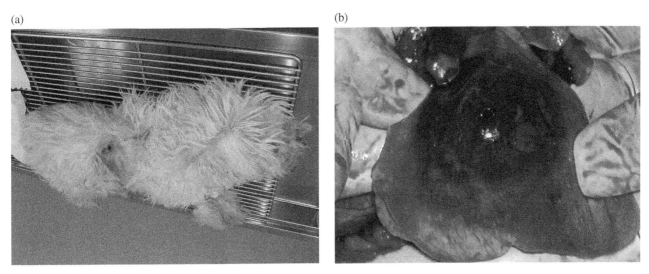

Figure 5.3   Photographs of a patient with a gunshot wound. (a) Photograph of patient on presentation. After clipping, a small entrance wound into the dorsal thoracic cavity can be seen. (b) Photograph of right cranial lung with bullet wound. *Source:* Courtesy of Gretchen Schoeffler, DVM, DACVECC.

(a)

(b)

(c)

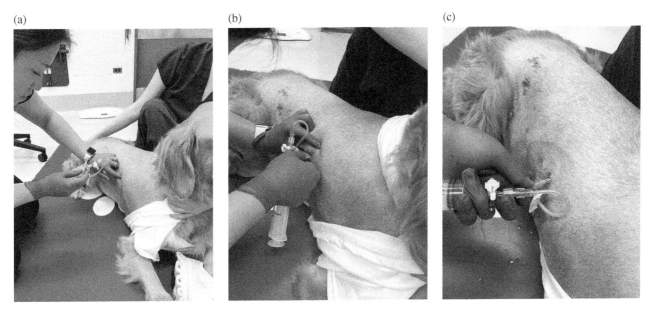

Figure 5.4   (a–c) Photographs of a thoracocentesis. Note the set-up including a syringe, three-way stopcock, large gauge (18–20 g) over the needle catheter or needle, and extension set. The site for thoracocentesis should always be sterilely prepped to avoid contamination into the chest cavity. *Source:* Courtesy of Nicole Buote, DVM, DACVS.

Stable and/or Chronic Wound Patients

Patients with chronic wounds typically present in a more stable clinical condition than those sustaining acute wounds. True cardiorespiratory stabilization and resuscitation of these patients is unlikely to be required unless the chronic wounds have resulted in systemic illness and/or sepsis. Initial examination should fully characterize the duration and severity of the wound, underlying comorbidities of the patient, and any other predisposing factors to wound healing impairment (see Chapter 4). Chronic wounds will have an underlying cause that has resulted in prolongation or cessation of the normal wound healing steps.

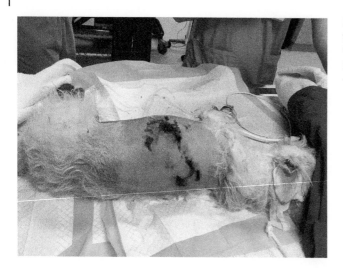

Figure 5.5 Photograph of a patient sustained severe trauma to the chest cavity from bite wounds. The full extent of these wounds was not visible until the patient was clipped. This patient was anesthetized for clipping and wound evaluation. *Source:* Courtesy of Nicole Buote, DVM, DACVS.

Overall, successful wound management throughout the healing process relies on a thorough understanding of the pathophysiology of the stages of wound healing, which is discussed in more detail in Chapter 2. Wounds typically heal in an orderly fashion through several stages of healing, namely the inflammatory phase, proliferation/repair phase, and maturation/remodeling phase [1]. Normal progression through these phases is dependent upon a variety of factors and any abnormalities resulting in prolongation of any of these stages will lead to delayed healing or possibly non-healing wounds [1]. Thus, identification of any systemic patient or local wound factor that may influence any part of the healing process is of utmost importance to maximize chances of successful wound healing.

Evaluation of Patient Factors

Systemic patient factors that may affect wound healing include preexisting comorbidities (such as endocrinopathies and cancer), nutritional intake, signalment of the animal, severity of systemic disease, medications, and certain therapeutics (Table 5.1). A functional immune system is required for normal progression of the stages of wound [1]. Thus, disease processes resulting in impaired immune function will result in delayed wound healing. Primary disease processes studied in veterinary and human patients that result in immunosuppression have been shown to delay wound healing by increasing risk of infection and prolonging the inflammatory phase [1–10]. Dogs and cats with endocrinopathies have been shown to be 8.2 times more likely to develop a postoperative wound infection in clean-contaminated wounds [2]. Humans with diabetes mellitus have been shown to have higher risks of postoperative wound infection as a result of altered bactericidal activity and opsonic activity as well as delayed healing as a result of hyperglycemia [3]. In humans, hyperglycemia has been shown to affect normal collagen production, decrease fibroblast proliferation, decrease differentiation and migration ability of keratinocytes, increase matrix metalloproteinases, and impair angiogenesis and vasculogenesis resulting in a hypoxic wound environment [4]. While these effects have not been demonstrated in veterinary patients, glycemic control during wound healing should remain a priority. Hyperadrenocorticism results in immunomodulatory changes due to excess serum glucocorticoid concentrations, decreasing the functionality of natural killer (NK) cells and decreasing T-lymphocyte production [5]. Additionally, increased serum glucocorticoid levels can reduce macrophage activity, fibroblast proliferation, and collagen synthesis as well as inhibit synthesis of matrix metalloproteinases, all of which are required for normal wound healing [1, 6, 7]. These negative effects of excessive glucocorticoid levels on wound healing have also been demonstrated to be mostly dose and time-dependent [7, 8]. Systemic uremia associated with chronic kidney disease or acute kidney injuries is also associated with inhibition of capillary and fibroblast proliferation as well as delayed granulation tissue formation and low rates of vascularization of wounds [9]. These findings may also be in part due to the chronic inflammatory state of chronic kidney disease patients [9].

Patients suffering from cancer can have systemic immunologic changes from neoplasia itself, or due to associated treatments such as chemotherapy or radiation therapy. Chemotherapeutics can have cytotoxic effects or inhibit normal cellular proliferation via antiproliferative or antimetabolic mechanisms [10]. Radiation therapy can also result in delayed wound healing primarily as a result of fibrotic microangiopathy, resulting in decreased oxygen supply to wounds, and may in itself

Table 5.1   Patient factors resulting in decreased wound healing.

Disease process	Pathophysiology
Endocrinopathies Diabetes mellitus	8.2× more likely to develop a postoperative wound infection in clean-contaminated wounds (Nicholson)
	Altered bactericidal activity and opsonic activity (Rayfield)
	Hyperglycemia decreases collagen production, fibroblast proliferation, differentiation, and migration ability of keratinocytes; increases matrix metalloproteinases; impairs angiogenesis and vasculogenesis leading to hypoxic wound environments (Baltzis)
Hyperadrenocorticism	Excess serum glucocorticoids decrease functionality of natural killer cells, T-lymphocyte production, macrophage activity, fibroblast proliferation, and collagen synthesis (Tobias, Nuutinen, Richardson)
Systemic disease Chronic kidney disease	Uremia is associated with inhibition of capillary and fibroblast proliferation, as well as delayed granulation tissue formation and decreased wound vascularization (Maroz)
Neoplasia	Immunologic alterations secondary to neoplastic cells
	Chemotherapeutics contribute to antiproliferative or antimetabolic mechanisms in normal cells (Franz)
	Radiation therapy results in fibrotic microangiopathy, leading to hypoxic wound environments (Franz)
Signalment Age	Dermal thickness, dermo-epidermal junction thickness, number of active hair follicles, and organization of microcirculation are decreased with increasing age (Gosain)
	Ultimate healing strength may be equivocal, though duration of healing is typically longer
Neuter status	Intact male dogs may be at higher risk of postoperative wound infections due to decrease in anti-inflammatory mediators (IL-2, IL-3, interferon-γ) due to androgenic hormones causing immunosuppression (Wichmann)
Size/breed	Larger dogs may have diminished derived fibroblast proliferative capacity (Li Y)
	Certain dogs are predisposed to having a thinner dermis (e.g., Greyhounds) which may result in decreased wound healing (Swaim)
Species	Cats have less collateral subcutaneous blood vessels compared to dogs, which results in slower second intention healing and worsened wound healing with subcutaneous tissue disruption (Bohling2, Balsa)
Medications Non-steroidal anti-inflammatories	Prolonged usage has been associated with prolonged bone healing as measured by radiographic findings (Gallaher, Al-Waeli)
Therapy Surgery and anesthesia	Longer duration of surgery and use of anesthetic gases results in immunosuppression of lymphocytes and decreased recruitment and function of neutrophils and natural killer cells (Frochlich, Dietz, Nicholson, Brand)
	Each additional hour of anesthesia results in a 30% greater risk of postoperative wound infections in clean procedures (Beal)

induce wounds secondary to radiation exposure [10]. Malnutrition has also been demonstrated to result in decreased wound healing. Decreased carbohydrates, fat, and protein intake in periods of increased energy requirements as a result of wounds can result in impaired leukocyte and fibroblast function, decreased collagen production, and prolonged inflammatory states [11]. In cancer patients, cancer cachexia as a result of elevated neoplasm cytokine levels results in hypoalbuminemia, reducing healing as well.

Patient signalment, including age, sex, breed, and species may also affect wound healing. Intact male dogs have been shown to be more predisposed to postoperative wound infections, suspected to be secondary to a decrease in anti-inflammatory mediators such as IL-2, IL-3, and interferon-γ as a result of androgenic hormones resulting in immunosuppression [12]. Older age has been historically associated with delayed wound healing, but whether or not this is secondary to the presence of secondary comorbidities rather than a true age-related specific pathology with wound healing is unknown. With increasing age, decreases in dermal thickness, dermo-epidermal junction thickness, number of active hair follicles, organization of microcirculation, and loss of dermally derived fibroblast proliferative capacity have been identified [13]. The healing process is typically longer in duration, although healing is obtained to a similar capacity. On a similar note, larger dogs may also have diminished dermally derived fibroblast proliferative capacity, and some breeds may be predisposed to having a thinner dermis (e.g., Greyhounds) [1, 14, 15]. Subcutaneous tissue disruption may result in delayed second intention healing, more so in cats compared to dogs as dogs may have larger numbers of collateral subcutaneous blood vessels compared to cats [16, 17]. Additionally, initial cutaneous perfusion in surgically created wounds was noted to be lower in cats than in dogs [18]. Lastly, cats undergoing primary wound repair have sutured wounds that are only half the strength of those compared to dogs at day 7, and second intention healing in cats noticeably produced less granulation tissue throughout stages of healing with a peripheral distribution rather than a central, potentially resulting in longer healing times for cats [18].

Severity of systemic illness also disrupts the balance between pro-inflammatory and anti-inflammatory mediators, leading to prolonged infection, decreased nutritional intake due to malaise, and overall negative outcomes. Medications used for treatments during periods of illness may also play a role in modulating the immune response, leading to prolonged healing times. Non-steroidal anti-inflammatory administration may have adverse effects on bone healing in regards to biomechanical properties, likely related to impairment of the inflammatory phase [19]. Dogs undergoing tibial fracture repairs that received carprofen for a full eight-week course were reported to have less radiographic healing compared to dogs receiving two weeks or no carprofen, though some studies demonstrate no changes to the bone based on micro-CT and histopathological analyses [20, 21]. Exogenous glucocorticoid administration will delay healing by the same mechanisms as discussed for hyperadrenocorticism. Other therapeutics such as chemotherapy and radiation therapy may result in prolonged healing times as aforementioned. Other considerations for contributions of therapeutics to delayed wound healing mostly regard surgical procedures and anesthesia in the context of postoperative wound infection rates. Prolonged surgical and anesthesia times have been demonstrated in multiple studies to increase the risk of postoperative wound infections as a result of multiple factors. Immunosuppression of lymphocytes has been associated with duration of surgery, and anesthetic gases can decrease the recruitment and function of both neutrophils and NK cells, increasing the risk of postoperative wound infections [2, 22–24]. In clean surgical procedures in dogs and cats, a 30% greater risk of postoperative wound infection is associated with each additional hour of anesthesia [25].

Evaluation of Wound Factors

Local wound factors include wound perfusion, tissue viability, presence of wound fluid, infection, and mechanical factors including movement and tension [1, 10]. Poor wound perfusion decreases oxygen delivery needed for adequate neutrophil function and progression of wound healing. Certain injuries, such as crush and shearing injuries, can cause severe perfusion compromise. Systemic factors as discussed previously can also decrease wound perfusion due to systemic hypotension and critical illness. The most important factor dictating oxygen diffusion in a wound bed is the partial pressure of oxygen (PO_2) in the wound bed rather than the amount of oxygen bound to hemoglobin entering the wound bed [1]. Thus, if cardiac output is maintained, wound bed hypoxia will not occur despite significant anemia (even down to a hematocrit of 15–18%) [26]. Perfusion should also be considered in the context of general anesthesia as anesthetic drugs can cause profound vasodilation and hypotension. Perfusion should be maintained while under general anesthesia via intravenous fluid administration. Postoperative complications such as hypothermia or pain resulting in vasoconstriction should be corrected as soon as possible to maximize perfusion.

The majority of acute open wounds will have a degree of contamination, defined as the presence of nonreplicating organisms within a wound. This should be differentiated from true wound infection, which is classified as the presence of microorganisms $\geq 10^5$ per gram of tissue [1]. This differentiation is difficult to establish in reality and is largely based on timing, with six hours since wounding being considered the "golden period" as the time it takes bacteria to replicate to levels that increase the chance of infection. Wounds considered infected have been shown to result in visible incisional complications (dehiscence, necrosis, purulent discharge) in 50–100% of cases if primarily closed [27]. While low levels of bacteria can benefit wound healing by promoting initial inflammation, failure to adequately regulate the degree of contamination will result in the transition from simple bacterial colonization to critical colonization, a point at which bacterial replication has begun to affect the healing process in the absence of a host response [28, 29]. Critical colonization is considered the stage immediately prior to wound infection, which signifies progressive bacterial replication that has also resulted in host systemic inflammatory responses. This prolongs the inflammatory phase of healing through a variety of mechanisms, including reducing adequate clearance of bacteria through consumption of complement proteins and decreased chemotaxis. Tissue damage is propagated through the production of cytotoxic enzymes and free oxygen radicals. The proliferative phase is also altered, with decreased fibroblast proliferation, aberrant and disorganized collagen production, increased collagen breakdown, and ultimately decreased wound strength [30]. Similarly, presence of necrotic or non-viable tissue and debris within the wound bed prolongs the inflammatory phase. Debridement can aid in decreasing bacterial contamination and improving tissue viability to aid in progression to the proliferative phase.

Accumulations of serum or blood within a wound can delay healing by increasing distances that normal signaling and inflammatory molecules need to travel, serve as a media for bacterial proliferation, and in rare circumstances cause local pressure necrosis if accumulation is significant [1]. Adherence to Halsted's principles of meticulous hemostasis and obliteration of dead space should help minimize hematoma and seroma formation after surgical procedures Additionally, excessive tension, motion, or pressure at the wound site should be considered when selecting the type of surgical wound closure technique. These factors can lead to dehiscence of the sutures and ischemia and necrosis of the skin surrounding the wound and are often involved in the delayed healing of chronic wounds (Figure 5.6a–d). Motion or excessive pressure at the wound site may warrant use of additional external coaptation, negative pressure wound therapy, or advanced tension-relieving suture techniques (e.g., releasing incisions, pre-placed mattress sutures, etc.) (Figure 5.7a,b), particularly in the initial postoperative setting. Presence of excessive granulation tissue should be noted and addressed by debridement or resection to prevent obstruction of epithelization.

Initial Treatment

As previously described, immediate wound care should focus on adequate analgesia, decreasing current contamination, and preventing further contamination. In unstable patients, this may simply require brief flushing with a readily available irrigant, coverage with sterile lubricant or antibiotic ointment, and covering the wound with a bandage while stabilization is performed. Once the patient has been stabilized and analgesia provided, further wound therapy and exploration can commence.

Wound Preparation

Wound preparation and irrigation of the wound are often the first steps in wound exploration. Once definitive wound therapy is considered, the bandage or cover should be removed. The surrounding wound area should be clipped and prepped in an aseptic manner. The wound itself should be protected during this time by filling the wound with sterile water-soluble lubricant or moistened sterile gauzes or laparotomy sponges. These techniques create a barrier between the wound and fur/hair and debris that is removed during the clipping and cleaning process. Scrub preparations should not contain detergents as these can be cytotoxic to open wounds. Antiseptics should be diluted prior to usage [1, 31, 32]. Dilute (0.05–0.1%) chlorhexidine or dilute (0.1–0.01%) povidone–iodine is recommended [1, 17, 32]. A thorough discussion of cleansing solutions is found in Chapter 6.

Wound Irrigation

After aseptic preparation, irrigation of the wound can be performed to remove gross contamination from the wound bed. The type of fluid used for lavage is less important than the amount of fluid utilized. In fact, multiple studies have demonstrated that irrigation of wounds with tap water versus sterile saline does not have significant impacts on wound infection [33, 34]. Ideal irrigation pressures have not been defined, though a balance between contamination removal and local tissue damage, contaminant dissemination, and edema caused by irrigation should be considered. The exact pressure at which injury to tissues occurs also has not been defined; however, some studies suggest a pressure greater than 70 psi can result in tissue trauma [35]. Typical recommendations for irrigation pressures depends on the degree of contamination; high-pressure irrigation (>5–8 psi) can be considered for highly contaminated wounds, while low-pressure irrigation (≤5 psi) is considered for minimally contaminated wounds [1]. A consistent pressure of 7–8 psi can be generated by attaching a 16–22-gauge needle to a fluid administration set and 1 l fluid bag, and pressurizing the fluid bag to 300 mmHg [36]. No irrigation technique has been demonstrated to be superior to any other in a variety of studies [35, 37]. The amount of irrigation historically utilized is approximately 50 ml per centimeter of wound length in human studies, though no current veterinary studies have evaluated a standard volume of irrigation to utilize [38]. Several different wound flushing setups include utilizing an 18-gauge needle to perforate the cap of a sterile saline bottle, open-line saline bag flushing, and pressure-bag saline flushing (Chapter 6).

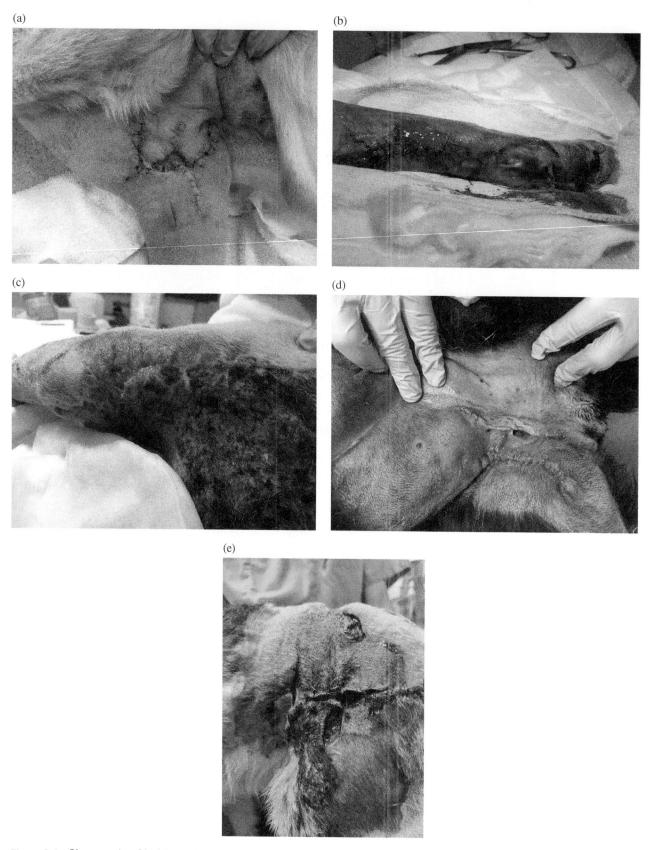

Figure 5.6 Photographs of incisional dehiscence. (a) Photograph of a patient with an incisional dehiscence after a tumor was removed on the medial aspect of the thoracic limb. There is evidence that this incision has been addressed previously as there are sutures and skin staples present. This is a difficult area to close due to tension and constant movement. This incision also has evidence of necrotic (gray tissue) but the underlying tissue in the open wound appears to have granulation tissue present. (b) Photograph of a dehiscence on the medial surface of a cat's thoracic limb paw. There is moderate exudate present and dehiscence of the incision distally with tissue necrosis. (c) Photograph of a caudal thigh incision with dehiscence in the middle section. The tissue appears healthy and this was most likely due to tension in this high motion area. (d) Photograph of a previous inguinal incision with tissue necrosis and dehiscence. The necrotic tissue appears gray and thin. This site is notoriously difficult to close due to tension and the potential (dead) space that occurs with dissection. (e) Photograph of significant dehiscence and progression of necrosis after closure of bite wounds. *Source:* Courtesy of Nicole Buote, DVM, DACVS.

Figure 5.7 (a) Photograph of a
patient with a modified Robert-Jones
bandage to cover a wound.
(b) Photograph of releasing incisions
to aid in primary closure of a wound.
Source: Courtesy of Nicole Buote,
DVM, DACVS.

(a)

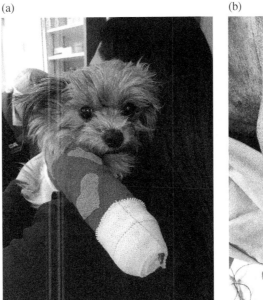

(b)

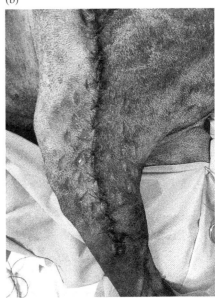

Complications associated with wound irrigation are minimal. However, puncture wounds should not be flushed directly until the remainder of the wound is opened to prevent flushing of debris deeper into the wound. Additionally, severely hemorrhagic wounds should be flushed carefully to prevent disruption or dislodgement of major clots.

Decision-Making for Primary Closure

Following wound preparation, the wound should be thoroughly evaluated to determine the appropriate course of action and ultimate goal of wound therapy. Primary closure or secondary closure at this time should be determined. This decision is heavily influenced by considering patient and local wound factors as previously mentioned. In the majority of acute wound settings, primary closure is typically not performed as the wound is often grossly contaminated and may require additional time to progress and declare itself. Closing a wound too early may result in dehiscence of the wound and further patient morbidity. Surgically created, clean, or clean-contaminated wounds with minimal contamination are good candidates for primary closure, particularly if sustained within the purported "golden period" [1, 17]. In most cases, primary closure is not chosen, and delayed primary closure, secondary closure, or second intention is considered. These are discussed more in-depth in Chapter 4.

Debridement

Surgical Debridement

Regardless of the ultimate wound closure method chosen, initial wound management should consist of wound debridement, which can be classified into two categories: surgical or nonsurgical [1]. The goal of initial wound debridement is to remove foreign contamination as well as non-viable or necrotic tissue [1, 17]. Removal of these tissues will speed up the inflammatory process and decrease the potential for infection (Table 5.2). Wound exploration, particularly for puncture wounds, should be performed to assess the degree and severity of underlying tissue trauma (Figure 5.8). It is important not to force hemostats or cotton-tipped applicators deeper than the edges of the wound. While drain placement is important if gravity-dependent pocketing is present, a good rule of thumb is to avoid making a wound worse or more extensive just to place a drain. Surgical debridement utilizes surgical excisional debridement and can consist of either complete en bloc debridement or layered debridement. En bloc debridement (Figure 5.9) involves removal of the entire wound edge (full thickness tissue removal), converting it to a controlled surgical wound [1, 17]. This can be considered for small wounds or in regions where enough surrounding tissue is available for closure. En bloc debridement is also performed when clearly

Table 5.2   Wound debridement instrumentation and techniques.

Puncture wound exploration

Technique	Instrumentation required
• Gently grasp the edges of puncture with forceps and place hemostats/CTAs within wound. • Sweep the hemostats in a 360° fashion paying particular attention to any ventral or gravity-dependent pocketing. • Be careful NOT to force the hemostats or CTAs into tissue thereby creating a deeper wound. • If a sufficiently large gravity-dependent wound is present consider placement of a drain or umbilical tape to allow for continued drainage (see Figure 5.8)	Mosquito hemostats Cotton-tipped applicators (CTAs) Adson/Brown-Adson forceps ±Penrose drain ±Umbilical tape

En-bloc wound debridement

Technique	Instrumentation required
• In cases where en-bloc debridement is to be followed by immediate closure of the wound, aseptic technique of the surrounding region must be followed. This includes draping of the area with sterile four-quarter drapes and meticulous preparation of the tissue. • Following skin preparation and draping, the necrotic or unhealthy tissue will be sharply excised 2-3 mm from the declared edge with a #10 blade so that healthy bleeding tissue is visualized (see Figure 5.9) • If the wound is deemed ready to be closed, appropriate suture is used to close the wound in multiple layers • If the wound requires delay (granulation tissue growth for skin graft placement), an appropriate dressing and bandage (tie-over, modified Robert Jones) is applied	Sterile drapes Penetrating towel clamps Adson/Brown-Adson forceps Blade handle #10 blades Sterile gauze (3×3 or 4×4) Suture for closure OR Wound dressing and bandage

Layered wound debridement

Technique	Instrumentation required
• Gently grasp the edges of the wound and with a #10 or #15 blade scrape the edges or top layer of tissue (see Figure 5.10) • STOP debriding when bleeding or healthier tissue is observed • Leave questionable tissue in situ to re-evaluate at next bandage change/wound assessment • Place appropriate dressing over wound depending on phase of healing and patient factors	Adson/Brown-Adson forceps Blade handle #10, #15 blades Sterile gauze (3×3 or 4×4) Wound dressing

necrotic tissue is present, regardless of the size of the wound, as leaving it in situ will only delay healing. In more extensive wounds, debridement of visibly necrotic or non-viable tissue is usually performed through repeated layered or serial debridements over several days (Figure 5.10). Removal of necrotic tissue layer by layer allows identification of healthy underlying tissue which facilitates early healing. The ultimate goal of wound management is to have a well-vascularized clean wound bed to help facilitate wound healing prior to definitive closure, typically by a two- to three-layered technique. Deeper fascial and subcutaneous layers are sutured together with absorbable suture to allow tension relief of more superficial layers. Sequentially superficial layers are sutured together, with the skin finally being apposed with absorbable or non-absorbable suture under minimal tension.

Serial surgical debridement in contaminated wounds from crushing and shearing injuries will allow tissues to declare themselves. Care should be taken to avoid excessive removal of tissue that may be healthy; excessive debridement, particularly of subcutaneous tissues, has been demonstrated to slow wound healing in dogs and cats by decreasing wound perfusion, rate of granulation tissue formation, and potential wound infection [16, 18]. If serial debridement is to be performed prior to definitive closure, open wound management with bandages and dressings are instituted in between debridements (see Chapters 8, 10, and 12).

Nonsurgical Debridement

Nonsurgical debridement consists of a variety of mechanisms, including mechanical debridement, enzymatic debridement, and autolytic debridement. Mechanical debridement utilizes adherent bandages, typically gauze, either in a wet-to-dry or dry-to-dry manner, that stick to the wound bed. Removal of the bandage subsequently results in removal of associated

Figure 5.8 Photographs of wound explore. The hemostat is being used to probe the inner aspects of this bite wound to determine the full extent of damage to the deeper layers. *Source:* Courtesy of Nathan Peterson, DVM, MS, DACVECC.

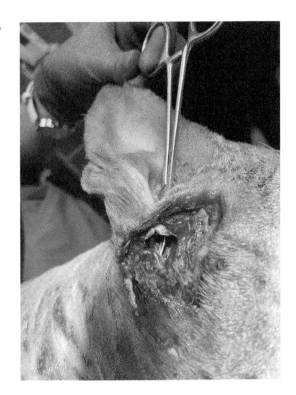

(a)

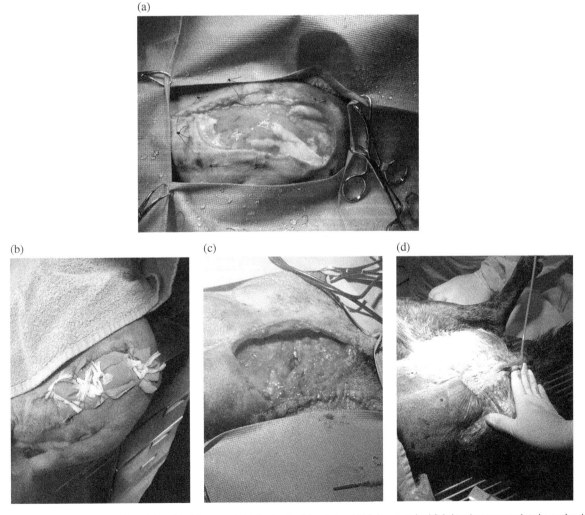

(b)　　　　　　　　　　(c)　　　　　　　　　　(d)

Figure 5.9 Examples of en-bloc debridement. (a,b) Patient with a lateral thigh wound which has been completely excised. A tie-over bandage was placed after excision due to tension. (c,d) An inguinal wound was sharply debrided and a negative pressure (vacuum) bandage applied. *Source:* Courtesy of Nicole Buote, DVM, DACVS.

(a)

(b)

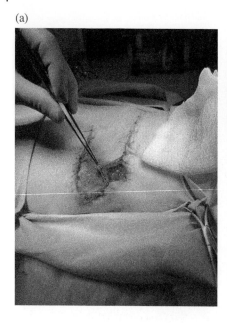
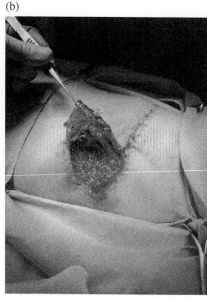

Figure 5.10 Photograph of a patient with distal necrosis of an axial pattern flap. (a) The necrotic tissue was gently grasped at the edge of the incision and lifted to determine what layer of tissue required debridement. (b) The skin and some of the subcutaneous tissue easily lifted off from the deeper layers. The visibly unhealthy tissue was removed but serial evaluations were performed and more tissue at the edges and deep were removed at subsequent visits. *Source:* Courtesy of Nicole Buote, DVM, DACVS.

debris and often the superficial layer of the wound bed. These methods have largely fallen out of favor due to their highly nonselective means of debridement and patient discomfort [1, 39, 40].

Topical agents applied as dressings for nonsurgical debridement are discussed in depth in Chapters 7 and 8. Briefly, enzymatic debridement utilizes topical agents that typically contain enzymes such as collagenases, trypsin, papain, or urea which selectively break down non-viable tissues [1, 17]. Hyperosmotic agents such as hypertonic saline (20%), sugar, and honey-soaked dressings facilitate more autolytic debridement, utilizing the patient's own natural debridement mechanisms and also largely spare healthy tissue. Certain debridement agents, such as honey and silver-based products, are also bactericidal or have an inhibitory effect on bacterial growth. Additionally, given their hyperosmolarity, exudate and edema may also be reduced. Care during application of these must be exercised to not cause desiccation of surrounding tissue. Numerous enzymatic and autolytic debridement products currently exist and the choice to utilize one particular product over another largely depends on the etiology and stage of the wound, available product choices, and clinician familiarity with products available. Furthermore, comparisons between debridement products and dressings largely remain challenging given a variation in the duration of wounds (acute versus chronic) and etiology of wounds (bite wounds versus lacerations versus burns, etc.). Negative pressure wound therapy has also been increasingly commonly used in the acute wound setting and is discussed in detail in Chapter 10 [1, 41–43].

In most cases, acute infected open wounds will require a combination of serial surgical debridement and topical wound bed management strategies. This allows for serial assessment as the wound continues to declare itself over time, maximizing the health of the underlying wound bed prior to definitive closure (Figure 5.11).

Drain and Bandage Placement

Regardless of the type of initial wound therapy chosen, drains and bandages can be incorporated into ongoing wound management. Primary closure of acute wounds with an active or passive drain can help improve chances of closure success by decreasing dead space and the incidence of seroma/hematoma formation, as well as provide drainage for fluid. Specific details regarding the advantages and disadvantages of different drains are discussed in Chapter 9. Drains are typically left in place until the fluid production has decreased or plateaued, often within three to five days [1].

Bandages typically consist of three layers: a primary or contact layer, a secondary or intermediate layer, and a tertiary or outer layer. The most commonly utilized bandages in context of wounds are modified Robert-Jones bandages and tie-over bandages (Figure 5.12). The location and extensiveness of the wound largely dictate the type of bandage being utilized. Modified Robert-Jones bandages are typically used when wounds are present on the middle to distal limbs, whereas tie-over bandages can be utilized in all regions of the body. Detailed discussions regarding these bandages are found in Chapter 12.

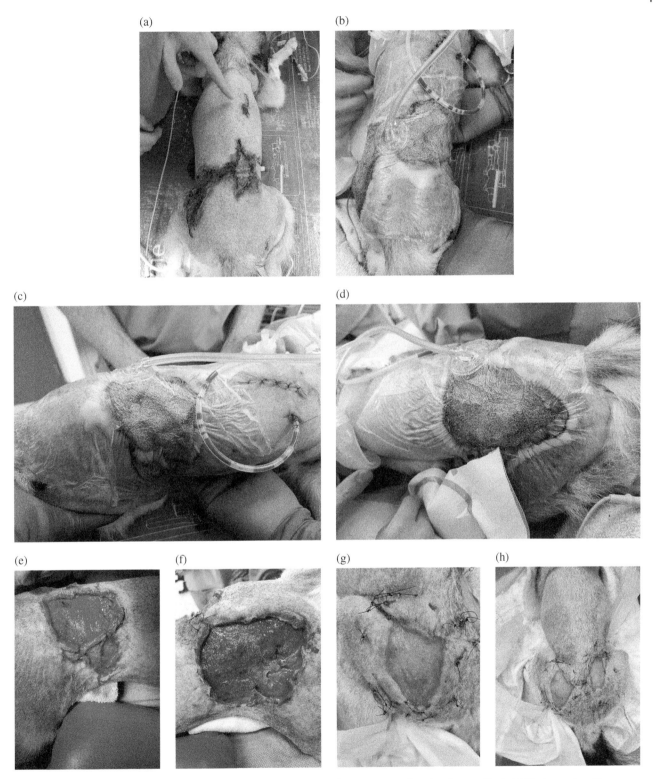

Figure 5.11   Photographs of serial wound debridement and bandaging over seven days in a burn patient. (a) Photographs of burn wounds at initial evaluation. (b–d) Initially these wounds were managed with a negative pressure (vacuum) bandage. (e,f) Right and left lateral wounds after three days with the vacuum bandage in place. Patient was then placed in tie-over bandages with a hydrocolloid dressing. (g,h) Photographs after three days in a tie-over bandage with a hydrocolloid dressing. *Source:* Courtesy of Colin Chik, DVM.

Bandages are commonly utilized in the initial wound management setting. Understanding safe and predictable bandage strategies is important in any practice dealing with wounds. The contact layer is in direct contact with the wound and typically contains the dressing utilized for nonsurgical debridement in the acute wound setting. The type of dressing placed in the contact layer changes over time and is largely selected based on the amount and type of exudate the wound is producing [1, 17]. In the acute setting, wounds are expected to be largely contaminated with purulent exudate; thus typical initial antimicrobial agents most utilized in clinical practice are silver-based products and honey. A variety of mechanisms have been proposed for honey's antimicrobial effects, including the production of hydrogen peroxide with subsequent cytotoxic free radicals. Honey also contains other phytochemicals which may have some degree of antimicrobial effects. Silver has also been utilized for its bactericidal properties in its ionized form and has been applied both as a topical ointment in silver sulfadiazine or incorporated into silver-impregnated dressings [44–46]. Controversies exist on silver's role in the acute wound phase, with some studies suggesting no overt benefit while others describe improvement in outcomes [43]. In the acute infected wound setting, either option is likely to be rewarding, however in burn wounds, several systematic reviews comparing honey with silver sulfadiazine demonstrated a benefit of honey over silver in healing time for burn wounds [47, 48]. If mechanical debridement is necessary, laparotomy sponges or gauze can be placed on top of the dressings to facilitate a modified wet-to-dry bandage (Figure 5.13). The intermediate layer, which is typically cast padding or cotton, keeps the contact layer in place, absorbs additional exudate, and provides pressure on the wound. The outer layer provides protection for the other bandage layers in the form of cohesive elastic wraps (Vetwrap) or waterproof surgical drapes [1, 17].

(a)

(b)

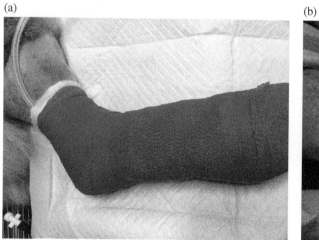
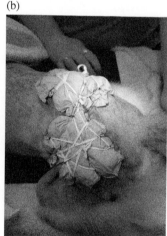

Figure 5.12 Photographs of common bandaging techniques. (a) Photograph of a modified Robert Jones on pelvic limb for a wound. *Source:* Photograph courtesy of Nicole Buote, DVM, DACVS. (b) Photograph of a tie-over bandage from patient in Figure 5.11. *Source:* Courtesy of Colin Chik, DVM.

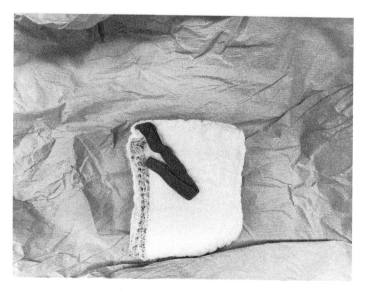

Figure 5.13 Photograph of lap sponge and blue drape commonly used to cover the primary and secondary layer of a tie-over bandage. *Source:* Courtesy of Nicole Buote, DVM, DACVS.

References

1 Tobias, K.M. and Johnston, S.A. (2018). *Veterinary Surgery*. St. Louis, MI: Elsevier Inc.

2 Nicholson, M., Beal, M., Shofer, F. et al. (2002). Epidemiologic evaluation of postoperative wound infection in clean-contaminated wounds: a retrospective study of 239 dogs and cats. *Vet. Surg.* 31 (6): 577–581.

3 Rayfield, E.J., Ault, M.J., Keush, G.T. et al. (1982). Infection and diabetes: the case for glucose control. *Am. J. Med.* 72 (3): 439–450.

4 Baltzis, D., Eleftheriadou, I., and Veves, A. (2014). Pathogenesis and treatment of impaired wound healing in diabetes mellitus: new insights. *Adv. Ther.* 31 (8): 817–836.

5 Masera, R.G., Staurenghi, A., Sartori, M.L. et al. (1999). Natural killer cell activity in the peripheral blood of patients with Cushing's syndrome. *Eur. J. Endocrinol.* 140 (4): 299–306.

6 Nuutinen, P., Riekki, R., Parikka, M. et al. (2003). Modulation of collagen synthesis and mRNA by continuous and intermittent use of topical hydrocortisone in human skin. *Br. J. Dermatol.* 148 (1): 39–45.

7 Richardson, D.W. and Dodge, G.R. (2003). Dose-dependent effects of corticosteroids on the expression of matrix-related genes in normal and cytokine-treated articular chondrocytes. *Inflamm. Res.* 52 (1): 39–49.

8 Sandrini, S., Setti, G., Bossini, N. et al. (2009). Steroid withdrawal five days after renal transplantation allows for the prevention of wound-healing complications associated with sirolimus therapy. *Clin. Transplant.* 23 (1): 16–22.

9 Maroz, N. and Simman, R. (2013). Wound healing in patients with impaired kidney function. *J. Am. Coll. Clin. Wound Spec.* 5 (1): 2–7.

10 Franz, M.G., Robson, M., Steed, D. et al. (2008). Guidelines to aid healing of acute wounds by decreasing impediments of healing. *Wound Repair Regen.* 16 (6): 723–748.

11 Stechmiller, J.K. (2010). Understanding the role of nutrition and wound healing. *Nutr. Clin. Pract.* 25 (1): 61–68.

12 Wichmann, M.W., Zellweger, R., DeMaso, C.M. et al. (1996). Mechanism of immunosuppression in males following trauma-hemorrhage. Critical role of testosterone. *Arch. Surg.* 131 (11): 1186–1191.

13 Gosain, A. and DiPietro, L.A. (2004). Aging and wound healing. *World J. Surg.* 28 (3): 321–326.

14 Li, Y., Deeb, B., Pendergrass, W. et al. (1996). Cellular proliferative capacity and life span in small and large dogs. *J. Gerontol. A Biol. Sci. Med. Sci.* 51 (6): B403–B408.

15 Swaim, S.F., Bradley, D.M., Vaughn, D.M. et al. (1993). The greyhound dog as a model for studying pressure ulcers. *Decubitus* 6 (2): 32–35, 38–40.

16 Bohling, M.W., Henderson, R.A., Swaim, S.F. et al. (2006). Comparison of the role of the subcutaneous tissue in cutaneous wound healing in the dog and cat. *Vet. Surg.* 35 (1): 3–14.

17 Balsa, I.M. and Culp, W.T.N. (2015). Wound care. *Vet. Clin. North. Am. Small Anim. Pract.* 45 (5): 1049–1065.

18 Bohling, M.W., Henderson, R.A., Swaim, S.F. et al. (2004). Cutaneous wound healing in the cat: a macroscopic description and comparison with cutaneous wound healing in the dog. *Vet. Surg.* 33 (6): 579–587.

19 Farii, H.A., Farahdel, L., Frazer, A. et al. (2021). The effect of NSAIDs on postfracture bone healing: a meta-analysis of randomized controlled trials. *OTA Int.* 4 (2): e092.

20 Gallaher, H.M., Butler, J.R., Wills, R.W. et al. (2019). Effects of short- and long-term administration of nonsteroidal anti-inflammatory drugs on osteotomy healing in dogs. *Vet. Surg.* 48 (7): 1318–1329.

21 Al-Waeli, H., Reboucas, A.P., Mansour, A. et al. (2021). Non-steroidal anti-inflammatory drugs and bone healing in animal models - a systematic review and meta-analysis. *Syst. Rev.* 10 (1): 201.

22 Fröhlich, D., Rothe, G., Schwall, B. et al. (1997). Effects of volatile anaesthetics on human neutrophil oxidative response to the bacterial peptide FMLP. *Br. J. Anaesth.* 78 (6): 718–723.

23 Dietz, A., Heimlich, F., Daniel, V. et al. (2000). Immunomodulating effects of surgical intervention in tumors of the head and neck. *Otolaryngol. Head Neck Surg.* 123 (1 Pt 1): 132–139.

24 Brand, J.M., Kirchner, H., Poppe, C. et al. (1997). The effects of general anesthesia on human peripheral immune cell distribution and cytokine production. *Clin. Immunol. Immunopathol.* 83 (2): 190–194.

25 Beal, M.W., Brown, D.C., and Shofer, F.S. (2000). The effects of perioperative hypothermia and the duration of anesthesia on postoperative wound infection rate in clean wounds: a retrospective study. *Vet. Surg.* 29 (2): 123–127.

26 Jensen, J.A., Goodson, W.H. 3rd, Vasconez, L.O. et al. (1986). Wound healing in anemia. *West J. Med.* 144 (4): 465–467.

27 Tobin, G.R. (1984). Closure of contaminated wounds. Biologic and technical considerations. *Surg. Clin. North Am.* 64 (6): 639–652.

28 Wysocki, A.B. (2002). Evaluating and managing open skin wounds: colonization versus infection. *ACCN Clin. Issues* 13 (3): 382–397.

29 White, R.J., Cooper, R., and Kinglsey, A. (2001). Wound colonization and infection: the role of topical antimicrobials. *Br. J. Nurs.* 10 (9): 563–578.

30 Jones, S.G., Edwards, R., and Thomas, D.W. (2004). Inflammation and wound healing: the role of bacteria in the immuno-regulation of wound healing. *Int. J. Low Extrem. Wounds* 3 (4): 201–208.

31 Liu, J.X., Werner, J., Kirsch, T. et al. (2018). Cytotoxicity evaluation of chlorhexidine gluconate on human fibroblasts, myoblasts, and osteoblasts. *J. Bone Joint Infect.* 3 (4): 165–172.

32 van Meurs, S.J., Gawlitta, D., Heemstra, K.A. et al. (2014). Selection of an optimal antiseptic solution for intraoperative irrigation: an in vitro study. *J. Bone Joint Surg. Am.* 96: 285–291.

33 Moscati, R.M., Mayrose, J., and Reardon, R.F. (2007). A multicenter comparison of tap water versus sterile saline for wound irrigation. *Acad. Emerg. Med.* 14 (5): 404–409.

34 Huang, C. and Choong, M. (2019). Comparison of wounds' infection rate between tap water and normal saline cleansing: a meta-analysis of randomised control trials. *Int. Wound J.* 16 (1): 300–301.

35 Lewis, K. and Pay, J.L. (2022). *Wound Irrigation.* Treasure Island, FL: StatPearls Publishing.

36 Gall, T. and Monnet, E. (2010). Evaluation of fluid pressures of common wound-flushing techniques. *Am. J. Vet. Res.* 71 (11): 1384–1386.

37 Chatterjee, J.S. (2005). A critical review of irrigation techniques in acute wounds. *Int. Wound J.* 2 (3): 258–265.

38 Chisholm, C.D., Cordell, W.H., Rogers, K. et al. (1992). Comparison of a new pressurized saline canister versus syringe irrigation for laceration cleansing in the emergency department. *Ann. Emerg. Med.* 21 (11): 1364–1367.

39 Nicks, B.A., Ayello, E.A., Woo, K. et al. (2010). Acute wound management: revisiting the approach to assessment, irrigation, and closure considerations. *Int. J. Emerg. Med.* 3 (4): 399–407.

40 Armstrong DG, Meyr AJ, Collins KA et al. Basic principles of wound management. UpToDate 2022.

41 Nolff, M.C. (2021). Filling the vacuum: role of negative pressure wound therapy in open wound management in cats. *J. Feline Med. Surg.* 23 (9): 823–833.

42 Nolff, M.C., Albert, R., Reese, S., and Meyer-Linderberg, A. (2018). Comparison of negative pressure wound therapy and silver-coated foam dressings in open wound treatment in dogs: a prospective controlled clinical trial. *Vet. Comp. Orthop. Traumatol.* 31 (4): 229–338.

43 Demaria, M., Stanley, B.J., Hauptman, J.G. et al. (2011). Effects of negative pressure wound therapy on healing of open wounds in dogs. *Vet. Surg.* 40 (6): 658–669.

44 Dissemond, J., Böttrich, J.G., Braunwarth, H. et al. (2017). Evidence for silver in wound care - meta-analysis of clinical studies from 2000-2015. *J. Dtsch. Dermatol. Ges.* 15 (5): 524–535.

45 Leaper, D.J. (2006). Silver dressings: their role in wound management. *Int. Wound J.* 3 (4): 282–294.

46 Heggers, J., Goodheart, R.E., Washington, J. et al. (2005). Therapeutic efficacy of three silver dressings in an infected animal model. *J. Burn Care Rehabil.* 26 (1): 53–56.

47 Aziz, Z. and Hassan, B.A.R. (2017). The effects of honey compared to silver sulfadiazine for the treatment of burns: a systematic review of randomized controlled trials. *Burns* 43 (1): 50–57.

48 Lindberg, T., Andersson, O., Palm, M. et al. (2015). A systematic review and meta-analysis of dressings used for wound healing: the efficiency of honey compared to silver on burns. *Contemp. Nurse* 51 (2-3): 121–123.

6

Cleansing Solutions

Julia P. Sumner

Small Animal Specialist Hospital, Sydney, Australia

It is often stated that the number of bacteria required to establish an infection in a wound is 10^6 per gram of tissue [1–5]; however, the severity of tissue damage, ischemia, and the presence of foreign material can greatly decrease this number. For example, wounds that are contaminated with certain types of soil (such as inorganic clay fractions) require just 100 bacteria per gram of tissue to establish an infection [1]. Wound irrigation mechanically removes foreign material and reduces bacterial numbers and is therefore considered a critical step in the prevention and management of wound infection [1–6].

When managing an open wound, irrigation should initially be used for mechanical debridement of foreign material, debris, exudate, and bacteria [1]. Subsequently, irrigation should be performed at each bandage change to remove surface contaminants and decrease bacterial numbers. The most appropriate lavage solution may vary depending on the phase of wound healing and the degree of contamination [1–6].

Wound cleansing can be achieved via high or low pressure. High-pressure lavage of 8 pounds per square inch (psi) is most easily achieved using a 19G or 18G needle and a 35-ml syringe [1, 5]. Connecting a syringe to a bag of intravenous fluid solution and a 19G needle via a 3-way stopcock provides an easy and convenient way to administer large volumes at pressure (Figure 6.1). High-pressure lavage is most suitable for heavily contaminated or dirty wounds to reduce bacterial loads [1, 5]. High-pressure lavage, while very effective, should be used judiciously because excessive high pressure can lead to contamination of the surrounding area with bacteria or edema of the tissues making them more susceptible to infection [1]. In addition, continued, unnecessary high-pressure lavage can damage fragile new tissue around the wound leading to delays in healing [7].

Low-pressure lavage methods (around 0.5 psi) include bathing and showering [1, 5]. This can practically be achieved by puncturing multiple holes in the top of a sterile saline bottle with an 18G needle and using it to lavage the wound (Figure 6.2). This is the most suitable method for cleaning wounds and will remove surface contaminants and large foreign bodies but is not as effective at removing gross contaminants or bacteria as high-pressure lavage [1].

While it is well established that cleansing solutions are an essential part of wound therapy, there remains some debate as to the most ideal fluid to use. The perfect solution would have a similar tonicity to living cells, be non-toxic, and be cost effective [7, 8]. The most widely available cleansing solutions include water, saline, or other intravenous fluid preparations, and antiseptics. There is no strong evidence that antiseptic cleansing solutions reduce infection and may actually delay healing in some cases due to cytotoxicity [9, 10]. Most, however, have not been shown to clearly impede healing, so they may be useful in infected or heavily contaminated wounds especially in the light of immerging resistance to antibiotics [11]. Once granulation tissue is developed in the wound bed, antiseptic cleansing solutions are no longer indicated as granulation tissue is very resistant to infection, and the presence of antiseptics may impede healing during this stage of wound healing [1–5].

Cleansing Solutions

A wide variety of wound cleansing solutions exist (Table 6.1), all with advantages and disadvantages depending on the type and stage of wound healing.

Techniques in Small Animal Wound Management, First Edition. Edited by Nicole J. Buote.
© 2024 John Wiley & Sons, Inc. Published 2024 by John Wiley & Sons, Inc.
Companion website: www.wiley.com/go/buote/wounds

(a)

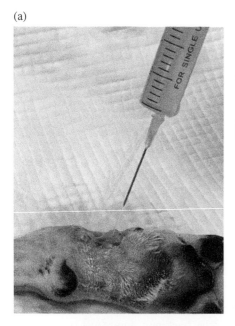

(b)

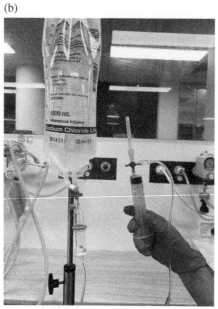

Figure 6.1 Photographs of wound flush setups using a needle or catheter and syringe. (a) A 20-ml syringe and 18-gauge needle being used to flush a wound; (b) an 18-g catheter, 35-ml syringe, three-way stopcock, and 1 l bag of fluids for flushing; (c) flush setup being used for a patient with a severe wound on the lateral flank. *Source:* Courtesy of Julia Sumner, BVSc, DACVS.

(c)

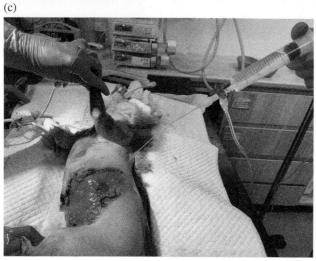

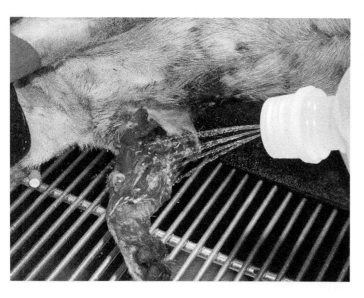

Figure 6.2 Photograph of a wound being flushed with a sterile saline bottle with holes created by an 18 g needle. *Source:* Courtesy of Julia Sumner, BVSc, DACVS.

Table 5.1 Cleansing solutions.

Examples	Dilution	Advantages	Warnings	Disadvantages	Appropriate usage
Tap water	NA	Cheap, readily available in large quantities	NA	Not sterile or isotonic. May result in surface contamination or cytotoxicity	Initial lavage of heavily contaminated or infected wounds in the inflammatory phase
0.9% saline, LRS, Hartman's, etc	NA	Isotonic, isosmotic, sterile	NA	May cause edema in large quantities. 0.9% saline is acidic and may be cytotoxic	Appropriate for all phases of wound healing
Gluconate or diacetate solution only	0.05%: 1 part 2% solution to 40 parts sterile water or electrolyte solution	Immediate action, binds to skin and mucous membranes resulting in residual effect; good choice for oral wounds	Do not use on eye, meninges, or within inner ear	Resistance reported in some gram-negative sp. Serratia has colonized hospital solutions	Initial lavage of heavily contaminated or infected wounds in the inflammatory phase
Povidone-iodine	1%: 1 part 10% povidone–iodine to 9 parts sterile water or electrolyte solution	Wide bactericidal action	Do not use in large wounds, burns, body cavities, or neonates. Do not use in patients with renal, thyroid problems or metabolic acidosis. Cytotoxic to cells involved in wound healing	Systemic absorption may lead to toxicity in patients. Residual activity only lasts 4–8 h. Inactivated by the presence of organic matter	Initial lavage of heavily contaminated or infected wounds in the inflammatory phase without the aforementioned exceptions.
Triz-EDTA	NA	Synergistic effects with aminoglycosides and penicillins to improve bactericidal effect. Effective against biofilms	NA	NA	Contaminated or infected wounds. Not needed after granulation tissue established.
Triclosan	NA	Most effective against gram-positive bacteria	MRSA recently reported to be resistant to its use	Less effective than chlorhexidine and povidone-iodine	Contaminated or infected wounds
Alcohol	Optimal action above 60% concentration	Works synergistically with chlorhexidine by reducing alcohol evaporation and prolonging effect	Painful in open wounds	Highly cytotoxic	Not recommended for wound lavage
Hydrogen Peroxide	3% solution	Forms foam on contact filling all bacteria, fungi, yeast, viruses, prions, ad spores	Do not use under pressure or in areas of poor drainage	Highly cytotoxic	Initial lavage only if superficial wounds with suspected anaerobic or gram-negative bacterial infection.
Dakin's solution	0.125–0.25%	Used for chemical debridement of wounds during WWI	Painful in open wounds	Highly cytotoxic, highly irritant	Not recommended
Vinegar White or distilled	0.5–1% solution (up to 2%) as a wound lavage or soak	Gram-positive and gram-negative bacteria Creates an unfavorable environment for Pseudomonas sp. by lowering pH thereby effective for MDR infections	NA	Painful at concentrations above 2%	Contaminated or infected wounds especially those with Pseudomonas sp.

Tap Water

Tap water is readily available, is cheap, and can be delivered via a shower head attached to a grated table at a comfortable temperature [1, 4, 5, 12–14]. Potential negatives to using tap water include that it is not isotonic, is not sterile, and can cause surface contamination. It is also cytotoxic to fibroblasts due to its alkaline pH, hypotonicity, and the presence of various trace minerals [4, 15]. For this reason, tap water is best used for the initial debridement of heavily contaminated wounds (e.g., road rash, old wounds contaminated with soil, hair, or plant material) where the need for large quantities of lavage is necessary to effectively reduce the bacterial load and remove foreign debris. As wound healing progresses and wound contamination decreases, a more isotonic lavage solution is recommended.

Isotonic Intravenous Crystalloid Fluid Preparations (e.g., 0.9% Saline, Lactated Ringer's Solution, Hartman's Solution, Plasmalyte, Normosol)

These physiologic fluids are isotonic, iso-osmotic, and sterile, making them less likely to damage the cells involved in wound healing [1]. They have the most ubiquitous use for all wound types. They can be used to lavage contaminated or infected wounds and reduce bacterial load via mechanical debridement. They are also suitable for lavage of clean contaminated or clean wounds during the repair phase as they are sterile and not thought to be cytotoxic [15].

When used in large quantities, isotonic lavage solutions can result in edema delaying wound healing [1, 4]. In addition, the pH of 0.9% saline is around 5.5 and may be cytotoxic due to its lack of buffering system and acidic pH [8].

Antiseptic Solutions

Unlike tap water and isotonic intravenous fluid preparations, antiseptics provide an antibacterial action. Their use is controversial because it is likely that the physical action of lavage, rather than the product itself, leads to the removal of debris, contaminants, and unwanted exudate from a wound bed [1, 16]. Typically, antiseptics are only indicated in the irrigation of heavily contaminated or infected wounds. Once granulation tissue is present in the wound, irrigation with antiseptics is rarely necessary and should be discontinued due to their potential cytotoxicity.

Chlorhexidine

Chlorhexidine is a biguanide antiseptic widely used in veterinary hospitals for surgical hand preparation, disinfection, lavage of oral wounds, and surgical skin preparation. Chlorhexidine comes as a solution (diacetate or gluconate) and as

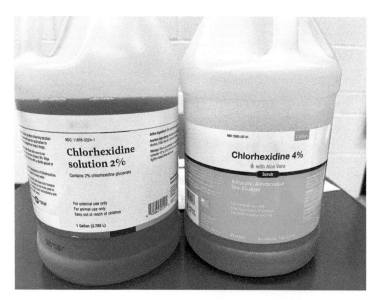

Figure 6.3   Photograph of chlorhexidine bottles. The solution (blue) on the left is appropriate for lavage. The scrub (pink) on the right is most commonly used for skin preparation. *Source:* Courtesy of Nicole Buote, DVM, DACVS.

a scrub (Figure 6.3) [1, 7, 17]. Chlorhexidine has a wide spectrum of anti-microbial activity by damaging both the inner and outer bacterial cell membranes. It is most effective against gram-positive bacteria [17]. Some gram-negative bacteria will be resistant to chlorohexidine. Most notably – nosocomial infections in both human and veterinary hospitals have been reported secondary to multidrug-resistant *Serratia* sp. That were identi-fied to be chlorhexidine resistant and colonizing chlorhexidine prepara-tions throughout the affected hospitals [18]. Chlorhexidine is also less effective against fungi and tubercle bacilli and inactive against bacterial spores [17, 18].

Chlorhexidine has an immediate bactericidal action and is not made ineffective by the presence of organic matter. It has a strong affinity for binding to skin and mucous membranes, resulting in a residual effect and making it a good choice for lavage of oral wounds [1]. Toxicity, systemic absorption, and hypersensitivity to chlorhexidine are rarely reported in both human and veterinary medicine. Despite this, chlorhexidine should never be used in the eyes, inner ear, or meninges [1, 4, 7].

Chlorhexidine for lavage should be in the diacetate or gluconate form in a 0.05% solution (1 part 2% solution to 40 parts water) (Figure 6.4). Chlorhexidine scrub should not be used for wound lavage [4].

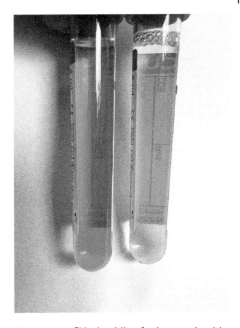

Figure 6.4   Chlorhexidine for lavage should be diluted by 1 part 2% solution to 40 parts water. The test tube on the left has straight 2% chlorhexidine gluconate, while the test tube on the right has the appropriate dilution for lavage. *Source:* Courtesy of Nicole Buote, DVM, DACVS.

Iodine

Povidone–iodine is a complex of a 1-vinyl-2-pyrrolidinone polymer and a halogen-releasing agent [17]. When the complex comes in contact with organic matter such as skin, free iodine is slowly released, resulting in cell death via attacks on bacterial key proteins, nucleotides, and fatty acids [17, 19]. Because it is activated on contact, povidone–iodine is largely rendered inactive in environments where large amounts of nontarget organic material are present such as pus, red blood cells, white blood cells, necrotic tissue, exudate, or fat [1, 4, 17, 19].

Iodine has a broad spectrum of activity against gram-positive and gram-negative bacteria, fungi, and protozoa [4, 11, 17]. Povidone–iodine is systemically absorbed via the skin, mucous membranes, and via large wounds, body cavities, and severe burns. Its bactericidal activity only lasts four to eight hours [17]. Povidone–iodine is toxic to cells essential to wound healing including lymphocytes, granulocytes, monocytes, fibroblasts, and neutrophils [17, 19, 20]. In both veterinary and human patients, povidone–iodine has been linked to renal failure and thyroid malfunction. Neonates are particularly sen-sitive to absorption which can lead to transient hypothyroidism. In addition, povidone–iodine is acidic and systemically absorbed and can therefore lead to worsening metabolic acidosis in susceptible patients [1, 4, 17, 19–21].

Hypersensitivity reactions have been reported in both veterinary and human patients. A detergent form is also available but should not be used for wound irrigation as it is irritating [4].

It has been found that dilute solutions of povidone–iodine are actually more bactericidal than full-strength solutions because more free iodine is present. When considering povidone–iodine as a lavage solution, it should be used at 1% (one part 10% povidone–iodine to nine parts sterile water or electrolyte solution to yield 0.1% free iodine) [4] (Figure 6.5). All organic matter needs to be removed prior to lavage (such as blood, exudate, or organic soil).

Others

Triz-EDTA

Triz-EDTA is a commercially available combination of tromethamine edetate disodium dihydrate buffered with trometh-amine hydrochloride and deionized water. It has efficacy against *Pseudomonas aeruginosa*, *E. coli*, and *Proteus vulgaris* [4]. In addition, Triz-EDTA has been shown to work synergistically with antimicrobials to reduce the minimal inhibitory concentration and the minimal bactericidal concentration. Triz-EDTA has also been shown to be effective against bio-films [4]. Triz-EDTA may be a suitable wound lavage agent for contaminated or infected wounds but is likely not necessary once granulation is well established.

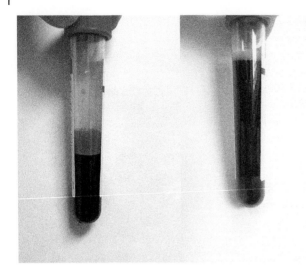

Figure 6.5 Iodine is also used most commonly as a dilution (one part 10% povidone–iodine to nine parts sterile water or electrolyte solution). The test tube on the right is straight 10% povidone–iodine while the test tube on the left has the appropriate dilution for lavage. *Source:* Courtesy of Nicole Buote, DVM, DACVS.

Triclosan

Triclosan is a diphenyl ether that has a broad spectrum of antimicrobial activity particularly against gram-positive bacteria. It is also effective against some viruses and fungi. It works by halting fatty acid biosynthesis within the cells disrupting a multitude of cellular processes [1, 17, 19]. It can be found in soaps, surgical scrubs, hand washes, and mouthwashes and has been used for MRSA decontamination protocols in human hospitals. It is less effective than chlorhexidine and povidone–iodine at reducing bacterial numbers. Recent reports of resistance of MRSA to triclosan have restricted its use in commercial products [17].

Alcohol

Alcohol causes cell lysis and protein coagulation and denaturation leading to death. Alcohol and chlorhexidine can work synergistically by slowing the rate of alcohol evaporation and thereby increasing antimicrobial efficacy [17].

Alcohol is effective against bacteria, mycobacterium, fungi, and viruses but not against spores. Alcohol effectiveness is concentration-dependent and is optimal above 60% [22]. It is highly cytotoxic and not typically recommended for wound lavage.

Hydrogen Peroxide

Hydrogen peroxide is a highly potent antiseptic agent with activity against bacteria, viruses, protozoa, spores, and prions [17]. Hydrogen peroxide rapidly converts into a foam of water and oxygen when it contacts tissue catalases found in wound tissue. It rapidly crosses the cell membrane leading to oxidative damage of the cell wall and disruption of many of the cellular processes [1, 4, 17].

Hydrogen peroxide has no residual effect and does not penetrate tissue. It is highly cytotoxic to all cells so its use is perhaps limited to a one-time use in an infected wound [4, 20]. The foaming action of hydrogen peroxide may have an additional mechanical debridement effect. Hydrogen peroxide should never be used under pressure or in situations where drainage is not adequate because the expansile foam forces between tissue plains create emphysema and enlarge the wound [4].

Sodium Hypochlorite (Dakin's Solution)

This solution was popular during WWI for chemical debridement of wounds. It has a pH of 11 and is significantly cytotoxic even at dilutions of 0.125–0.25%. It is no longer recommended due to its irritant effects [4].

Acetic Acid (Vinegar)

Vinegar was first described by Hippocrates in the fifth century BCE as an antiseptic to promote wound healing [23]. Acetic acid works by lowering the pH and by breaching the cytoplasmic membrane to lower the internal pH and denature cellar proteins. Acetic acid is nontoxic and is bactericidal against gram-positive and gram-negative bacteria [23]. White or distilled vinegar can be used at a 0.5–1% solution as a wound lavage or used to soak gauze for the contact layer of bandages. Concentrations as high as 2% have been used to treat burns in humans, but higher concentrations lead to significant pain upon application [23]. Vinegar has been used in humans to treat superficial wounds colonized with multidrug-resistant strains of *Pseudomonas aeruginosa*, leg ulcers, ear infections, and for soaks to reduce bioburden on dentures and contact lenses. *In vitro* trials have demonstrated cytotoxicity to epithelial cells until day 8; however, this has not been repeated in human or animal models. Vinegar is therefore a useful consideration in infected or contaminated wounds in the face of multidrug resistance to antibiotics [23, 24].

References

1 Atiyeh, B.S., Dibo, S.A., and Hayek, S.N. (2009). Wound cleansing, topical antiseptics and wound healing. *Int. Wound J.* 6: 420–430.

2 Fowler, D. and Williams, J.M. (ed.) (1999). Chapter 5: Open wound management. In: *Manual of Canine and Feline Wound Management and Reconstruction*, pp. 37–46. Cheltenham: British Small Animal Veterinary Association.

3 Pavletic, M.M. (2010). *Atlas of Small Animal Wound Management and Reconstructive Surgery*, 3e. Ames, IA: Wiley-Blackwell.

4 Swaim, S.F. and Henderson, R.A. (ed.) (1997). Chapter 3: wound dressing materials and topical medications. In: *Small Animal Wound Management*, 2e, pp. 53–85. Baltimore: Williams & Wilkins.

5 Hosgood, G. (2017). Chapter 76: Open wounds. In: *Veterinary Surgery Small Animal*, 2e (ed. K.M. Tobias and S.A. Johnstson), pp. 1410–1421. Elsevier Saunders: St. Louis.

6 Bianchi, J. (2000). The cleansing of superficial traumatic wounds. *Br. J. Nurs.* 9 (Suppl 19): S28–S38.

7 Main, R.C. (2008). Should chlorhexidine gluconate be used in wound cleansing? *J. Wound Care* 17: 112–114.

8 Horrocks, A. (2006). Prontosan wound irrigation and gel: management of chronic wounds. *Br. J. Nurs.* 15: 122–128.

9 Wilson, J.R., Mills, J.G., Prather, I.D. et al. (2005). A toxicity index of skin and wound cleansers used on in vitro fibroblasts and keratinocytes. *Adv. Skin Wound Care* 18: 373–378.

10 Cooper, M.L., Laxer, J.A., and Hansbrough, J.F. (1991). The cytotoxic effects of commonly used topical antimicrobial agents on human fibroblasts and keratinocytes. *J. Trauma* 31: 775–784.

11 Leaper, D.J. and Durani, P. (2008). Topical antimicrobial therapy of chronic wounds healing by secondary intention using iodine products. *Int. Wound J.* 5: 361–368.

12 Fernandez, R. and Griffiths, R. (2008). Water for wound cleansing. *Cochrane Database Syst. Rev.* 23: CD003861.

13 Moscati, R.M., Reardon, R.F. et al. (1998). Wound irrigation with tap water. *Acad. Emerg. Med.* 5: 1076–1080.

14 Svoboda, S.J., Owens, B.D. et al. (2008). Irrigation with potable water versus normal saline in a contaminated musculoskeletal wound model. *J. Trauma* 64: 1357–1359.

15 Towler, J. (2001). Cleansing traumatic wounds with swabs, water or saline. *J. Wound Care* 10: 231–234.

16 Smith, R.G. (2005). A critical discussion of the uses of antiseptics in acute traumatic wounds. *J. Am. Podiatry Med. Assoc.* 95: 148–153.

17 Williamson, D.A., Carter, G.P., and Howden, B.P. (2017). Current and emerging topical antibacterials and antiseptics: agents, action and resistance patterns. *Clin. Microbiol. Rev.* 30 (3): 827–860.

18 Allen, J.L., Doidge, N.P., Bushell, R.N. et al. (2022). Healthcare-associated infections caused by chlorhexidine-tolerant *Serratia marcescens* carrying a promiscuous IncH12 multi-drug resistance plasmid in a veterinary hospital. *PLoS One* 17 (3): e0264848.

19 McDonnell, G. and Russell, A.D. (1999). Antiseptics and disinfectants: activity, action and resistance. *Clin. Microbiol. Rev.* 12: 147–179.

20 Thomas, G.W., Rael, L.T., Bar-Or, R. et al. (2009). Mechanisms of delayed wound healing by commonly used antiseptics. *J. Trauma* 66: 82–91.

21 Noda, Y., Fujii, K. et al. (2009). Critical evaluation of cadexomer-iodine ointment and povidone-iodine sugar ointment. *Int. J. Pharm.* 372: 85–90.

22 Morton, H.E. (1950). The relationship of concentration and germicidal efficiency of ethyl alcohol. *Annu. N. Y. Acad. Sci.* 53: 191–196.

23 Nitin, S. and Raghuveer, C. (2016). A review of the therapeutic applications of vinegar. *Sch. J. Appl. Med. Sci.* 4: 3971–3976.

24 Pye, C.C., Singh, A., and Weese, S.J. (2014). Evaluation of the impact of tromethamine edetate disodium dihydrate on antimicrobial susceptibility of *Pseudomonas aeruginosa* in biofilm *in vitro*. *Vet. Dermatol.* 25 (2): 120. e34.

7

Topicals

Nicole J. Buote

Department of Clinical Sciences, Cornell University, Ithaca, NY, USA

Topical wound therapy is initiated frequently for wound management. In daily life, scrapes and minor injuries are commonly treated with triple antibiotic ointments, a familiar topical treatment. The use of topicals can be considered either as a protective barrier for the wound or as an active treatment for the wounded tissue. Many topicals listed in this chapter have also been incorporated into dressings discussed in Chapter 8, but they can be found as separate treatments as described below.

The primary goal of many topicals is to encourage moist wound healing [1–3]. The term "moist wound healing" refers to the use of specific bandaging techniques that help retain moisture levels in the wounded tissues. This has been shown to enhance wound healing if done appropriately [1, 4, 5]. Transepidermal water loss (TEWL), which is a measurement of water molecule transfer across the skin, can be assessed to determine tissue health. In normal undamaged skin, the TEWL is between 4 and $9\,g/m^2/h$ but this can increase to over $80\,g/m^2/h$ in partial or full-thickness wounds [6]. Moisture vapor transmission rate (MVTR) is a similar measurement for bandage material and relates to the occlusiveness of a bandage. A bandage with a low MVTR denotes low water loss and higher moisture retention at the wound surface. Previous studies have shown positive wound healing and lower infection rates with low MVTR bandages [7, 8] but increased bandage changes [9] are also required many times to decrease possible complications. A detailed review of different wound dressings as related to MVTR is discussed in Chapter 8. The topicals discussed in this chapter have a low MVTR due to their gaseous, liquid, or semi-solid formulation (Table 7.1).

Hydrogels

Mechanism of Action

As their name implies, hydrogels are a type of water-based gel treatment. Polymers, such as polyvinyl alcohol, polyethylene glycol or polyacrylates, and humectants are combined with water (90–95%) to form this amorphous gel which can contribute moisture to tissues. These gels can also absorb fluid in certain formulations and the primary mechanism of action in wound therapy is to encourage a moist wound environment and autolytic debridement. This environment facilitates migration of fibroblasts and keratinocytes speeding up healing. Hydrogels possess excellent biocompatibility which allows their use on wounds without any significant adverse reactions. While hydrogels can create a protective barrier for wounds, they can also allow exchange of fluids, oxygen, and nutrients. Hydrogels can also encourage autolytic debridement by creating a welcoming environment for macrophages. Hydrogels are available in various forms including gels or films but this discussion will focus on gels.

Specific Directions for Use

Hydrogels are applied directly to the wound with a gloved finger or application tube. Their application is nonpainful and cooling. Many are sold as single-use applications and are sterile initially (Figure 7.1). If remaining gel is stored, it is not considered sterile. These gels must be in direct contact with the wounded tissue and covered with a secondary dressing to

Techniques in Small Animal Wound Management, First Edition. Edited by Nicole J. Buote.
© 2024 John Wiley & Sons, Inc. Published 2024 by John Wiley & Sons, Inc.
Companion website: www.wiley.com/go/buote/wounds

Table 7.1 Commonly used topicals in veterinary medicine.

Type of topical	Name of specific product(s)	Stage of wound healing	Indications	Tips/notes
Hydrogel	Amorphous gels: Curafil Gel; Kendall Wound Care; Medline Skintegrity; Smith & Nephew Intrasite gel; Curafil, Nu-Gel, BioDres, Aquacel, Aquasorb	Inflammatory, proliferative (all stages)	• Provides additional moisture • Encourages autolytic debridement • Partial-thickness wounds (abrasions) • Promotes epithelialization	• Best for wounds with minimal to no exudate, eschars • Applied over granulation tissue (NOT intact skin)
Zinc-oxide hydrophilic pastes	McKesson Hydrophilic Wound Dressing with Zinc plus Vitamins A and B6; Coloplast Triad Hydrophilic Wound Dressing Paste; Balmex Diaper rash cream	Inflammatory, early proliferative	• Encourages autolytic debridement • Moisture retention	• Best for burns, water barrier, eschars • Can be used on wound and peri-wound skin • NOT for infected wounds
Honey/sugar	Manuka; Derma Science Medihoney; First Honey Manuka Honey Ointment; self-formulated dressing	Inflammatory, early proliferative	• Antibacterial (hydrogen peroxide content, hyperosmotic effect, low pH, and inhibin content) • Encourages autolytic debridement • Osmotic diuretic (decreases edema) • Encourages granulation tissue and epithelialization	• Best for wounds prior to granulation tissue or multi-drug resistant wounds
Nitrofurazone	Squire Laboratories Fura-Zone; VetOne Nitrofurazone ointment	Inflammatory, (infected)	• Antibacterial for sensitive bacteria	• Hypersensitivity reactions • Possible carcinogenic
Triple antibiotic (neomycin, polymyxin b, bacitracin)	Neosporin®; Dynarex triple antibiotic; Safetec triple antibiotic	Inflammatory (infected)	• Antibacterial for sensitive bacteria	• Best for prevention not treatment • petrolatum base decreases contraction
Silver sulfadiazine	Silver Sulfadiazine 1% (Ascend Laboratories LLC) SSD (Dr. Reddy's Laboratories)	Inflammatory (infected)	• Burn wounds before epithelialization • Antibiotic prophylaxis (silver ions) • Burn wound sepsis treatment • BEST for *Pseudomonas* spp.	• Hypersensitivity reactions (hematologic reactions and dermatologic reactions) • Decreases epithelialization • Propylene glycol toxicity if ingested • Not indicated if patient allergic to sulfonamides
Nitrous oxide	Noxsana® Restore gel	Inflammatory, proliferative	Healing surgical incisions Open or infected wounds	Do not use on actively hemorrhaging wounds Limited studies in clinical veterinary patients

(a) (b)

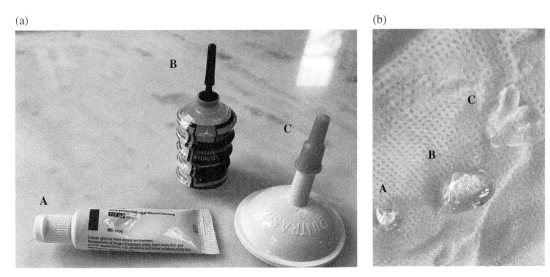

Figure 7.1   (a) Photograph of different hydrogel formulations (A-Kendall Wound Care; B-Medline Skintegrity; C-Smith & Nephew Intrasite gel). (b) Photograph of contents of the hydrogels in 1A. *Source:* Courtesy of Nicole Buote, DVM, DACVS.

prevent their transfer to the absorptive layers of the bandage. Most commonly, they are covered with a non-adherent or vapor permeable polyurethane film or foam (see Chapter 8) and when first employed the bandage should be changed every three to four days to ensure the gel has not dried. Depending on the amount of wound exudate produced, these bandages may be left in place for up to five to seven days. To remove hydrogels from the wound surface, gentle irrigation with saline and or moistened gauze is performed.

Indication(s)

These topicals are especially helpful for dry wounds such as eschars, or wounds in the early reparative stage (granulation tissue present). Hydrogels can also encourage autolytic debridement in necrotic/infected wounds by maintaining the moist environment allowing cellular activities (by macrophages, fibroblasts) to proceed efficiently but this is not their primary use.

Hydrogels can also be used to fill deep wounds due to their semi-solid nature and allow for non-painful removal of secondary dressings which is beneficial to patients. Hydrogels have been studied in varying canine wound models and found to have discordant effects on wound contraction: increasing contraction for limb wounds but delaying contraction in trunk wounds [10, 11].

Contraindications/Complications

While some hydrogels are able to absorb fluid [12], the majority are not recommended in highly exudative wounds due to the concern for maceration of tissue if excessive moisture is not appropriately withdrawn to secondary bandage layers. They should not be applied to intact skin due to concern for maceration and pure hydrogels are not recommended for grossly infected wounds as they do not provide any specific antimicrobial effects seen with other topicals/dressings.

Zinc-Oxide Hydrophilic Pastes

Mechanism of Action

The most common formulation of zinc for wound treatment is topical zinc-oxide ointments or creams. There is very little peer-reviewed research on the effects of zinc-oxide topicals in veterinary literature with the most common uses being reported for equine wounds and moist dermatitis (diarrhea-induced) [13]. Zinc oxide-based ointments or creams act as a physical barrier to water absorption and have been reported to reduce bacterial infections in mild dermatitis by inhibiting the adhesion and penetration of microorganisms [14]. According to one review on the use of zinc-containing compounds, zinc-oxide has sunscreening abilities, anti-inflammatory activities, antibacterial activities (especially against *Staph aureus*), and anti-odor properties [15].

Most zinc-oxide pastes are occlusive and do not allow anything to pass through them. Hydrophilic pastes are reported to encourage endogenous wound fluid to spread evenly across the wound surface, creating a moist environment, and facilitating autolytic debridement. Depending on the vehicle product, (for example, carboxymethyl cellulose) zinc-oxide pastes can also absorb low to moderate levels of wound exudate.

Specific Directions for Use

Hydrophilic pastes are applied directly from the tube or by using a gloved finger. Some hydrophilic zinc-oxide pastes are specifically designed for use on wet surfaces (Triad) and therefore dry and do not need to be covered with a secondary bandage, however in veterinary patient's self-removal of the paste must be considered. Spread the paste evenly over the wound to the thickness of a dime. If the wound is covered, adherent (dry gauze) or non-adherent (Telfa, Covidien™) dressings can be applied over it depending on the amount of expected exudate.

If the zinc-oxide dries to the wound, a commercial wound cleanser (not saline) will need to be used to remove it as it is not soluble in saline. Use a pH-balanced wound cleanser to soften the paste, and gently wipe to remove without scrubbing. Hydrophilic pastes can stay in place for five to seven days, depending on the amount of exudate produced.

Indication(s)

Hydrophilic pastes facilitate autolytic debridement to help manage necrotic tissue such as slough and eschar. Pastes can be applied to wounds and peri-wound skin without maceration. These pastes are commonly used in human medicine for local management of partial- and full-thickness pressure and venous stasis ulcers, moist dermatitis, and first and second-degree burns.

Contraindications/Complications

While no serious side effects have been reported in many decades of use [14] of zinc-oxide pastes, they are generally thought to be contraindicated for infected wounds and third-degree burns.

Honey/Sugar

Mechanism of Action

Honey is probably the most commonly used topical agent in veterinary wound care currently, and there are multiple formulations of honey (liquid, semi-solid, and dressing-impregnated) available to clinicians (Figure 7.2). Granulated sugar can also be used in wound management but is uncomfortable for the patient and requires wound exudate to liquify the granules to recreate the same effects. Manuka honey is the most well-known of all and originates from the *Leptospermum* spp. of bee [16]. It has been shown to inhibit the growth of *S. aureus* within eight hours of contact, but studies of other honey varieties also show promise [17]. Multiple processes work to create a positive wound environment when honey is used as a topical. The known mechanisms of action for honey include (i) Antimicrobial effects, (ii) Hyperosmotic effects, (iii) Autolytic debridement, and (iv) Encouragement of granulation tissue/epithelialization (Table 7.2) [2, 18–21].

Antibacterial Effects

The antimicrobial effects of honey are the most researched and are explained by multiple functions. Honey produces hydrogen peroxide at a low concentration (0.003%) by oxidation of glucose, which is damaging to bacteria but does not create the cytotoxicity seen with standard hydrogen peroxide solutions (3%). Hydrogen peroxide is also oxidized to produce oxygen-derived free radicals which harm bacteria. There are also nonperoxide antimicrobial effects (NPAB) brought on by components such as phenols and organic acids which produce an acidic pH (3.2–4.5) which is discouraging to bacterial growth. Originally the creation of hydrogen peroxide was thought to be the most important antibacterial effect but recent work has illustrated methylglyoxal and not hydrogen peroxide, might be the main antibacterial agent (Albaridi). Methylglyoxal is created by conversion of dihydroacetone which is found in the nectar of Manuka flowers. The inhibine

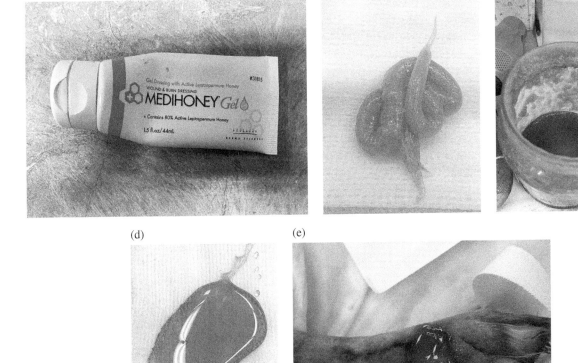

(a) (b) (c)

(d) (e)

Figure 7.2 (a,b) Photographs of Medihoney® topical ointment. (c,d) Photograph of multiuse tub of honey. Note the crystallization around the edges of the tub. As the honey ages and is exposed to air over time it becomes thicker, granular, and more opaque. (e) Photograph of honey within a canine pes wound. *Source:* Courtesy of Nicole Buote, DVM, DACVS.

Table 7.2 Mechanism of action of honey.

Mechanism of action	
Antimicrobial	Hyperosmolality
	Hydrogen peroxide production (inhibine)
	Oxygen-derived free radicals
	Methylglyoxal
	NPAB → acidic pH
Hyperosmotic	Dehydrate microorganisms
	Draw exudate, debris out of wound
	Decrease tissue edema
Autolytic debridement	Moist wound environment
	Migration of macrophages
	Exudation
Granulation/epithelialization	Nutrition for fibroblasts, epithelial cells
	Antioxidant effects
	Stimulation of B- and T-cells
	Cytokine release

effect/number is a term used to define the antibacterial activity of honey and is enumerated in medical-grade honey. These numbers are related to the dilution to which the honey will retain its inherent antimicrobial activity (5–25 v/v%) [21, 22]. Some honey producers also use a scale for rating the potency of Manuka honey, the Unique Manuka Factor (UMF™) but research has not shown a clear connection between the UMF rating and antimicrobial activity [23]. The hyperosmolality of honey also produces an inhospitable environment for bacteria through dehydration. This effect can be bactericidal or static depending on the type and concentration of bacteria present.

Hyperosmotic Effects

The dehydrating effects of honey on bacterial cell walls are responsible for a mild antibacterial result but this property more importantly reduces tissue edema and can be helpful in the early phase of healing at drawing out wound exudate and contaminated debris. These effects cannot debride/dissolve gross contamination per se therefore honey is best not to be used as a sole debridement topical in those cases.

Autolytic Debridement Effects

Honey is an excellent topical to create a moist wound environment. As discussed previously, a moist environment allows for efficient transfer of nutrients and migration of cells responsible for debridement (macrophages), improving phagocytic activity. Because honey can draw wound fluid out of the tissues, bandage changes must be timed to ensure maceration of the peri-wound tissues does not occur.

Granulation/Epithelialization Effects

Honey also has anti-inflammatory effect due to its antioxidant content which is known to stimulate granulation tissue and epithelialization. The high glucose content can also provide nutrition to cells promoting angiogenesis, growth of fibroblasts, and mobilization of epithelial cells. Honey has also been reported to expedite wound healing by stimulation of B- and T-lymphocyte proliferation and cytokine release from monocytes, which may encourage granulation tissue formation and epithelialization.

Specific Directions for Use

Honey is applied directly from the single-use tube, incorporated into a dressing, or by using a tongue depressor from a multi-use jar. Spread the honey evenly over the wound and then cover the wound with an adherent (dry gauze) or non-adherent dressings depending on the amount of expected exudate.

For removal, gently wash the exudate with sterile saline or tap water and gently wipe to remove without scrubbing. Honey bandages can stay in place for two to four days, depending on the amount of exudate produced.

Indication(s)

Because honey facilitates autolytic debridement and a moist wound environment and claims many antimicrobial activities, it can be used in many wound scenarios. Having said that, while it *can* be used in almost any stage of healing, there are times it will work best and times it will not. Chronic wounds have actually been shown in some human studies to stall with the use of honey, therefore early acute wounds are the clearest indication of a honey application [24–26]. And while there might be some supportive effects for epithelialization, other topicals (hydrogel) and dressings (see Chapter 8) may have similar or improved outcomes without the chance for tissue maceration and frequent bandage changes. This author usually recommends using honey after gross contamination is gone, and before granulation tissue is present or in the case of multi-drug resistant wound infections. As granulation tissue is usually resistant to bacteria, many of the activities of honey are not needed past this point.

While randomized clinical trials in human medicine have found equivocal results, many veterinary case reports or case series show improved wound healing in patients randomized to honey treatment groups [25, 27, 28] but very little rigorous data exists [29]. The only prospective randomized controlled study of acute superficial wounds in dogs as of June 2023, investigated a proprietary honey hydrogel and reported no significant differences in wound contraction or histologic scores between the honey and control groups [30]. Other recent work has illustrated other topicals (herbal preparation – moist exposed burn ointment) may have superior results in immunocompromised dogs [31]. A scoping review of medicinal uses of honey in animals concluded that high-quality peer-reviewed research is needed to provide sound data for the efficacy of honey in clinical practice [32]. There have been studies illustrating no difference between honey types but the majority of research centers around Manuka honey therefore it is the most widely used [16, 17, 33, 34].

Contraindications/Complications

Honey is not appropriate in the face of gross contamination and purulent material as the antibacterial action will be reduced when honey is diluted by body fluids at the site of infection. Granulated sugar is also not effective in highly exudative wounds because of dilution and may require three to four times daily bandages. In keeping with the hyperosmotic effects, honey bandages can become extremely exudative so they are not recommended in wounds that are already highly exudative.

While sugar and honey have been shown to produce no systemic side effects, sugar bandages are painful to apply and remove and should not be used after granulation tissue is present. One review by Majtan et al. illustrated concern with the use of honey in chronic diabetic ulcers due to the production of advanced glycation end-products [35].

Antimicrobials (Nitrofurazone, Triple Antibiotic, Silver Sulfadiazine)

Nitrofurazone

Mechanism of Action
Nitrofurazone ointment is a topical antibiotic medication in the class of drugs known as nitrofuran antibiotics. Nitrofurans are synthetic chemotherapeutic agents with a broad antimicrobial spectrum. Nitrofurazone acts by interfering with the bacterial cell's ability to synthesize proteins and DNA, ultimately leading to bacterial cell death [36]. The exact details of its mechanism of action are not completely understood, but several processes contribute to its antibacterial activity. Firstly, nitrofurazone is converted into reactive intermediates in the presence of bacterial enzymes. These intermediates generate reactive oxygen species (ROS), such as superoxide radicals and hydroxyl radicals. ROS can cause significant damage to bacterial cells by targeting their DNA, proteins, and other essential cellular components. This oxidative stress disrupts the normal functioning of bacteria and ultimately leads to their destruction. Secondly, nitrofurazone also interferes with the bacterial cell membrane by disrupting its integrity and inhibition of ATP synthesis.

Specific Directions for Use

Nitrofurazone most commonly comes as a bright green/yellow ointment and is applied by gloved finger from a multiuse jar onto the surface of the wound (Figure 7.3). A thin layer is applied and the wound is then covered with a non-adherent or absorptive bandage. Depending on the amount of exudate created by the wound, the bandage will need to be changed every three to four days.

Indication(s)

Nitrofurazone has broad-spectrum activity against various bacteria, including both gram-positive and gram-negative organisms. Nitrofurazone is used for infected burns or skin grafts in human medicine [36–38]. It is effective against common pathogens such as *Staphylococcus aureus*, *Streptococcus pyogenes*, *Escherichia coli*, and *Aerobacter aerogenes*. The best indication would be for a wound that cultures a sensitive bacterium.

Contraindications/Complications

Hypersensitivity reactions (inflammation, itching to the peri-wound skin) have been reported in people [39] with application of nitrofurazone and concerns regarding carcinogenesis have encouraged many clinicians to use other antibacterial ointments [40]. In 2002, the FDA banned the use

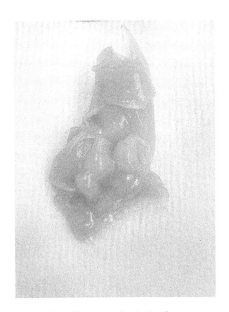

Figure 7.3 Photograph of nitrofurazone ointment. *Source:* Courtesy of Nicole Buote, DVM, DACVS.

of oral nitrofurans in food-producing animals due to health risks but topical use continues to be allowed. The antibacterial potency is diminished in the presence of pus or blood so overtly infected wounds are not effectively treated. Wounds infected with *Pseudomonas aeruginosa, Proteus* spp., and *Streptococcus faecalis* should not be treated with Nitrofurazone as these bacteria are usually resistant [37]. In a study on full-thickness wounds in rats, the authors found that the use of nitrofurazone caused delay in wound healing and had a negative effect on epithelialization [41].

Triple Antibiotic (Neomycin, Polymixin B, and Bacitracin)

Mechanism of Action

Triple antibiotic in veterinary medicine is usually a mixture of several closely related cyclic polypeptide antibiotics that have both bacteriostatic and bactericidal properties depending on the concentration of the drug and the susceptibility of the microorganism. Bacitracin, one component of triple antibiotic ointment, is absorbed through the wound and prevents the transfer of mucopeptides into the cell walls of various bacteria. This in turn inhibits bacterial cell wall synthesis and, ultimately, bacterial proliferation. Bacitracin also inhibits proteases and other enzymes involved in altering bacterial cell membrane function and inhibits bacterial cell wall synthesis [42, 43]. Interestingly, bacitracin was discovered in the United States in 1945 from a leg injury of a seven-year-old girl named Margaret Tracey. The United States Food and Drug Administration (FDA) approved the use of bacitracin in 1948 for the short-term prevention and treatment of both acute and chronic localized skin infections.

Specific Directions for Use

Triple antibiotic is usually applied by gloved finger from a multiuse tube onto the surface of the wound. A thin layer is applied, and the wound is then covered with a non-adherent or absorptive bandage (Figure 7.4). Depending on the amount of exudate created by the wound, the bandage will need to be changed every three to four days.

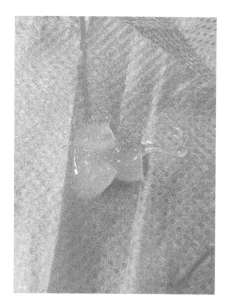

Figure 7.4 Photograph of triple antibiotics ointment. *Source:* Courtesy of Nicole Buote, DVM, DACVS.

Indication(s)

Triple antibiotic ointment is most commonly used for minor injuries in both human and veterinary medicine. The most common use in the author's practice is as a layer over free mesh skin grafts to prevent adherence of the graft to the primary contact layer/dressing and as a preventative against infection. While triple antibiotic may treat some infections, the best use for it is for small superficial acute wounds that can be easily covered with a bandage as the petrolatum base will attract dust and dirt. Many gram-positive bacteria, including *Staphylococcus* spp., *Streptococcus* spp., *Corynebacterium* spp., *Clostridium* spp., *and Actinomyces* spp., are reportedly susceptible to triple antibiotic ointment but, most gram-negative organisms and *Pseudomonas* spp. are resistant [44]. The petrolatum base is also occlusive and therefore does not allow for free transport of oxygen and fluid from the wound.

Contraindications/Complications

While not reported in veterinary patients, allergic reactions including hives, swelling, and fever have been reported in human medicine [45, 46] and bacitracin was named the "contact allergen of the year" in 2003 by the American Contact Dermatitis Society [47]. These formulations are not effective against fungal or viral infections and can lead to bacterial resistance if used inappropriately. Topical application is also not recommended over large areas of the body [42].

Zinc found in most formulations of triple antibiotic may stimulate epithelialization in some wounds but the petroleum base has been shown to decrease epithelialization [48] therefore its use should be infrequent in most wound management scenarios.

Silver Sulfasalazine

Mechanism of Action

Silver sulfadiazine (SSD) is a sulfa-derived heavy metal topical antibiotic medication [49]. Unlike other sulfa drugs, SSD does not inhibit folic acid synthesis as its antibacterial mechanism. Instead, these effects are due to the silver ions in the formulation. The exact mechanism of action is not

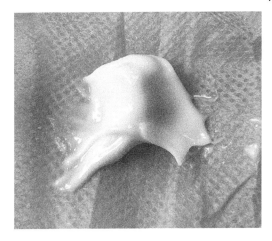

Figure 7.5   Photograph of silver sulfadiazine cream. *Source:* Courtesy of Nicole Buote, DVM, DACVS.

known but increases in cell wall permeability through the impairment of DNA replication, modification of the lipid cell membrane, and/or the formation of free radicals have been theorized [50, 51].

Specific Directions for Use

SSD is a white thick cream typically applied with a gloved finger to non-adherent dressings in a thick layer (1/16″) and then covered with a light soft padded bandage (Figure 7.5). Each tub or tube of ointment should only be used for one patient. As the silver ions act superficially, there is limited absorption through eschars [52]. Application is cooling and well tolerated by patients. Care must be taken to avoid mucosal contact as increased absorption can occur therefore patients should not be allowed to lick SSD. Bandages are changed daily based on exudate production.

Indication(s)

SSD is most commonly used for management of burn wounds in veterinary medicine but its use can be expanded to chronic wounds as well. In human medicine, SSD is a common antibacterial prophylaxis agent as well as treatment for burn sepsis. Topical agents used for antibacterial prophylaxis control microbe colonization in the wound and attempt to prevent the development of wound infection. SSD is effective against gram-positive and gram-negative bacteria, some yeasts, and *Pseudomonas aeruginosa*, which is a common cause of burn wound infections. Recently the quality of previous clinical trials highlighting the effectiveness of SSD against *Pseudomonas* have been called into question [53].

Contraindications/Complications

This topical treatment is safe and well tolerated with few side effects. Hematologic effects are the most commonly reported side effects in human medicine, including agranulocytosis, aplastic anemia, hemolytic anemia, and leukopenia but they have not been specifically reported in clinical veterinary patients [54–56]. Dermatologic reactions including pruritis, skin discoloration, and skin photosensitivity have also been reported in human.

In human studies, SSD can slow reepithelization and application should be discontinued once epithelialization is expected [57]. A pseudoeschar or thick adherent film has been reported with repeated use, making assessment of the wound more difficult, and surgical removal of this layer can be painful [53, 58].

The use of SSD should be avoided if possible in patients with a known previous reaction to sulfonamide drugs. Propylene glycol is present in the most common formulations of SSD ointment and while this additive is less toxic than ethylene glycol possible side effects include depression, weakness, involuntary muscle movements, polydipsia/

polyuria, hypotension, and seizures. Lactic acidosis and Heinz body anemia (especially in cats) can develop hours after ingestion so any ingestion of SSD should be reported [59].

Oxygen

Mechanism of Action

Oxygen is required for multiple steps during the phases of wound healing on an intracellular level. Increased oxygen levels in tissue are essential for the production of ROS which are utilized by white blood cells (neutrophils and macrophages) to debride wounds [60, 61]. Oxygen levels also affect the quality of new blood vessel ingrowth, growth factor activation, and collagen formation [62, 63]. Oxygen transport into wounded tissue can occur through diffusion when oxygen molecules move from areas of high partial pressure to areas of low partial pressure [60]. Topical oxygen can increase oxygen levels in a wound bed over 4× within four minutes without a hyperbaric chamber in one study [64]. Topically applied oxygen has the benefit of circumventing the dependence on local microvasculature for oxygen delivery to the healing tissues.

Specific Directions for Use

While there are multiple modalities for delivery of oxygen, including inspired and topical, Chapter 13 discussed hyperbaric oxygen therapy so this section will only discuss topical methods. Topical applications can also be categorized as intermittent or continuous, but all methods must ensure humidification of the oxygen to avoid desiccation of the wound. Intermittent topical oxygen typically uses high concentration oxygen (~93%) applied using a bag or boot sealed around the wound. One of the commercial systems for intermittent application uses a cyclic pressure controller to create varied pressure between 0 and 50 mmHg which has been shown to improve diffusion into the wound. This oxygen is supplied by a high-flow oxygen concentrator. A typical regimen for intermittent topical oxygen application is 90 minutes a day, 3–5 days a week [60].

Continuously applied topical oxygen (CDO) is applied to the wound by a wearable electrochemical oxygen generator. Currently, there are two different CDO systems that use a compression-plate oxygen generator. One system uses a fixed flow of oxygen through tubing connected to a wheel-shaped diffusion membrane placed under a moist wound dressing. The other uses an integrated oxygen diffusion dressing which is available in many sizes and does not require other bandage/dressing coverage. This system also provides feedback on wound bed pressure and allows for variability in oxygen flow rate. A typical regimen for continuous oxygen therapy application is 24 hours a day, 7 days a week [60].

Indication(s)

Topically applied oxygen is used in human medicine for a variety of wound types including: diabetic ulcers, vascular ulcers, postoperative infections, burns, skin grafts, and prevention of wound dehiscence's. Some clinicians will also supplement other wound management strategies in chronic wounds as well. In human wound, care assessment for arterial insufficiency is very important as this alone can be the cause of reduced wound healing progress. There are no clinical studies in veterinary patients using topical oxygen applications to date but hopefully, this will be investigated in the future.

Contraindications/Complications

Contraindications for topical oxygen include the presence of necrotic tissue or any dressing or ointment (petrolatum-based especially) that would prevent the oxygen molecules from being applied to the wound tissue.

There are no known risks to patients and no serious adverse side effects reported in human literature to date [60].

Nitrous Oxide

Mechanism of Action

Nitrous oxide (NO) is a diatomic gas responsible for many important physiological processes throughout the body. Recent work studying the effects of endogenous and exogenous NO on wound healing has shown promising results [65–67]. NO appears to affect wound healing through multiple mechanisms of action depending on the stage

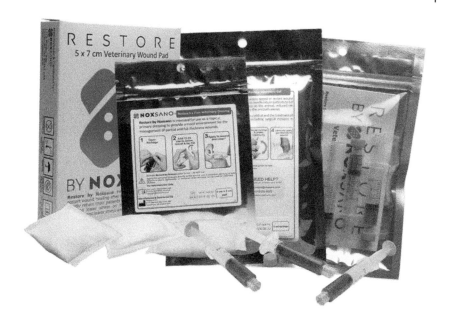

Figure 7.6 Photograph of Nitric Oxide gel kit (Restore, Noxsano). *Source:* Courtesy of Jacob Adams.

of the wound. During the inflammatory stage, NO regulates cytokines such as IL-8, TGF-B1, and encourages migration of monocytes and neutrophils into the wound. Once in the proliferative phase, NO is reported to improve proliferation of keratinocytes, protect endothelial cells from apoptosis, and mediate the actions of vascular endothelial growth factor (VEGF). In the last phase of wound healing (maturation), NO is involved in fibroblast production and collagen deposition [65].

Specific Directions for Use

One commercial system available for use in veterinary patients (Noxsano®) has two formulations including a gel-based product and a wound pad. When using the wound gel (Restore™), tap water or saline is added to the dry mixture and mixed thoroughly. This gel is then applied to the wound or incision (Figure 7.6). An occlusive dressing can be applied over the gel to extend NO activity. Depending on secondary dressing, environmental conditions, the gel is reported to remain active for up to one week. Most veterinarians choose to leave the gel in place for two to four days.

Indication(s)

Reported indications for nitric oxide treatment includes healing surgical incisions or infected open wounds [65, 66]. To date, only one experimental veterinary study [67] has been performed which illustrated that the time to first granulation tissue was shorter and there was a higher contraction rate for NO-treated wounds when compared to control wounds.

Contraindications/Complications

The only known contraindication to NO wound treatments is in actively hemorrhaging wounds as nitric oxide is a vasodilatory compound that could intensify bleeding. No adverse side effects or reactions have been reported in human or experimental animal literature.

Miscellaneous Topicals

Multiple other topical substances have been reported in the literature (Table 7.3) but their use has not been rigorously investigated in veterinary medicine on clinical patients.

Table 7.3 Summary of miscellaneous topical treatments for wounds.

Substance	Proposed mechanism of action	Specific instructions for use	Indications	Concerns	References
Maltodextrin-ascorbic acid	Stimulated repair by increasing collagen turnover and TGF-β1 expression	Daily topical Application of maltodextrin -Ascorbic acid powder Covered with sterile gauze and noncompressive bandage	Tissue repair of **chronic wounds** by changing the stage of inflammation and modifying collagen turnover Directly through fibroblast response	None	[68, 69]
Maltodextrin Silver (Alginex, DeRoyal Industries) Maltodextrin (Multidex, DeRoyal Industries)	Chemotactant for wbc, macrophages, and fibroblasts (debridement antibacterial effects). Fibroblasts promote collagen formation, gel form also provides a moist environment	Daily application of gel, powder or foam depending on amount of exudate	Antibiotic-resistant or chronic wounds	None	
Acemannan/*Aloe vera*	Stimulates macrophages to secrete interleukin-1 (IL-1) and tumor necrosis factor-alpha (TNF-α) which stimulate proliferation of fibroblasts, development of epidermal cells, and collagen deposition.	Daily topical application with coverage by a bandage	Excessively exudative wounds (drying effect) Cell proliferation stimulated late (day 42) Recommended for full-thickness burns in pigs Lacerations, ulcers, abrasions Enhances contraction and epithelialization of paw wounds in dogs and stimulates granulation tissue formation over exposed bone	Delays granulation tissue formation	[13, 70–72]
Tripeptide copper complex	Activator of tissue remodeling growth factor, chemotactic agent Direct angiogenic effect by eliciting migration of inflammatory cells and enhancing mobility of the endothelium.	Intra-articular injections were given from week 2, once a week, for four weeks Daily topical application with bandage	Increased neovascularization increased epithelialization and collagen deposition accelerated wound contraction Improving the acute wound environment by increasing proteinases.	None	[73–77]
Chitosan (native hydrogel) Polymeric biomaterial obtained by the deacetylation of chitin from crustacean shells	Promote hemostasis (platelet adhesion and aggregation), antibacterial (disrupting cell walls, cell membranes) Promotes proliferation of granulation tissue (secretion of TGF-β, PDGF, and IL-1)	Most commonly a component of hydrogel dressings/gels	Burns, infected, chronic wounds	Do not use in patients with shellfish allergies	[78, 79]
Becaplermin 0.01% Regranex® gel homodimeric protein	Platelet-derived growth factor Promotion of chemotactic recruitment and the proliferation of cells	Applied once daily	Diabetic ulcers Chronic wounds	Not useful in wounds with gross debris and necrotic tissue	[80, 81]

References

1 Campbell, B.G. (2006). Dressings, bandages, and splints for wound management in dogs and cats. *Vet. Clin. North Am. Small Anim. Prac.* 36 (4): 759–791.

2 Hosgood, G. (2018). Open wounds. In: *Veterinary Surgery: Small Animal Expert Consult*, 2e (ed. S.A. Johnston and K.M. Tobias), 1410–1421. St. Louis, MO: Elsevier Health Sciences (US).

3 Nuutila, K. and Eriksson, E. (2021). Moist wound healing with commonly available dressings. *Adv. Wound Care* 10: 685–698.

4 Geng, J., Cai, Y., Lu, H. et al. (2023). Moist dressings in the treatment of pressure injuries: a network meta-analysis. *J. Tissue Viability* 32 (2): 213–227.

5 Yamashita, Y., Ohzuno, Y., Saito, Y. et al. (2023). Autoclaving-triggered hydrogelation of chitosan-gluconic acid conjugate aqueous solution for wound healing. *Gels* 9 (4): 280.

6 Seaman, S. (2002). Dressing selection in chronic wound management. *J. Am. Podiatr. Med. Assoc.* 92 (1): 24–33.

7 Bolton, L.L., Monte, K., and Pirone, L.A. (2000). Moisture and healing: beyond the jargon. *Ostomy Wound Manage.* 46 (Suppl 1A): 51S–62S.

8 Hutchinson, J.J. and Lawrence, J.C. (1991). Wound infection under occlusive dressings. *J. Hosp. Infect.* 17 (2): 83–94.

9 Slavkovic, M., Zivanovic, D., Dučić, S. et al. (2023). Comparison of negative pressure wound therapy (NPWT) and classical wet to moist dressing (WtM) in the treatment of complicated extremity wounds in children. *Children* 10 (2): 298.

10 Morgan, P.W., Binnington, A.G., Miller, C.W. et al. (1994). The effect of occlusive and semi-occlusive dressings on the healing of acute full-thickness skin wounds on the forelimbs of dogs. *Vet. Surg.* 23 (6): 494–502.

11 Ramsey, D.T., Pope, E.R., Wagner-Mann, C. et al. (1995). Effects of three occlusive dressing materials on healing of full-thickness skin wounds in dogs. *Am. J. Vet. Res.* 56 (7): 941–949.

12 Kannon, G.A. and Garrett, A.B. (1995). Moist wound healing with occlusive dressings: a clinical review. *Dermatol. Surg.* 21 (7): 583–590.

13 Dart, A.J., Dowling, B.A., and Smith, C.L. (2005). Topical treatments in equine wound management. *Vet. Clin. North Am. Equine Prac.* 21 (1): 77–89.

14 Hebert, A. (2021). A new therapeutic horizon in diaper dermatitis: novel agents with novel action. *Int. J. Womens Dermatol.* 7 (4): 466–470.

15 Abendrot, M. and Kalinowska-Lis, U. (2018). Zinc-containing compounds for personal care applications. *Int. J. Cosmet. Sci.* 40 (4): 319–327.

16 Nolan, V.C., Harrison, J., Wright, J.E.E., and Cox, J.A.G. (2020). Clinical significance of Manuka and medical-grade honey for antibiotic-resistant infections: a systematic review. *Antibiotics* 9 (11): 766.

17 Tan, H.T., Rahman, R.A., Gan, S.H. et al. (2009). The antibacterial properties of Malaysian tualang honey against wound and enteric microorganisms in comparison to Manuka honey. *BMC Complement Altern. Med.* 9: 34.

18 Singh, A. and Weese, J.S. (2018). Wound infections and antimicrobial use. In: *Veterinary Surgery: Small Animal Expert Consult*, 2e (ed. S.A. Johnston and K.M. Tobias), 148–155. St. Louis, MO: Elsevier Health Sciences (US).

19 French, V.M., Cooper, R.A., and Molan, P.C. (2005). The antibacterial activity of honey against coagulase-negative staphylococci. *J. Antimicrob. Chemother.* 56: 228.

20 Bang, L.M., Buntting, C., and Molan, P. (2003). The effect of dilution on the rate of hydrogen peroxide production in honey and its implications for wound healing. *J. Altern. Complement Med.* 9: 267.

21 Albaridi, N.A. (2019). Antibacterial potency of honey. *Int. J. Microbiol.* 2019: 2464507. https://doi.org/10.1155/2019/2464507.

22 White, J.W. Jr., Subers, M.H., and Schepartz, A.I. (1963). The identification of inhibine, the antibacterial factor in honey, as hydrogen peroxide and its origin in a honey glucose-oxidase system. *Biochim. Biophys. Acta* 73: 57.

23 Girma, A., Seo, W., and She, R.C. (2019). Antibacterial activity of varying UMF-graded Manuka honeys. *PLoS One* 14 (10): e0224495. https://doi.org/10.1371/journal.pone.0224495.

24 Bardy, J., Slevin, N.J., Mais, K.L. et al. (2008). A systematic review of honey uses and its potential value within oncology care. *J. Clin. Nurs.* 17: 2604.

25 Jull, A., Walker, N., Parag, V. et al. (2008). Randomized clinical trial of honey-impregnated dressings for venous leg ulcers. *Br. J. Surg.* 95: 175.

26 Wijesinghe, M., Weatherall, M., Perrin, K. et al. (2009). Honey in the treatment of burns: a systematic review and meta-analysis of its efficacy. *N. Z. Med. J.* 122: 47.

27 Jull AB, Rodgers A, Walker N. Honey as a topical treatment for wounds. *Cochrane Database Syst. Rev.* 2008;(4) [CD005083]. https://doi.org/10.1002/14651858.CD005083.

28 Kodie, D.O., Oyetayo, N.S., Aina, O.O., and Eyarefe, O.D. (2022). Nigeria bee honey-enhanced adherence, neovascularisation and epithelisation of full-thickness skin autografts on distal extremities of dogs. *BMC Vet. Res.* 18 (1): 94.

29 Brennan, M. and Belshaw, Z. (2020). Does Manuka honey improve the speed of wound healing in dogs? *Vet. Rec.* 187 (1): 30.

30 Repellin, R.L., Pitt, K.A., Lu, M. et al. (2021). The effects of a proprietary Manuka honey and essential oil hydrogel on the healing of acute full-thickness wounds in dogs. *Vet. Surg.* 50 (8): 1634–1643.

31 Alshehabat, M., Hananeh, W., Ismail, Z.B. et al. (2020). Wound healing in immunocompromised dogs: a comparison between the healing effects of moist exposed burn ointment and honey. *Vet. World* 13 (12): 2793–2797.

32 Vogt, N.A., Vriezen, E., Nwosu, A., and Sargeant, J.M. (2021). A scoping review of the evidence for the medicinal use of natural honey in animals. *Front. Vet. Sci.* 7: 618301. https://doi.org/10.3389/fvets.2020.618301.

33 Willix, D.J., Molan, P.C., and Harfoot, C.G. (1992). A comparison of the sensitivity of wound-infecting species of bacteria to the antibacterial activity of Manuka honey and other honey. *J. Appl. Bacteriol.* 73 (5): 388–394. https://doi.org/10.1111/j.1365-2672.1992.tb04993.x.

34 Ranzato, E., Martinotti, S., and Burlando, B. (2012). Epithelial mesenchymal transition traits in honey-driven keratinocyte wound healing: comparison among different honeys. *Wound Repair Regener.* 20 (5): 778–785.

35 Majtan, J. (2011). Methylglyoxal-a potential risk factor of Manuka honey in healing of diabetic ulcers. *Evid. Based Complement Alternat. Med.* 2011: 295494. https://doi.org/10.1093/ecam/neq013.

36 Le, V.V.H. and Jasna, R.J. (2021). Nitrofurans: revival of an "old" drug class in the fight against antibiotic resistance. *PLoS Pathog.* 17 (7): e1009663. https://doi.org/10.1371/journal.ppat.1009663.

37 Mercer, M.A. Nitrofurans Use in Animals. Rahway, NJ: Merck & Co. https://www.merckvetmanual.com/pharmacology/antibacterial-agents/nitrofurans-use-in-animals (accessed 20 May 2023).

38 Coffey, R.P., Rice, T.L., and Thomson, P.D. (1991). Effect of blood and serum on in vitro antibacterial activity of nitrofurazone. *Am. J. Hosp. Pharm.* 48 (7): 1496–1499. https://doi-org.proxy.library.cornell.edu/10.1093/ajhp/48.7.1496.

39 Bagheri, T., Fatemi, M.J., Hosseini, S.A. et al. (2017). Comparing the effects of topical application of honey and nitrofurazone ointment on the treatment of second-degree burns with limited area: a randomized clinical trial. *Med. Surg. Nurs. J.* 5 (4): 22–30.

40 IARC. (1990). IARC Working Group on the Evaluation of Carcinogenic Risks to Humans. Pharmaceutical Drugs. Lyon: International Agency for Research on Cancer (IARC Monographs on the Evaluation of the Carcinogenic Risks to Humans, No. 50). Nitrofural (Nitrofurazone). https://www.ncbi.nlm.nih.gov/books/NBK526235 (accessed 20 May 2023).

41 Saydam, M., Yilmaz, S., Seven, E. et al. (2006). The effects of topically applied nitrofurazone and rifamycin on wound healing. *Wounds Compendium Clin. Res. Prac.* 18 (3): https://www.hmpglobballearningnetwork.com/site/wounds/article/5471.

42 Nguyen, R., Khanna, N.R., Safadi, A.O. et al. (2023). Bacitracin topical. In: *StatPearls*. Treasure Island, FL: StatPearls Publishing https://www.ncbi.nlm.nih.gov/books/NBK536993.

43 Stone, K.J. and Strominger, J.L. (1971). Mechanism of action of bacitracin: complexation with metal ion and C_{55}-isoprenyl pyrophosphate. *Proc. Natl. Acad. Sci.* 68 (12): 3223–3227.

44 Johnson, B.A., Anker, H., and Meleney, F.L. (1945). Bacitracin: a new antibiotic produced by a member of the B. subtilis group. *Science* 102 (2650): 376–377.

45 Katz, B.E. and Fisher, A.A. (1987). Bacitracin: a unique topical antibiotic sensitizer. *J. Am. Acad. Dermatol.* 17 (6): 1016–1024.

46 Saryan, J.A., Dammin, T.C., and Bouras, A.E. (1998). Anaphylaxis to topical bacitracin zinc ointment. *Am. J. Emerg. Med.* 16 (5): 512–513.

47 Sood, A. and Taylor, J.S. (2003). Bacitracin: allergen of the year. *Am. J. Contact Dermatol.* 14 (1): 3–4.

48 Lee, A.H., Swaim, S.F., McGuire, J.A., and Hughes, K.S. (1987). Effects of nonadherent dressing materials on the healing of open wounds in dogs. *J. Am. Vet. Med. Assoc.* 190 (4): 416–422.

49 Oaks, R.J. and Cindass, R. (2023). Silver sulfadiazine. In: *StatPearls*. Treasure Island, FL: StatPearls Publishing https://www.ncbi.nlm.nih.gov/books/NBK556054.

50 Fox, C.L. and Modak, S.M. (1974). Mechanism of silver sulfadiazine action on burn wound infections. *Antimicrob. Agents Chemother.* 5 (6): 582–588.

51 Durán, N., Durán, M., de Jesus, M.B. et al. (2016). Silver nanoparticles: a new view on mechanistic aspects on antimicrobial activity. *Nanomedicine* 12 (3): 789–799.

52 Modak, S.M., Sampath, L., and Fox, C.L. (1988). Combined topical use of silver sulfadiazine and antibiotics as a possible solution to bacterial resistance in burn wounds. *J. Burn Care Rehabil.* 9 (4): 359–363.

53 Lo, S.F., Hayter, M., Chang, C.J. et al. (2008). A systematic review of silver-releasing dressings in the management of infected chronic wounds. *J. Clin. Nurs.* 17 (15): 1973–1985.

54 Hadrup, N., Sharma, A.K., and Loeschner, K. (2018). Toxicity of silver ions, metallic silver, and silver nanoparticle materials after in vivo dermal and mucosal surface exposure: a review. *Regul. Toxicol. Pharm.* 98: 257–267.

55 Fong, J., Wood, F., and Fowler, B. (2005). A silver coated dressing reduces the incidence of early burn wound cellulitis and associated costs of inpatient treatment: comparative patient care audits. *Burns* 31: 562.

56 MacPhail, C. and Radlinsky, M.A. (2019). Surgery of the integumentary system. In: *Small Animal Surgery*, 5e (ed. T.W. Fossum), 179–204. Philadelphia, PA: Elsevier Health Sciences (US).

57 Aziz, Z., Abu, S.F., and Chong, N.J. (2012). A systematic review of silver-containing dressings and topical silver agents (used with dressings) for burn wounds. *Burns* 38 (3): 307–318.

58 Storm-Versloot, M.N., Vos, C.G., Ubbink, D.T., and Vermeulen, H. (2010). Topical silver for preventing wound infection. *Cochrane Database Syst. Rev.* (3): CD006478. https://doi.org/10.1002/14651858.

59 American College of Veterinary Pharmacists (2011). Propylene Glycol [Internet], Bartlett, TN, USA. https://vetmeds.org/pet-poison-control-list/propylene-glycol/#!form/PPCDonations (accessed 20 May 2023).

60 Oropallo, A. and Andersen, C.A. (2023). Topical oxygen. In: *StatPearls*. Treasure Island, FL: StatPearls Publishing https://www.ncbi.nlm.nih.gov/books/NBK574579.

61 Gordillo, G.M. and Sen, C.K. (2003). Revisiting the essential role of oxygen in wound healing. *Am. J. Surg.* 186 (3): 259–263.

62 Schreml, S., Szeimies, R.M., Prantl, L. et al. (2010). Oxygen in acute and chronic wound healing. *Br. J. Dermatol.* 163 (2): 257–268.

63 Oropallo, A.R., Serena, T.E., Armstrong, D.G., and Niederauer, M.Q. (2021). Molecular biomarkers of oxygen therapy in patients with diabetic foot ulcers. *Biomolecules* 11 (7): 925. https://doi.org/10.3390/biom11070925.

64 Fries, R.B., Wallace, W.A., Roy, S. et al. (2005). Dermal excisional wound healing in pigs following treatment with topically applied pure oxygen. *Mutat. Res.* 579 (1–2): 172–181.

65 Pinto, R.V., Carvalho, S., Antunes, F. et al. (2022). Emerging nitric oxide and hydrogen sulfide releasing carriers for skin wound healing therapy. *ChemMedChem* 17 (1): e202100429. https://doi.org/10.1002/cmdc.202100429.

66 Krausz, A. and Friedman, A.J. (2015). Nitric oxide as a surgical adjuvant. *Future Sci. OA* 1 (1): FSO56. https://doi.org/10.4155/fso.15.56.

67 Rodriguez-Diaz, J.M., Wallace, M.L., Emond, S.A., and Howerth, E.W. (n.d.). Effect of hydrocolloid-nitric oxide wound dressings on wound healing in dogs. *Proceedings of the 22nd Annual Scientific Meeting of the Society of Veterinary Soft Tissue Surgery* (15–17 June 2023). Jacksonville Beach, FL, USA.

68 Salgado, R.M., Cruz-Castañeda, O., Elizondo-Vázquez, F. et al. (2017). Maltodextrin/ascorbic acid stimulates wound closure by increasing collagen turnover and TGF-β1 expression in vitro and changing the stage of inflammation from chronic to acute in vivo. *J. Tissue Viability* 26 (2): 131–137.

69 Hartzell, L.D., Havens, T.N., Odom, B.H. et al. (2014). Enhanced tracheostomy wound healing using maltodextrin and silver alginate compounds in pediatrics: a pilot study. *Respir. Care* 59 (12): 1857–1862.

70 Iacopetti, I., Perazzi, A., Martinello, T. et al. (2020). Hyaluronic acid, Manuka honey and Acemannan gel: wound-specific applications for skin lesions. *Res. Vet. Sci.* 129: 82–89.

71 Maenthaisong, R., Chaiyakunapruk, N., Niruntraporn, S., and Kongkaew, C. (2007). The efficacy of Aloe vera used for burn wound healing: a systematic review. *Burns* 33 (6): 713–718.

72 Liu, C., Cui, Y., Pi, F. et al. (2019). Extraction, purification, structural characteristics, biological activities and pharmacological applications of Acemannan, a polysaccharide from Aloe vera: a review. *Molecules* 24 (8): 1554. https://doi.org/10.3390/molecules24081554.

73 Fu, S.C., Cheuk, Y.C., Chiu, W.Y. et al. (2015). Tripeptide-copper complex GHK-Cu (II) transiently improved healing outcome in a rat model of ACL reconstruction. *J. Orthop. Res.* 33 (7): 1024–1033.

74 Gul, N.Y., Topal, A., Cangul, I.T., and Yanik, K. (2008). The effects of topical tripeptide copper complex and helium-neon laser on wound healing in rabbits. *Vet. Dermatol.* 19 (1): 7–14.

75 Cangul, I.T., Gul, N.Y., Topal, A., and Yilmaz, R. (2006). Evaluation of the effects of topical tripeptide-copper complex and zinc oxide on open-wound healing in rabbits. *Vet. Dermatol.* 17 (6): 417–423.

76 Canapp, S.O. Jr., Farese, J.P., Schultz, G.S. et al. (2003). The effect of topical tripeptide-copper complex on healing of ischemic open wounds. *Vet. Surg.* 32 (6): 515–523.

77 Swaim, S.F., Vaughn, D.M., Kincaid, S.A. et al. (1996). Effect of locally injected medications on healing of pad wounds in dogs. *Am. J. Vet. Res.* 57 (3): 394–399.

78 Feng, P., Yang, L., Ke, C. et al. (2021). Chitosan-based functional materials for skin wound repair: mechanisms and applications. *Front. Bioeng. Biotechnol.* 9: 650598. https://doi.org/10.3389/fbioe.2021.650598.

79 Mohan, K., Ganesan, A.R., Muralisankar, T. et al. (2020). Recent insights into the extraction, characterization, and bioactivities of chitin and chitosan from insects. *Trends Food Sci. Technol.* 105: 17–42. https://doi.org/10.1016/j.tifs.2020.08.016.

80 Papanas, N. and Maltezos, E. (2008). Becaplermin gel in the treatment of diabetic neuropathic foot ulcers. *Clin. Interv. Aging* 3 (2): 233–240.

81 Margolis, D.J., Bartus, C., Hoffstad, O. et al. (2005). Effectiveness of recombinant human platelet-derived growth factor for the treatment of diabetic neuropathic foot ulcers. *Wound Repair Regener.* 13: 531–536.

8

Wound Dressings

Nicole J. Buote

Department of Clinical Sciences, Cornell University, Ithaca, NY, USA

Moist Wound Healing

As discussed in Chapter 7, moist wound environments have been shown to encourage wound healing through multiple different physiological mechanisms. While the number of wound dressings continues to grow, the general characterization of these primary contact layers can be helpful in determining which type of dressing to use at what point in wound healing. No one dressing is best all the time in every case. As a brief description, moist wound healing includes topicals and dressings that have a low moisture vapor transmission rate (MVTR), meaning low water loss and high moisture retention, on the wound surface. These dressings may decrease infection rates and encourage autolytic debridement and epithelialization but also increase the number of bandage changes as maceration of surrounding tissue can occur [1–3]. Dressings with a MVTR of $<35\,g/m^2/h$ are typically considered moisture retentive with hydrocolloids averaging 11 compared to weaved gauze averaging 67 [4]. One of the benefits of dressings that have a MVTR close to the transepidermal water loss measurement of uninjured skin (4–$9\,g/m^2/h$) is stability of moisture across adjacent uninjured skin and the wound bed.

The mechanisms that improve wound healing in a moist environment are multifactorial. Wound fluid has been shown to provide proteases, protease inhibitors, growth factors, and cytokines that aid in cell proliferation and repair [4, 5]. When fluid is allowed to remain in contact with the wound bed, white blood cells can perform autolytic debridement of microscopic debris and bacteria [1, 6]. When occlusive dressings are used to contain wound fluid, a low oxygen tension occurs which encourages collagen formation and discourages bacterial growth [7, 8]. Waterproof moisture retentive dressings (MRDs) also create a barrier against nosocomial bacterial contamination, urine, feces, or other environmental products. Interestingly, MRDs such as hydrogels have been associated with less scarring [9, 10] and decreased aerosolization of bacteria during bandage changes [11].

Characterization of Dressings

A continuous onslaught of new wound dressing products awaits any veterinarian treating wounds in clinical practice [4, 12–14]. The complexity of when to choose what dressing and for which patient leads many clinicians to give up and treat all the wounds, at every stage, with one or two products (honey most times). While stocking every product mentioned in this chapter would be unreasonable, the author encourages clinicians to have access to one dressing from each category and to note that many dressings do have multiple uses and therefore can be used in multiple scenarios.

In this chapter, primary contact wound dressings are defined as any physical dressing (not liquid or semisolid) that is placed directly onto a wound surface. These dressings can be categorized in many ways, but we will classify them as adherent, non-adherent, absorbent, moisture retentive, antimicrobial, bioelectric, and xenograft based on previous references (Table 8.1). The use of the descriptor semiocclusive denotes that a material is permeable to gas but not water or bacteria. Many dressings not included in this discussion exist and will be invented, but the author has tried to include the most commonly used dressings sited in veterinary literature and through decades of experience.

Techniques in Small Animal Wound Management, First Edition. Edited by Nicole J. Buote.
© 2024 John Wiley & Sons, Inc. Published 2024 by John Wiley & Sons, Inc.
Companion website: www.wiley.com/go/buote/wounds

Table 8.1 Characteristics of primary wound dressings.

Dressing type	Adherent (Y/N)	Fluid absorption features	Debridement type	Notes	Best wound type
Woven gauze and lap sponges	Yes (unless soaked)	Absorbs	Mechanical	– Adherence can remove healthy tissue (nonselective) – Can be used as a secondary layer for highly exudative wounds – Not recommended for use as a primary contact layer in majority of wounds – Require daily bandage changes	Grossly contaminated Moderately exudative
Non-adherent Dry porous Semiocclusive (Telfa)	N	Minimal	N/A	– Each side covered in non-adherent film surrounding a lightly absorbent cotton pad	Primarily sutured wounds Small, granulated wounds if used with a hydrogel Minimally exudative
Non-adherent Petrolatum-impregnated Semiocclusive (Adaptic)	N	None-flows through to secondary layer	N/A	– Tissue ingrowth a concern if not covered in occlusive ointment – Petrolatum may decrease epithelialization	Primarily sutured wounds Skin grafts Minimally exudative
Hypertonic saline (Molnlycke Mesalt®, Kendall Curasalt™)	Yes (unless soaked)	Absorbs	Desiccation (osmotic debridement)	– Create osmotic effect drawing fluid from wound (nonselective debridement) – Decreases wound tissue edema – Only use with highly exudative wounds	Infected or necrotic Highly exudative
Calcium alginate	Yes (until turns into a gel)	Absorbs	Autolytic	– Derived from seaweed – Felt-like sheet turns into a gel – Hemostatic – Antibacterial effects from autolytic debridement and trapping bacteria in gel – Gel may appear purulent (not infection)	Moderate to highly exudative Infected (not necrotic)
Hydrocolloid foams	N	Absorbs	Autolytic	– Can be placed over other dressings for improved moisture retention	Inflammatory phase (encourages formation of granulation tissue) Mildly exudative (can be used as a secondary layer)
Hydrocolloid + polyurethane sheet Occlusive (Coloplast, Comfeel)	N	Absorbs	Autolytic	– Protects the wound from friction – Blocks entry of exogenous bacteria – Change when fluid-filled blister appears	Superficial wounds (split-thickness skin graft donor site) Granulation tissue needed Epithelialization needed – stimulate angiogenesis and collagen synthesis

Dressing	Antimicrobial	Absorption	Debridement	Properties	Indications
Polyurethane foam (Kendall hydrophilic foam; Mölnlycke Mepilex)	N	Absorbs	Autolytic	- Soft and absorbent - If becomes dry can incorporate tissue and damage wound when removed	Moderate to Highly exudative (can be used as a secondary layer) Full-thickness inflammatory phase wounds Mild protection against pressure Epithelialization needed
Polyurethane film (3M Tegaderm)	Y	None	Autolytic	- Transparency allows for wound monitoring - Wound fluid may appear purulent (not infection)	
Silver impregnated foam (Genewel Medifoam® Silver; Smith & Nephew Allevyn® AG; Mölnlycke Mepilex AG; Ferris Polymem® Silver)	N	Absorbs	Autolytic	- Antibacterial effects due to silver ions and autolytic effects - Tissue ingrowth can occur with some pore sizes	Infected wounds (especially *Staph, Pseudomonas, Enterococcus,* and *Candida*) Wounds at high risk for becoming infected Chronic wounds in which matrix metalloproteinase may be present
Honey impregnated dressing (Medihoney® Calcium alginate + honey dressing or honey colloid; First Honey® dressings, bandages)	N	Minimal (depending on formulation)	Autolytic	- Antibacterial (hydrogen peroxide content, hyperosmotic effect, low pH, and inhibin content) - Encourages autolytic debridement - Osmotic diuretic (decreases edema) - Encourages granulation tissue and possibly epithelialization	- Best for wounds prior to granulation tissue or multidrug-resistant wounds - Mildly exudative depending on formulation
PHMB (Covidien Curity™ AMD strips or sponges, Kendall AMD foam)	N	Moderate	Possible autolytic if moist wound environment promoted	- Antiseptic action leads to reduction in DNA replication and cell wall damage - No known bacterial resistance - Possible carcinogen	- Best for wounds with confirmed infections - Causes mild cytotoxicity to normal healing cells so best to be discontinued when infection cleared
Nitric oxide producing dressing (Noxsano restore wound pad)	N	Minimal (depending on formulation)	Autolytic	- Regulates cytokines (IL-8, TGF-B1) - Supports migration of monocytes and neutrophils - Mediates the actions of vascular endothelial growth factor (VEGF) - Involved in fibroblast production and collagen deposition	- Surgical incisions - Infected open wounds - Inflammatory phase - Do not use in actively bleeding wounds

(Continued)

Table 8.1 (Continued)

Dressing type	Adherent (Y/N)	Fluid absorption features	Debridement type	Notes	Best wound type
Bioelectric (Vomaris, Procellera Antimicrobial wound dressing)	N	None-minimal	None	- Antibacterial properties (disrupt electrostatic interactions for bacterial adhesion to surfaces; generate hypochlorous acid) - Prevention of biofilm formation - Increase keratinocyte migration and epithelialization	- Chronic and infected wounds - Wounds that epithelialization is needed (healthy granulation beds) - Split-thickness skin graft donor sites
Xenograft-porcine small intestinal submucosa (PSIS) (Avalon Medical, SIS+; Vetrix® BioSIS)	Incorporates	None-minimal (depends on thickness)	None	- Acellular biodegradable sterile bioscaffold - As the scaffold degrades, cytokines and growth factors are released which promote wound healing	- Should not be used in infected wounds - No evidence of significant wound healing advantages when used in acute cutaneous wounds
Xenograft-Cod skin (Kerecis MariGen™)	Incorporates	Low	Autolytic	- Available commercially as an acellular product - Contains Omega-3 fatty acids, collagen, elastin, laminin, lipids, fibrin, proteoglycans, and glycosaminoglycans - Creates a bacterial barrier - Pain-modulating effects.	- Should not be used in infected wounds - Burn patients - Inflammatory phase - Early or late repair phase - Best-suited for wounds after granulation tissue present
Xenograft-Tilapia skin	N	None	Autolytic	- Not available commercially - Stimulate proliferation and differentiation of fibroblasts and keratinocytes - Presence of piscidin 3 and 4 (antimicrobial activity) - Excellent adherence to wound surface (supports a moist wound environment) and - Decreases the chance of bacterial colonization	- Should not be used in infected wounds - Burn patients - Inflammatory phase - Early or late repair phase - Best-suited for wounds after granulation tissue present
Xenograft – Wharton's jelly matrix (Sanatela Matrix)	Incorporates	None-minimal	None	- Acellular extracellular matrix - Contains collagen, fibronectin, hyaluronic acid, and sulfated proteoglycan - Contains growth factors (IGF-1, FGF, TGF-βI, EGF).	- Should not be used in infected wounds - Best suited for wounds after granulation tissue observed to speed the rate of epithelialization and decrease scar tissue formation

Adherent Dressings – Woven Gauze and Lap Sponges

Mechanism of Action

Woven gauze (Figure 8.1) is one of the most common primary contact dressings used in veterinary medicine. Gauze has the capacity to absorb its own weight in exudate [15]. In recent years, wet-to-dry bandages have been discouraged due to their non-selective debridement and because the MVTR of moistened gauze is not low enough to classify these dressings as moisture retentive [4, 16]. In order for wet-to-dry bandages to remove debris, the wound surface must dry to some degree, which is counter to a moist wound healing environment.

Indications

Even with the disadvantages of woven gauze, they still have an important place in wound care. In the author's opinion, their use in highly exudative or contaminated wounds is still appropriate as a primary or secondary layer. Gauze and lap sponges (Figure 8.2) can absorb exudate efficiently, and their use is cost effective. Their use in the first days of wound management to remove grossly visible debris and purulent or serous exudate is still performed at many institutions.

Contraindications

Woven gauze or lap sponges as a primary layer should be avoided in minimally exudative wounds, infected wounds that would be better treated with an antibacterial dressing, and in wounds with healthy granulation tissue as the material is drying and could damage healthy tissue when removed.

Specific Directions for Use

Sterile gauze and lap sponges should be used for wound dressings if possible, even if the wound appears grossly contaminated to avoid additional bacteria from entering the wound. One report found that within 30 seconds of adding saline to gauze, the material can become contaminated with environmental bacteria; therefore, sterile technique should be followed [17]. Packages are opened, and sterile saline is applied to moisten the gauze. The gauze/lap sponges should be wrung out slightly by a sterilely gloved hand so that they are not dripping wet before being applied to the wound. In cases of highly exudative wounds, dry gauze/lap sponges can be applied, but this is a rare occurrence. Bandage changes must be done on a regular basis depending on the amount of exudate or debris being produced. It is a delicate balance between ensuring the wound does not dry out but also is not overly saturated. In the author's experience, these bandages need to be changed at a minimum of once per day but sometimes require changes two to three times a day.

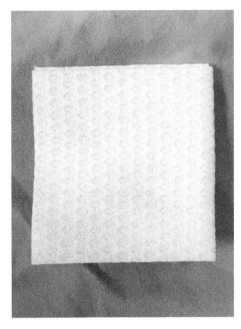

Figure 8.1 Photograph of a commonly used 3 × 3 in woven gauze. Some brands have a radio-opaque thread inserted which is helpful if the patient ingests the bandage material. Gauze can be used as a primary layer (during debridement) or as a secondary absorptive layer. *Source:* Courtesy of Nicole Buote, DVM, DACVS.

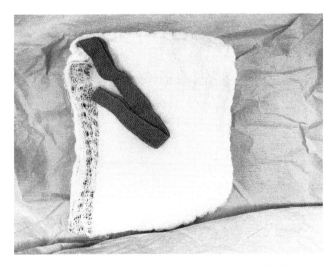

Figure 8.2 Photograph of lap sponges used in many highly exudative wounds as a primary layer (during wet-to-dry debridement) or as a secondary wicking layer. *Source:* Courtesy of Nicole Buote, DVM, DACVS.

Complications

Removal of healthy healing tissue and desiccation of the wound bed are the two most notable complications of using woven gauze/lap sponges as a primary layer for wounds. Special attention must be paid when determining when to change these dressings based on the wound environment.

Non-adherent Semiocclusive (Porous-Dry or Petrolatum-Impregnated)

Mechanism of Action

Non-adherent semiocclusive primary dressings are gentle on healing tissues but are minimally absorptive. The porous nature allows exudate to transfer to secondary layers; therefore, they should be covered by gauze, lap sponges, or hydrophilic foam if the wound is still creating moderate exudate. Regardless of their classification, these dressings can become adherent if exudate dries into the dressing or if tissue grows into the pores of the dressing; therefore, attention should be paid to using them at the appropriate stage of wound healing. These dressings can be further classified into dry forms (Telfa™) and petrolatum-impregnated (Adaptic™).

Dry Form – consists of a layer of absorbent material within a perforated thin film sleeve which decreases adhesion and allows exudate to be absorbed by the central layer or a secondary layer if needed (Figure 8.3).

Petrolatum-Impregnated – gauze impregnated by a petrolatum mixture. Larger pore sizes allow for more effective transfer of exudate through to secondary layers but also increase the chance of tissue ingrowth and adherence (Figure 8.4).

Indications

Dry Form – best used for superficial wounds in the late reparative phase with healthy granulation tissue present and low exudative wounds. They can also be used to cover sutured wounds for added protection.

Petrolatum-Impregnated – best suited for the early repair phase when moderate to significant exudate is produced, as a covering for mesh skin grafts and sutured incisions. The author primarily uses these dressings over meshed free skin grafts due to their low adherence and their ability to transfer exudate to secondary layers.

(a)

(b)

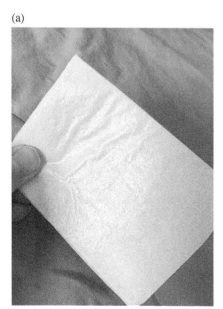
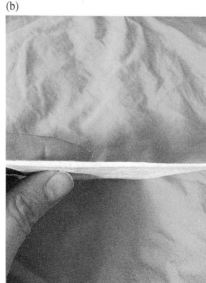

Figure 8.3 Photographs of a non-adherent Telfa pad. (a☺) Note the shine on the outer surface of the pad indicates the non-adherent coating; (b) side view of the pad shows a thin layer of absorbent material within the coated perforated film sleeve. This is an example of a "dry" non-adherent. *Source:* Courtesy of Nicole Buote, DVM, DACVS.

Figure 8.4 Photographs of a 5 × 9-in double-layer non-adherent Adaptic® dressing. (a,b) Note the large pore size and the shiny (petrolatum) coating. This is an example of a "petrolatum-impregnated" non-adherent dressing. *Source:* Courtesy of Nicole Buote, DVM, DACVS.

(a)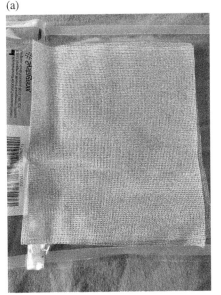

(b)

Contraindications

Dry Form – Do not use with highly exudative wounds as tissue maceration may occur. It is also not recommended for use in full-thickness open wounds or infected wounds as purulent exudate may be too gelatinous to traverse the pores.

Petrolatum-Impregnated – Do not use in full-thickness open wounds or infected wounds. Petrolatum is utilized to decrease tissue adherence, but some studies have theorized that some formulations delay epithelialization; therefore, their use should also be avoided once epithelialization has occurred [18, 19]. Wounds with exuberant granulation tissue should be avoided as the wide mesh can encourage tissue ingrowth.

Specific Directions for Use

These dressings should be placed on wounds after cleansing (if necessary) and can be placed with or without other topical dressings (antibiotic, hydrogel, etc.). Both dressings required some type of covering to keep them in place. This is most commonly a light, soft-padded bandage, but adhesive polyurethane films can also be used. Usually, these dressings are changed every five to seven days, but this depends on the stage of healing. If the dressing is adhering to the underlying tissue, the bandage should be changed more frequently or its use discontinued.

Complications

The most important complications seen with these dressings are tissue ingrowth and tissue desiccation/maceration. Appropriate placement and monitoring can decrease the rate of these complications. If a petrolatum-impregnated dressing becomes dry to the underlying wound, saline soaking may not aid in its removal as the material is hydrophobic, but saline may dissolve the exudate holding the dressing to the wound.

Absorbent

Absorbent dressings act in various ways to remove exudate from the wound surface. While gauze and lap sponges are also absorbent, the following dressings augment this characteristic with other advantages.

Hypertonic Saline

Mechanism of Action
Hypertonic saline dressings are formulated to include 20% sodium chloride [4]. They produce an osmotic effect drawing fluid from the wound bed into the dressing material. This effect can lead to desiccation of the wound bed if used inappropriately but can also decrease tissue edema which in turn improves perfusion.

Indications
Because the osmotic effects can lead to bacterial cell wall desiccation and cell death (osmotic debridement), these dressings are best suited for infected or highly exudative wounds. These dressings are absorptive but also antibacterial due to their osmotic debridement effect.

Contraindications
Osmotic debridement is not selective; therefore, healthy granulation tissue can also become damaged during this process.

Specific Directions for Use
These dressings are woven gauze squares or ribbons impregnated with sodium chloride. They usually require changes every one to two days due to the amount of exudate produced and can be placed within crevices or cavities and cut to size. They must be covered with an absorptive secondary layer.

Complications
Once the wound is cleared of infection, these dressings should be removed due to the risk of damage to healthy reparative tissue.

Calcium Alginate

Mechanism of Action
Calcium alginate hydrophilic dressings are one of the most versatile dressings available for wound care. These dressings are able to absorb 20–30 times their weight in fluid making them a great choice for highly exudative wounds [4]. They are derived from seaweed, using calcium, and sodium salts from alginic acid as their primary ingredients [20] and are manufactured as felt pads most commonly (Figure 8.5).

The felt dressings are transformed into a gel-like substance when sodium ions in wound exudate are exchanged with the calcium ions in the dressing [4]. This gel covers the wound bed, preserves a moist wound environment, and supports

(a)

(b)

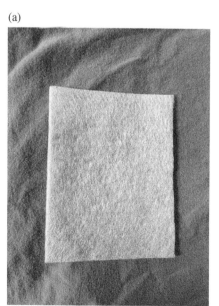

Figure 8.5 Photographs of a calcium alginate dressing. (a) Note the soft felt-like weave to this dressing; (b) close-up view highlights the materials weave which allows exudate to be absorbed and pass through to secondary layers as needed. This felt will be completely absorbed or turn into a yellow-red gel which is commonly mistaken for infectious exudate. *Source:* Courtesy of Nicole Buote, DVM, DACVS.

autolytic debridement, but the gel can appear like purulent exudate during bandage changes. Other than supporting autolytic debridement, the gel also exerts antibacterial properties by capturing bacteria so they cannot contaminate the wound [21, 22]. Calcium alginate also has hemostatic properties because calcium ions released from the dressing can activate prothrombin [23]. Some formulations have zinc added to the dressing, which supplements the hemostatic properties and encourages epithelialization.

Indications

Calcium alginate dressings can be used at many phases of wound healing due to their absorptive, moisture retentive, and antibacterial properties. These dressings can help wounds transition from the inflammatory phase to the repair phase because they promote autolytic debridement and encourage granulation tissue formation. They can be used in infected wounds as well due to their antibacterial properties.

Contraindications

As with any absorptive dressing, calcium alginates can dehydrate wound tissue if adequate exudate is not produced, or they are not premoistened. Minimal to no exudate wounds should not have calcium alginate applied as well as wounds that are grossly necrotic as autolytic debridement will not be sufficient in those cases.

Specific Directions for Use

These pads can be cut to size, placed within cavities and crevices, and are soft to the touch. Place these dressings into the wound bed dry and ensure good contact with the underlying wound but avoid contact with the peri-wound skin. If the wound is not exudative, it is best to moisten the dressing with saline to avoid eschar formation. If exudate production is significant, cover the dressing with an absorptive secondary layer (hydrophilic foam, lap sponges, etc.). Transformation into a gel usually requires two to four days depending on the wound phase; therefore, changes are not performed until exudate begins to strike through the outer layers.

The gel may appear purulent, and a foul odor may be present during bandage changes, but this is not evidence of infection. The gel may be gently cleansed from the wound with sterile saline, and fragments of dressing have been shown to break down into calcium ions and simple sugars, so they do not elicit a foreign body reaction [24].

Complications

In theory, if a patient suffers from a seaweed allergy, they may have a hypersensitivity reaction to these dressings. This has never been reported in veterinary medicine but has been reported in humans [25]. While calcium alginate felt dressings are soft, there have been reports in people of a burning sensation when placed in dry or minimally exudative wounds [26]. If these dressings are allowed to dry completely, a calcium eschar can form which is uncomfortable and can be difficult to remove without considerable rehydration.

Moisture Retentive Dressings

Polyurethane Foam

Mechanism of Action

Polyurethane foams are available as sheets in multiple thicknesses and sizes. They are soft and compressible and are usually created from polyurethane polymers (Figure 8.6). There are multiple different formulations with some having a MVTR as low as $33 \, g/m^2/h$ and others eight times that [6]. Due to these differences, it is important to check the manufacturer's label before purchase or use if a MRD is required. They can create an environment for autolytic debridement but are not as effective for necrotic or infected wounds as alginates or hydrocolloids.

Indications

Most commercially available foams are moisture retentive and highly absorptive making them useful in highly exudative wounds. They are especially valuable in wounds transitioning to the late repair phase (promoting epithelialization), so they are commonly placed after granulation tissue has formed. These foams create a moist wound environment by absorbing excess exudate but do not dry wounds out as long as some exudate is present or if they are premoistened with sterile saline.

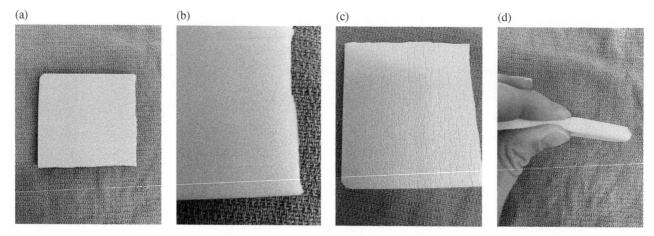

Figure 8.6 Photographs of a hydrocellular foam dressing. (a) This foam was originally 4 × 4 in but had been cut to size for a wound; (b) close up of the foam side which will be placed into the wound bed – note the small pore size which is excellent for absorbing exudate but preventing tissue ingrowth; (c) close up of the polyurethane film backing of this dressing – this feature provides a waterproof and breathable outer layer that protects the wound from environmental contamination; (d) these bandages are soft and compressible making them extremely comfortable for the patient. *Source:* Courtesy of Nicole Buote, DVM, DACVS.

Contraindications

Specific Directions for Use: The foam pads can be cut to size and come in a variety of formulations depending on the manufacturer. Some foam pads have a "top sheet" (Kendall™ Hydrophilic Foam) that prevents strike-through while allowing moisture vapor transmission. Some foams come with a silicone adhesive layer which is laid onto the surface of the wound (Mepilex®). This silicone surface helps the foam adhere to the skin but not to the wound bed; therefore, overlapping the wound edges by 2 cm is recommended to prevent peri-wound maceration.

Unlike calcium alginate dressings, foam dressings can overlap the peri-wound skin as they are strongly wicking and can remove any excess fluid that may macerate the adjacent healing tissue. While soft and absorbent, these dressings still need to be covered with a secondary layer if the wound is over a bony prominence or is highly exudative. Foams can also act as a secondary absorptive layer for other primary dressings. These dressings can be in place for three to seven days depending on the amount of exudate and the presence of strikethrough.

Complications

The only known complication to foam dressings is in cases of desiccation where tissue becomes incorporated into the material and is damaged during removal. Careful monitoring of the wound and rehydration of the foam prior to removal, if necessary, eliminates this complication.

Polyurethane Film

Mechanism of Action

Polyurethane films are semiocclusive thin dressings that allow transmission of water vapor to the environment or a secondary dressing. They usually have a MVTR of 12.5–33 g/m²/h making them moisture retentive and supportive of autolytic debridement [4, 27].

Indications

These dressings are non-absorptive; therefore, they are indicated only in wounds with minimal to no exudate such as abrasions or sutured wounds. Due to their MVTR, they can promote epithelialization in the late repair phase, especially if placed as a secondary layer to support moisture retention. These dressings also act as a barrier to environmental contamination and moisture.

Contraindications

These films are not intended for open, full-thickness or highly exudative wounds, as they are not absorptive and peri-wound tissue may become macerated quickly in these cases. These films should not be used in infected wounds as other primary dressings are more appropriate. Consideration of the discomfort with removal should be given when placing these dressings on sensitive or fragile skin.

Specific Directions for Use

These films have an adhesive perimeter, but veterinary patients' hair growth interferes with application without clipping adjacent fur. Polyurethane films are transparent allowing for wound monitoring after application (Figure 8.7). The film should cover the wound and 1–2 cm of adjacent peri-wound skin. Due to the adhesive nature of these films, they can be uncomfortable when removed. Changing these dressings occurs when exudate begins to leak, usually every three to seven days depending on the wound type [15]. As with calcium alginates, the wound exudate may turn a white or yellow color, and this is not indicative of infection but autolytic debridement.

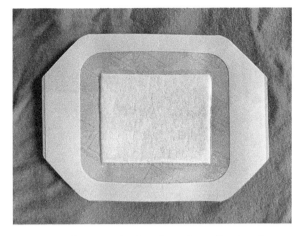

Figure 8.7 Photograph of a polyurethane film dressing (Tegaderm) with a non-adherent pad. This type of dressing is commonly placed over a sutured incision or superficial abrasion to prevent environmental contamination. *Source:* Courtesy of Nicole Buote, DVM, DACVS.

Complications

There are polyurethane films manufactured for use over intra-venous catheters that have a high MVTR and should not be confused with wound dressings. Those films create a dry environment and would lead to desiccation. The author has seen hypersensitivity reactions to the adhesives of these dressings in some patients. These reactions have been easily treated with topical antihistamines and time.

Hydrocolloid

Mechanism of Action

Hydrocolloids have many potential uses in wound management for veterinary patients. These dressings are usually produced as semi-sheer sheets with a backing impermeable to fluid, gas, and bacteria. Hydrocolloids are created from absorbent and elastomeric components which create a gel when contacting wound fluid [4, 13, 22, 27]. Formulations usually consist of moisture absorbing sodium carboxymethylcellulose (CMC) particles encapsulated in a synthetic adhesive/elastomer matrix (Coloplast, Comfeel®). The outer film is sometimes a semipermeable polyurethane film. These dressings are occlusive and create a moist and thermally insulated environment. The average MVTR of solid hydrocolloid dressings is less than $12.5 \, g/m^2/h$ meaning they are highly moisture retentive. They cannot, however, absorb large quantities of wound exudate. Hydrocolloids provide a moist wound environment that promotes autolytic debridement when adequate wound exudate is present.

Indications

Hydrocolloid dressings are best suited for wounds in the early repair phase as they stimulate angiogenesis and collagen synthesis, encouraging epithelialization [13]. Examples include sutured wounds, superficial partial-thickness wounds (split-thickness grafts), or wounds with healthy granulation tissue needing epithelialization. Hydrocolloids come in many different forms including foams, thin films, and those combined with alginates or other antimicrobials (Figure 8.8). Because they create a barrier to fluids, they are a good choice in areas that may be contaminated by feces or urine. One study by Abramo et al., investigating a hydrocolloid/polyurethane film dressing (Coloplast, Comfeel) on surgical wounds found it helped to avoid contamination and encourage epithelialization [28]. Two studies described the use of hydrocolloids in second-intention wound healing in cats, which are known to have decreased healing rates compared to dogs [29, 30]. The first study reported a subjectively accelerated formation of granulation tissue (p < 0.01) in the hydrocolloid-treated wounds [29]. The other study compared a hydrocolloid/polyurethane film dressing (Coloplast, Comfeel) to a semiocclusive dressing and observed no significant differences in subjective clinical evaluation or in planimetry. While no specific wound healing benefits were detected, the authors did note the hydrocolloid group did not require daily bandage changes, which simplified wound care and decreased cost [30].

(a)

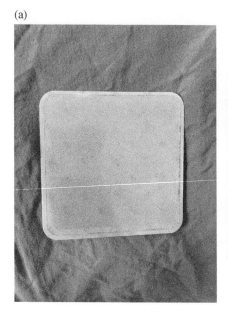

(b)

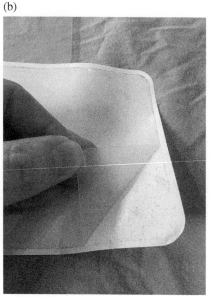

Figure 8.8   Photographs of a thin hydrocolloid dressing. (a) This dressing has a clear protective film and a sticky backing which will stick to the peri-wound skin around the wound bed. (b) This dressing is very thin and therefore not absorptive but does maintain a moist wound environment. It will "bubble" when excessive exudate forms underneath it alerting the clinician it needs to be changed. *Source:* Courtesy of Nicole Buote, DVM, DACVS.

Contraindications

Hydrocolloids are not suited to highly exudative wounds as the high moisture retention qualities will lead to maceration of adjacent skin. Hydrocolloids should not be used in infected wounds as their antimicrobial properties are mild (autolytic debridement), and the hypoxic environment they create may encourage anaerobic bacterial growth [31]. Using hydrocolloids in the late reparative phase may lead to delays in contraction so transitioning to other dressings once epithelialization is underway is advised.

Specific Directions for Use

When using a hydrocolloid foam or thin sheet, the material may be cut to a size slightly larger than the wound allowing overlap onto peri-wound skin. Hydrocolloids are adhesive even to damp tissues usually, but gentle pressure is required to attach the dressing to the peri-wound skin. Removal of a hydrocolloid dressing should not be done until a fluid-filled blister is noted above the wound, usually between three and seven days after placement. Removal at this point should not damage the wound because the dressing has partially dissolved into a gel. As with calcium alginate and polyurethane films, the gel may have a mild odor and a purulent appearance, but this is not an indication of infection.

Complications

Complications associated with hydrocolloid dressings include maceration or desiccation if wound environments are not monitored appropriately. Inappropriate placement over infected wounds may lead to worsening wound health, and delayed contraction can be seen if placed in the late reparative phase.

Antimicrobial

Antimicrobial dressings (AMDs) are a popular addition to wound management strategies. These dressings usually combine porous materials with agents that prevent infiltration of bacteria from the environment or eliminate organisms in the wound. The most commonly added antimicrobial agents are silver, honey, and polyhexamethylene biguanide (PHMB), but many other dressings can have antimicrobial effects as described in this chapter. The dressings in this section should be used for wounds with a confirmed infection or wounds in which an infection could be disastrous. Iodine-releasing dressings that act as s antiseptics exist but concerns over hypersensitivities and toxicities, especially in large wounds, make them less practical so they are not discussed.

Mechanism of Action

Silver-impregnated foams are available in many formulations including those used in negative pressure wound therapies (NPWTs), foams, combined with alginates, and rolls/pads (see Chapter 10) [13, 21, 22, 32, 33]. The antibacterial processes for silver-impregnated dressings may utilize silver sulfate particles or silver sulfadiazine within the polyurethane foam. Some dressings have a silicone wound contact layer, while others may have a polyurethane film [33]. When wound fluid contacts the silver components, silver ions are released which rupture bacterial cell walls, bind to bacterial enzymes arresting respiratory and nutritional processes, and disrupt bacterial replication. Silver ions may also decrease inflammation in the wound by reducing matrix metalloproteinase activity [6].

Indications

Silver-impregnated dressings are best suited for infected wounds, wounds that are at high risk of becoming infected, or chronic wounds in which matrix metalloproteinases may be active. These dressings can be effective against *Staphylococcus, Pseudomonas, Enterococcus,* and *Candidiasis* and produce less bacterial resistance and fewer adverse reactions [4, 33]. Silver dressings have also been shown to promote granulation tissue and epithelialization [33]. An experimental study by Lee et al. compared physicochemical and structural properties of available silver dressings and found all tested materials had excellent bactericidal effects against *Staphylococcus aureus* and *Pseudomonas aeruginosa* [33]. Veterinary studies relating to silver-based dressings have compared them to NPWT [34–36], or investigated their use for biofilm treatment [37], or as implant coatings [38].

Contraindications

Specific contraindications to the use of silver-impregnated wounds relate to the phase of healing and wound type. These dressings should not be used in wounds that are acute and without evidence of or risk for infection as the risk of resistance (while low) does exist. Depending on the type of silver dressing, the appropriate formulations should be used to maintain proper wound moisture balance.

Specific Directions for Use

As many different formulations of silver-impregnated dressings exist, it is important to follow manufacturer recommendations. In those dressings with a silicone adhesive layer (Mepilex Ag), counterintuitively, the adhesive layer must be applied to the wound surface (Figure 8.9). The silicone does not adhere to the wound surface but does gently adhere to the

(a)
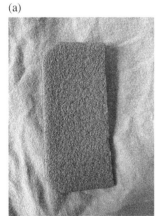
(b)
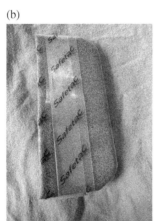
(c)
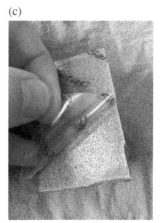
(d)
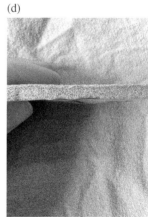

Figure 8.9 Photographs of a Mepilex Ag polyurethane foam impregnated with silver. (a) Note the soft appearance of the outer surface of the dressing. (b,c) The dressing has an adhesive silicone coating which needs to be placed toward the wound bed. This covering will stick to the peri-wound skin to protect it from exudate and maceration but will not stick to the wound bed. While it seems counterintuitive, the coating is also permeable to allow exudate to be absorbed by the foam. (d) Side view of the foam to illustrate the absorptive quality of this material. *Source:* Courtesy of Nicole Buote, DVM, DACVS.

peri-wound skin preventing it from becoming macerated in highly exudative scenarios. Overlap the wound edges by ~2 cm to facilitate security of the dressing, and change the bandage every three to seven days based on exudate level.

Complications

The only known complication to silver dressings is in cases of desiccation where tissue becomes incorporated into the material and is damaged during removal. Careful monitoring of the wound eliminates this complication.

Honey-Impregnated Dressings

Mechanism of Action

A detailed description of the antibacterial and anti-inflammatory mechanisms of honey is discussed in Chapter 7. Briefly, the antibacterial effects are due to the hydrogen peroxide and methylglyoxal content, the hyperosmotic effect, the low wound bed pH that is created, and the support for autolytic debridement honey provides by maintaining a moist wound environment. Promotion of granulation tissue occurs due to honey's antioxidant and glucose content as well as immunomodulating effects [13, 39, 40].

Indications

Honey has been incorporated into hydrocolloid, calcium alginate, and gauze formulations (Figure 8.10). Medical-grade honey dressings are best suited for wounds prior to granulation tissue or multidrug-resistant wounds, but honey has also been added to commercially available bandages marketed for cuts, scrapes, abrasions, and minor burns. The author uses these dressings most commonly during the inflammatory phase and early repair phase to maximize the anti-inflammatory and antimicrobial benefits but opts to discontinue their use once a healthy granulation bed exists or epithelialization has begun.

Contraindications

Honey dressings are not appropriate in the face of gross contamination and purulent material as the antibacterial action will be reduced when honey is diluted by body fluids at the site of infection. Honey dressings can encourage exudate creation due to the hyperosmotic effects, so they are combined with absorptive materials (foams, alginates) in many formulations. If combined with hydrocolloids which are not highly absorptive, they should only be placed on superficial minimally exudating wounds.

(a)

(b)

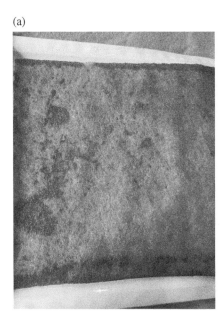 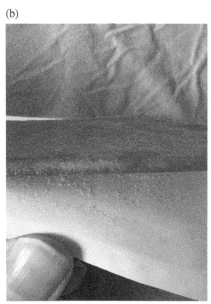

Figure 8.10 Photographs of a MediHoney® honey + calcium alginate dressing. (a) This dressing is sticky to the touch and firm and not particularly absorptive as the weave is saturated with honey. It will soften as exudate is absorbed but is uncomfortable until that point. The dressing can partially dissolve and turn into a purulent appearing gel depending on the amount of exudate the wound produces. (b) The side view illustrates the rigidity of the dressing and lack of absorptive qualities compared to other dressings. *Source:* Courtesy of Nicole Buote, DVM, DACVS.

Specific Directions for Use

If foam or alginate formulations are applied, the dressing should be cut to the size of the wound unless a silicone or other coating is present to prevent maceration of the peri-wound tissue. The honey alginate dressing is firm and not comfortable until it softens with exudate absorption. If the wound is full-thickness or highly exudative, an absorptive secondary layer must be placed to wick away wound fluid. Honey dressings should be changed every three to five days depending on exudate level.

Complications

The only known complication to honey dressings is in cases of desiccation or maceration. Careful monitoring of the wound eliminates this complication.

Polyhexamethylene Biguanide (PHMB)

Mechanism of Action

AMD in human wound care commonly utilize the antiseptic PHMB. The mechanism of action was initially thought to center around the ability of this cationic agent to destabilize bacterial cytoplasmic membranes irreversibly [4, 13]. Newer research concluded that PHMB does not create pores in the cell membrane as previously theorized, but instead translocation of PHMB across the bilayer may take place through binding to phospholipids. Once inside the cell, this polymer may effectively bind to DNA and block the replication process [41]. No known resistances have developed to PHMB meaning this compound has broad-spectrum control even against MRSA and vancomycin-resistant *Enterococcus*.

Indications

The best use for 0.2% PHMB dressings is for wounds with confirmed infections. Wounds with MRSA, vancomycin-resistant *Enterococcus*, gram+ and gram− bacteria, fungi, and yeast infections are candidates for treatment with PHMB. One *in vitro* veterinary study investigating PHMB-impregnated dressings illustrated a reduced number or elimination of bacterial pathogens within and underneath the dressing [42]. When the infection is cleared, this dressing should be discontinued.

Contraindications

These dressings should not be used in clean or non-infected wounds. Depending on the formulation, they may be mildly or moderately absorptive, but these dressings should not be used in grossly contaminated or necrotic wounds. While some studies report that PHMB does not negatively impact epithelization, there is known cytotoxicity to normal fibroblasts suggesting these bandages should not be used once infection is controlled.

Specific Directions for Use

PHMB dressings are available in rolls, gauze bandages, or impregnated into polyurethane foams. Follow manufacturer recommendations regarding placement and wound monitoring. In general, the antimicrobial effects can be seen for up to seven days. Dressing changes should be based on exudate production or peri-wound health.

Complications

No specific dressing-related complications have been reported in veterinary medicine. In human pharmaceuticals, there has been a carcinogenic warning attached to PHMB at doses higher than 0.3%, and in California, there is a Cancer and Reproductive Harm warning labeled on these products.

Bioelectric Dressings

Bioelectric dressings (BEDs) have been used in human medicine for diabetic ulcers, pressure sores, and burn injuries for many years. In veterinary medicine, they have been investigated for use in acute and chronic wounds. When skin is damaged, a change in the transepithelial resting electric potential occurs, stimulating cell migration and reepithelialization [12, 43, 44]. Wound fluid provides the conduction medium for microcurrents (2–10 mA) that are created at the edges of the wound, but this current only extends ~1–2 mm from the wound edge [45]. BEDs need to recreate this current across the entire wound to speed up wound healing.

Mechanism of Action

Most BEDs (Figure 8.11) mimic the physiologic currents created at wound edges by generating microcurrents on the wound surface in the presence of a conductive medium. Physiologic benefits of this dressing include antibacterial properties [43–48], prevention of biofilm formation [49], optimization of the moist wound environment, increase in keratinocyte migration (galvanotaxis) [50], and epithelialization [51, 52]. The antibacterial properties may be related to the fact that bacteria rely on electrostatic interactions for adhesion to surfaces and that electrical currents generate hypochlorous acid in *in vitro* studies [48].

One type of BED is a microcell battery-impregnated dressing (BED) such as the Procellera Antimicrobial wound dressing (Vomaris, Tempe, AZ, USA) which consists of a polyester substrate with embedded elemental silver and zinc microcell batteries. This dressing uses the generated electric fields from an open-circuit potential but has no direct current (DC) flow. These dressings are easy to apply and comfortable to wear. A second type of BED is the printed electroceutical dressing (PED) which uses DC with a battery pack as a source of electric potential. To the author's knowledge, no commercially available PED is on the market currently. The use of a DC has been shown to have inhibitory effects against gram+ and gram− bacteria, and one case report in a cat and a dog illustrated resolution of chronic infections and eventual wound healing [48].

Multiple studies on animal models have been performed to test BEDs [45, 48, 52]. One review reported encouraging wound healing results with DC and BEDs [45] but there were variable results. Studies tested different methods and polarities leading to faster rates of reepithelialization, increased wound collagen content, and improved angiogenesis in some but no improvement or even deleterious effects in others.

Indications

Studies in clinical veterinary patients (equine, canine, feline) have reported positive outcomes in traumatic chronic or infected wounds [46, 48, 53]. These clinical studies were retrospective and did not include control groups, but the wounds had failed typical management by the time a BED or PED was employed. The author has used these dressings on chronic and infected wounds in clinical cases with success and anecdotally agrees that epithelialization also seems to occur at a faster rate when the dressing is applied to healthy granulation tissue. BEDs have also been used in human medicine to cover skin graft donor sites and have been shown to produce faster healing, improved scarring, and improved patient subjective outcomes [51].

(a)   (b)   (c)

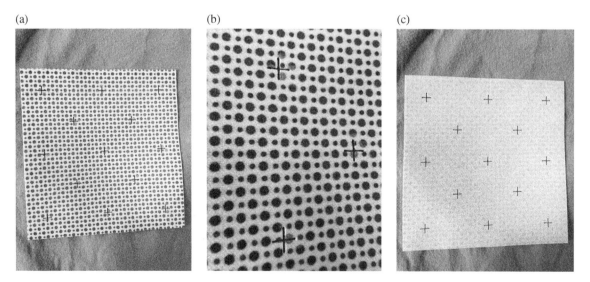

Figure 8.11 Photographs of a bioelectric dressing (Procellera). (a) The dressing can be cut to size and fenestrated as needed but manufacturer-placed fenestrations are present upon removal from the sterile packaging. (b) Close-up view of the silver and zinc microcells is visible on the surface of the dressing that should be in contact with the wound bed. (c) Outer surface of the dressing should be covered by a secondary layer to ensure adequate contact between the dressing and the wound bed. *Source:* Courtesy of Nicole Buote, DVM, DACVS.

There are no specific contraindications to the use of BED or PED, but the best use for them is in wounds in the late repair phase (after granulation tissue has formed) and with chronic or infected wounds. These bandages do require hydrogel or fluid to conduct electricity so any wound that must remain dry should not have a BED applied.

Directions for use of BEDs are described below; the author could not find a commercially available PED for use in veterinary patients. It is very important to moisten the dressing on battery (dot) side with saline, sterile water, or sterile amorphous water-based hydrogel. A hydrogel is supplied by the manufacturer, but this specific product is not necessary. Hydrogels are used as they will not evaporate as quickly, allowing the dressing to remain in place for up to seven days. Saline or water is also an excellent conductive medium, but these dry out more quickly and will require periodic remoistening if the wound is not creating sufficient exudate. Be careful not to oversaturate the dressing or wound maceration can occur. Place the dressing battery (dot) side down on the wound. Ensure contact with the wound. If the wound is a deep cavity, be sure to place material over the dressing to hold contact between the dressing and wound surface. You can cut the dressing to size, but the manufacturer recommends including 1–2 cm of dressing overlap on the wound edge.

The dressing is minimally absorptive so always cover it with a secondary dressing. If the wound is mildly exudative, a semiocclusive dressing can be applied (Tegaderm™). If the wound is highly exudative, an absorptive layer (hydrocolloid foam, gauze, lap sponges) can be applied. Dressing change frequency is determined by the amount of wound exudate produced. The dressing can remain in place for up to seven days if it is a low-exudative wound. If the wound is highly exudative, dressings can be changed every three to four days. If the dressing becomes adhered to the wound bed, moisten the dressing with sterile saline or water until it can be gently peeled away.

No complications have been reported with the use of BED in animal models or clinical reports. Tissue necrosis at the positive polarity [54], severe tissue reaction around electrodes [55], and delayed wound healing at the negative polarity [56] have been noted in experimental studies of PED dressings.

Xenograft Dressings

Xenograft dressings have been studied in many animal models and periodic clinical studies and include porcine small intestinal submucosa (PSIS), Wharton's jelly (WJ), and fish skin grafts. These dressings are theorized to supply collagen or growth factors to heal wounds, but clinical results are varied. Extracellular matrix dressings (PSIS, WJ) provide structural proteins, growth factors, cytokines, and their inhibitors in physiologic proportions [4, 27].

Porcine Small Intestinal Submucosa (PSIS)

Mechanism of Action
PSIS dressings are available in multiple formulations and thicknesses (Figure 8.12). Sheets can be delivered dry and then moistened or wet. These dressings are considered a bioscaffold and are acellular, biodegradable, and sterile. When placed in the wound, the scaffold is reportedly invaded by polymorphonuclear and mononuclear cells [57], and by day 3, angiogenesis occurs. As the scaffold degrades, cytokines and growth factors are released which promote wound healing. Studies have shown that the degradation products are chemotactic for repair cells, stimulate angiogenesis, and have antibacterial properties [58, 59].

Indications
In human medicine, PSIS bioscaffolds may be indicated in the inflammatory phase to encourage granulation tissue formation [22], but this has not been seen in experimental veterinary studies. Case reports and anecdotal evidence have described successful treatment of clinical wounds [27]. At this time, the author does not recommend its use in cutaneous wounds but has used it as an adjunct in abdominal procedures (bladder, hernia, and intestinal repairs).

(a)

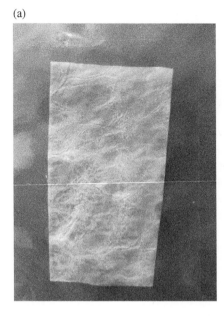

(b)

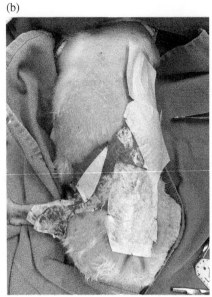

Figure 8.12 Photographs of porcine small intestinal submucosa (PSIS) dressings. (a) Single-ply dressing (Avalon Medical, SIS+™) in sterile packaging. This thickness will become a wet tissue paper consistency when moistened. (b) Patient with two different thicknesses of PSIS dressing applied to a large burn wound. In the center of the wound, single-layer sheets can be seen melting into the underlying wound bed while other locations have 4-ply sheets sutured to the wound edges. *Source:* Courtesy of Nicole Buote, DVM, DACVS.

Contraindications: Acute full-thickness wounds have not been shown to benefit from PSIS application [60, 61]. One experimental study in canines reported delayed contraction, decreased epithelialization, and increased acute inflammation after implantation compared to control wounds [61]. The other study investigating acute open wounds with bone exposure also reported no significant differences in wound healing between control wounds and wounds treated with PSIS. PSIS dressings should not be placed on infected wounds.

Specific Directions for Use

PSIS dressings should be cut to overlap the skin edges by ~1 cm. If using dry sheets, they should be rehydrated in sterile saline before application if the wound bed is not particularly moist. Sheets come in single, double, and 4-ply thickness. Depending on the thickness, the sheet may "melt" quickly to the consistency of tissue paper when wet so the author would recommend placing the sheet over the wound and then wetting it. The sheet can be sutured to the wound edges, but it is important that there is good contact between the wound bed and the PSIS (BC). If the wound is highly exudative, it is recommended that the sheet be fenestrated and a non-adherent or MRD placed over it. In theory, the PSIS is incorporated into the wound and is not removed at subsequent bandage changes. A purulent-appearing discharge can be seen at the first bandage change (days 3–4 post-placement), but this is not an indication of infection. Usually, bandages are changed every three to four days, and PSIS is only replaced or added to the wound until granulation tissue is observed [4].

Complications

No specific dressing-related complications have been reported with PSIS in veterinary medicine. The major disadvantages of PSIS are the cost and the lack of studies reporting evidence of improvement in wound healing.

Wharton's Jelly

Mechanism of Action

WJ is a gelatinous substance that rests between the amniotic epithelium and umbilical vessels. This substance contains high levels of proteoglycans and collagen and few mesenchymal stem cells (MSCs) [62]. Dressings with MSCs or that can attract MSCs have the advantage of applying multipotent cells directly into wounds and reportedly increase angiogenesis, increase epithelization, and decrease scar formation [63, 64]. MSC can be harvested from numerous anatomical locations including bone marrow, adipose tissue (ASC), and the umbilical cord. MSCs from adipose and bone marrow supplied in gel form have been previously investigated in veterinary wound models, but WJ has recently been applied to a sheet wound dressing [65]. After undergoing a patented processing technique that removes all cells, the remaining acellular extracellular matrix contains natural substances that support MSC colonization and replication including collagen, fibronectin, hyaluronic acid, and sulfated proteoglycan, as well as several growth factors, including insulin-like growth factor 1 (IGF-I), FGF, TGF-βI, and epidermal growth factor (EGF). These substances should recruit MSCs to the wound bed to assist in healing, thereby providing an advantage over pure collagen dressings (PSIS, fish skin grafts).

Indications

In human medicine, WJ seeded on the human acellular amniotic membrane has been successfully used to treat chronic, nonhealing diabetic ulcers [66]. In veterinary medicine, case reports of two dogs and one horse described successful treatment of chronic nonhealing wounds [67, 68] and an experimental controlled trial in acute wounds illustrated a higher percent epithelialization and better histologic repair scores in WJ-treated wounds compared to controls [65]. The improved histologic repair score was determined by evidence of increased fibroblast proliferation, collagen density, and neovascularization. Kierski et al. concluded that the WJ dressing is most useful once granulation tissue appears to speed the rate of epithelialization and decrease scar tissue formation [65].

Contraindications

In the one experimental study on acute wounds in veterinary medicine, there was not any advantage to the use of WJ dressings in the early inflammatory phase of healing (before granulation tissue); however, the application did not appear to inhibit this phase of wound healing either. Highly exudative wounds may require frequent reapplication of WJ dressings, which may be cost-prohibitive.

Specific Directions for Use

Application of WJ dressings should be performed after appropriate cleansing of the wound bed (Figure 8.13). As with PSIS, WJ dressings are incorporated into the wound bed and should not be removed at subsequent bandage changes. Additional dressings can be applied over the previous dressing if none is visible. The matrix comes as a felt-like sheet that melts into moist wound beds. If the wound bed is dry, a small amount of sterile saline or hydrogel can be applied. The WJ dressing should then be covered with a non-adherent (Telfa) bandage or an absorptive (hydrophilic foam) bandage if the wound is highly exudative. As the WJ dressing is incorporated, a purulent fluid may appear, but this is not indicative of infection. Bandage changes are timed based on exudate production to ensure a moist wound environment is maintained, usually every three to five days.

Complications

No specific wound-related complications have been reported with WJ dressing application. The reported WJ dressing [65] appeared biocompatible and was well-tolerated by the participants.

Figure 8.13 Photographs of novel Whart'n's jelly (WJ) dressing (Sanatela™ Matrix). (a) 2 × 2 cm sterile dressing – note the open weave formulation which is very soft and fragile. This dressing can tear easily during manipulation. (b) WJ dressing in a canine acute wound study – the dressing is saturated by blood or exudate easily, similar to calcium alginate, and becomes incorporated into the wound bed. *Source:* Courtesy of Nicole Buote, DVM, DACVS.

(a)
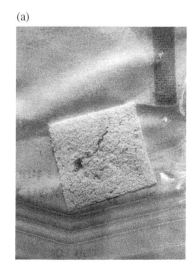

(b)
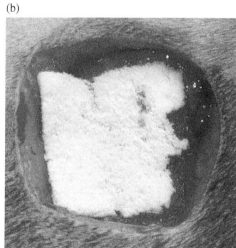

The use of fish skin grafts for the treatment of burns and other wounds has been studied in human medicine for many years. The first report for the treatment of a burn with tilapia skin was in a pediatric patient, followed by multiple randomized controlled studies describing multiple benefits [69–72]. North Atlantic cod skin grafts have also been reported to speed epithelialization in multiple human studies [73, 74]. In veterinary medicine, case reports and case series have also investigated the use of these dressings [75–78].

Mechanism of Action

Tilapia – Morphologic studies on tilapia skin have found similarities to human skin such as a deep dermis of thick, organized collagen fibers arranged in similar orientation. Studies suggest tilapia skin can induce EGF and fibroblast growth factor expression from its own collagen, stimulating the proliferation and differentiation of fibroblasts and keratinocytes from the host wound [79]. Other advantageous mechanisms include the presence of peptides found in tilapia skin (piscidin 3 and 4) which have also been shown to have antimicrobial activity [80, 81]. Another reported benefit to tilapia skin is excellent adherence to wound surfaces which supports a moist wound environment and decreases the chance of bacterial colonization [72].

Cod – North Atlantic cod skin is available for use in wound healing after a patented process that is reported to create an acellular product that maintains Omega-3 fatty acids, collagen, elastin, laminin, lipids, fibrin, proteoglycans, and glycosaminoglycans [78]. The reported advantages of Omega-3 fatty acids in this dressing are the proposed theory that this substance creates a bacterial barrier and has pain-modulating effects [74]. This graft is known to become incorporated into the wound bed over the first two weeks which accelerates epithelialization. This graft is also similar to mammalian skin and has been shown to provide an effective antimicrobial barrier and intrinsic anti-inflammatory properties [74, 82–84].

Indications

Tilapia – The most recognized indication for tilapia grafts is treatment of burn patients. In one study, burn patients randomized to tilapia skin graft showed faster reepithelialization and reduced pain scores compared to conventional treatment with silver sulfadiazine cream [70]. A study on collagen hydrogels created from tilapia skin also showed significantly accelerated wound healing in deep second-degree burns in a mouse model [85]; therefore, veterinary burn patients would be the prime candidates for these dressings. In theory, these dressings could also be used for wounds in the inflammatory phase and early or late repair phase, but there are currently no randomized controlled trials in veterinary medicine to support this use. The author has used tilapia in full-thickness wounds in multiple canine patients, but anecdotally, the best results have been seen after granulation tissue was present.

Cod – As discussed above, cod fish skin grafts have been investigated in human and veterinary studies. One prospective double-blind acute full-thickness skin biopsy study compared these grafts to human amnionic/chorionic membrane dressings and found a faster healing time [74]. A study by Mauer et al. on cod skin grafts used for the management of a variety of wounds in dogs and cats found the application helpful in most cases but this was not a controlled trial [78]. In theory, cod grafts could be used in the same instances as tilapia grafts: burns, inflammatory phase, and early or late repair phase.

Contraindications

The use of fish skin grafts in actively or grossly infected wounds is contraindicated. In human medicine, they are almost exclusively used for partial-thickness (burn) wounds, but veterinarians have used them for full-thickness wounds with some success.

Specific Directions for Use

Tilapia – There is no commercially available tilapia graft to date; therefore, the method for the application of tilapia grafts in veterinary medicine varies (Figure 8.14). Multiple human studies reporting different sterilization and storage techniques for fish skin exist, and veterinary references also outline potential techniques [71, 75, 86]. The author follows a similar technique as previously published [75] for the creation of these grafts, which can be found in Table 8.2. A published protocol based on human studies and the authors' experience applying fish skin grafts are provided in Table 8.3 [12]. The wound should not have active purulent or necrotic debris present at the time of graft placement.

(a)

(b)

(c)

(d)

(e)

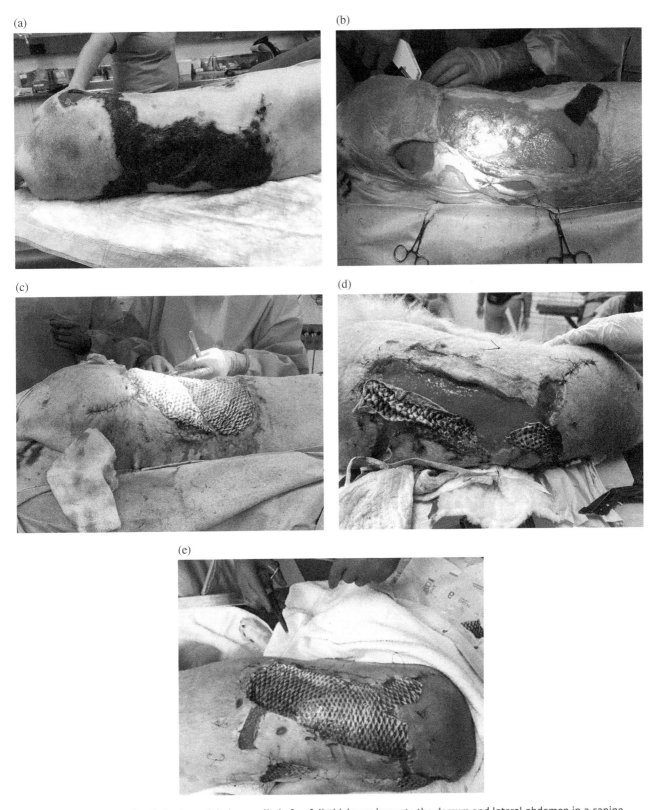

Figure 8.14   Photographs of tilapia graft being applied after full-thickness burns to the dorsum and lateral abdomen in a canine patient. (a) Necrotic eschar present over significant portion of right lateral flank, caudal dorsum, and left flank. (b) Appearance of the right-sided wound after sharp debridement and placement of a NPWT bandage for a total of four days. Healthy granulation tissue is covering the wound bed at this time. (c) Placement of first tilapia graft on the right-sided wound. Tilapia was placed on the left side as well and a hydrophilic foam dressing can be seen on the left patient covering the graft on that side. Stay sutures for a tie-over bandage are being applied to hold the grafts in place. (d) Appearance of tilapia graft and wound at the first dressing change. Note that the granulation tissue is more robust and closer to the surface of the wound edge. Moderate contraction of the wound edges has occurred. A portion of the graft has been incorporated into the wound, but the majority was easily removed as this wound was highly exudative. (e) Appearance of patient with second application of tilapia graft in place. *Source:* Courtesy of Nicole Buote, DVM, DACVS.

Table 8.2 Sterilization and storage for Tilapia skin grafts.

1) Fresh tilapia is acquired from a fish market and skinned with a sterile #10 blade.

   *Frozen tilapia can be used but it must be allowed to thaw completely before skinning

2) Lavage skins with sterile saline.

3) Place in a 2% chlorhexidine solution for 90 min.

4) Lavage with sterile saline.

5) Place in a 100% glycerol: 2% chlorhexidine solution at a 3:1 ratio for 60 min.

6) Lavage with sterile saline.

7) Massage skins with 100% glycerol solution for 5 min, and then place in 100% glycerol solution for another 60 min.

8) Lavage with sterile saline.

9) Swab each skin and submit for aerobic and anaerobic cultures.

   *Be sure cultures are negative before using them on patients

10) Place skins in packaging and place in freezer until needed.

Table 8.3 Application of Tilapia skin grafts to wounds.

1) Lavage and clean the wound – no necrotic tissue or active purulent debris can be present.

2) Place sterile hydrogel or wound gel in a thin layer on wound bed.

3) Place tilapia graft with pigmented scales facing outward.

4) Place more hydrogel on the surface of the graft to ensure moisture is maintained.

5) Place an absorbent hydrophilic foam over tilapia graft.

6) Cover with a soft padded bandage.

7) Check the bandage every 2–3 d.

   - If excessive exudate is present, remove graft, clean, and reapply new graft.
   - If graft is well-adhered, reapply hydrogel and new absorbent layer and rebandage.

8) To remove tilapia graft, saline or tap water can be used to gently lift up or disperse graft tissue. Petrolatum jelly can also be used to loosen the graft from the wound edges if deemed necessary.

Cod – Commercially available cod skin dressings exist and have the benefit of being readily available and freeze-dried with a shelf life of three years (Figure 8.15). All wounds must be appropriately cleaned before placement, and aseptic technique employed when handling the graft. After removing the graft from its sterile packaging, it must be rehydrated with a room-temperature saline (0.09% NaCl) solution for one minute. Then the graft is cut to fit the size of the wound and fenestrated (if necessary) with a scalpel to allow for exudate to pass through to secondary layers. The graft is applied with the scale pattern up and pressed into the wound bed to assure appropriate contact. The graft can be sutured to the wound edges (Figure 8.16) and is then covered with a non-adherent dressing (Telfa) or absorptive dressing (hydrocolloid foam) to optimize exudate management [78].

Bandage changes are performed based on the amount of exudate produced. The cod skin graft is not removed, but reapplication can occur if epithelialization is not occurring after incorporation. If the graft is not fully incorporated after two weeks of application, the wound is debrided again, and another cod skin graft is reapplied. Once epithelialization along the wound edges is observed, reapplication is not necessary [78].

Complications

These fish grafts appear to have a noninfectious microbiota which allows their successful use without irradiation, but experimental and clinical studies in veterinary medicine must be performed. To date, no adverse effects from tilapia or cod grafts have been reported in people or in animal studies.

(a) (b) (c)

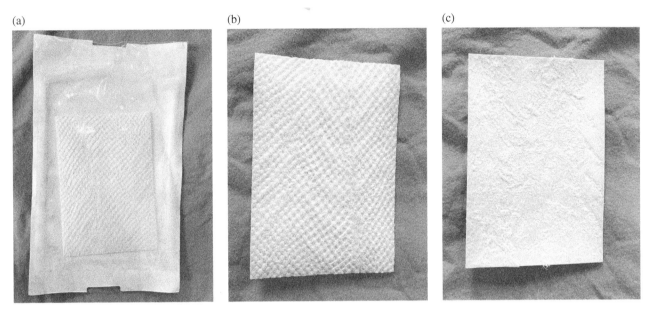

Figure 8.15   Photographs of a 7 × 10 cm North Atlantic cod skin graft (Kerecis® Omega-3 VET). (a) These grafts come in individual sterilized packages. (b) Note the scale side is supposed to face outwards. (c) The opposite smoother side should be placed in contact with the wound bed after rehydrating the graft in sterile saline. *Source:* Courtesy of Nicole Buote, DVM, DACVS.

Figure 8.16   Photographs of cod skin graft (Kerecis Omega-3 VET) being used in a clinical case. (a) Graft being soaked in sterile saline before application. (b) Graft applied to wound and held in place with skin staples. *Source:* Courtesy Daniel Spector, DVM, DACVS.

(a) (b)

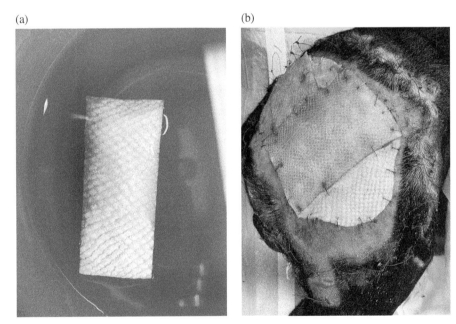

Miscellaneous

Nitrous Oxide

Mechanism of Action

Nitrous oxide (NO) has been discussed in detail in Chapter 7, as it is also available as a wound gel. Briefly, NO appears to affect wound healing through multiple mechanisms of including regulation of cytokines (IL-8, TGF-B1), supporting migration of monocytes and neutrophils, improving proliferation of keratinocytes, protecting endothelial cells from apoptosis, and mediating the actions of vascular endothelial growth factor (VEGF). In the last phase of wound healing (maturation), NO is involved in fibroblast production and collagen deposition [87].

(a)

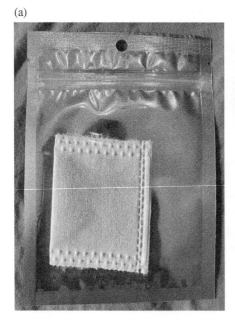

(b)

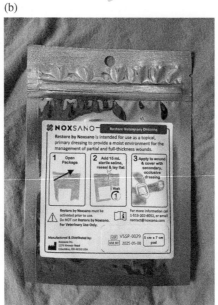

Figure 8.17 Photographs of a 5 × 7 cm nitric oxide dressing (Restore by Noxsano). (a) The dressing comes in an individual pouch in which saline or tap water is poured to rehydrate the pad. (b) Instructions on the pouch explain that for this size pad, 15 ml of liquid is placed into the pouch and allowed to soak in for one minute. *Source:* Courtesy of Nicole Buote, DVM, DACVS.

Indications

Reported indications for NO treatment include healing surgical incisions or infected open wounds [87, 88]. To date, only one experimental veterinary study [89] has been performed which illustrated that the time to first granulation tissue was shorter and there was a higher contraction rate for NO-treated wounds when compared to control wounds.

Contraindications

The only known contraindication to NO wound treatments is in actively hemorrhaging wound as nitric oxide is a vasodilatory compound which could intensify bleeding.

Specific Directions for Use

One commercial system available for use in veterinary patients (Noxsano®) has a NO-based wound pad (Figure 8.17). When using the wound pad (Restore™), the sterile pouch is opened, and the pad is hydrated with the amount of tap water or saline indicated on the front of the pouch. This pad is allowed to soak in the fluid for one minute, and the pad is gently massaged to ensure the fluid is distributed. The pad is then applied to the wound or incision, and an occlusive dressing (Tegaderm) is applied. Depending on secondary dressing, the wound environment, and patient factors, the pad is reported to remain active for up to one week. Most veterinarians choose to leave the pad in place for two to four days.

Complications

No adverse side effects or reactions have been reported in human or experimental animal literature to date. If the pad is allowed to dry, damage to the underlying wound tissue could occur but this complication can be eliminated with appropriate wound monitoring.

References

1 Bolton, L.L., Monte, K., and Pirone, L.A. (2000). Moisture and healing: beyond the jargon. *Ostomy Wound Manage.* 46 (Suppl 1A): 51S–62S.

2 Hutchinson, J.J. and Lawrence, J.C. (1991). Wound infection under occlusive dressings. *J. Hosp. Infect.* 17 (2): 83–94.

3 Slavkovic, M., Zivanovic, D., Dučić, S. et al. (2023). Comparison of negative pressure wound therapy (NPWT) and classical wet to moist dressing (WtM) in the treatment of complicated extremity wounds in children. *Children* 10 (2): 298.

4 Campbell, B.G. (2006). Dressings, bandages, and splints for wound management in dogs and cats. Dressings, bandages, and splints for wound management in dogs and cats. *Vet. Clin. North Am. Small Anim. Pract.* 36 (4): 759–791.

5 Nuutila, K. and Eriksson, E. (2021). Moist wound healing with commonly available dressings. *Adv. Wound Care* 10: 685–698.

6 Seaman, S. (2002). Dressing selection in chronic wound management. *J. Am. Podiatr. Med. Assoc.* 92 (1): 24–33.

7 Varghese, M.C., Balin, A.K., Carter, D.M., and Caldwell, D. (1986). Local environment of chronic wounds under synthetic dressings. *Arch. Dermatol.* 122 (1): 52–57.

8 Henry, M., Byrne, P., and Dinn, E. (1988). Pilot study to investigate the pH of exudate on varicose ulcers under DuoDERM. In: *Beyond Occlusion: Wound Care Proceedings* (ed. T.J. Ryan), 67–70. London: Royal Society of Medicine.

9 Hadley, H.S., Stanley, B.J., Fritz, M.C. et al. (2013). Effects of a cross-linked hyaluronic acid based gel on the healing of open wounds in dogs. *Vet. Surg.* 42 (2): 161–169.

10 Jones, J. (2005). Winter's concept of moist wound healing: a review of the evidence and impact on clinical practice. *J. Wound Care* 14 (6): 273–276.

11 Lawrence, J.C. (1994). Dressings and wound infection. *Am. J. Surg.* 167 (1A): 21S–24S.

12 Buote, N.J. (2022). Updates in wound management and dressings. *Vet. Clin. North Am. Small Anim. Pract.* 52 (2): 289–315.

13 Davidson, J.R. (2015). Current concepts in wound management and wound healing products. *Vet. Clin. North Am. Small Anim. Pract.* 45 (3): 537–564.

14 Stashak, T.S., Farstvedt, E., and Othic, A. (2004). Update on wound dressings: indications and best use. *Clin. Tech. Equine Pract.* 3: 148–163. https://doi.org/10.1053/j.ctep.2004.08.006.

15 Campton-Johnson, S. and Wilson, J. (2001). Infected wound management: advanced technologies, moisture-retentive dressings, and die-hard methods. *Crit. Care Nurs. Q.* 24 (2): 64–77.

16 Hosgood, G. (2018). Open wounds. In: *Veterinary Surgery: Small Animal Expert Consult*, 2e (ed. S.A. Johnston and T. DAKM), 1410–1421. St. Louis, MO: Elsevier Health Sciences (US).

17 Popovich, D.M., Alexander, D., Rittman, M. et al. (1995). Strike-through contamination in saturated sterile dressings: a clinical analysis. *Clin. Nurs. Res.* 4 (2): 195–207.

18 Lee, A.H., Swaim, S.F., McGuire, J.A., and Hughes, K.S. (1987). Effects of nonadherent dressing materials on the healing of open wounds in dogs. *J. Am. Vet. Med. Assoc.* 190 (4): 416–422.

19 Eaglstein, W.H. and Mertz, P.M. (1980). "Inert" vehicles do affect wound healing. *J. Invest. Dermatol.* 74 (2): 90–91.

20 Fletcher, J. (2005). Understanding wound dressings: alginates. *Nurs. Times* 101 (16): 53–54.

21 Minsart, M., Van Vlierberghe, S., Dubruel, P., and Mignon, A. (2022). Commercial wound dressings for the treatment of exuding wounds: an in-depth physico-chemical comparative study. *Burns Trauma* 21 (10): tkac024.

22 Boateng, J. and Catanzano, O. (2015). Advanced therapeutic dressings for effective wound healing—a review. *J. Pharm. Sci.* 104 (11): 3653–3680.

23 Segal, H.C., Hunt, B.J., and Gilding, K. (1998). The effects of alginate and non-alginate wound dressings on blood coagulation and platelet activation. *J. Biomater. Appl.* 12 (3): 249–257.

24 Casey, G. (2000). Modern wound dressings. *Nurs. Stand.* 15 (5): 47–51.

25 McCarthy, S., Dvorakova, V., O'Sullivan, P., and Bourke, J.F. (2018). Anaphylaxis caused by alginate dressing. *Contact Dermatitis* 79 (6): 396–397.

26 Hollinworth, H. and Collier, M. (2000). Nurses' views about pain and trauma at dressing changes: results of a national survey. *J. Wound Care* 9 (8): 369–373.

27 Fahie, M.A. and Shettko, D. (2007). Evidence-based wound management: a systematic review of therapeutic agents to enhance granulation and epithelialization. *Vet. Clin. North Am. Small Anim. Pract.* 37 (3): 559–577.

28 Abramo, F., Argiolas, S., Pisani, G. et al. (2008). Effect of a hydrocolloid dressing on first intention healing surgical wounds in the dog: a pilot study. *Aust. Vet. J.* 86 (3): 95–99.

29 Tsioli, V., Gouletsou, P.G., Galatos, A.D. et al. (2016). Effects of two occlusive, hydrocolloid dressings on healing of full-thickness skin wounds in cats. *Vet. Comp. Orthop. Traumatol.* 29 (4): 298–305.

30 Tsioli, V., Gouletsou, P.G., Galatos, A.D. et al. (2018). The effect of a hydrocolloid dressing on second intention wound healing in cats. *J. Am. Anim. Hosp. Assoc.* 54 (3): 125–131.

31 Pudner, R. (2001). Hydrocolloid dressings in wound management. *J. Comm. Nurs. Online* 15 (4): www.jcn.co.uk/journals/issue/04-2001/article/hydrocolloid-dressings-in-wound-management (accessed 2 May 2023).

32 Kotz, P., Fisher, J., McCluskey, P. et al. (2009). Use of a new silver barrier dressing, ALLEVYN Ag in exuding chronic wounds. *Int. Wound J.* 6 (03): 186–194.

33 Lee, S.M., Park, I.K., Kim, Y.S. et al. (2016). Superior absorption and retention properties of foam-film silver dressing versus other commercially available silver dressing. *Biomater. Res.* 6 (20): 22.

34 Nolff, M.C., Fehr, M., Bolling, A. et al. (2015). Negative pressure wound therapy, silver coated foam dressing and conventional bandages in open wound treatment in dogs. A retrospective comparison of 50 paired cases. *Vet. Comp. Orthop. Traumatol.* 28 (1): 30–38.

35 Nolff, M.C., Fehr, M., Reese, S., and Meyer-Lindenberg, A.E. (2017). Retrospective comparison of negative pressure wound therapy and silver-coated foam dressings in open-wound treatment in cats. *J. Feline Med. Surg.* 19 (6): 624–630.

36 Nolff, M.C., Albert, R., Reese, S., and Meyer-Lindenberg, A. (2018). Comparison of negative pressure wound therapy and silver-coated foam dressings in open wound treatment in dogs: a prospective controlled clinical trial. *Vet. Comp. Orthop. Traumatol.* 31 (4): 229–238.

37 Swanson, E.A., Freeman, L.J., Seleem, M.N., and Snyder, P.W. (2014). Biofilm-infected wounds in a dog. *J. Am. Vet. Med. Assoc.* 244 (6): 699–707.

38 Pagès, G., Hammer, M., Grand, J.G., and Irubetagoyena, I. (2022). Long-term outcome of tibial plateau leveling osteotomy using an antimicrobial silver-based coated plate in dogs. *PLoS One* 17 (8): e0272555.

39 Albaridi, N.A. (2019). Antibacterial potency of honey. *Int. J. Microbiol.* 2 (2019): 2464507. https://doi.org/10.1155/2019/2464507.

40 Vogt, N.A., Vriezen, E., Nwosu, A., and Sargeant, J.M. (2021). A scoping review of the evidence for the medicinal use of natural honey in animals. *Front. Vet. Sci.* 18 (7): 618301. https://doi.org/10.3389/fvets.2020.618301.

41 Sowlati-Hashjin, A., Carbone, P., and Karttunen, M. (2020). Insights into the polyhexamethylene biguanide (PHMB) mechanism of action on bacterial membrane and DNA: a molecular dynamics study. *J. Phys. Chem. B* 124 (22): 4487–4497.

42 Lee, W.R., Tobias, K.M., Bemis, D.A., and Rohrbach, B.W. (2004). In vitro efficacy of a polyhexamethylene biguanide impregnated gauze dressing against bacteria found in veterinary patients. *Vet. Surg.* 33 (4): 404–411.

43 McCaig, C.D., Rajnicek, A.M., Song, B., and Zhao, M. (2005). Controlling cell behavior electrically: current views and future potential. *Physiol. Rev.* 85: 943–978.

44 Foulds, I.S. and Barker, A.T. (1983). Human skin battery potentials and their possible role in wound healing. *Br. J. Dermatol.* 109 (5): 515–522.

45 Ashrafi, M., Alonso-Rasgado, T., Baguneid, M., and Bayat, A. (2016). The efficacy of electrical stimulation in experimentally induced cutaneous wounds in animals. *Vet. Dermatol.* 27 (4): 235–e257.

46 Maijer, A., Gessner, A., Trumpatori, B., and Varhus, J.D. (2018). Bioelectric dressing supports complex wound healing in small animal patients. *Top. Companion Anim. Med.* 33 (1): 21–28.

47 Kim, H., Makin, I., Skiba, J. et al. (2014). Antibacterial efficacy testing of a bioelectric wound dressing against clinical wound pathogens. *Open Microbiol. J.* 8: 15–21.

48 Heald, R., Salyer, S., Ham, K. et al. (2022). Electroceutical treatment of infected chronic wounds in a dog and a cat. *Vet. Surg.* 51 (3): 520–527.

49 Banerjee, J., Ghatak, P.D., Roy, S. et al. (2015). Silver-zinc redox-coupled electroceutical wound dressing disrupts bacterial biofilm. *PLoS One* 10 (3): e0119531.

50 Sheridan, D.M., Isseroff, R.R., and Nucitelli, R. (1996). Imposition of a physiologic DC electric current alters the migratory response of human keratinocytes on extracellular matrix molecules. *J. Invest. Dermatol.* 106 (4): 642–646.

51 Blount, A.L., Foster, S., Rapp, D.A., and Wilcox, R. (2012). The use of bioelectric dressings in skin graft harvest sites: a prospective case series. *J. Burn Care Res.* 33 (3): 354–357.

52 Harding, A.C., Gil, J., Valdes, J. et al. (2012). Efficacy of a bio-electric dressing in healing deep, partial-thickness wounds using a porcine model. *Ostomy Wound Manage.* 58 (9): 50–55.

53 Varhus, J.D. (2014). A novel bioelectric device enhances wound healing: an equine case series. *J. Equine Vet. Sci.* 34: 421–430.

54 Carey, L.C. and Lepley, D. (1962). Effect of continuous direct electric current on healing wounds. *Surg. Forum* 13: 33–35.

55 Steckel, R.R., Page, E.H., Geddes, L.A., and Van Vleet, J.F. (1984). Electrical stimulation on skin wound healing in the horse: preliminary studies. *Am. J. Vet. Res.* 45 (4): 800–803.

56 Stromberg, B.V. (1988). Effects of electrical currents on wound contraction. *Ann. Plast. Surg.* 21 (2): 121–123.

57 Badylak, S.F. (2002). The extracellular matrix as a scaffold for tissue reconstruction. *Semin. Cell Dev. Biol.* 13 (5): 377–383.

58 Sarikaya, A., Record, R., Wu, C.C. et al. (2002). Antimicrobial activity associated with extracellular matrices. *Tissue Eng.* 8 (1): 63–71.

59 Badylak, S.F. (2004). Xenogeneic extracellular matrix as a scaffold for tissue reconstruction. *Transpl. Immunol.* 12 (3–4): 367–377.

60 Winkler, J.T., Swaim, S.F., Sartin, E.A. et al. (2002). The effect of porcine-derived small intestinal submucosa product on wounds with exposed bone in dogs. *Vet. Surg.* 31 (6): 541–551.

61 Schallberger, S.P., Stanley, B.J., Hauptman, J.G., and Steficek, B.A. (2008). Effect of porcine small intestinal submucosa on acute full-thickness wounds in dogs. *Vet. Surg.* 37 (6): 515–524.

62 Taghizadeh, R.R., Cetrulo, K.J., and Cetrulo, C.L. (2011). Wharton's jelly stem cells: future clinical applications. *Placenta* 32: S311–S315.

63 Oryan, A., Alemzadeh, E., Mohammadi, A.A., and Moshiri, A. (2019). Healing potential of injectable Aloe vera hydrogel loaded by adipose-derived stem cell in skin tissue-engineering in a rat burn wound model. *Cell Tissue Res.* 377 (2): 215–227.

64 Joseph, A., Baiju, I., Bhat, I.A. et al. (2020). Mesenchymal stem cell-conditioned media: a novel alternative of stem cell therapy for quality wound healing. *J. Cell. Physiol.* 235 (7–8): 5555–5569.

65 Kierski, K., Buote, N.J., Rishniw, M. et al. (2023). Novel extracellular matrix wound dressing shows increased epithelialization of full thickness skin wounds in dogs. *Am. J. Vet. Res.* https://doi.org/10.2460/ajvr.23.05.0105.

66 Hashemi, S.S., Mohammadi, A.A., Kabiri, H. et al. (2019). The healing effect of Wharton's jelly stem cells seeded on biological scaffold in chronic skin ulcers: a randomized clinical trial. *J. Cosmet. Dermatol.* 18 (6): 1961–1967.

67 Lanci, A., Merlo, B., Mariella, J. et al. (2019). Heterologous Wharton's jelly derived mesenchymal stem cells application on a large chronic skin wound in a 6-month-old filly. *Front. Vet. Sci.* 6: 9. https://doi.org/10.3389/fvets.2019.00009.

68 Ribeiro, J., Pereira, T., Amorim, I. et al. (2014). Cell therapy with human MSCs isolated from the umbilical cord Wharton jelly associated to a PVA membrane in the treatment of chronic skin wounds. *Int. J. Med. Sci.* 11 (10): 979–987.

69 Costa, B.A., Lima Junior, E.M., de Moraes Filho, M.O. et al. (2019). Use of tilapia skin as a xenograft for pediatric burn treatment: a case report. *J. Burn Care Res.* 40 (5): 714–717.

70 Lima Júnior, E.M., de Moraes Filho, M.O., Costa, B.A. et al. (2020). Innovative burn treatment using tilapia skin as a Xenograft: a phase II randomized controlled trial. *J. Burn Care Res.* 41 (3): 585–592.

71 Lima Júnior, E.M., de Moraes Filho, M.O., Costa, B.A. et al. (2020). Lyophilized tilapia skin as a xenograft for superficial partial thickness burns: a novel preparation and storage technique. *J. Wound Care* 29 (10): 598–602.

72 Lima Júnior, E.M., de Moraes Filho, M.O., Costa, B.A. et al. (2021). Nile tilapia fish skin–based wound dressing improves pain and treatment-related costs of superficial partial thickness burns: a phase III randomized controlled trial. *Plast Reconstr. Surg.* 147 (5): 1189–1198.

73 Fiakos, G., Kuang, Z., and Lo, E. (2020). Improved skin regeneration with acellular fish skin grafts. *Engineer. Regener.* 1: 95–101. https://doi.org/10.1016/j.engreg.2020.09.002.

74 Kirsner, R.S., Margolis, D.J., Baldursson, B.T. et al. (2020). Fish skin grafts compared to human amnion/chorion membrane allografts: a double-blind, prospective, randomized clinical trial of acute wound healing. *Wound Repair Regener.* 28 (1): 75–80.

75 Choi, C., Linder, T., Kirby, A. et al. (2021). Use of a tilapia skin xenograft for management of a large bite wound in a dog. *Can. Vet. J.* 62 (10): 1071–1076.

76 Ibrahim, A., Soliman, M., Kotb, S., and Ali, M.M. (2020). Evaluation of fish skin as a biological dressing for metacarpal wounds in donkeys. *BMC Vet. Res.* 16 (1): 472.

77 Dawson, K.A., Mickelson, M.A., Blong, A.E., and Walton, R.A.L. (2021). Management of severe burn injuries with novel treatment techniques including maggot debridement and applications of acellular fish skin grafts and autologous skin cell suspension in a dog. *J. Am. Vet. Med. Assoc.* 260 (4): 428–435.

78 Mauer, E.S., Maxwell, E.A., Cocca, C.J. et al. (2021). Acellular fish skin grafts for the management of wounds in dogs and cats: 17 cases (2019–2021). *Am. J. Vet. Res.* 83 (2): 188–192.

79 Chen, J., Gao, K., Liu, S. et al. (2019). Fish collagen surgical compress repairing characteristics on wound healing process in vivo. *Mar. Drugs* 17 (1): 1–12.

80 Peng, K.C., Lee, S.H., Hour, A.L. et al. (2012). Five different piscidins from Nile tilapia, Oreochromis niloticus: analysis of their expressions and biological functions. *PLoS One* 7 (11): e50263. https://doi.org/10.1371/journal.pone.0050263.

81 Pan, C.Y., Tsai, T.Y., Su, B.C. et al. (2017). Study of the antimicrobial activity of tilapia piscidin 3(TP3) and TP4 and their effects on immune functions in hybrid tilapia (*Oreochromis* spp.). *PLoS One* 12 (1): e0169678. https://doi.org/10.1371/journal.pone.0169678.

82 Baldursson, B.T., Kjartansson, H., Konrádsdóttir, F. et al. (2015). Healing rate and autoimmune safety of full-thickness wounds treated with fish skin acellular dermal matrix versus porcine small-intestine submucosa: a noninferiority study. *Int. J. Low Extrem. Wounds* 14 (1): 37–43.

83 Magnusson, S., Baldursson, B.T., Kjartansson, H. et al. (2017). Regenerative and antibacterial properties of acellular fish skin grafts and human amnion/chorion membrane: implications for tissue preservation in combat casualty care. *Mil. Med.* 182 (S1): 383–388.

84 Magnússon, S., Baldursson, B.T., Kjartansson, H. et al. (2015). Decellularized fish skin: characteristics that support tissue repair. *Laeknabladid.* 101 (12): 567–573.

85 Ge, B., Wang, H., Li, J. et al. (2020). Comprehensive assessment of nile tilapia skin (*Oreochromis niloticus*) collagen hydrogels for wound dressings. *Mar. Drugs* 18 (4): 178.

86 Ibrahim, A., Hassan, D., Kelany, N. et al. (2020). Validation of three different sterilization methods of tilapia skin dressing: impact on microbiological enumeration and collagen content. *Front. Vet. Sci.* 7: 597751. https://doi.org/10.3389/fvets.2020.597751.

87 Pinto, R.V., Carvalho, S., Antunes, F. et al. (2022). Emerging nitric oxide and hydrogen sulfide releasing carriers for skin wound healing therapy. *ChemMedChem* 17 (1): e202100429. https://doi.org/10.1002/cmdc.202100429.

88 Krausz, A. and Friedman, A.J. (2015). Nitric oxide as a surgical adjuvant. *Future Sci. OA* 1 (1): FSO56. https://doi.org/10.4155/fso.15.56.

89 Rodriguez-Diaz JM, Wallace ML, Emond SA, Howerth EW. (n.d.). Effect of hydrocolloid-nitric oxide wound dressings on wound healing in dogs [abstract]. *Proceedings of the 22nd Annual Scientific Meeting of the Society of Veterinary Soft Tissue Surgery* (15–17 June 2023). Jacksonville Beach, FL.

9

Drains: How and When to Place Them

Angela C. Banz

VCA Northwest Veterinary Specialists, Clackamas, OR, USA

Drains can be useful tools in veterinary medicine for managing traumatic wounds, contaminated wounds, and surgical wounds. Drains allow evacuation of fluid and/or air from the tissues in order to improve wound conditions and promote healing. Potential space created by surgical interventions or trauma, also known as "dead space," allows accumulation of fluids such as blood, serum, and purulent material to accumulate between tissue planes. This fluid can provide a potential medium for bacteria which is not easily reached by the immune system or antimicrobial therapy. Tissue expansion by fluid accumulation can also lead to pain and compromised tissue perfusion and is associated with delayed wound healing by preventing tissue planes from adhering to each other.

The use of drains is not innocuous, however, and prudent use with adherence to Halstead's Principles is important. Drains are generally classified as passive or active depending on their mechanism of action.

Passive Drains

Passive drains simply channel fluids from the wound by relying on gravity, body movements, overflow, and pressure differentials between the tissue and the exterior. They are open, allowing fluid to flow through or around the drain and exit the wound. Passive drains are inexpensive, readily available, and easy to place.

The most common passive drain used in veterinary medicine is the Penrose drain, which is a radiopaque collapsible latex rubber tube available in multiple sizes (Figure 9.1). Other materials can also be used as passive drains, such as silastic or silicon tubing and umbilical tape. Penrose drains are best for superficial locations such as subcutaneous spaces or between superficial muscle layers in cases of trauma. Penrose drains function by drainage along the surface area (outside) of the material; minimal drainage occurs through the center of the drain. Specific indications include bite wounds, in surgical sites where dead space cannot otherwise be alleviated and there is anticipated fluid production. They are best for smaller wounds or those where fluid accumulation is expected to be minimal or resolve within a few days (Table 9.1). Passive drains are contraindicated in body cavities, as they allow retrograde air and bacteria into the cavity and increase risk of visceral herniation.

Passive drains must be exited in a gravity-dependent location to maximize drainage. Exit passive drains through a separate stab incision as opposed to the primary incision, as this minimizes incidence of wound infection and delayed healing of the primary wound. *Never place any type of drain directly under an incision as this may lead to decreased perfusion of the tissues and dehiscence.* Tubing should remain free from kinks and should be adequately secured to prevent early dislodgement or migration into the wound. The smallest diameter drain is preferred to help minimize complications. The exit incision should be in the ventralmost area and large enough to prevent obstruction of the flow from the drain by the skin. Allowing the drain to have a second exit point is not recommended, as it does not increase drainage, provides an additional

Techniques in Small Animal Wound Management, First Edition. Edited by Nicole J. Buote.
© 2024 John Wiley & Sons, Inc. Published 2024 by John Wiley & Sons, Inc.
Companion website: www.wiley.com/go/buote/wounds

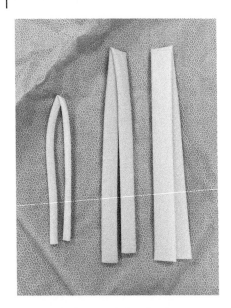

Figure 9.1 Penrose drains of various sizes-from left to right ¼″, ½″, 1″.
Source: Courtesy of Nicole Buote DVM, DACVS.

site where healing will need to occur, and potentially increases chances for infection. <u>Ensure that the drain is not incorporated into wound closure sutures.</u>

Placement of Passive Drains

Placement of the drain depends on the depth of the wound/space being closed. If the drain is placed into a deeper region (deep to muscle), no proximal tacking suture is possible therefore maintaining position is achieved by closing the overlying tissues. If the drain is placed in a more superficial wound (subcutaneous region), it can be tacked dorsally/proximally to the skin with an interrupted suture. This can be done with visualization in some cases but many times that is not possible. Using a different colored suture to secure the drain is helpful for drain removal to eliminate accidental early removal of the incision sutures as drains are commonly removed three to five days after placement. When the dorsal/proximal aspect of the wound space is not visible, the drain can be placed blindly (Figure 9.2, Video 9.1 ☉). Percutaneous drain placement is accomplished by grasping the corner of the drain with a Kelly or Mosquito hemostat, the hemostats are then directed from inside the wound or the proposed ventral exit incision with tips upward toward the skin, and the suture passed percutaneously into the drain adjacent to the hemostat tip blindly by feel of the needle next to the hemostat tip. Pulling on the drain from the exit site while holding onto the suture will allow you to evaluate for suture purchase of the drain prior to tying the external knot. If the drain is being placed for dead space without a large open wound (bite wounds), the easiest way to exit the drain is to place hemostats through one of the wounds (after probing) to the most ventral point and using a blade, create a small opening for the tips of the hemostat. Then a second set of hemostats can be grasped and pulled dorsally to the original opening to pull the drain through (Video 9.2 ☉). If the purchase is appropriate tie the knot. To exit a Penrose drain, there are two common methods. If the wound or incision is open, the end of the drain can be grasped within a hemostat which is tunneled to a gravity-dependent (usually the ventral most) location at least 1 cm from the primary incision. The hemostat tip is pressed upward against the skin at the desired exit point, and a surgical blade is used to create a hole slightly wider than the Penrose drain. The hemostat and drain are then pushed through the created incision and secured at one or two of the skin edges with interrupted sutures (Figure 9.3). Umbilical tape can also be used to keep an incision made at the most distal aspect of a wound open to allow for passive drainage. The umbilical tape is placed through the created incision and out a stab incision nearby and tied in a loose knot (Figure 9.4). This can be gently manipulated 2–3× daily to keep the incision open and express fluid from the wound.

If the drain tears or is removed by the patient inadvertently, radiographs to assess for residual drain in the wound are performed. The drain is a foreign body and if pieces remain in the tissue, they must be removed. Drain type, location, size, and details on method of securing the drain must be recorded in the patient's medical record so that missing or broken drains are readily identified.

Table 9.1 Advantages and disadvantages to passive drains.

Advantages	Disadvantages
Inexpensive	Should not be placed in thoracic or abdominal cavities
Easy to place	Not ideal for large wounds as drainage can be inconsistent
Easy to remove	Cannot be used for deep wounds as they require gravity for drainage
	Can be messy if not covered in a bandage
	Cannot monitor volume of fluid drainage

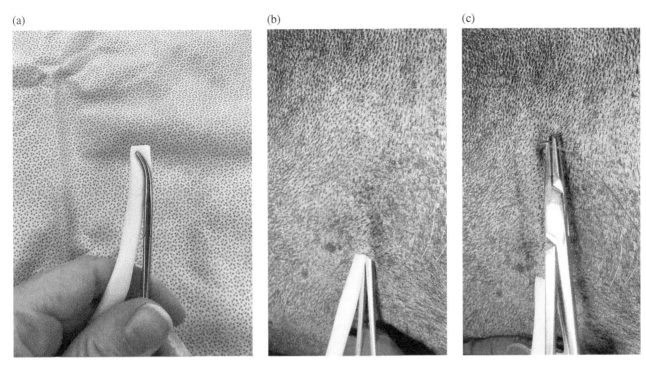

Figure 9.2   Placement of a Penrose drain blindly. (a) Grasping the Penrose drain with a hemostat. (b) Tunneling the drain under the skin to a dorsal location. (c) Percutaneously grasping the Penrose drain by feeling for the edge of the hemostat. *Source:* Courtesy of Nicole Buote DVM, DACVS.

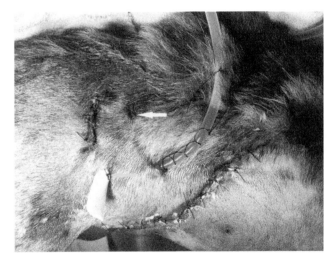

Figure 9.3   Severe bite wounds on the abdomen and right flank of a dog. Patient is in left lateral recumbency and the head of the patient is to the right of the picture. Smaller wound closed with Penrose drain and larger wound required a Jackson Pratt drain. Note the sutures placed at the proximal (yellow arrow) and distal (green arrow) aspect of the Penrose drain. *Source:* Courtesy of Angela Banz DVM, DACVS.

Postoperative Care

Some clinicians prefer to cover passive drains with a bandage to help minimize contamination of the wound site and for environmental cleanliness, particularly in clean surgical wounds. The placement of a drain will convert the wound from a clean to a clean-contaminated site in cases of surgically created wounds (mass removals). The bandage should be changed prior to seeing "strike-through," which is the saturation of a bandage with fluid that wets both the inner and outer surfaces. If bandages are not changed in a timely fashion, fluid accumulation may lead to maceration of the tissues. Bandaging also prevents the owner or clinician from assessing the incisions/wounds and ensuring the exit site is open; therefore, their use is not always appropriate. In some locations, bandaging may be impossible or increase potential complications and owners should be cautioned to keep the site clean and avoid activities that lead to contamination.

(a)

(b)

(c)

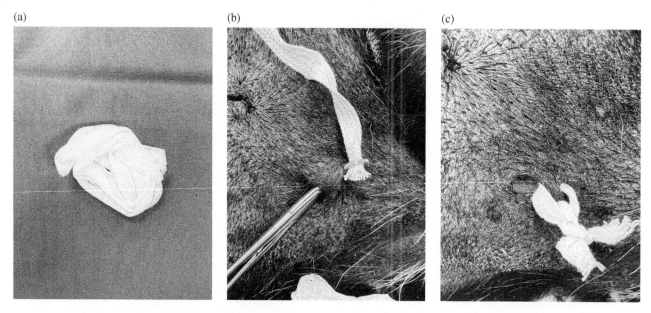

Figure 9.4   Umbilical tape used for drainage. (a) Umbilical tape. (b) Umbilical tape being passed through ventral exit incision out of an adjacent stab incision. (c) Umbilical tape tied and exited the ventral incision to maintain an open incision for drainage. *Source:* Courtesy of Nicole Buote DVM, DACVS.

Patients should wear an Elizabethan collar or other protective device to prevent licking or inadvertent removal of the drain if they are not covered. Tissue fragments, fibrin clots, contraction of the exit hole, or improper drain size selection can contribute to drain failure. Bacteria can enter and colonize the wound, as passive drains expose the wound to the outer environment. Infection risk is increased if the end of the drain is overly long, contacts fur, if drain is left in place too long, or if aseptic technique is not followed.

The drain is left in place for generally three to five days depending on the volume of fluid exiting the area [1]. They can be removed as early as 48 hours if drainage is minimal. Latex incites an inflammatory response, and the drain should not be left in place longer than it benefits the patient. If left in place too long, the risk of infection is higher, and it may create a persistent epithelialized tract. To remove passive drains, the sutures that secure the drain in place are cut and the drain is gently pulled out of the exit incision in one quick, smooth motion. Visually inspect the drain after removal to ensure that it was removed completely. The drain exit site is left open for continued draining and healing by second intention. Warm compress can be performed for two to three days after drain removal to promote any additional drainage if needed.

Closed-Suction/Active Drains

Active drain systems work by utilizing negative pressure to pull fluid through the tube placed in the potential space into an external reservoir. Also known as closed-suction drains, these include compressible reservoirs such as the Jackson Pratt drain, or rigid reservoirs such as Surgivac, Redovac, and Snyder Hemovac. They are a closed system and therefore provide multiple advantages over passive drains (Table 9.2).

The most significant of these advantages include improved apposition of tissue due to the suction effect and ability to monitor for changes in fluid character and volume. Although considerably more expensive than Penrose drains, they are superior for the treatment of larger wounds, clean surgical beds, and under surgical flaps. Active drains also allow flexibility when choosing the exit site as it is not limited to a gravity-dependent location. These types of drains create continuous suction until the reservoir is filled with air or fluid. Continuous suction is preferred over intermittent suction (intermittent percutaneous drainage of seromas for example), as it minimizes opportunities for bacterial proliferation and decreased tissue adherence from the accumulation of static fluid.

Common indications for closed suction drains are large wounds where the potential space is created by large mass removals, avulsion bite wounds, excision of necrotic tissue; in areas where skin is loose and motion is high such as the

Table 9.2   Advantages and disadvantages to active drains.

Advantages	Disadvantages
Clean environment for owners (fluids contained within reservoir)	More expensive
Eliminate maceration of skin (fluid is not draining directly onto skin)	±Require sedation for removal if placed in deep or sensitive region
Decreased contamination risk	±Hospitalization required until removal
More effective drainage of fluid and air due to suction action	
Allow for objective monitoring of fluid volume	

(a)   (b)

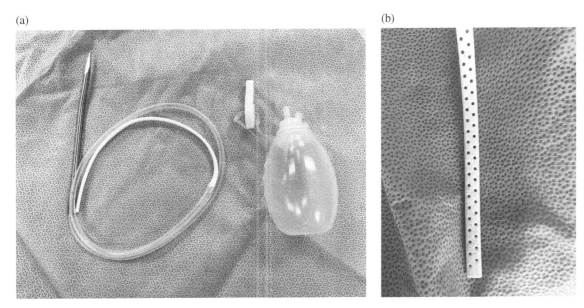

Figure 9.5   Components of a closed suction (JP) drain. (a) A 7mm wide fenestrated drain (white) with a trocar attached to non-fenestrated (clear) tubing to aid in placement. The bulb reservoir to the left holds 100 ms of fluid. (b) Close-up of fenestrated tubing. *Source:* Courtesy of Nicole Buote, DVM, DACVS.

axilla or inguinal regions; areas of high incidence of infection such as bite wounds, abscesses, foxtail tracts; under axillary pattern skin flaps; and to primarily treat seromas. Closed suction drains are also commonly utilized in the management of septic peritonitis.

Closed suction drains are comprised of three main components: fenestrated drain, non-fenestrated tubing, and suction bulb (Figure 9.5). The fenestrated drain is inserted into the cavity/potential space and is attached to the non-fenestrated tubing exiting the site. It is important that all of the fenestrated drain is covered by tissue so that an air-tight seal can be produced. The non-fenestrated tubing is then attached to the vacuum device (suction bulb). The most commonly used drain in veterinary medicine is the Jackson Pratt drain, commonly referred to as a JP drain. Initially developed as a "brain drain" by Navy surgeons Drs. Jackson and Pratt to provide a sterile, closed reservoir with gentle suction to treat subdural hematomas and for postoperative drainage of craniotomies, it is made of medical-grade multi-fenestrated silicone rubber which is minimally inflammatory and decreases intraluminal clotting. These drains have small internal ridges to help prevent collapse of the walls of the tubing, and are soft, increasing patient comfort and decreasing adjacent tissue damage compared to more rigid drains [2]. The fenestrated tubing has a radiopaque line to aid in assessment of positioning or if suspected fragments are left after removal. The tubing is attached to a "grenade" suction bulb that is compressed by hand to evacuate air through an open vent hole (Video 9.3 ◉). The grenade has a one-way valve that prevents retrograde movement of fluid.

Placement of Closed-Suction Drains

To place a closed suction drain, choose the exit site in an area of healthy skin where it will be easy to empty and manage the reservoir, comfortable for the patient while minimally impeding function, and is easiest to secure. Jackson Pratt drains are available with or without an attached trocar for placement. If no trocar is included, Kelly or Mosquito hemostats are tunneled from inside the wound with the tips directed up toward the skin at the proposed exit site, and an incision is made directly over the tips with a scalpel blade, taking care to ensure the hole is no larger than the drain tubing. Open the tips of the forceps enough to interlock a second pair of hemostats externally and pull the tips of the external hemostats into the wound via the first pair of hemostats. Gently grasp the tip of the end of the non-fenestrated tubing and pull the tubing through the exit hole. The entire fenestrated end should be within the wound bed and engaging the deepest part of the wound. The end of the fenestrated tubing can be cut to accommodate the size of the wound. Secure the external non-fenestrated tubing in place with a purse string around the exit hole to ensure a tight seal, leaving the ends long enough to use the same suture for a fingertrap pattern along the tubing for security (Video 9.4 ☉). Identify the desired direction of the tubing for best positioning to prevent kinking and place an interrupted suture or secure with a suture through adding a surgical tape butterfly (Figure 9.6). Ensure that the drain is not caught in the wound closure sutures and that it does not lie directly under a significant portion of the incision. When a trocar is included, pass the trocar from inside the wound externally at the desired exit site and secure as described (Figure 9.7). Trim the external tubing to a length that allows convenient manipulation of the grenade. Securely attach the tubing to the grenade port with the one-way valve. Once the wound is closed and an air-tight seal is achieved, activate the suction by closing the evacuation port while compressing the grenade. Negative pressure is exerted through the tubing and into the wound as the reservoir naturally expands to its original shape. Higher suction may be generated by rolling the grenade from its apex to base compared to squeezing by hand [3]. The drain may quickly fill with air and/or fluid after initial placement from residual air and fluid in the wound bed. If the grenade will not hold negative pressure, ensure that the grenade is securely attached to the tubing, the evacuation port is closed, the incision and drain exit sites are air-tight, and that there are no tears or holes in the external tubing.

Postoperative Care

In vitro studies have shown that compressible reservoirs quickly lose suction pressure as they fill to 20–30% capacity. After that point, suction pressure decreases gradually until the reservoir is filled. Some units lose all suction pressure before they are full, although the grenade bulb type has been shown to maintain some suction pressure even when filled [3]. Because of this decline in suction pressure, a larger reservoir should be chosen if a sizable amount of drainage is expected, and it is ideal that any reservoir be emptied by the time it is half full. To empty the grenade, hands should be thoroughly cleaned or gloved and the evacuation port on the grenade cleaned with alcohol. Attach a sterile syringe to the port and withdraw the

(a)

(b)

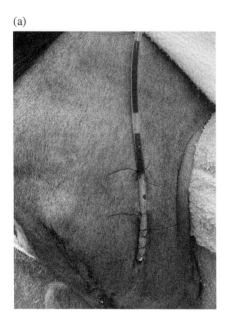
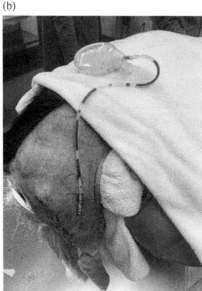

Figure 9.6 Photographs of a Jackson Pratt drain in place on the caudal thigh of a dog after large lipomatous mass removal. (a) Secured with a purse-string and fingertrap suture and two additional interrupted sutures. (b) Close-up of the fingertrap pattern. *Source:* Courtesy of Angela Banz DVM, DACVS.

(a)   (b)

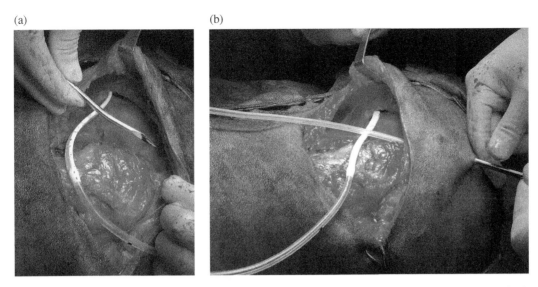

Figure 9.7   Photographs of a trocar-style closed suction drain placement. (a) The fenestrated end is within the wound cavity and (b) the trocar is used to advance the external drain component through the skin at the planned exit site. *Source:* Courtesy of Angela Banz DVM, DACVS.

contents or the fluid can be dispensed into a graduated cylinder or bowl by squeezing the grenade and allowing the fluid to flow through the evacuation port (Video 9.5 🔵). Close the evacuation port with the attached plug or plug it with a sterile intermittent injection port. The amount and character of the fluid is recorded.

"Homemade" active drains can also be created when there is no commercially available drain in the hospital, or the size and site of the wound dictate smaller diameters than commercially available. For smaller sites, tubing from a butterfly needle can be adapted for this purpose. The syringe adapter tip of a butterfly needle can be cut off and the desired length of the tubing fenestrated and placed into the wound bed (Figure 9.8, Video 9.6 🔵). Placement of the fenestrated end is as described above with Mosquito hemostat technique. The needle end is then inserted into a negative suction (Vacutainer®) blood tube to create suction. The negative suction tube is secured to the butterfly by using ½ inch medical tape in a figure of 8 pattern around the butterfly (Figure 9.9). The blood tube should be exchanged when it is 1/3 to ½ full. Another option is to attach a large syringe to a fenestrated tube implanted as a drain with the plunger pulled back to apply the desired

Figure 9.8   Components of a butterfly needle drain. (a) Photograph of a 21 gauge × ¾" needle with 0.8 × 19 mm tubing. The syringe adapter is removed and the tubing fenestrated on alternating sides. (b) Close-up of the fenestrations. *Source:* Courtesy of Nicole Buote DVM, DACVS.

(a)   (b)

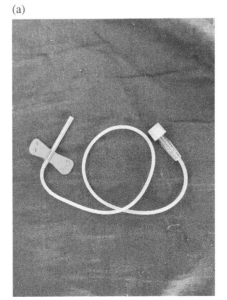
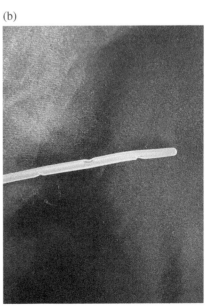

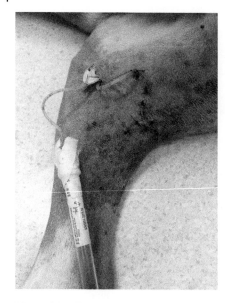

Figure 9.9 Example of a closed suction drain made from butterfly catheter and negative suction blood tube. The needle of the butterfly enters the tube cap and tape is used to secure the tube to the drain setup. *Source:* Courtesy of Angela Banz DVM, DACVS.

level of suction, and a needle or safety pin placed across the plunger to maintain it in position where desired suction is created. The pin is then removed from the end of the syringe for emptying. A three-way stopcock placed between the syringe and tubing facilitates emptying of the syringe [1]. Drains can be secured to the patient with bandages or netting (Figure 9.10).

No consensus has been reached on the timing of drain removal with regard to duration of placement or quantity of fluid produced. Generally, drains are retained until drainage has dropped significantly, reached a plateau, decreased to less than 25–50 cc/day [4, 5], or production is <0.2 ml/kg/hour (4.8 ml/kg/day) [6]. Most closed suction drains are removed between 3- and 7-days post-placement. If fluid production remains high, consideration for maintaining the drain is weighed against risk of infection or delayed tissue healing on an individual patient basis. Drains left in too long may be difficult to remove or promote a tract formation impeding healing. Early removal, when possible, may decrease chances for surgical site infection, but may increase seroma formation (see Chapter 3). Infection rates after clean procedures receiving closed suction drains have been reported to be 15 times higher than similarly classified surgical cases where drains were not placed [7].

Drains can usually be removed in the fully awake patient depending on location and patient demeanor. Distraction of the patient with attention or treat while it is removed can aid in patient compliance. The restraining sutures are cut, and drain is pulled in one smooth motion in the orientation of the internal portion of the drain. A linear clot commonly accompanies the end of the drain as it is pulled. Drain removal can create a short-lived pain response therefore sedation or pain medication can be warranted. The drain hole is left open to heal by second intention and covered with a dressing, as drainage may continue for two to three days.

Complications related to closed suction drains include loss of negative pressure (from wound dehiscence, perforation of the tubing, disconnected reservoir), early removal by the patient, infection (Figure 9.11), clogging, hemorrhage, migration, and rarely tissue necrosis from pressure of very hard/stiff drain [5] or excessive negative pressure. Due to potential for seeding of tumor cells along the tissues, drains should be used sparingly in neoplastic resection sites and should exit close to the surgical wound in a location that would be amenable to further treatment by resection or included in the radiation field if clean margins were not obtained [8].

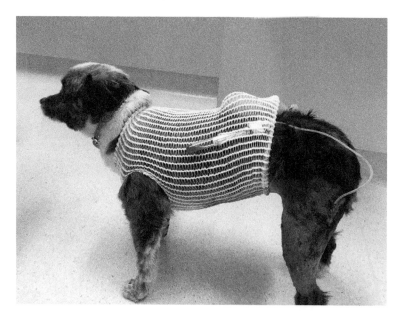

Figure 9.10 A dog with a butterfly drain placed in a wound on the left lateral thigh. A Jackson Pratt drain was placed on the right flank. Burn netting was used to create a t-shirt to help secure the drain reservoirs to the patient. *Source:* Courtesy of Angela Banz DVM, DACVS.

Figure 9.11 Patient with partial necrosis of wound and evidence of infection. The drain had an increase in volume of production and was thick and cloudy character. Cytology confirmed infection with extracellular and intracellular bacteria. *Source:* Courtesy of Angela Banz DVM, DACVS.

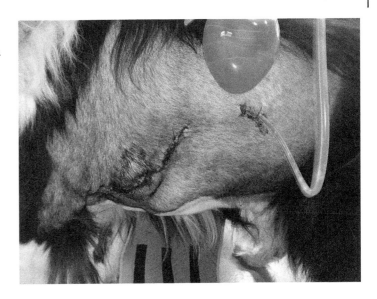

References

1 Pavletic, M.M. (1999). Chapter 4 – common complications in wound healing. In: *Atlas of Small Animal Reconstructive Surgery*, 2e. Philadelphia, PA, USA: WB Saunders.

2 Jackson, F.E. and Pratt, R.A. (1972). Silicone rubber "brain drain". *Z. Neurol.* 201: 92–94.

3 Halfacree, Z.J., Wilson, A.M., and Baines, S.J. (2009). Evaluation of in vitro performance of suction drains. *Am. J. Vet. Res.* 70: 283.

4 Janis, J.E., Khansa, L., and Khansa, I. (2016). Strategies for postoperative seroma prevention: a systematic review. *Plast. Reconstr. Surg.* 138 (1): 240–252.

5 Makama, J.G. and Ameh, E.A. (2008). Surgical drains: what the resident needs to know. *Nigerian J. Med.* 17 (3): 244–250.

6 Shaver, S. and Hunt, G.B. (2014). Evaluation of fluid production and seroma formation after placement of a closed suction drains in clean subcutaneous surgical wounds of dogs: 77 cases (2005-2012). *J. Am Vet. Med. Assoc.* 245 (2): 211–215.

7 Bristow, P.C., Halfacree, Z.J., and Baines, S.J. (2015). A retrospective study of the use of active suction wound drains in dogs and cats. *J. Small Anim. Prac.* 56 (5): 325–330.

8 Lascelles, B.D.X. (2007). Strategic planning in oncological surgery. In *Proceedings of British Small Animal Veterinary Association: 50th Annual Congress,* Birmingham, UK (12–15 April 2007).

10

Vacuum-Assisted Bandages (Negative Pressure Wound Therapy)

Kathryn A. Pitt[1] and Bryden J. Stanley[2]

[1] *Wanderlust Veterinary Services: Academic and Private Practice Locum*
[2] *Animal Surgical Center of Michigan, Flint, MI, USA*

Physiology

Negative pressure wound therapy (NPWT) is a treatment modality that has become widely adopted for a broad range of clinical applications. NPWT is also known by many other names including "vacuum-assisted closure," "subatmospheric pressure therapy," and "topical negative pressure therapy" [1].

NPWT refers to the application of a vacuum evenly distributed across the surface of a wound, typically through a foam dressing. An open-cell, polyurethane or polyvinyl alcohol foam is conformed to the wound and sealed from the environment with occlusive drapes that adhere to the surrounding skin. Specialized access tubing connects the dressing to a programmable vacuum pump, which subjects the entire wound to an evenly distributed negative pressure. Wound exudate is collected into a canister attached to the pump (Figure 10.1). Depending on the unit used, the level of vacuum may be programmable, ranging from 75 to 150 mmHg with 125 mmHg being commonly used for open wounds [2]. NPWT can be continuously, cyclically, or intermittently applied [3].

Many different mechanisms to ameliorate wound healing have been attributed to NPWT, even when scientific validation has been lacking (Table 10.1). Purported effects of NPWT include increased fibroplasia through microdeformation, enhanced angiogenesis, reduction of wound bacterial load, decreased interstitial edema, increased blood flow to the wound, decreased hematoma/seroma formation, and increased expression of various cytokines and growth factors [4–7].

Increased Granulation Tissue

An animal model by Fabian et al. [8] created an ischemic wound using four full-thickness wounds on each ear of 41 male New Zealand white rabbits. On each rabbit, one ear was dressed for use with NPWT and the other ear was used as the control, identically dressed but without NPWT components. The rabbits were then separated into four treatment groups:

Group One had NPWT with no suction and no hyperbaric oxygen therapy
Group Two had NPWT dressing with hyperbaric oxygen therapy but no suction
Group Three had NPWT dressing with suction but no hyperbaric oxygen therapy
Group Four had NPWT dressing with both negative pressure and hyperbaric oxygen therapy.

Statistical significance was found in comparison of NPWT dressing to suction and NPWT dressing alone for peak granulation tissue and granulation tissue gap both with and without use of hyperbaric oxygen. Hyperbaric oxygen alone did not significantly affect the rate of healing; however, NPWT dressing with suction was found to significantly affect the rate of healing.

Wounds treated with NPWT with suction demonstrated a significantly smaller tissue gap and a significantly greater mean peak granulation tissue than control wounds.

Techniques in Small Animal Wound Management, First Edition. Edited by Nicole J. Buote.
© 2024 John Wiley & Sons, Inc. Published 2024 by John Wiley & Sons, Inc.
Companion website: www.wiley.com/go/buote/wounds

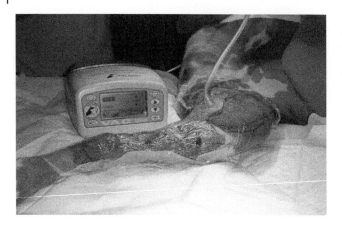

Figure 10.1 NPWT applied to the wound. An open-cell foam is conformed to the wound and sealed from the environment with occlusive drapes. Tubing connects the dressing to a programmable vacuum pump. Wound exudate is collected in a canister attached to the machine/pump. *Source:* Courtesy of Bryden J. Stanley, BVMS, MVETSC, MACVSC, DACVS.

Table 10.1   Mechanisms to ameliorate wound healing attributed to NPWT.

Increased granulation tissue

Reduced bacterial load

Increased blood flow

Decreased hematoma and seroma formation

Increased cytokines/growth factors

Microdeformation with *in-vitro* modeling

Morykwas et al. [4] not only looked at the effects of NPWT on formation of granulation tissue, but they also examined differences caused by varying levels of subatmospheric pressure. In a swine model, they were able to look at multiple different wound treatments on the same animal. Each of four pigs was subjected to −25, −125, and −500 mmHg. They noted that by day 8, wounds treated with −125 mmHg had fully granulated. At this same time point, wounds treated with −25 mmHg had only granulated 21.2% and wounds treated with −500 mmHg had granulated 5.9%. Therefore, it was concluded that wounds treated with −125 mmHg had a significant increase in the rate of granulation tissue formation when compared with other subatmospheric pressures.

Another recent study by Malmsjo et al. [9] also looked at the effects of varying levels of subatmospheric pressure on granulation tissue formation. Peripheral wounds in a swine model were treated for 72 hours with continuous NPWT (−80 mmHg), intermittent NPWT (0 to −80 mmHg), or variable NPWT −10 to −80 mmHg). It was concluded that both intermittent NPWT and variable NPWT resulted in more granulation tissue than continuous NPWT. However, it was also noted that intermittent NPWT caused more discomfort and pain to the patient; therefore, the use of variable NPWT should be researched further. Jacobs et al. [10] used a rodent model to investigate whether NPWT promotes the formation of granulation tissue and healing. Wound closure rates were calculated as a percentage of initial wound size. Statistically significant wound closure rates were found at all time points in the experimental group, and by Day 7 the NPWT treated wounds histologically had well-organized collagen fibers and fibroblast proliferation when compared to the control wounds.

Reduced Bacterial Load

Early studies implied that NPWT could reduce bacterial wound load [5]. Weed et al. [11] provided a clinical retrospective report on the effects of NPWT on bacterial load in 25 patients. Using serial wound cultures, they concluded that there was not a consistent effect of NPWT on bacterial load. In fact, bacterial load increased significantly with the use of NPWT and remained in the range of 10^4–10^6 bacteria/gram of tissue. A randomized trial by Moues et al. [12] looked at 54 patients in need of open wound management before closure. Wounds were randomized to NPWT or moistened gauze therapy. Biopsies were collected to quantify the bacterial load of the wounds. The total bacterial load was comparable in both therapies; however, there was a difference in bacterial species found in the wounds. There was significantly more *Staphylococcus aureus* and significantly less non-fermentative gram-negative bacilli in NPWT-treated wounds. Since its invention, researchers have hypothesized that NPWT will decrease the bacterial load in wounds. To date, there is no robust scientific evidence to support this claim.

Increased Blood Flow

Wackenfors et al. [13] used laser Doppler to measure microvascular blood flow to an inguinal wound of pigs during NPWT. Varying levels of subatmospheric pressure were used (−50 to −200 mmHg). They noted that NPWT increased microvascular blood flow a few centimeters from the wound edge. Blood flow was decreased in the immediate proximity of NPWT, and an area of hypoperfusion was noted. This area increased with increased negative pressures and was especially prominent in the subcutaneous tissues when compared to the muscle. They concluded that soft and dense tissues react differently to NPWT and that a lower subatmospheric pressure during treatment may be more beneficial for soft tissue (−75 mmHg for soft tissue as compared −100 mmHg for dense tissue).

Wackenfors et al. [14] produced another study using a similar model. However, in this model, they focused on wounds of the peristernal thoracic area as opposed to the inguinal area. This model resulted in the same conclusions: NPWT increases microvascular blood flow to the soft tissue and muscle surrounding the wound. A hypoperfused zone was noted in the immediate proximity of NPWT and was larger at greater negative pressures. NPWT induces a change in microvascular blood flow that is dependent on the type of tissue, distance from the wound, and pressure applied.

In a randomized, prospective study, Chen et al. [15] used a rabbit animal model to look at blood flow and edema of skin wounds. They examined the effects of NPWT versus the control in 32 rabbits. Round full-thickness skin defects were made on the dorsal portion of each ear. At different time points, a microcirculation microscope and image pattern analyses were used to observe the variation in wound microcirculation through a detective window. They determined that NPWT promoted capillary blood flow velocity, increased capillary caliber, and blood volume. It was also noted that NPWT stimulated angiogenesis and endothelial proliferation, narrowed endothelial spaces, and restored the integrity of the capillary basement membrane. Another animal model by Lindstedt et al. [16] looked specifically at the effects of NPWT on the blood flow to the myocardium. Laser Doppler velocimetry was used to analyze the microvascular blood flow before and after application of NPWT of −25 and −50 mmHg. It was found that both subatmospheric pressures of NPWT significantly increased the microvascular blood flow in normal, ischemic, and reperfused myocardium. A follow-up study using higher levels of subatmospheric pressure (−75 and −150 mmHg) did not induce microvascular blood flow changes [17].

Another animal model used by Petzina et al. [18] examined the effects of NPWT on peristernal soft tissue blood flow after internal mammary artery harvesting. The effect of NPWT was investigated on the left side, where the internal mammary artery had been removed, and the right side, where the internal mammary artery was intact. Blood flow to the left side was decreased when the left internal mammary artery was surgically removed; however, skin blood flow was not affected. NPWT induced an immediate and similar increase in wound edge blood flow on both sides at both −75 and −125 mmHg. A prospective, randomized study by Timmers et al. [19] looked at the effects of varying subatmospheric pressures on cutaneous blood flow of healthy intact forearm skin using two different foam types (black polyurethane foam and white polyvinyl alcohol foam). Continuous negative pressure was used at a range of −25 to −500 mmHg. Non-invasive laser Doppler probes, incorporated into the dressing, were used to measure blood flow. A significant increase in cutaneous blood flow was noted in both foams up to a subatmospheric pressure of −300 mmHg, with a fivefold increase with the polyurethane foam, and a threefold increase with the polyvinyl alcohol foam.

While other studies have focused on increased circulation to the wound edge, Ichioka et al. [20] focused on blood flow in the wound bed. An intravital microscope-video-computer system was used to visualize the preserved vessels in the wound bed. Three varying subatmospheric pressures were used (−125, −500, and 0 mmHg). It was noted that wound bed circulation was significantly decreased when subatmospheric pressures of −500 mmHg were used, whereas wound bed circulation was significantly increased with −125 mgHg. The control group (0 mmHg) showed no changes in blood flow during the observation period.

Decreased Hematoma and Seroma Formation

Chintamani et al. [21] used a prospective, randomized clinical study to compare the amount and duration of drainage between varying subatmospheric pressures following modified radical mastectomy. About 50 patients were part of the full suction group ($700\,g/m^2$) and 35 patients were in the half-suction group ($350\,g/m^2$). The two groups were comparable in age, weight, and extent of operation. There was not a significant difference between the two treatment groups in regard to seroma formation. However, the half-suction group did have the NPWT removed earlier, and they had a significantly shorter hospital stay without any increase in postoperative morbidity.

Increased Cytokines/Growth Factors

Kilpadi et al. [22] used a swine model to investigate the effect of NPWT on inflammatory cytokine levels. Interleukin (IL)-6, -8, 10, and transforming growth factor-β1 were analyzed using ELISA. Levels were measured at the time of wound creation and hourly for four hours. They noted that there was a significantly earlier and greater peak of IL-10 and maintenance levels of IL-6 compared with control wounds. Labler et al. [23] described a prospective, clinical, nonrandomized study on wounds treated with NPWT. They looked at 32 patients with traumatic wounds that required temporary coverage. About 16 patients were treated with NPWT and the other 16 with Epigard® (Medisave Medical Products, Germany). At each bandage change, wound fluid was collected and IL-6 and -8, vascular endothelial growth factor (VEGF), and fibroblast growth factor-2 were measured by ELISA. Significantly higher levels of Interleukin-8 and VEGF were noted in wound fluid from NPWT-treated patients. Additionally, histologic examination of biopsies (using CD31 and von Willebrand factor immunohistochemistry) indicated significantly more neovascularization in NPWT-treated patients.

Microdeformation with *In-Vitro* Modeling

In-vitro research has suggested that only cells that are able to stretch will respond to growth factors, whereas cells that are confined and unable to stretch are more likely to undergo apoptosis rather than proliferate [24, 25]. Saxena et al. [6] used a computer-based *in-vitro* model to explore the effect of NPWT on microdeformation of cells. In Saxena's model, the pressure, pore diameter, and pore fraction volumes were all altered to assess the effects of NPWT on material deformations. This model showed deformations of 5–20% strain with NPWT, which are consistent with previous results shown to promote cellular proliferation. The authors hypothesized that tissue deformation caused by the application of NPWT causes individual cells to stretch, which thereby promotes cellular proliferation in the microenvironment of the wound.

Table 10.2   Indications for NPWT.

Acute, subacute, and traumatic wounds
Acute surgical wounds that are managed open
Physiologic degloving injuries
Necrotizing fasciitis or vasculitis
Abscesses
Burn wounds
Chronic, non-healing wounds
Multiple wounds
Dehisced incisions
Skin flaps
Skin grafts
Closed surgical incisions
Treatment of myofascial compartment syndrome

Indications of NPWT

Experience with NPWT in veterinary medicine is not as extensive as in human medicine; the literature consists of a controlled study, several case series, some reviews, and many case reports in a variety of species including dogs, cats, horses, a tiger, a tortoise, and a rhinoceros [26–52]. NPWT has also been reported successfully in avians [53]. There are several different commercially available NPWT systems on the market, several of which have penetrated the veterinary market [3]. For example, KCI Animal Health has two veterinary-specific units, V.A.C. Simplicity™ and V.A.C. Freedom™ and Infinity Medical has the Curato®. Given the widespread use of NPWT in human and veterinary medicine, it is important to develop robust guidelines and protocols for different indications [54].

The indications for NPWT are wide and varied (Table 10.2) [49, 55]. Even with the use of NPWT, the previously established principles of wound management should still be followed. These involve thorough cleansing of the periwound and wound, debridement of necrotic and devitalized tissues and copious, and pressured lavage [56, 57]. The main tenets of open wound management (Cleanse, Débride, Lavage, Dress) should never be forgotten, regardless of the dressing that is placed over the wound.

NPWT is an appropriate treatment for acute, subacute, and traumatic wounds, including anatomic degloving and shear wounds with exposed bone [58]. One of the earliest veterinary reports was a clinical case series evaluating outcomes in 15 dogs with traumatic extremity open wounds [27]. The modality has been shown to be well tolerated and allows for several days between dressing changes in the inflammatory phase, where previously daily bandage changes were indicated. It is often utilized to shorten the time period to surgical closure, but can also be used in the proliferative phase [49]. Time to healing in dogs when NPWT is employed is significantly shortened compared to both non-adhesive impregnated gauze dressings and highly absorbent foam dressings [40]. Overall, these studies show that NPWT is a valuable mechanical adjunct to healing in large, complicated wounds, providing a "a bridge to reconstruction." In addition to the enhanced wound healing effects of NPWT, the distinct logistical advantage of the prolonged time between dressing changes (up to 72 hours), compares favorably to the traditional daily wet-to-dry dressing for open wounds still in the inflammatory phase.

Several studies have additionally shown the feasibility and beneficial effects of NPWT in securing and enhancing acceptance of free full-thickness skin grafting in dogs and cats [27, 34, 44, 45, 50]. Not only does granulation tissue appear earlier in the interstices of the meshed graft, but the open meshes close more rapidly, and percentage of graft "take" is higher. There is also better early adhesion of the graft to the recipient bed when under NPWT and decreased reported seroma formation. It appears that NPWT can be used to optimize graft survival and may be especially valuable for large grafting procedures where immobilization is challenging.

NPWT can also be used in acute surgical wounds that are managed open [42], physiologic degloving injuries, necrotizing fasciitis [43], vasculitis, abscesses, burns [37], chronic wounds, multiple wounds (bit wounds, stab wounds), dehisced incisions (including over exposed orthopedic implants), high-risk skin flaps and closed incisions [29, 36, 41, 46, 48], open septic abdomens [30, 52], over closed surgical incisions [41, 48], and to help with myofascial compartment syndrome.

There are certain wound conditions that are not suited for NPWT in veterinary medicine (Table 10.3). Contraindications include poor periwound skin condition, necrotic or clearly devitalized tissue, coagulopathy, exposed major blood vessels, open joints, neoplasia, unexplored draining tracts, untreated osteomyelitis, exposed joints/tendons, very small wounds, and lack of overnight monitoring. Before managing a wound, make sure to assess the patient's overall cardiovascular, respiratory and neurologic status, look for comorbid conditions, contraindications, and administer an appropriate level of analgesia.

Table 10.3 Contraindications for NPWT.

Poor periwound skin condition
Necrotic or clearly devitalized tissue
Coagulopathy
Exposed major blood vessels
Open joint
Neoplasia
Unexplored draining tracts
Untreated osteomyelitis
Very small wounds
Lack of overnight care if patient to be hospitalized

Description of Technique

Preparation Tips

NPWT can be time-consuming and sometimes challenging to apply initially but becomes much easier once practiced. Proper preparation during the initial application can improve the quality of the seal on the periwound skin and save time and frustration later.

The periwound skin should be clipped and prepped with a minimum of 3–5 cm margins, and often a larger margin is desired. This margin allows adequate area for contact of the adhesive drape.

The wound should be cleansed, debrided, and lavaged prior to the application of NPWT. Make sure to use alcohol as the last cleansing agent on the periwound skin as it is an effective defatting and drying agent.

The periwound skin needs to be completely dry prior to the application of the adhesive drape. Moisture will weaken the adhesion of the drape and significantly increase the risk of leakage. A hairdryer on low setting can be used to ensure the periwound skin is completely dry.

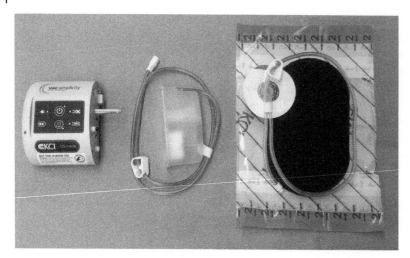

Figure 10.2 Prior to anesthetizing the patient and applying the NPWT dressing, ensure that the machine is fully charged and that all required equipment is gathered together (machine/pump-left, unused canister-middle, occlusive drapes, and open-cell foam-right).
Source: Courtesy of Bryden J. Stanley, BVMS, MVETSC, MACVSC, DACVS.

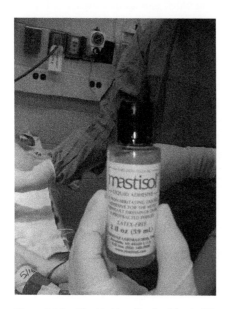

Figure 10.3 Liquid skin adhesive Mastisol® (Eloquest Healthcare®, Ferndale, MI).
Source: Courtesy of Bryden J Stanley, BVMS, MVETSC, MACVSC, DACVS.

Remember that the foam being used must be porous (open-cell or reticulated). Closed-cell foam mattress material is occlusive and will cause wound maceration; it is therefore contraindicated.

Primary application of NPWT is typically performed when the patient is under general anesthesia. Reapplication/dressing changes can generally be performed with sedation alone. Aseptic technique should be maintained throughout any dressing application. There is a learning curve associated with NPWT. Complications with dressing leakage or pump alarm systems will decrease as the team becomes more familiar with the system.

Application of NPWT

1) Prior to anesthetizing the patient and applying the NPWT dressing, ensure that the machine is fully charged and that all required equipment is gathered together (Figure 10.2). Place the reservoir canister with the canister tubing onto the machine.
2) Check the periwound area to ensure that the area is clipped, clean, and absolutely dry.
3) A thin coating of liquid skin adhesive can be applied to the prepared 3–5 cm periwound area and allowed to dry for a few minutes. If there are uneven surfaces, such as between the digits or in skin folds, stoma paste, or hydrocolloid gels can be molded to help make the dressing airtight (Figure 10.3).
4) Next, the foam dressing should be cut to the shape of the wound. If properly sized, the dressing should fit just inside the wound edge to avoid compression of the adjacent periwound skin edge. If the wound is large and/or irregular, the foam dressing can be roughly secured to the wound edge with a few skin staples or cut strips of adhesive drape to prevent dislodgement while the adhesive drape is applied (Figure 10.4a–e).
5) Once the foam is in place, seal the whole wound area with the impermeable, adhesive drapes. These drapes typically come sandwiched between two layers to facilitate placement. Avoid wrinkles or folds in the adhesive drape, when possible, as they can track air from the environment and compromise the integrity of the dressing (Figure 10.5a,b). Adhesive drape placement is easier with two operators.
6) Once the drape is in place, cut an approximately 2 cm round hole in the sheet exposing a small area of the foam dressing. Place the proprietary, adhesive-fenestrated disc with associated evacuation tubing over the hole (Figure 10.6).
7) Immediately connect the evacuation tubing to the tubing on the reservoir canister of the programmable vacuum pump and set either continuous or intermittent negative pressure to the sealed wound, between −80 to −125 mmHg (Figure 10.7). Once powered on, if there are no leaks, the dressing should contract noticeably and become very firm and "raisin-like" (Figure 10.8) to the touch.

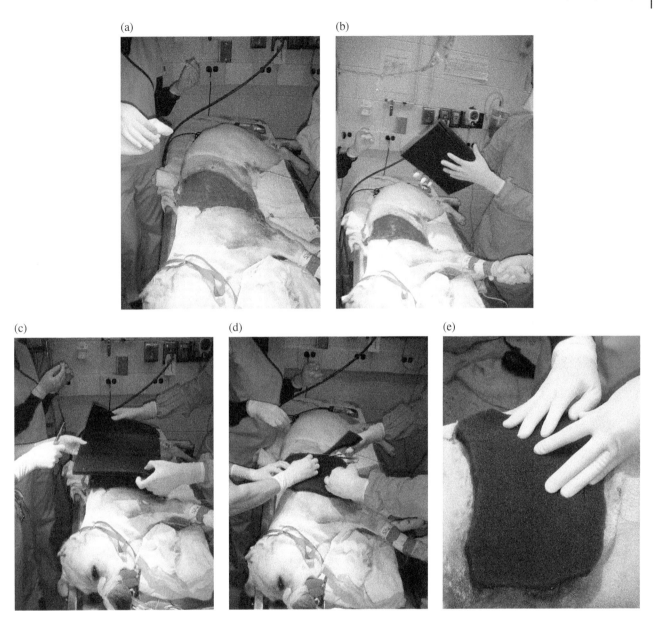

Figure 10.4 (a) The periwound skin is clipped and cleaned and liquid skin adhesive is applied sparingly. (b–d) The foam dressing is removed from the packaging and cut to the shape of the wound. (e) Ensure that the dressing fits just inside the wound edge to avoid compression of the adjacent periwound skin edge. *Source:* Courtesy of Bryden J. Stanley, BVMS, MVETSC, MACVSC, DACVS.

If the seal is airtight, as the pump approaches the preset vacuum level, it becomes quiet and only activates on an intermittent basis, to maintain the vacuum. Listen closely to the dressing for sounds of leakage (a low, moist whistling sound) – more adhesive draping may be required. Continue to place adhesive drape to cover any leaking areas.

If the wound is on a limb, the NPWT dressing can be covered with a soft, padded bandage, coiling a length of the evacuation tubing into the bandage layers to provide a safety loop (Figure 10.9). With trunk wounds, the dressing can be left unbandaged. Allow adequate tubing to extend from the bandage to the patient's dorsum throughout full range of motion if patient is ambulatory.

The pump should never be disconnected from the patient while in place. When the patient needs to go on walks/go outside, the pump should be disconnected from the charger and brought with the patient. With large dogs, the pump can be inserted into a vest and worn; with small dogs and cats, it should reside immediately outside the cage, and transported with the dog when ambulating.

(a)
(b)

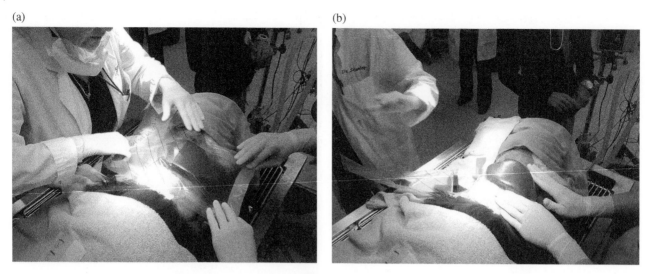

Figure 10.5   (a) Seal the wound area with the impermeable, adhesive drapes. (b) Avoid wrinkles or folds in the adhesive drape when possible. *Source:* Courtesy of Bryden J. Stanley, BVMS, MVETSC, MACVSC, DACVS.

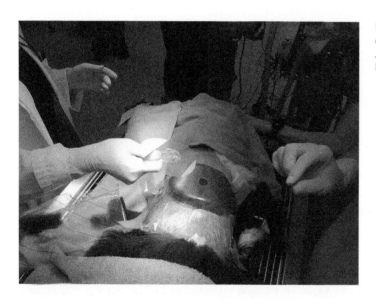

Figure 10.6   A 2 cm round hole is cut in the sheet exposing a similarly sized area of the foam dressing. *Source:* Courtesy of Bryden J. Stanley, BVMS, MVETSC, MACVSC, DACVS.

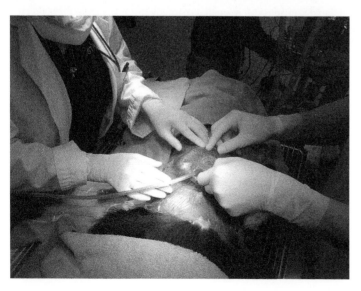

Figure 10.7   Adhesive fenestrated disc with associated evacuation tubing is placed over the hole. *Source:* Courtesy of Bryden J. Stanley, BVMS, MVETSC, MACVSC, DACVS.

Dressing integrity and machine function should be checked regularly during the period of use. The animal should be either continually monitored in an intensive care unit or checked every two hours. If the vacuum is lost for more than several hours, the dressing becomes occlusive and wound maceration will result and therefore the bandage should be changed.

Postoperative Care

NPWT is redressed every 48–72 hours and typically requires only 1–3 dressing changes before a healthy bed of granulation tissue is evident. If the dressing is on left in place for longer than 72 hours, granulation tissue may grow into the interstices of the foam. This causes damage to the delicate vascular components of the granulation tissue when the bandage is ultimately changed and increased discomfort to the patient. Each dressing change takes approximately 15 minutes and can be performed under sedation or brief anesthesia.

When a dressing change is performed, it is important to note that the entire dressing and adhesive drapes do NOT need to be removed. Continued removal of an adhesive drape that has been reinforced with liquid skin adhesive will cause recurrent and unnecessary damage to the periwound skin. To prevent continued damage, it is advised to remove just the portion of the dressing that is covering the foam primary layer. Generally, a scalpel blade is used to cut the drape directly around the edges of the foam to allow its removal (Figure 10.10a,b). This method not only prevents unnecessary skin damage, but it also enhances adhesion of the newly applied dressing and decreases complications with leakage. Following light wound cleansing, and placement of the new foam dressing, the adhesive drapes are placed over the new foam and cover the original drapes on the periwound skin. If a bandage is placed over the dressing, it is useful to create a "window" in the bandage so that the actual foam dressing can be palpated, and confirmed that it is still firm and "raisin-like."

Outcomes/Complications

Complications associated with NPWT systems are generally minor and will decrease as the team becomes familiar with the modality (Table 10.3). One of the most common challenges is loss of vacuum. This is most common area of high motion such as the digits. The motion and crevices can make it difficult to form a seal due to drape detachment. As previously mentioned, meticulous

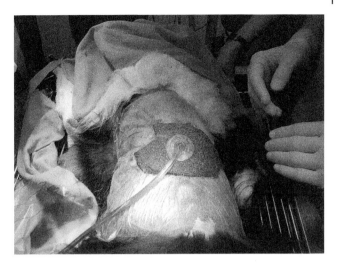

Figure 10.8 When the NPWT is activated, the foam dressing is suctioned down and becomes firm to the touch. *Source:* Courtesy of Bryden J. Stanley, BVMS, MVETSC, MACVSC, DACVS.

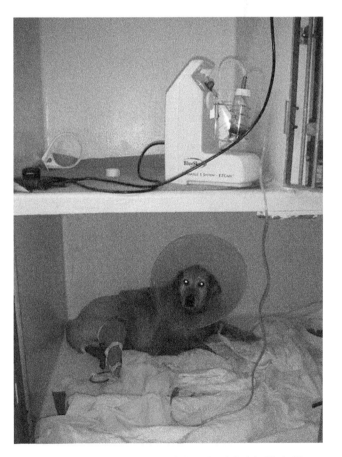

Figure 10.9 NPWT has been applied to the right hindlimb. The adhesive dressing has been covered with a soft, padded bandage. The evacuation tubing has been coiled in the bandage to provide a safety loop. *Source:* Courtesy of Bryden J. Stanley, BVMS, MVETSC, MACVSC, DACVS.

(a)   (b)

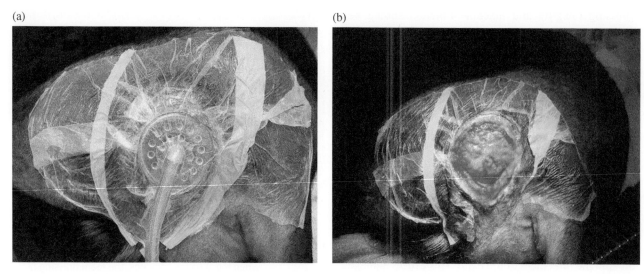

Figure 10.10   (a) Continued removal of an adhesive drape will cause recurrent and unnecessary damage to the periwound skin. (b) To prevent continued damage, remove just the portion of the dressing that is covering the foam primary layer with a scalpel blade. *Source:* Courtesy of Bryden J. Stanley, BVMS, MVETSC, MACVSC, DACVS.

attention to clipping and cleansing the periwound skin, using a spray adhesive, and creating a dam across the uneven surfaces (such as interdigital areas) with stoma paste is important for avoiding complications with loss of vacuum [49]. Pumps are designed to alarm with loss of pressure due to disruption of the occlusive dressing. In this case, either reinforce the dressing with more adhesive drapes or change the dressing as soon as possible (within two to four hours) to prevent wound maceration. To prevent leakage of the dressing, be meticulous during original dressing placement. Additionally, patients can cause their own set of complications by chewing or kinking the tubing. Making sure that E-collars are placed appropriately and the patients are adequately confined can prevent these complications [49].

References

1 Hunter, J.E., Teot, L., Horch, R., and Banwell, P.E. (2007). Evidence-based medicine: vacuum-assisted closure in wound care management. *Int. Wound J.* 4 (3): 256–269.

2 Peinemann, F. and Sauerland, S. (2011). Negative-pressure wound therapy: systematic review of randomized controlled trials. *Deutsches Arzteblatt Int.* 108 (22): 381–389.

3 Glass, G.E. and Nanchahal, J. (2012). The methodology of negative pressure wound therapy: separating fact from fiction. *J. Plast. Reconstr. Aesthetic Surg.* 65 (8): 989–1001.

4 Morykwas, M.J., Faler, B.J., Pearce, D.J., and Argenta, L.C. (2001). Effects of varying levels of subatmospheric pressure on the rate of granulation tissue formation in experimental wounds in swine. *Ann. Plast. Surg.* 47 (5): 547–551.

5 Morykwas, M.J., Argenta, L.C., Shelton-Brown, E.I., and McGuirt, W. (1997). Vacuum-assisted closure: a new method for wound control and treatment: animal studies and basic foundation. *Ann. Plast. Surg.* 38 (6): 553–562.

6 Saxena, V., Hwang, C.-W., Huang, S. et al. (2004). Vacuum-assisted closure: microdeformations of wounds and cell proliferation. *Plast. Reconstr. Surg.* 114: 1086–1096.

7 Xie, X., McGregor, M., and Dendukuri, N. (2010). The clinical effectiveness of negative pressure wound therapy: a systematic review. *J. Wound Care* 19 (11): 490–495.

8 Fabian, T.S., Kaufman, H.J., Lett, E.D. et al. (2000). The evaluation of subatmospheric pressure and hyperbaric oxygen in ischemic full-thickness wound healing. *Am. Surgeon* 66 (12): 1136–1143.

9 Malmsjo, M., Gustafsson, L., Lindstedt, S. et al. (2012). The effects of variable, intermittent, and continuous negative pressure wound therapy, using foam or gauze, on wound contraction, granulation tissue formation, and ingrowth into the wound filler. *Eplasty* 12: e5.

10 Jacobs, S., Simhaee, D.A., Marsano, A. et al. (2009). Efficacy and mechanisms of vacuum-assisted closure (VAC) therapy in promoting wound healing: a rodent model. *J. Plast. Reconstr. Aesthetic Surg.* 62 (10): 1331–1338.

11 Weed, T., Ratliff, C., and Drake, D.B. (2004). Quantifying bacterial bioburden during negative pressure wound therapy: does the wound VAC enhance bacterial clearance? *Ann. Plast. Surg.* 52 (3): 276–279; discussion: 9–80.

12 Moues, C.M., Vos, M.C., van den Bemd, G.J. et al. (2004). Bacterial load in relation to vacuum-assisted closure wound therapy: a prospective randomized trial. *Wound Repair Regener.* 12 (1): 11–17.

13 Wackenfors, A., Sjogren, J., Gustafsson, R. et al. (2004). Effects of vacuum-assisted closure therapy on inguinal wound edge microvascular blood flow. *Wound Repair Regener.* 12 (6): 600–606.

14 Wackenfors, A., Gustafsson, R., Sjogren, J. et al. (2005). Blood flow responses in the peristernal thoracic wall during vacuum-assisted closure therapy. *Ann. Thoracic Surg.* 79 (5): 1724–1730; discussion: 30–31.

15 Chen, S.Z., Li, J., Li, X.Y., and Xu, L.S. (2005). Effects of vacuum-assisted closure on wound microcirculation: an experimental study. *Asian J. Surg.* 28 (3): 211–217.

16 Lindstedt, S., Malmsjo, M., and Ingemansson, R. (2007). Blood flow changes in normal and ischemic myocardium during topically applied negative pressure. *Ann. Thoracic Surg.* 84 (2): 568–573.

17 Lindstedt, S., Malmsjo, M., Sjogren, J. et al. (2008). Impact of different topical negative pressure levels on myocardial microvascular blood flow. *Cardiovasc. Revascul. Med.* 9 (1): 29–35.

18 Petzina, R., Gustafsson, L., Mokhtari, A. et al. (2006). Effect of vacuum-assisted closure on blood flow in the peristernal thoracic wall after internal mammary artery harvesting. *Euro. J. Cardio Thoracic Surg.* 30 (1): 85–89.

19 Timmers, M.S., Le Cessie, S., Banwell, P., and Jukema, G.N. (2005). The effects of varying degrees of pressure delivered by negative-pressure wound therapy on skin perfusion. *Ann. Plast. Surg.* 55 (6): 665–671.

20 Ichioka, S., Watanabe, H., Sekiya, N. et al. (2008). A technique to visualize wound bed microcirculation and the acute effect of negative pressure. *Wound Repair Regener.* 16 (3): 460–465.

21 Chintamani, S.V., Singh, J., Bansal, A., and Saxena, S. (2005). Half versus full vacuum suction drainage after modified radical mastectomy for breast cancer- a prospective randomized clinical trial [ISRCTN24484328]. *BMC Cancer* 5: 11.

22 Kilpadi, D.V., Bower, C.E., Reade, C.C. et al. (2006). Effect of vacuum assisted closure therapy on early systemic cytokine levels in a swine model. *Wound Repair Regener.* 14 (2): 210–215.

23 Labler, L., Rancan, M., Mica, L. et al. (2009). Vacuum-assisted closure therapy increases local interleukin-8 and vascular endothelial growth factor levels in traumatic wounds. *J. Trauma* 66 (3): 749–757.

24 Chen, C.S., Mrksich, M., Huang, S. et al. (1998). Micropatterned surfaces for control of cell shape, position, and function. *Biotechnol. Progr.* 14 (3): 356–363.

25 Huang, S., Chen, C.S., and Ingber, D.E. (1998). Control of cyclin D1, p27(Kip1), and cell cycle progression in human capillary endothelial cells by cell shape and cytoskeletal tension. *Mol. Biol. Cell* 9 (11): 3179–3193.

26 Adkesson, M.J., Travis, E.K., Weber, M.A. et al. (2007). Vacuum-assisted closure for treatment of a deep shell abscess and osteomyelitis in a tortoise. *J. Am. Vet. Med. Assoc.* 231 (8): 1249–1254.

27 Ben-Amotz, R., Lanz, O.I., Miller, J.M. et al. (2007). The use of vacuum-assisted closure therapy for the treatment of distal extremity wounds in 15 dogs. *Vet. Surg.* 36 (7): 684–690.

28 Bertran, J., Farrell, M., and Fitzpatrick, N. (2013). Successful wound healing over exposed metal implants using vacuum-assisted wound closure in a dog. *J. Small Anim. Prac.* 54 (7): 381–385.

29 Bristow, P.C., Perry, K.L., Halfacree, Z.J., and Lipscomb, V.J. (2013). Use of vacuum-assisted closure to maintain viability of a skin flap in a dog. *J. Am. Vet. Med. Assoc.* 243 (6): 863–868.

30 Buote, N.J. and Havig, M.E. (2012). The use of vacuum-assisted closure in the management of septic peritonitis in six dogs. *J. Am. Anim. Hosp. Assoc.* 48 (3): 164–171.

31 Cioffi, K.M., Schmiedt, C.W., Cornell, K.K., and Radlinsky, M.G. (2012). Retrospective evaluation of vacuum-assisted peritoneal drainage for the treatment of septic peritonitis in dogs and cats: 8 cases (2003-2010). *J. Vet. Emerg. Crit. Care* 22 (5): 601–609.

32 Demaria, M., Stanley, B.J., Hauptman, J.G. et al. (2011). Effects of negative pressure wound therapy on healing of open wounds in dogs. *Vet. Surg.* 40 (6): 658–669.

33 Gemeinhardt, K.D. and Molnar, J.A. (2005). Vacuum-assisted closure for management of a traumatic neck wound in a horse. *Equine Vet. Educ.* 17 (1): 27–33.

34 Guille, A.E., Tseng, L.W., and Orsher, R.J. (2007). Use of vacuum-assisted closure for management of a large skin wound in a cat. *J. Am. Vet. Med. Assoc.* 230 (11): 1669–1673.

35 Harrison, T.M., Stanley, B.J., Sikarskie, J.G. et al. (2011). Surgical amputation of a digit and vacuum-assisted-closure (V.A.C.) management in a case of osteomyelitis and wound care in an eastern black rhinoceros (Diceros bicornis michaeli). *J. Zoo Wildlife Med.* 42 (2): 317–321.

36 Lafortune, M., Fleming, G.J., Wheeler, J.L. et al. (2007). Wound management in a juvenile tiger (Panthera tigris) with vacuum-assisted closure (V.A.C. Therapy). *J. Zoo Wildlife Med.* 38 (2): 341–344.

37 Mullally, C., Carey, K., and Seshadri, R. (2010). Use of a nanocrystalline silver dressing and vacuum-assisted closure in a severely burned dog. *J. Vet. Emerg. Crit. Care* 20 (4): 456–463.

38 Nolff, M.C., Fehr, M., Reese, S., and Meyer-Lindenberg, A.E. (2016). Retrospective comparison of negative-pressure wound therapy and silver-coated foam dressings in open-wound treatment in cats. *J. Feline Med. Surg.* 19 (6): 624–630.

39 Nolff, M.C., Pieper, K., and Meyer-Lindenberg, A. (2016). Treatment of a perforating thoracic bite wound in a dog with negative pressure wound therapy. *J. Am. Vet. Med. Assoc.* 249 (7): 794–800.

40 Nolff, M.C., Fehr, M., Bolling, A. et al. (2015). Negative pressure wound therapy, silver coated foam dressing and conventional bandages in open wound treatment in dogs. A retrospective comparison of 50 paired cases. *Vet. Compar. Orthopaedics Traumatol.* 28 (1): 30–38.

41 Nolff, M.C., Flatz, K.M., and Meyer-Lindenberg, A. (2015). Preventive incisional negative pressure wound therapy (Prevena) for an at-risk-surgical closure in a female Rottweiler. *Schweiz Arch. Tierheilkd.* 157 (2): 105–109.

42 Nolff, M.C., Layer, A., and Meyer-Lindenberg, A. (2015). Negative pressure wound therapy with instillation for body wall reconstruction using an artificial mesh in a dachshund. *Aust. Vet. J.* 93 (10): 367–372.

43 Nolff, M.C. and Meyer-Lindenberg, A. (2015). Necrotising fasciitis in a domestic shorthair cat--negative pressure wound therapy assisted debridement and reconstruction. *J. Small Anim. Prac.* 56 (4): 281–284.

44 Nolff, M.C. and Meyer-Lindenberg, A. (2015). Negative pressure wound therapy augmented full-thickness free skin grafting in the cat: outcome in 10 grafts transferred to six cats. *J. Feline Med. Surg.* 17 (12): 1041–1048.

45 Or, M., Van Goethem, B., Kitshoff, A. et al. (2017). Negative pressure wound therapy using polyvinyl alcohol foam to bolster full-thickness mesh skin grafts in dogs. *Vet. Surg.* 46 (3): 389–395.

46 Or, M., Van Goethem, B., Polis, I. et al. (2015). Pedicle digital pad transfer and negative pressure wound therapy for reconstruction of the weight-bearing surface after complete digital loss in a dog. *Vet. Compar. Orthopaedics Traumatol.* 28 (2): 140–144.

47 Owen, L.J., Hotston Moore, A., and Holt, P.E. (2009). Vacuum-assisted wound closure following urine-induced skin and thigh muscle necrosis in a cat. *Vet. Compar. Orthopaedics Traumatol.* 22: 417–421.

48 Perry, K.L., Rutherford, L., Sajik, D.M., and Bruce, M. (2015). A preliminary study of the effect of closed incision management with negative pressure wound therapy over high-risk incisions. *BMC Vet. Res.* 11: 279.

49 Pitt, K.A. and Stanley, B.J. (2014). Negative pressure wound therapy: experience in 45 dogs. *Vet. Surg.* 43 (4): 380–387.

50 Stanley, B.J., Pitt, K.A., Weder, C.D. et al. (2013). Effects of negative pressure wound therapy on healing of free full-thickness skin grafts in dogs. *Vet. Surg.* 42 (5): 511–522.

51 Nolff, M.C. (2021). Filling the vacuum: role of negative pressure wound therapy in open wound management in cats. *J. Feline Med. Surg.* 23 (9): 823–833.

52 Spillbeen, A.L., Robben, J.H., Thomas, R. et al. (2017). Negative pressure therapy versus passive open abdominal drainage for the treatment of septic peritonitis in dogs: a randomized, prospective study. *Vet. Surg.* 46 (8): 1086–1197.

53 Knapp-Hoch, H. and de Matis, R. (2014). Clinical technique: negative pressure wound therapy - general principles and use in avian species. *J. Exotic Pet Med.* 23: 56–66.

54 Newton, K., Wordsworth, M., Allan, A.Y., and Dumville, J.C. (2017). Negative pressure wound therapy for traumatic wounds. *Cochrane Database Syst Rev.* (1): CD012522. https://doi.org/10.1002/14651858.CD012522. PMICD: PMC6472626.

55 Kirkby, K.A., Wheeler, J.L., Farese, J.P. et al. (2010). Surgical views: vacuum-assisted wound closure: clinical applications. *Compendium* 32 (3): E1–E6; quiz: E7.

56 Broughton, G. 2nd, Janis, J.E., and Attinger, C.E. (2006). A brief history of wound care. *Plast. Reconstr. Surg.* 117 (7 Suppl): 6S–11S.

57 Shepard, G.H. and Rich, N.M. (1972). Treatment of the soft tissue war wound by the American military surgeon: a historical resume. *Mil. Med.* 137 (7): 264–266.

58 Guy, H. and Grothier, L. (2012). Using negative pressure therapy in wound healing. *Nurs. Times.* 108 (36): 16, 8, 20.

11

Biologic Treatments

Subsection A: Medicinal Leech Therapy

Celine S. Kermanian[1] and Nicole J. Buote[2]

[1] *VCA West Los Angeles, Animal Hospital, Los Angeles, CA, USA*
[2] *Department of Clinical Sciences, Cornell University, Ithaca, NY, USA*

Anatomy and Physiology

A brief review of the history of MLT reveals that while they were quite popular in Medieval times for everything from headaches to humors their use declined precipitously in the late nineteenth century due to overuse and a lack of efficacy. In the late nineteenth century, hirudin, an anticoagulant found in the saliva of leeches was discovered and this created a scientifically supported role for leeches in human medicine [1–3]. The possible utilities of leeches have since been studied extensively, discovering more than 100 different bioactive compounds within their saliva. These compounds function through various distinct, yet cooperative processes.

Anatomy

There are more than 650 species of leeches in the world, but *Hirudo medicinalis* and *Hirudo verbena* are the most commonly used in the human medical field [4]. Leeches are a segmented hermaphroditic invertebrate (annelid worms) that commonly reach 20 cm in length when fully mature. Their appearance is marked by a dark brownish–green body color with a dorsal red or brown stripe (Figure 11.A.1). The caudal end of a leech is supplied with a large sucker on which it is used for crawling and attachment to various surfaced (Figure 11.A.2, Videos 11.A.1 🔊 and 11.A.2 🔊). The cranial or cephalad sucker is for feeding and consists of a tripartite jaw with 60–100 teeth, each with its own secretory opening. It is difficult to tell the cephalad and caudal aspects apart in most cases but the feeding cephalad sucker is smaller and tapered. Due to the anatomy of a leech jaw, a star or Y-shaped bite mark is left after MLT and the feeding site [5]. The intestinal tract of a leech comprises the jaw, a pharynx, an esophagus, crop, stomach, intestine, and hindgut [6]. Leeches can ingest a blood volume of almost 10 times their own weight and may not require feeding for up to one year after their last meal.

Physiology

Sanguivorous leeches use symbiotic bacteria, such as *Aeromonas* spp., which reside in their gut to help break down stored blood into different components for energy. The most famous bioactive compound found in leeches is hirudin, an anticoagulant responsible for inhibiting thrombin. Hirudin is an extremely effective anticoagulant due to three mechanisms: (i) it is not inactivated by platelet factors, (ii) it does not affect platelet function, and (iii) it can inactivate thrombin already bound to a thrombus [4]. Leech saliva is also known to carry anesthetics (a histamine-like substance), anti-aggregating substances like calin, vasoactive substances like histamine, and proteases such as collagenases and hyaluronidases which increase tissue permeability [1, 4, 7, 8]. The combination of these substances allows for the perforation of the skin to go unnoticed, the ingestion of blood without cessation, and increases the capillary flow of the

Techniques in Small Animal Wound Management, First Edition. Edited by Nicole J. Buote.
© 2024 John Wiley & Sons, Inc. Published 2024 by John Wiley & Sons, Inc.
Companion website: www.wiley.com/go/buote/wounds

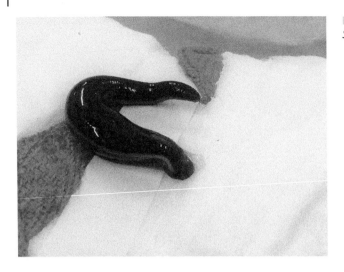

Figure 11.A.1   Photograph of a leech, *Hirudo medicinalis*. *Source:* Courtesy of Nicole Buote, DVM, DACVS.

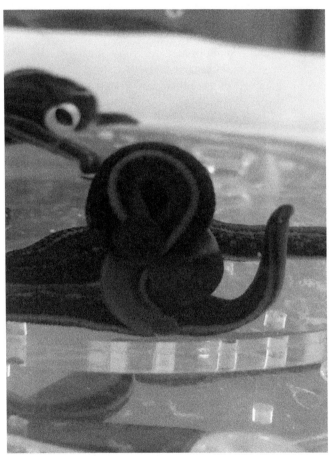

Figure 11.A.2   Photograph of a leech suctioned to side of plastic mobile home. *Source:* Courtesy of Nicole Buote, DVM, DACVS.

tissue bed by vasodilatation and thrombolysis. This mixture also explains the prolonged passive bleeding after withdrawal of the leech that is seen in all clinical cases.

Each leech can remove approximately 5–10 ml of blood per feeding and each site will continue to ooze an additional meal volume over the following 24–48 hours after detachment [4, 8].

An experimental study by Conforti et al., in pigs from 2002 reported 90% of passive bleeding after detachment occurs within the first five hours and laser Doppler illustrated increases in perfusion localized to the 16–20 mm diameter centered around the bite zone [9]. This zone correlated well with a return to normal skin color in these patients and skin color is still used today for monitoring of MLT efficacy.

Indications

Although the indications of MLT in human medicine are well-established, only a few reports have been published in veterinary medicine documenting their use and outcomes. The first report documented the successful use of MLT in a domestic shorthair care for treatment of polycythemia vera (PCV) when blood viscosity prevented phlebotomy treatments [8]. A second case report in a cat suffering from severe venous stasis of a paw after a constrictive wound also illustrated a favorable outcome and no complications of MLT were documented (Figure 11.A.3) [10]. The chapter authors have also

(a)　　　　　　　　　　(b)　　　　　　　　　　(c)

(d)　　　　　　　　　　(e)　　　　　　　　　　(f)

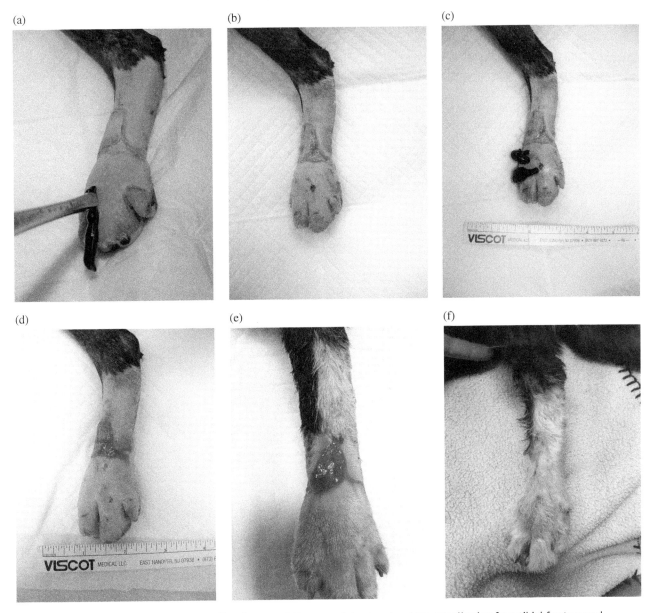

Figure 11.A.3　Photographs of cat who suffered a constrictive wound due to a bandage complication for a tibial fracture and underwent MLT daily for four days. (a) Paw on presentation after owner complained of pet becoming non-weight bearing on the limb and appearing painful on palpation of the bandage. A necrotic wound is visible on the dorsal aspect of the paw with distal swelling of the toes. The wound acted as 360° band around the tarsus. In this photograph, a leech is being placed on the paw with atraumatic forceps. (b) Three days post initiation of MLT. The distal paw swelling has decreased but is still present, the necrotic wound has been partially debrided, and healthy granulation tissue is present at the edges. A wound from a previous leech bite is seen on the center of the dorsal aspect of the paw. (c) MLT being instituted on day 3 post presentation. (d) Five days post initiation of MLT. Swelling of the toes continues to improve and all necrotic tissue from wound removed. No further MLT was performed. (e) Paw at 15 days post presentation. (f) Paw at 42 days post presentation. *Source:* Courtesy of Nicole Buote, DVM, DACVS.

seen leeches used successfully to decrease venous congestion after leashes, hair ties, bandages, and orthopedic procedures in the distal forelimb and hindlimbs – specifically, tarsal arthrodesis, metacarpal fracture repair, and tarsometatarsal luxation (Figure 11.A.4). A third case report described the use of leeches to address cervical and sublingual swelling in a dog with upper respiratory obstruction [11]. The only retrospective study performed in veterinary medicine examined the indications and outcomes of MLT in 12 patients and found that nearly 70% underwent treatment after reconstructive skin surgery while the remaining were for constrictive wounds [12]. In this cohort, 75% of patients showed clear improvement of the affected tissue and no major complications were reported [12]. In human medicine, leeches are frequently used with reconstructive surgeries including skin flaps and reimplantations to aid in treatment of venous congestion which can occur postoperatively [8, 10, 12–14]. A European review also discussed the usage of leeches in hip and elbow dysplasia, acute and chronic arthritis, and the treatment of scars [6]. *The main indication for MLT in the United States in human and veterinary practice is microvascular and reconstructive surgery, especially salvage of skin flaps whose viability is jeopardized by venous congestion and treatment of venous congestion from constrictive injuries* (Table 11.A.1).

Venous congestion occurs any time; there is an imbalance between arterial inflow and venous outflow. This leads to a stasis of blood within the capillary bed indicated by the dark purple skin color that is the hallmark of this condition. Decreases in venous outflow occur due to various causes including constrictive wounds (hair ties, chain, leashes, bandages), damage to venous structures during interventional or surgical procedures, and in reconstruction and

(a)

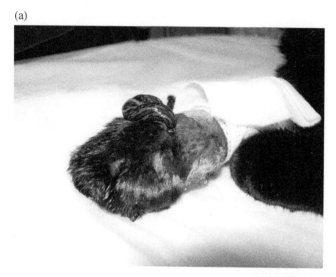

Figure 11.A.4 Photographs of patients undergoing MLT for venous congestion from constrictive wounds. Neither of these patients required sedation. (a) Cat in which an IV catheter pressure bandage had been left on inadvertently for many days after discharge. (b,c) Dog experienced wounds from bandage placed at the level of the carpus. (b) Pre-MLT, (c) Post-MLT, and primary closure of wound. *Source:* Courtesy of Nicole Buote, DVM, DACVS.

(b) (c)

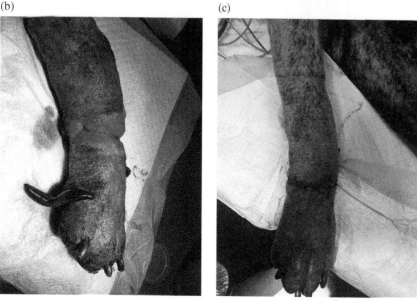

Table 11.A.1 Indications for MLT in veterinary medicine.

Cause	Pathophysiologic effect	Mechanism of action
Axillary or subdermal skin flap (dogs, cats)	Venous congestion	Removal of accumulated blood Decreased capillary blood pressure
Constrictive wound from bandages, ties, leashes (dogs, cats)	Venous congestion	Removal of accumulated blood Decreased capillary blood pressure
Swelling after orthopedic procedures to distal limbs: arthrodesis, luxation repairs, metacarpal fracture repair (dogs, cats)	Venous congestion	Removal of accumulated blood Decreased capillary blood pressure
Cervical region swelling and a sublingual hematoma (dog)	Upper airway obstruction Venous congestion	Removal of accumulated blood Decreased capillary blood pressure
Polycythemia vera (cat)	Increased blood viscosity	Decreased blood viscosity due to anticoagulant effect
[a]Arthritis of the hip, stifle, elbow, and shoulder (dogs, cats)	Inflammation	Unknown-presumed that bioactive agents in leech saliva dilate blood vessels and promote circulation to the injured body part
[a]Neuritis, discopathies, and spinal arthritis, and caudal equina syndrome (dogs, cats, horses)	Inflammation	Unknown-presumed that bioactive agents in leech saliva dilate blood vessels and promote circulation to the injured body part
[a]Tendonitis, ligament strain (dogs, cats, horses)	Inflammation	Unknown-presumed that bioactive agents in leech saliva dilate blood vessels and promote circulation to the injured body part
[a]Laminitis (horses)	Inflammation	Unknown-presumed that bioactive agents in leech saliva dilate blood vessels and promote circulation to the injured body part

[a] Proposed use but no validated studies in veterinary medicine.

reimplantation procedures because the thin walls of the low capacitance venules are easily collapsed [4, 15, 16]. When venous congestion occurs, decreased tissue perfusion leads to hypoxia, acidosis, arterial thrombi formation, and eventually tissue necrosis. Venous congestion leads multiple to physical exam findings such as skin discoloration, edema, brisk capillary return, and warmth in the tissue [17]. MLT is an excellent treatment for venous congestion because it allows for an alternative route or removal of congested venous blood allowing collapsed venules to recover, all while arterial perfusion continues [2, 7, 17]. Specifically, elimination of excessive accumulated blood decreases the capillary filling pressure and allows arterial capillary beds to reperfuse. For some types of reimplantation surgeries in human patients (ears), venous congestion is an accepted postoperative finding, and MLT is a standard treatment. MLT treatments must be continued until capillary flow is reestablished or constrictive injuries are resolved. Although one report briefly mentions, the use of MLT in veterinary medicine for treatment of arthritis, tendonitis, scars, and other conditions, no specific data was described regarding the presumed mechanism of action or outcomes so its use cannot be recommended until more data is presented [6].

Description of Technique

Diagnostic Tests

Prior to MLT, several diagnostic tests should be performed and a variety of additional patient data recorded (Table 11.A.2). The patient's vital parameters (temperature, heart rate, respiratory rate) should always be recorded prior to leech therapy. The minimum required diagnostic tests to be performed prior to leeching include pack cell volume (PCV) or hematocrit (HCT), total protein (TP), prothrombin time (PT), and partial thromboplastin time (PTT). Additional patient data that

Table 11.A.2   Table summarizing preoperative diagnostic tests, MLT technique, postoperative care, and postoperative diagnostic tests to be performed by clinicians during medicinal leech therapy.

Preoperative diagnostic tests	Patient vital parameters
	Patient CRT
	Patient PCV or HCT
	Patient TP
	Patient PT/PTT
	Tissue CRT
	Tissue temperature
	Tissue glucose, lactate
	Leech weights
	Culture of leech GI tract
MLT technique	Antibiotic prophylaxis
	Administer sedative medication, if indicated
	Prepare affected skin; remove all residue
	Cover surrounding skin
	Place leeches on affected tissue
	Encourage latching, if indicated
	Await spontaneous detachment of leeches
	Careful monitoring throughout feeding
Postoperative care	Passive oozing expected up to 24 h
	Wipe site every 15–30 min, until clotted
	Apply bandage if indicated and amenable
	Clean site with betadine or topical antibiotic
	Immerse leeches in 70% ethanol
	Apply leeches again when oozing stops
	Continue leeching until tissue appearance improves by 50%
Postoperative diagnostic tests	Patient vital parameters
	Patient CRT
	Patient PCV or HCT
	Patient TP
	Tissue CRT
	Tissue temperature
	Leech weights

could be recorded prior to MLT includes mucous membrane capillary refill time (CRT), CRT of the affected tissue, appearance and temperature of the affected tissue, antibiotics administered, glucose and lactate levels of the affected tissue, and time to treatment after original surgery or injury. Weight of all leeches prior to (and after) leeching should also be recorded as an additional method for quantification of blood loss. Use of photographs to document the appearance of the affected tissue before, during, and after treatments can be helpful and is very important, as is proper documentation of treatment progress in the patient's medical records.

During MLT, number of leech sessions, number of leeches used, length of leeching time, number of days between leechings, willingness or failure of leeches to feed, antibiotic therapy, patient's body position, room temperature, and whether or not the tissue was punctured should also be recorded. Need for blood transfusion should always be documented. Additionally, any complications associated with MLT, such as infection, leech migration, localized pruritus, hypersensitivity, anaphylaxis, fever or hyperthermia, need for sedation, or prerenal azotemia should be recorded.

The authors have provided a data collection form to be used by veterinary clinicians (Figure 11.A.5).

Medicinal Leech Therapy: Data Collection Form

Name	Date
DOB	Age
Breed	Species

Reason for MLT: _____   MLT Session #:_____   Days since previous MLT: _____

Pre-MLT

PCV Pre-MLT: [   ] %

Mucous Membrane CRT Pre-MLT: <2 seconds   ≤2 seconds

Tissue Glucose Pre-MLT: [   ] g/dL

Tissue Lactate Pre-MLT: [   ] g/dL

Tissue CRT Pre-MLT: <2 seconds   ≤2 seconds

PT/PTT Pre-MLT: /

Appearance of Tissue Pre-MLT:

| white | pale | red | purple | black |

Temperature of Tissue Pre-MLT: [   ] °F

Pre-MLT Leech Weight: _____ g

Post-MLT

PCV Post-MLT: [   ] %

Mucous Membrane CRT Post-MLT: <2 seconds   ≤2 seconds

Tissue CRT Post-MLT: <2 seconds   ≤2 seconds

Appearance of Tissue Post-MLT:

| white | pale | red | purple | black |

Temperature of Tissue Post-MLT: [   ] °F

Bandage Applied: Y / N

Post-MLT Leech Weight: _____ g

During MLT

Room Temperature: [   ] °F

Prick with 20-Gauge Needle: Y / N

Application of D5W to Tissue: Y / N

Willingness of Leech to Feed: Y / N

Comments: _____

_____

Temperature of Tissue During MLT: [   ] °F

Number of Leeches Used: [   ] leeches

Leeching Time: [   ] hours [   ] minutes

Need for sedation: Y / N

Patient Tolerance: tolerant / intolerant

Complications with MLT:

| leech migration | passive bleeding | hypersensitivity |

Comments: _____

_____

Blood transfusion required: Y / N

Figure 11.A.5   Data collection form created for use by veterinarians during medicinal leech therapy.

MLT Technique

Before MLT is initiated, culture of the leech gastrointestinal tract should be performed for optimal selection of antibiotic prophylaxis against *Aeromonas hydrophila,* the most common bacteria found in the leech gastrointestinal tract. Antibiotic prophylaxis must be administered during and for at least 24 hours after MLT has been completed in all patients [18]. Fluoroquinolones or third/fourth-generation cephalosporins have historically been the treatment of choice [18], as *Aeromonas hydrophila* produces β-lactamase, which often renders the first-generation cephalosporins and penicillins ineffective [19]. Trimethoprim-sulfamethoxazole has been shown to be as effective as ciprofloxacin in one study [20]. However, a study published in 2012 reported culture results of a person infected with *Aeromonas hydrophila* following MLT, which was resistant to ciprofloxacin [21]. A recent veterinary study found the most common antibiotic used in dogs and cats was amoxicillin-clavulanic acid [12]. Antibiotic selection should always be determined on a case-by-case basis and based on leech gut culture results. Upon delivery of leeches to the hospital, the authors recommend sacrificing one leech from the cohort for culture of its digestive tract and appropriate antibiotic selection. The leech must first be submerged in 70% ethanol for five seconds for purposes of euthanasia [22]. A 2–3 cm longitudinal incision is made on the ventral aspect of the leech using a #15 blade between its anterior and posterior suckers [23]. The leech's crop is dissected free from the surrounding skin and connective tissues and is pierced [23]. The intraluminal fluid may be aspirated with a positive-pressure pipette [23] or puncture site may be extended with iris scissors and the lumen of the crop swabbed with a culturette. The collected digestive tract sample should be submitted to a laboratory for aerobic and anaerobic culture and sensitivity testing.

When all diagnostic tests are complete and the patient is ready to undergo MLT, the affected skin should be prepared using chlorhexidine scrub, followed by saline. It is important to ensure all soap residue is adequately removed, as any remaining chlorhexidine may deter leeches from latching to the site. The tissue must be warm, as leeches feed at temperatures between 33 and 40 °C [24]. The areas surrounding the affected skin are subsequently covered with 4×4 in gauze or clear occlusive dressings to prevent leech migration. Each leech can decongest and increase perfusion to a ~2 cm^2 [9]. Thus, the number of leeches is determined based on the surface area of the affected tissue and leeches are placed on the lesion using atraumatic forceps. If reluctant to feed, the leeches are encouraged to latch by pricking the skin with a 25 gauge needle or applying a small amount of D5W or dextrose over the affected area [4]. Leeches can also be placed inside syringe casings or 3-ml syringes with the plungers removed, leaving the open ends inverted onto the skin and held in place to keep them at the attachment sites and promote latching (Figure 11.A.6).

Careful monitoring throughout the treatment is critical to ensure that leeches do not migrate to areas of healthy skin, incisions, or open wounds (Videos 11.A.3 ⊕ and 11.A.4 ⊕). Each leech will draw approximately 5–15 ml of blood over a period of 20–120 minutes [6]. Medically trained personnel, i.e., a clinician, veterinary student, veterinary technician, etc. should observe the patient and leeches throughout the duration of feeding. Once leeches are fully engorged, spontaneous detachment will occur. It is imperative not to forcefully remove leeches from the site while feeding, as their microscopic teeth may break off and be left in the wound, increasing the risk of infection. If a leech must be removed before spontaneous detachment, a small volume of isopropyl alcohol, saline, or vinegar can be placed on a cotton swab and applied gently to the head of the leech (the smaller side of the leech), which usually results in spontaneous detachment. Take care not to apply excessive amounts, however, as this may cause the leech to regurgitate blood and gastrointestinal contents, increasing the risk of infection. Because of a histamine-like substance that acts as a local anesthetic found in the saliva of leeches, the process is pain-free. Therefore, administration of sedative medications is typically not required, though some patients may require sedation due to temperament or anxiety.

(a)   (b)   (c)

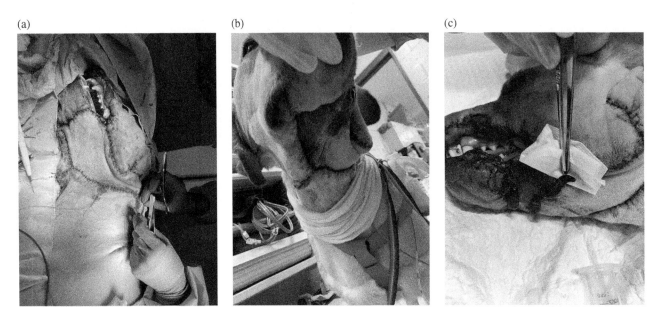

Figure 11.A.6   Patient with extensive skin loss over left lateral face and ventral chin/neck region from a dog bite. (a) Immediate postoperative caudal superficial epigastric flap for closure of chin/neck wound. (b) One day postoperatively venous congestion noticed at distal aspect of flap. (c) Leeches being applied to flap. This patient was mildly sedated for MLT due to the location being so close to the mouth. *Source:* Courtesy of Nicole Buote, DVM, DACVS.

Postoperative Care

Passive oozing of blood for up to 24 hours during the post-attachment period is expected and may account for an equal volume of blood loss as the active feeding itself (Figure 11.A.7). If there is continued passive bleeding or if passive bleeding is significant or messy, a soft padded bandage may be placed over the site, if amenable. Due to the anatomy of their anterior suckers, consisting of three half-moon-shaped jaws and sharp teeth, leeches will leave a characteristic Y-shaped bite at the site. The site should be wiped with a sterile saline-soaked gauze approximately every 15–30 minutes to determine if passive oozing has stopped. Betadine or topical antibiotic agents can be used to clean the site. Following MLT, all leeches that were used should be immersed in a container of 70% ethanol with a secure lid for euthanasia and should never be reused. Leeches should be subsequently disposed of as biohazardous waste.

New leeches are applied when passive bleeding has stopped; therefore, frequency of MLT often varies. In humans, leeches are applied everyone to eight hours on average, for a duration of days to weeks [13, 25, 26], which is a more aggressive protocol than the authors have performed or reported in the veterinary setting. In the authors' experience, leeching is

(a) (b) (c)
(d) (e) (f)

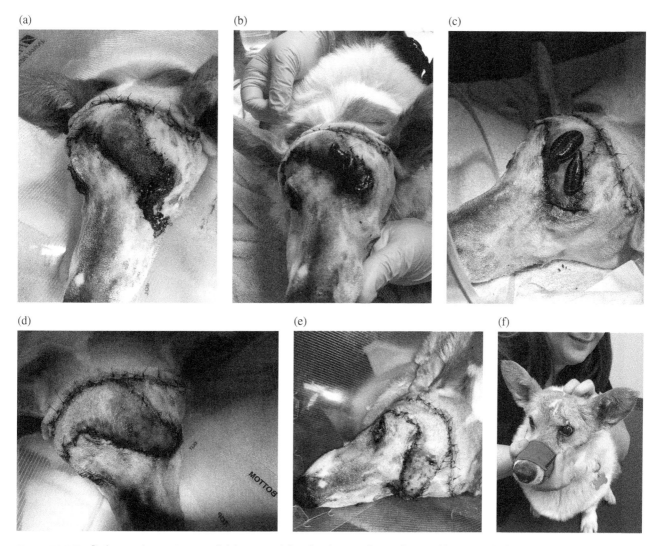

Figure 11.A.7   Patient underwent a superficial temporal flap for closure of wound created by removal of an upper eyelid mast cell tumor. (a) Day 1 postoperative a severely congested flap was identified. (b) Dorsal view of leeches applied day 1 postop to distal flap (first MLT). The patient was not sedated. (c) Lateral view of leeches applied day 2 postop to distal flap. (d) Day 2 postop immediately post-MLT some erythema remains but purple discoloration is gone (second MLT). Oozing from the bite wounds is visible. (e) Two hours post-MLT day 4 postop (fourth MLT) a normal color has returned to the majority of the flap. (f) Patient one month postop – the flap completely survived and patient experienced no complications with MLT. *Source:* Courtesy of Nicole Buote, DVM, DACVS.

practically performed once to twice daily as MLT is time-intensive. Leeching is continued until venous congestion has improved by 50%, which is easily confirmed by visual assessment. Decongestion is evidenced by improvement in the color (color change from deep purple to light pink), turgidity (skin palpates softer), and CRT of the affected tissue is less than two seconds. Improvement of venous congestion of a skin flap may occur as early as three to seven days following initial treatment and can take up to weeks or months thereafter [4].

Any remaining leeches that were not used may be stored in the hospital for extended periods of time, up to six months. Leeches should be maintained in cool, distilled water-lidded containers in the dark, such as a refrigerator. Water should be changed daily and, while leeches can survive for very long periods of time without ingesting blood, Hirudosalt should be added to their containers during daily water changes. Hirudosalt is free of iodine and is composed of sodium chloride, magnesium chloride, sodium sulfate, calcium chloride, and potassium chloride, important to leech health and creating physiologic osmolarity in the environment.

Following MLT, outcome data, including PCV and TP, mucous membrane CRT, affected tissue CRT, antibiotic therapy, appearance and temperature of the affected tissue, and whether a bandage was applied, should be documented (Table 11.A.2). Vital parameters should also be reassessed. Furthermore, weight of all leeches post-MLT should be recorded. This data has been incorporated into the data collection form in Figure 11.A.1. Vital parameters should subsequently be reevaluated every 4 hours for the first 24 hours following treatment and PCV and TP should be assessed at least twice daily during MLT.

Outcomes/Complications

Outcomes

To date, a paucity of objective information is available on clinical outcomes after MLT in the veterinary field. Nevertheless, the current veterinary literature holds promising results, similar to the outcomes seen in human medicine.

A recent single-institution retrospective assessment of clinical outcomes following MLT in nine dogs and three cats showed success in 75% of patients treated with MLT for venous congestion and necrosis in compromised skin flaps and wounds [12]. About 67% of patients in this study had venous congestion secondary to skin flaps and 33% had venous congestion caused by constrictive bandages, suggestive of the value of MLT not only in treating compromised skin flaps, but also for treatment of wounds in which skin perfusion has been compromised for other reasons [12]. The median number of MLT sessions in both dogs and cats was two sessions and time to complete healing ranged from 14 to 120 days with a mean of 41 days [12]. Total leeching time was reported for three cases with a mean of 2.2 hours. Neither sedative medications nor blood transfusions were required for any patients. Following MLT, six dogs (67%) and three cats (100%) visibly showed clear improvement of the affected tissue and healed completely, indicating that MLT may be an effective treatment option when conventional modalities have proven unsuccessful. This is the only retrospective study of MLT in the veterinary literature to date (Figures 11.A.8 and 11.A.9) [12].

There are only three additional reported clinical cases in veterinary medicine describing the use of MLT and favorable outcomes were achieved in treating all three patients with MLT [8, 10, 11]. One case documented success in treating a three-year-old female spayed domestic shorthair with a single session of MLT for polycythemia vera (PCV 79%) and secondary seizures, when causes of relative and secondary polycythemia were ruled out and initial phlebotomy was impossible due to hyperviscosity [8]. Leeching was successful in reducing the patient's PCV to 64% immediately following MLT and further to 56% 24 hours later, once passive bleeding had discontinued. A second case showed improved outcomes in treating venous stasis of the paw secondary to a constrictive wound in a one-year-old male castrated domestic shorthair [10]. Venous stasis was diagnosed approximately two weeks after placement of a bivalve cast for treatment of tibial and fibular fractures. Leech application in this case was performed once daily for four days and swelling of the paw subsequently significantly improved. A third case described the use of hirudotherapy for treatment of upper airway obstruction secondary to severe soft tissue swelling that was contiguous with the cervical region and a sublingual hematoma in a 10-month-old female Mastiff [11]. There were minimal changes to the patient's oropharyngeal swelling following 18 hours of medical management with intubation (total intravenous anesthesia maintained with propofol, fentanyl, and dexmedetomidine), oxygen supplementation, diphenhydramine, corticosteroid therapy, antimicrobial treatment, and gastrointestinal medications. Medicinal leeches were applied to the oral and ventral cervical swellings and sublingual swelling improved six to eight hours following treatment. Extubation was possible 44 hours post-intubation. Extubation and subsequent discharge

Figure 11.A.8   Cat undergoing MLT for venous congestion after an angularis oris flap performed to close a mass removal site. Patient was not sedated. *Source:* Courtesy of Nicole Buote, DVM, DACVS.

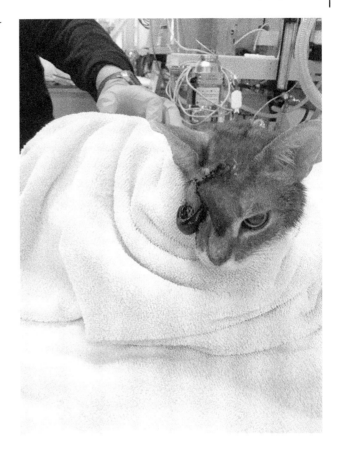

Figure 11.A.9   Photograph of MLT for venous congestion of a rotation flap on the medial elbow of a dog. *Source:* Courtesy of Nicole Buote, DVM, DACVS.

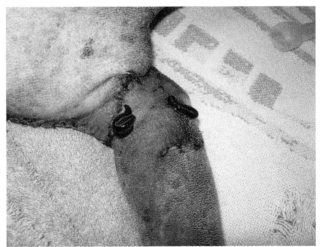

from hospital were hypothesized to have occurred more rapidly due to the adjunctive use of MLT [11]. There were no reported complications or adverse effects in any case [8, 10, 11].

While there is limited clinical data on MLT in veterinary medicine, the utility of MLT has been well-documented in human medicine for treatment of questionably viable skin flaps and reimplantations [13, 25–28]. Whitaker et al. found a 77.98% success rate in salvaging skin flaps using MLT in 277 cases, while 22.02% of tissues were deemed unsalvageable and required excision [25]. In another review of 39 human patients whose native skin and local flaps were treated with MLT, the total salvage rate was 90.9% and partial salvage rate was 9.1% [13]. In contrast, the same review found a total salvage rate of 33.3%, partial salvage rate of 33.3%, and total loss rate of 33.3% for regional and free flaps [13]. Other retrospective reviews in the human literature have reported 100% [27], 83.7% [26], and 62.5% [28] of total salvage rates following MLT.

Complications

The main reported complication associated with MLT is infection. The most common identified bacteria is *Aeromonas hydrophila*, which is a gram-negative rod that is a commensal organism of the leech digestive tract. It has high affinity for muscle tissue, with the potential to cause severe deep infections, septicemia, local tissue damage, flap failure, need for additional antibiotics, prolonged hospital stay, and rarely death [4, 19]. Other bacteria, including *Aeromonas veronii, Serratia marcescens, Proteus vulgaris, Morganella marganii, Aeromonas sobria,* and *Vibrio fluvialis* have also been reported [10, 25, 29]. In people, the incidence of infection associated with MLT has been reported from two to 36% [4]. Occurrence of leech-associated infection has not been reported in dogs and cats treated with MLT to date. Infection did not occur in any of the published clinical veterinary cases mentioned above [8, 10, 12]. Infections associated with MLT may resemble clostridial infections, presenting as cellulitis or local abscess with the production of gas [4, 19]. In a 1990 prospective study, which evaluated iatrogenic venous congestion of island abdominal skin flaps in 30 laboratory New Zealand White rabbits treated with MLT, an *Aeromonas hydrophila* infection was described similar to *Aeromonas* septicemia-toxemia syndrome in people, with an associated pneumonia and typhlitis [30]. The authors suggested that the two major contributing factors of *Aeromonas* septicemia in those rabbits were stress and excessive administration of prophylactic penicillin [30]. To minimize the risk of infection, all patients should be treated with prophylactic antibiotic therapy, as described above. Attempts to decontaminate the gut flora of leeches have proven unsuccessful and may lead to drug resistance and should therefore never be done [29]. If an infection is diagnosed following MLT, a second antibiotic should be added to the treatment protocol, based on culture and sensitivity results of the infected tissue. Deep, severe infections are treated with aggressive debridement and high doses of antibiotics in people. Survival of infected flaps has been shown to be less than 30% in the human literature [4].

Another common complication in humans following MLT is excessive blood loss requiring blood transfusions, which is the reason for which close patient monitoring and thorough documentation of progress in patients' medical records is necessary. One study reported 49.75% of cases in people who underwent MLT required blood transfusions following the procedure [25]. Tissue survival rate of 91.2% in patients who did not require blood transfusion was not significantly different when compared to 82.2% in patients who required blood transfusion, indicating that the need for a blood transfusion is not a negative prognostic indicator of flap survival [25]. Another study found 57.9% of human patients overall required blood transfusions and 74.1% in pedicled and free flaps [13]. An average of two to six transfusions in patients requiring blood transfusions has been reported in the human literature [13, 25]. While blood transfusions are frequently administered in people who have undergone MLT, blood transfusions are rarely administered in association with MLT in veterinary patients due to the use of fewer leeches during treatment and fewer total leeching sessions usually performed [10]. Despite findings of lower PCV post-MLT than had been measured before MLT in one study, with differences in PCV ranging from three to 16% and a mean of 7.5%, no patients required blood transfusions [12]. CRT in all patients included in the study was one second following MLT [12]. A clinical need for administration of blood transfusions following MLT has not been documented in any other veterinary reports [8, 10]. Nevertheless, prior to MLT, the clinician should ensure availability of blood products best suited for the patient being treated.

Transmission of blood-borne viruses between patients may occur if leeches are reused on more than one patient [10]. Other complications with MLT include leech migration, local hypersensitivity, anaphylaxis, scarring from the leech bite, psychologic aversion, and prerenal azotemia [4, 10, 13, 19, 25]. None of these have been reported in veterinary patients.

References

1 Zaidi, S.M.A., Jameel, S.S., Zaman, F. et al. (2011). A systematic overview of the medicinal importance of sanguivorous leeches. *Altern. Med. Rev.* 16: 59–65.

2 Porshinsky, B.S., Saha, S., Grossman, M.D. et al. (2011). Clinical uses of the medicinal leech: a practical review. *J. Postgrad. Med.* 57: 65–71.

3 Okka, B. (2013). Hirudotherapy from past to present. *Eur. J. Basic Med. Sci.* 3 (3): 61–65.

4 Green, P.A. and Shafritz, A.B. (2010). Medicinal leech use in microsurgery. *J. Hand Surg.* 35 (6): 1019–1021.

5 Abdualkader, A.M., Ghawi, A.M., Alaama, M. et al. (2013). Leech therapeutic applications. *Indian J. Pharm. Sci.* 75: 127–137.

6 Sobczak, N. and Kantyka, M. (2014). Hirudotherapy in veterinary medicine. *Ann. Parasitol.* 60 (2): 89–92.

7 Singh, A.P. (2010). Medicinal leech therapy (hirudotherapy): a brief overview. *Compliment. Ther. Clin. Pract.* 16: 213–215.

8 Nett, C.S., Arnold, P., and Glaus, T.M. (2001). Leeching as initial treatment in a cat with polycythemia vera. *J. Small Anim. Pract.* 42: 554–556.

9 Conforti, M.L., Connor, N.P., Heisey, D.M. et al. (2002). Evaluation of performance characteristics of the medicinal leech (*Hirudo medicinalis*) for the treatment of venous congestion. *Plast. Reconstr. Surg.* 109 (1): 228–235.

10 Buote, N.J. (2014). The use of medical leeches for venous congestion: a review and case report. *Vet. Comp. Orthop. Traumatol.* 27 (3): 173–178.

11 Trenholme, H.N., Masseau, I., and Reinero, C.R. (2021). Hirudotherapy (medicinal leeches) for treatment of upper airway obstruction in a dog. *J. Vet. Emerg. Crit. Care* 31: 661–667.

12 Kermanian, C.S., Buote, N.J., and Bergman, P.J. (2022). Medicinal leech therapy in veterinary medicine: a retrospective study. *J. Am. Anim. Hosp. Assoc.* 58 (6): 303–308.

13 Nguyen, M.Q., Crosby, M.A., Skoracki, R.J. et al. (2012). Outcomes of flap salvage with medicinal leech therapy. *Microsurgery* 32: 351–357.

14 Yantis, M.A., O'Toole, K.N., and Ring, P. (2009). Leech therapy. *Am. J. Nurs.* 109: 36–42.

15 Mommsen, J., Rodriguez-Fernandez, J., Mateos-Micas, M. et al. (2011). Avulsion of the auricle in an anticoagulated patient: is leeching contraindicated? A review and a case. *Craniomaxillofac. Trauma Reconstr.* 4: 61–68.

16 Freidman, J., Fabre, J., Netscher, D. et al. (1999). Treatment of acute neonatal vascular injuries-the utility of multiple interventions. *J. Pediatr. Surg.* 34: 940–945.

17 Weinfeld, A.B., Yuksel, E., Boutros, S. et al. (2000). Clinical and scientific considerations in leech therapy for the management of acute venous congestion: an updated review. *Ann. Plast. Surg.* 45: 207–212.

18 Elyassi, A.R., Terres, J., Rowshan, H.H. et al. (2013). Medicinal leech therapy on head and neck patients: a review of literature and proposed protocol. *Oral Surg. Oral Med. Oral Path Oral Radiol.* 116 (3): e167–e172.

19 Wells, M.D., Boyd, J.B., and Bowen, V. (1993). The medical leech: an old treatment revisited. *Microsurgery* 14 (3): 183–186.

20 Kruer, R.M., Barton, C.A., Roberti, G. et al. (2015). Antimicrobial prophylaxis during *Hirudo medicinalis* therapy: a multicenter study. *J. Reconstr. Microsurg.* 31: 205–209.

21 Patel, K.M., Svetska, M., Sinkin, J. et al. (2013). Ciprofloxacin- resistant *Aeromonas hydrophila* infection following leech therapy: a case report and review of the literature. *J. Plast. Reconstr. Aesthet. Surg.* 66: e20–e22.

22 Graf, J. (1999). Symbiosis of *Aeromonas veronii* Biovar sobria and *Hirudo medicinalis*, the medicinal leech: a novel model for digestive tract associations. *Infect. Immun.* 67 (1): 1–7.

23 Worthen, P.L., Gode, C.J., and Graf, J. (2006). Culture-independent characterization of the digetive-tract microbiota of the medicinal leech reveals a tripartite symbiosis. *Appl. Environ. Microbiol.* 72 (7): 4775–4781.

24 Whitaker, I.S., Cheung, C.K., Chahal, C.A.A. et al. (2005). By what mechanism do leeches help to salvage ischaemic tissues? A review. *Br. J. Plast. Surg.* 43: 155–160.

25 Whitaker, I.S., Oboumarzouk, O., Rozen, W.M. et al. (2012). The efficacy of medicinal leeches in plastic and reconstructive surgery: a systematic review of 277 reported clinical cases. *Microsurgery* 32: 240–250.

26 Herlin, C., Bertheul, N., Bekara, F. et al. (2017). Leech therapy in flap salvage: systematic review and practical recommendations. *Ann. Chir. Plast. Esthet.* 62 (2): e1–e13.

27 Koch, C.A., Olsen, S.M., and Moore, E.J. (2012). Use of the medicinal leech for salvage of venous congested microvascular free flaps of the head and neck. *Am. J. Otolaryngol. Head Neck Med. Surg.* 33 (1): 26–30.

28 Chepeha, D.B., Nussenbaum, B., Bradford, C.R. et al. (2002). Leech therapy for patients with surgically unsalvageable venous obstruction after revascularized free tissue transfer. *Arch. Otolaryngol. Head Neck Surg.* 128: 960–965.

29 Bibbo, C., Fritsche, T., Stemper, M. et al. (2013). Flap infection associated with medicinal leeches in reconstructive surgery: two new drug-resistant organisms. *J. Reconstr. Microsurg.* 29: 457–460.

30 Richerson, J.T., Davis, J.A., and Meystrik, R. (1990). *Aeromonas*, acclimation, and penicillin as complications when leeches are applied to skin flaps in rabbits. *Lab. Anim.* 24 (2): 147–150.

11

Biologic Treatments

Subsection B: Maggot Therapy
Megan Mickelson

College of Veterinary Medicine, University of Missouri, Columbia, MO, USA

Background/Physiology

Larval therapy consists of the application of live fly larvae to a wound bed. Typically *Lucilia* (*Phaenicia*) *sericata*, the green-bottle sheep blowfly, is disinfected in a lab and sterilized larvae are shipped overnight for clinical use [1] (Figures 11.B.1, 11.B.2, and 11.B.3). These are facultative maggots that require aerobic conditions and, thus, feeding is restricted to superficial layers of a wound only [2], unlike nonselective obligate feeders, such as the flesh fly (*Wohlfahrtia magnifica*) or screwworms (*Chrysomya bezziana, Cochliomyia hominivorax*), that are known to feed aggressively too deep, extending into normal tissues [3].

Historically, the use of maggots for treatment of battle wounds was reported in Mayan culture, up to and including the early 1900s [4]. With the advent of antibiotics, it was then employed for use in wounds less commonly, with a newer resurgence in certain areas of human medicine, especially with regard to antibiotic resistance and diabetic ulcers [5, 6]. The technique is now referred to as Maggot Debridement Therapy (MDT), while other names include biodebridement, biosurgery, and larval therapy [2, 7, 8].

The primary goals of MDT are to achieve debridement of necrotic tissue, reduce bacterial contamination, and enhance healthy granulation tissue, with reported success rates up to 80% [9–11].

MDT achieves these goals via multiple mechanisms, both mechanical and biochemical. Body spicules on the maggots themselves offer mechanical debridement [12]. A feeding mass is formed by aggregates of maggots using their mouth hooks to physically scrape their food source, causing further tissue abrasion. Two salivary glands release digestive enzymes and the pharynx functions as a pump to suck liquified food into the digestive system. Their saliva is composed of collagenases, carboxypeptidases A and B, leucine aminopeptidase, and serine proteases (trypsin-like and chymotrypsin-like enzymes, metalloproteinase, aspartyl proteinase) that function to breakdown necrotic tissues [13, 14]. Saliva also contains antibacterial substances that allow auto-disinfection and have demonstrated properties against *Staphylococcus aureus*, including multiple resistant isolates, *Streptococcus A and B*, various *Pseudomonas* species, and *Escherichia coli in vitro* [2, 15, 16]. Maggots secrete allantoin, ammonium bicarbonate, and urea that create an alkaline environment within the wound bed, leading to significant fluid exudate production and further inhibiting bacterial growth [2, 17]. Additional secretions, including phenylacetic acid, phenylacetaldehyde, and calcium carbonate have known bactericidal effects [14]. The physical movement and nature of crawling are thought to not only dislodge material aiding in mechanical debridement, but also to decrease the ability for bacteria to habituate alongside the effects of irrigation of wound fluid in the bed [2, 13]. A single maggot can digest 25 mg necrotic tissue in a 24 hour period [16, 18]. On a live host, the feeding stage is complete within three days and uncontained larvae would exit the wound into the environment.

With regards to increasing healthy granulation tissue, maggot secretions, and excretions have a proteolytic effect that can modify fibroblast adhesion and maintain cell viability *in vitro*, aiding in induction of granulation tissue formation [19–21]. The degradation of extracellular matrix components, such as fibronectin, into small fragments, enhances fibroblast-extracellular matrix interactions for debridement [13, 21]. Overall this leads to leukocyte adhesion, growth factor and

Techniques in Small Animal Wound Management, First Edition. Edited by Nicole J. Buote.
© 2024 John Wiley & Sons, Inc. Published 2024 by John Wiley & Sons, Inc.
Companion website: www.wiley.com/go/buote/wounds

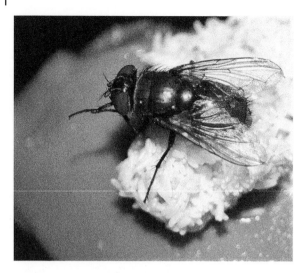

Figure 11.B.1 *Lucilia sericata* fly sitting on top of a cluster of eggs. *Source:* Courtesy of RA Sherman and the BioTherapeutics, Education and Research (BTER) Foundation.

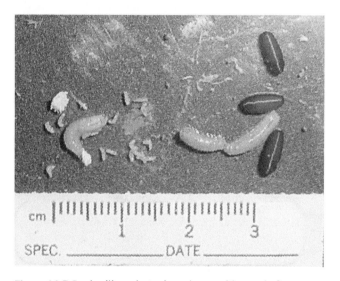

Figure 11.B.2 *Lucilia sericata* sizes shown with a scale for reference. Pictured are eggs, various larvae stages (first instars, third instars), and pupae (smallest to largest) from the medicinal maggot colony at University of California, Irvine, California. *Source:* Courtesy of RA Sherman and the BioTherapeutics, Education and Research (BTER) Foundation.

collagen production, and increased angiogenesis, macrophage responsiveness, fibrinolysis, and nitric oxide levels within the wound bed [22].

Tissue biopsies obtained post-application in chronic diabetic foot ulcer wounds in humans demonstrated progression from an inflammatory phase of wound healing on pre-MDT biopsy to a proliferative phase with presence of angiogenesis, granulation tissue, increased fibroblasts, and lack of bacteria on post-MDT biopsies [23].

Indications

Within human medicine, uses have been variable and the application has increased in more recent years, especially for more complicated and/or chronic wound scenarios. These include use in pressure wounds, burns, and chronic wounds or those deemed intractable to other therapies [12, 24–27]. MDT is commonly employed with diabetic ulcers [28, 29] and other chronic ulcers with or without osteomyelitis [4, 30–33]. Other reported uses include individuals with necrotic wounds, necrotizing fasciitis [10], pyoderma gangrenosum [34], chronic infection [27], fungal wounds, MRSA, or other antibiotic resistance [35, 36], and chemo extravasation [37] (Figures 11.B.4, 11.B.5, and 11.B.6).

MDT is utilized for areas where surgical debridement is considered challenging and in scenarios where avoidance of limb amputation and limb salvage may be able to be achieved with more successful debridement. Approximately 50–73% of human cases are reported to avoid limb amputation with the use of MDT over other techniques [8, 38–40].

Reports of the use of MDT remain limited in veterinary medicine to date. In the largest series of cases, MDT was used for wounds considered deep or challenging in two dogs, four cats, one rabbit, and 13 horses. These cases mostly consisted of application to problematic wounds, 86% of which had failed traditional therapies, in order to aid debridement (56%), control infection (43%), or treat technically challenging areas (29%) [41]. It was proposed to use MDT for limb salvage within veterinary medicine at the time [41]. Within small animal medicine specifically, reports are limited. A single case report describes its use for a particularly challenging burn injury in a dog [42]. One study reported the use of MDT for rabbits with chronic sores and ulcers treated with *Phormia regina* [43].

Most veterinary case reports have been in large animal medicine, including a buffalo [44], a bull with actinomyces [45], two donkeys [46, 47], and footrot in a sheep [48]. More literature exists regarding MDT in equine medicine with descriptions of its use in a large series of 108 horse hoof infection and another series of 41 horses treated for laminitis [49–52].

In general, MDT is oftentimes considered a last resort in wound therapy, but increased success when used earlier in the wounding process and in non-septic patients has been shown and, thus, MDT should be considered a second- or third-line treatment following initial surgical debridement instead [41].

Contraindications for the use of MDT include dry, necrotic wounds since maggots require moisture, fistulae or wounds open to a body cavity, wounds with important vasculature and/or nerves exposed due to the risk of bleeding or injury, highly exudative wounds that risk drowning or washing away maggots and diluting their digestive enzymes, and patients with fly larvae allergies or sepsis [2, 10].

Description of Technique

Application of MDT typically follows initial surgical debridement of grossly necrotic and devitalized tissues. The wound area is measured to calculate the amount of larvae needed. One technique is to perform a wound tracing or impression on a sterile plastic sheet or utilizing a hydrocolloid dressing. Maggots are applied as 5–10 maggots/cm^2 of wound and transferred when they measure between 1 and 3 mm long [2]. The number of maggots to order can be calculated via consultation with the company upon placement of the order.

Medical maggots have been regulated by the FDA as a medical device since 2004 [53] and sterile larvae are currently distributed in 12 labs through 20 countries [54]. For purchase within the United States, Irvine Medical Maggots™ (Monarch Labs, Maggot Therapy Laboratory, University of California) have been available since 1995

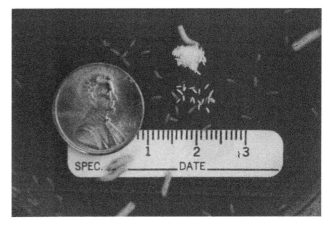

Figure 11.B.3 *Lucilia sericata* sizes shown with a scale and penny for reference. Pictured are eggs, various larvae stages (first instars, third instars), and pupae (smallest to largest) from the medicinal maggot colony at VA Medical Center, Long Beach, California. *Source:* Courtesy of RA Sherman and the BioTherapeutics, Education and Research (BTER) Foundation.

Figure 11.B.4   Human patient with IV extravasation of medication causing a wound on the antebrachium. MDT was instituted because the patient could not tolerate surgery. The wound is pictured before (a), after six weeks of treatment (b), after eight weeks of treatment (c) with MDT, and fully healed post-grafting four months following the initial wounding (d). *Source:* Courtesy of RA Sherman and the BioTherapeutics, Education and Research (BTER) Foundation.

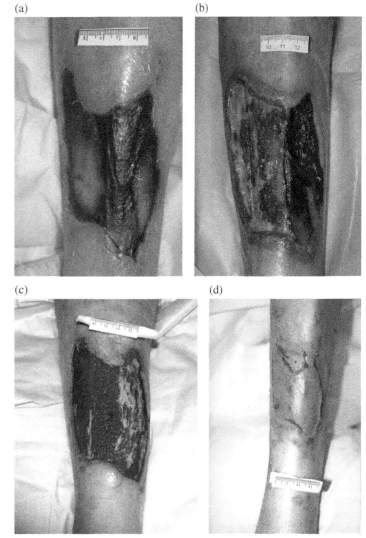

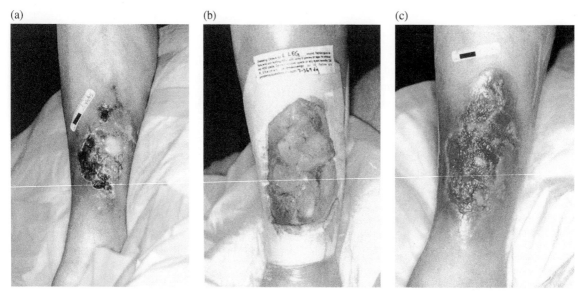

(a)   (b)   (c)

Figure 11.B.5   Human patient with a wound on the distal leg before treatment (a), with bandaging for MDT in place (b), and granulation tissue present post-MDT treatment (c). *Source:* Courtesy of RA Sherman and the BioTherapeutics, Education and Research (BTER) Foundation.

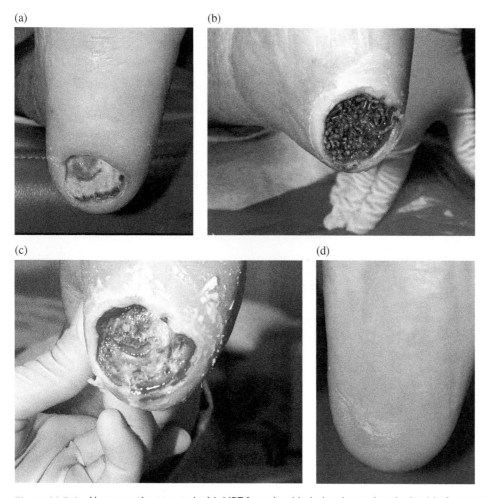

(a)   (b)

(c)   (d)

Figure 11.B.6   Human patient treated with MDT for a decubital ulcer located at the heal before treatment (a), with maggots in place at bandage change (b), granulation tissue progress during (c), and afterward when fully healed (d). *Source:* Courtesy of RA Sherman and the BioTherapeutics, Education and Research (BTER) Foundation.

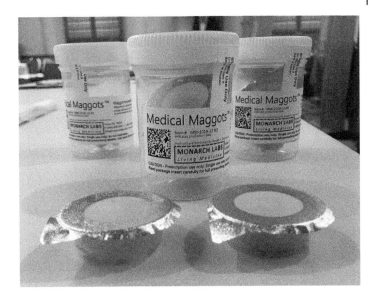

Figure 11.B.7 Vials of medical maggots as shipped from Monarch Labs in Irvine, California. Once the container is opened, it will be applied to the wound bed free-form. *Source:* Courtesy of RA Sherman and the BioTherapeutics, Education and Research (BTER) Foundation.

and within the United Kingdom, they are available from BioMonde® since 2005 (www.zoobiotic.co.uk). Maggots are supplied and applied as either "free range" directly to the wound bed individually or "contained" in bio bags, where maggots are located within a pouch of hydrophilic polyurethane foam (BioMonde®) that provides indirect contact within the dressing [2]. Contained maggots may be less effective because the maggots cannot use their mouth hooks directly on the wound bed for mechanical debridement [10], although no difference was noted in humans with a possible decrease in patient discomfort using biobags [17]. As of publication, cost for one vial of approximately 350 disinfected maggots cost $250 per vial from the US company which would cover a $35\,cm^2$ wound area (Figure 11.B.7). BioMonde® ships throughout Europe (Hamburg, BioMonde® GmbH) but can no longer ship to the US at the time of publication. The website aids customers with sizing and delivery is expected within one to two days of dispatch, with BioBag® costs between £250 and £350 in the UK (Figures 11.B.8, 11.B.9, and 11.B.10).

Once ordered and applied to the wound bed, placement of a semipermeable, porous dressing with dacron or nylon chiffon for breathability and retention of maggots at the wound bed is recommended [1, 44, 55]. The primary layer can be sutured or stapled in place or applied using an adhesive dressing or ostomy paste, as is more commonly done in people. The initial dressing should be covered gently with gauze to collect wound exudate. This outer layer is changed as needed for strikethrough (Figures 11.B.11, 11.B.12, 11.B.13, and 11.B.14). Maggots are left in place until considered "full" where they appear swollen and engorged up to 1 cm in size, generally after two to four days on the wound bed (Figure 11.B.15). At this time, they can no longer remove necrotic debris. Maggots are removed via gentle lavage from the wound bed and can be reapplied until complete debridement is achieved; therefore, the number of total cycles of MDT utilized will vary by the individual wound [11] (Figure 11.B.16, Video 11.B.1 ☉). Application may require sedation or general anesthesia in veterinary medicine depending upon patient temperament and current wound discomfort similar to any other form of debridement and dressing changes. See Figures 11.B.17 and 11.B.18 for an example of a canine patient with a severe burn injury.

Post-Procedural Care

Following application of larvae to the wound, the patient should remain calm and may require sedation in order to avoid damage to the dressings or self-removal in the case of veterinary patients. It is important to ensure proper management of pain and discomfort, as physical discomfort has been reported in people and the single canine reported [8, 31, 40, 42, 56], although it is possible to reduce and control discomfort with proper analgesia regimens [57].

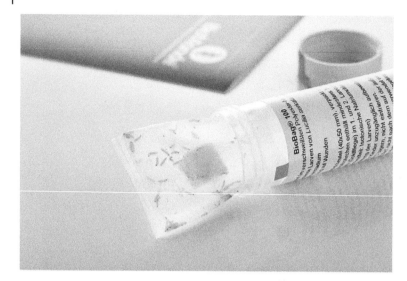

Figure 11.B.8 Pictured is the BB100 4 × 5 cm Biobag® containing larvae within the shipment vial as it would appear upon arrival within 24–48 hours of ordering. Measurements taken for ordering the proper size should allow for full wound bed coverage with some overlap of the Biobag onto the wound margins. The calculator on the company's website aids in size measurement ordering. *Source:* Courtesy of BioMonde®.

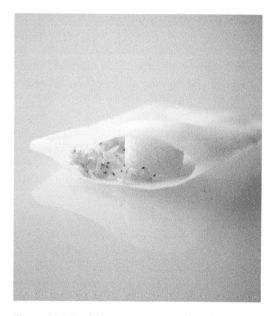

Figure 11.B.9 A close-up cross-sectional image of the opened BB100 Biobag containing larvae. The larvae are contained within a heat-sealed polyester pouch to be delivered as a contained system onto the patient's wound bed. The sterile polyvinyl alcohol foam spacer is designed to allow for continued larval movement throughout debridement for up to four days. Larvae are approximately 4 mm at this time prior to placement in the wound. *Source:* Courtesy of BioMonde®.

Outcomes/Complications

Given the limited number of cases reported in veterinary medicine, it is difficult to predict patient outcomes. No adverse events have been reported, but patients with sepsis can succumb to disease [41]. Overall success rates in people are 80–90% [25, 32, 58] with limb and digit salvage rates of 50–73% [8, 38–40]. When evaluating chronic wounds of less than three months' duration that failed to progress in a large metanalysis (n = 580) comparing MDT to standard hydrogel dressings in people, faster and more effective debridement, faster granulation tissue formation, and increased reduction in wound surface area were reported with MDT. There was no impact on disinfection of bacterial growth on the wound bed or complete healing rate and no serious adverse effects were reported [59].

Major benefits of MDT include its noninvasive nature of debridement, along with potentially improved rates of debridement, granulation tissue formation, and potential advantages in infected wounds.

MDT is considered very effective with faster, potentially expedited debridement times when compared to control hydrogel dressings [12, 56]. When used for chronic ulcers in people, 90% are considered fully debrided within one week (two to three cycles of MDT) [60]. A faster time to wound healing and superior granulation rates have been documented in some studies with chronic wounds and ulcers in humans [12, 61–64], with one showing a sevenfold increase in granulation with the use of MDT over control wounds [65]. However, other studies have not found increased granulation tissue formation to be the case [16]. When used for chronic wounds with or without osteomyelitis in people, a reduction in amputation rates is reported; with up to 73% avoiding amputation procedures [39, 40, 60, 63]. One study reported that patients were twice as likely to have an amputation without the use of MDT incorporated into their treatment regimen [66]. When comparing vacuum-assisted closure (VAC) to MDT in patients with ischemic wounds, 92% of those with MDT healed completely with a toe amputation rate of 7.7% compared to 17% completely healed with a foot and/or toe(s) amputation rate of 70% in VAC cases [67].

Reports on antibacterial properties especially with regards to resistant infections show mixed outcomes, with reduced rates of infection by two weeks post-MDT in some studies compared to conventional treatment [60] with no

Figure 11.B.10   A close-up image of the smallest size Biobag on a scalpel blade for reference. The BB50 measures 2.5 × 4 cm. *Source:* Courtesy of BioMonde®.

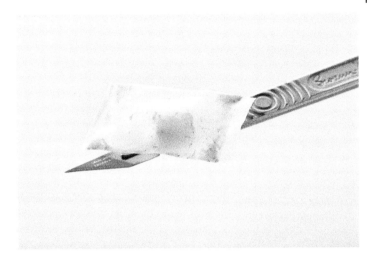

significant difference found in others [63]. Some studies report that patients are infection-free longer [64] and have a reduced bacterial burden compared to controls in diabetic foot ulcers in people [68]. MDT may reduce overall antimicrobial usage in wounds, with patients having more antibiotic-free days compared to control groups [16, 66, 69, 70].

Within veterinary medicine, it is difficult to assess cost-effectiveness given limited case reports; however, the cost in human medicine compared to hydrogel dressings has been shown to be cheaper [71], accounting for nursing care costs and frequency of dressing changes [65]. Some people are sent home as outpatient for MDT. However, in veterinary medicine, these patients would require inpatient management given the specific bandaging needs compared to dressings that may allow for outpatient care. If a faster healing time can be achieved, it may still be more cost-effective with more wound-free days, as reported in people compared to hydrogel [2, 72].

Reported complications with the use of MDT include irritation and itching which have been reported in horses [50] and physical discomfort reported that can be controlled with analgesia [8, 31, 40, 42, 56, 57]. Hypersensitivity reactions are thought to be very rare and ammonia toxicity described from absorption of maggot excretions into the bloodstream is rare if appropriate numbers of larvae are applied and monitored compared to cases with infestation or those with extreme wound-to-patient size ratios [2, 3]. Bleeding has been reported to be mild in up to 10% of cases [40, 58].

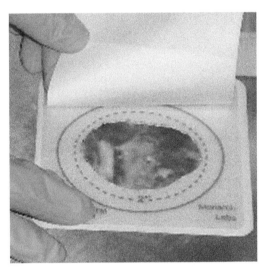

Figure 11.B.11   LeFlap™ primary dressing for confinement of medical maggots during application of MDT. It consists of a dual layer of woven polyester affixed to an adhesive hydrocolloid dressing. The hydrocolloid portion is cutout in the center to match the patient's wound size prior to applying the maggots to the wound bed and folding down the mesh layer. A breathable absorbent dressing, such as gauze is placed on top of the primary layer and changed as needed for strikethrough. *Source:* Courtesy of RA Sherman and the BioTherapeutics, Education and Research (BTER) Foundation.

Within human medicine, a significant limitation is both health professional and patient attitude and response to MDT, with a substantial psychologic impact at play. Oftentimes, there is an initial patient aversion, including repulsion and anxiety which has been shown to frequently resolve throughout the course of treatment [70, 73, 74]. This general negative attitude toward wounds with maggots is possibly an assumed association with death in humans [16]. Similar concerns are unlikely to be a factor in veterinary medicine; however, owners may have similar attitudes toward MDT treatment in their pets.

Logistical limitations include planning ahead to order the larvae, which typically arrive overnight within 24–48 hours. In veterinary medicine, specific limitations could include patient compliance with self-removal and the possible need for sedation and/or anesthesia during application. Other forms of debridement may allow for outpatient therapy, whereas MDT likely requires inpatient management.

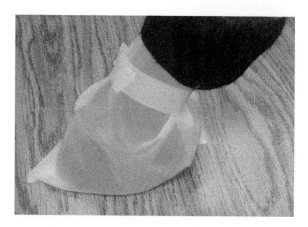

Figure 11.B.12 LeSoc™ primary dressing for confinement of medical maggots during application of MDT in an equine foot wound. These are composed of fixed-weave polyester stockings that can be utilized for complicated 3-dimensional wound surfaces. *Source:* Courtesy of RA Sherman and the BioTherapeutics, Education and Research (BTER) Foundation.

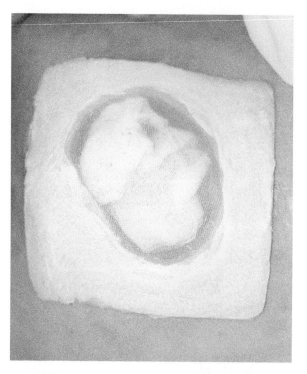

Figure 11.B.13 MDT dressing pictured covering a wound on the hip of a human patient allowing for confinement of the medical maggots. *Source:* Courtesy of RA Sherman and the BioTherapeutics, Education and Research (BTER) Foundation.

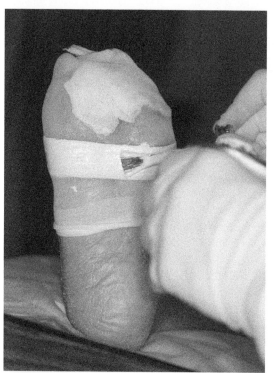

Figure 11.B.14 MDT dressing using nylon stocking to confine the medical maggots during MDT for a foot wound in a human patient. The stockings are secured using adhesive hydrocolloid dressing and glued in place. *Source:* Courtesy of RA Sherman and the BioTherapeutics, Education and Research (BTER) Foundation.

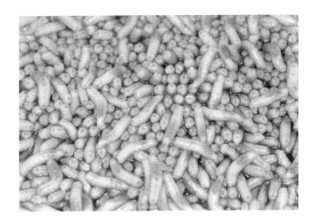

Figure 11.B.15 *Lucilia sericata* third instar larvae pictured with the prominent dark spot indicating a full crop following feeding. *Source:* Courtesy of RA Sherman and the BioTherapeutics, Education and Research (BTER) Foundation.

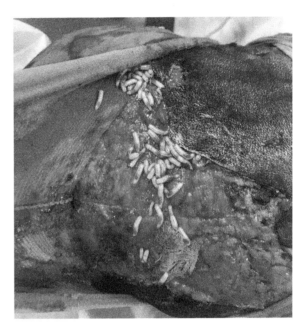

Figure 11.B.16 Close-up view of maggots demonstrating engorgement at the time of removal three days following initial application in a canine patient with severe burn injury along the dorsum. Note the mesh nylon dressing being reflected cranially (to the left) to reveal the maggots in place within the wound bed on the patient's dorsum. *Source:* Courtesy of Megan Mickelson, DVM, DACVS-SA.

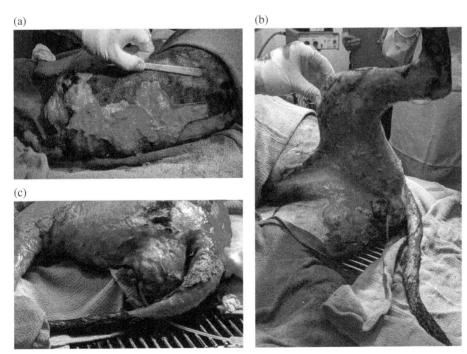

Figure 11.B.17 Wound appearance prior to MDT in a canine patient with severe burn injuries (a-dorsum, b-groin, c-left pelvic limb, and perianal and perivulvar region). Following sharp surgical debridement of the eschar on the dorsum, MDT was applied. MDT was utilized 10 days post-burn due to the extent of surgical debridement that had been required leading up to that point and the technically challenging location of the affected area around the perineum and vulva. For maintenance given the location of the injury, the patient has both a fecal and urinary catheter in place. *Source:* Courtesy of Megan Mickelson, DVM, DACVS-SA.

(a)

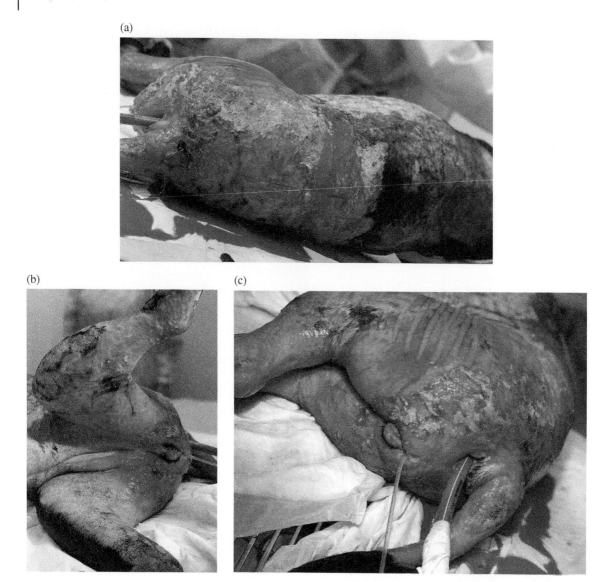

(b)

(c)

Figure 11.B.18   Wound appearance post-MDT two days following initial application in the canine from Figure 11.B.2 (a-dorsum, b-groin, c-left pelvic limb, and perianal and perivulvar region). There is significant improvement in the granulation bed and increased absence of necrotic tissue within the wound bed, especially surrounding the perivulvar and perianal regions where maggots seemed to congregate preferentially under the dressings. *Source:* Courtesy of Megan Mickelson, DVM, DACVS-SA.

References

1 Sherman, R.A. and Wyle, F.A. (1996). Low-cost low-maintenance rearing of maggots in hospitals, clinics, and schools. *Am. J. Trop. Med. Hyg.* 54: 38–41.

2 Jones, G. and Wall, R. (2008). Maggot-therapy in veterinary medicine. *Res. Vet. Sci.* 85: 394–398.

3 Hall, M.J.R. and Wall, R. (1995). Myiasis of humans and domestic animals. *Adv. Parasitol.* 35: 257–234.

4 Baer, W.S. (1931). The treatment of chronic osteomyelitis with the maggot (larva of the blowfly). *J. Bone Joint Surg.* 13: 438–475.

5 Bunkis, J., Gherini, S., Walton, R.L. et al. (1985). Maggot therapy revisited. *Western J. Med.* 142: 554–556.

6 Church, J.C. (1996). The traditional use of maggots in wound healing, and the development of larva therapy (biosurgery) in modern medicine. *J. Alter. Complement. Med.* 2: 525–527.

7 Sherman, R.A. (2000). Maggot therapy: the last five years. *Bull. Euro. Tissue Repair Soc.* 8: 97–98.

8 Sherman, R.A. (2002). Maggot therapy for foot and leg wounds. *Int. J. Lower Extremity Wounds* 1: 135–142.

9 Gottrup, F. and Jorgensen, B. (2011). Maggot debridement: an alternative method for debridement. *Open Access J. Plast. Surg.* 11: 290–302.

10 Steenvoorde, P., Jacobi, C.E., Van Doorn, L. et al. (2007). Maggot debridement therapy of infected ulcers: patient and wound factors influencing outcome-a study on 101 patients with 117 wounds. *Ann. R. Coll. Surg. Engl.* 89 (6): 596–602.

11 Sylvia, A. and Steenvoorde, P. (2011). Maggot debridement therapy. *Proc. Neth. Entomol. Soc. Meet.* 22: 61–66.

12 Moya-Lopez, J., Costela-Ruiz, V., Garcia-Recio, E. et al. (2020). Advantages of maggot debridement therapy for chronic wounds: a bibliographic review. *Adv. Skin Wound Care* 33: 515–525.

13 Chambers, L., Woodrow, S., Brown, A.P. et al. (2003). Degradation of extracellular matrix components by proteinases from the greenbottle larva *Lucilia sericata* used for the clinical debridement of non-healing wounds. *Br. J. Dermatol.* 148: 14–23.

14 Dholaria, S., Dalal, P., Shah, N. et al. (2014). Maggots debridement therapy (MDT). *Gujarat Med. J.* 69: 1.

15 Kerridge, A., Lappin-Scott, H., Stevens, J.R. et al. (2005). Antibacterial properties of larval secretions of the blowfly, *Lucilia sericata*. *J. Med. Vet. Entomol.* 19: 333–337.

16 Sherman, R.A. (2014). Mechanisms of maggot-induced wound healing: what do we know, and where do we go from here? *Evid. Based Complement. Alternat. Med.* 2014: 592419.

17 Blake, F.A.S., Abromeit, N., Bubenheim, M. et al. (2007). The biosurgical wound debridement: experimental investigation of efficiency and practicability. *Wound Repair Regener.* 15 (5): 756–761.

18 Choudhary, V., Choudary, M., Pandey, S. et al. (2016). Maggot debridement therapy as primary tool to treat chronic wound of animals. *Vet. World* 9: 403–409.

19 Prete, P.E. (1997). Growth effects of *Phaenicia sericata* larval extracts on fibroblasts: mechanism for wound healing by maggot therapy. *Life Sci.* 60: 505–510.

20 Horobin, A.J., Shakesheff, K.M., Woodrow, S. et al. (2003). Maggots and wound healing: an investigation of the effects of secretions from *Lucilia sericata* larvae upon interactions between human dermal fibroblasts and extracellular matrix components. *Br. J. Dermatol.* 148: 923–933.

21 Nigam, Y., Dudley, E., and Bexfield, A. (2010). The physiology of wound healing by the medicinal maggot, *Lucilia sericata*. *Adv. Insect Physiol.* 39: 39–81.

22 Cornell, R.S., Andrew, J., Meyr, J. et al. (2010). Debridement of the non-infected wound. *J. Vasc. Surg.* 52 (12): 31–36.

23 Steenvoorde, P., Calame, J.J., and Oskam, J. (2006). Maggot-treated wounds follow normal wound healing phases. *Int. Soc. Dermatol.* 45: 1479–1480.

24 Sherman, R.A., Shapiro, C.E., and Yang, R.M. (2007). Maggot therapy for problematic wounds: uncommon and off-label applications. *Adv. Skin Wound Care* 20 (11): 602–610.

25 Mumcuoglu, K.Y., Ingber, A., Gilead, L. et al. (1999). Maggot therapy for the treatment of intractable wounds. *Int. J. Dermatol.* 38: 623–627.

26 Bazalinski, D., Kozka, M., Karnas, M., and Wiech, P. (2019). Effectiveness of chronic wound debridement with the use of larvae of *Lucilia sericata*. *J. Clin. Med.* 8: 1845. https://doi.org/10.3390/jcm8111845.

27 Sherman, R.A. (2002). Maggot versus conservative debridement therapy for the treatment of pressure ulcers. *Wound Repair Regener.* 10: 2008–2014.

28 Jafari, A., Hosseini, S.V., Hemmat, H.J., and Khazaraei, H. (2022). *Lucilia sericata* larval therapy in the treatment of diabetic chronic wounds. *J. Diabetes Metabolic Disord.* 21: 305–512.

29 Paul, A.G., Ahmand, N.W., Lee, H.L. et al. (2009). Maggot debridement therapy with *Lucilia cuprina*: a comparison with conventional debridement in diabetic foot ulcers. *Int. Wound J.* 6: 36–46.

30 Livingston, S.K. (1936). The therapeutic active principle of maggots with a description of its clinical application in 567 cases. *J. Bone Joint Surg.* 18: 751–756.

31 Mudge, E., Price, P., Walkley, N. et al. (2014). A randomized controlled trial of larval therapy for the debridement of leg ulcers: results of a multicenter, randomized, controlled, open, observer blind, parallel group study. *Wound Repair Regener.* 22: 43–51.

32 Wolff, H. and Hansson, C. (2003). Larval therapy-an effective method for ulcer debridement. *Clin. Exp. Dermatol.* 28: 137.

33 Syam, K., Shaheer, A.J., Khan, S., and Unnikrishnan, N.P. (2021). Maggot debridement therapy for chronic leg and foot ulcers: a review of randomized controlled trials. *Adv. Skin Wound Care* 34: 603–607.

34 Dozier, L., Ceresnie, M., Habashy, J., and Kerdel, F. (2022). Improvement of refractory pyoderma gangrenosum with adjunctive maggot debridement therapy. *Int. J. Dermatol.* https://doi.org/10.1111/ijd.16531.

35 Kaplun, O., Pupiales, M., and Psevdos, G. (2019). Adjuvant maggot debridement therapy for deep wound infection due to methicillin-resistant *Staphylococcus aureus*. *J. Glob. Infect. Dis.* 11 (4): 165–167.

36 Bowling, F.L., Salgammi, E.V., and Boulton, A.J. (2007). Larval therapy: a novel treatment in eliminating methicillin-resistant *Staphylococcus aureus* from diabetic foot ulcers. *Diabetes Care* 30: 370–371.

37 Bazalinski, D., Przybek-Mita, J., Kucharzewski, M., and Wiech, P. (2021). Using maggot debridement therapy in treatment of necrosis in the forearm caused by docetaxel extravasation: a case report. *Iran. J. Parasitol.* 16 (4): 703–710.

38 Sherman, R.A., Sherman, J., Gilead, L. et al. (2001). Maggot debridement therapy in outpatients. *Arch. Phys. Med. Rehabil.* 82: 1226–1229.

39 Jukema, G.N., Menon, A.G., Bernards, A.T. et al. (2002). Amputation-sparing surgery by nature: maggots revisited. *Clin. Infect. Dis.* 35: 1566–1571.

40 Steenvoorde, P., Jacobi, C.E., and Oskam, J. (2005). Maggot debridement therapy: free-range or contained? An in-vivo study. *Adv. Skin Wound Care* 18 (8): 430–435.

41 Sherman, R.A., Stevens, H., Ng, D. et al. (2007). Treating wounds in small animals with maggot debridement therapy: a survey of practitioners. *Vet. J.* 173: 138–143.

42 Dawson, K.A., Mickelson, M.A., Blong, A.E., and Walton, R.A.L. (2022). Management of severe burn injuries with novel treatment techniques including maggot debridement and applications of acellular fish skin grafts and autologous skin cell suspension in a dog. *J. Am. Vet. Med. Assoc.* 260 (4): 428–435. https://doi.org/10.2460/javma.20.10.0579.

43 Kocisova, A., Conkova, E., Pistl, J., and Toporcak, J. (2003). First non-conventional veterinary treatment of skin infections with blowfly larvae (*Calliphoridae*) in Slovakia. *Bull. Vet. Inst. Pulawy* 47: 487–490.

44 Iversen, E. (1996). Methods of treating injuries of work animals. *Buffalo Bull.* 15: 34–37.

45 Dicke, R.J. (1953). Maggot treatment of actinomycosis. *J. Econ. Entomol.* 46: 706–707.

46 Bell, N.J. and Thomas, S. (2001). Use of sterile maggots to treat panniculitis in an aged donkey. *Vet. Rec.* 149 (25): 768–770.

47 Thiemann, A. (2003). Treatment of a deep injection abscess using sterile maggots in a donkey: a case report. *World Wide Wounds* http://www.worldwidewounds.com/2003/november/Thiemann/Donkey-Maggot-therapy.html. Retrieved on May 3, 2023.

48 Kocisova, A., Pistl, J., Link, R. et al. (2006). Maggot debridement therapy in the treatment of foot rot and foot scald in sheep. *Acta Vet. Brno* 75: 277–281.

49 Morrison, S.E. (2005). How to use sterile maggot debridement therapy for foot infections in the horse. *Proceedings of the Annual Convention of the American Association for Equine Practitioners*, pp. 461–467. Seattle, WA: AAEP.

50 Morrison, S. (2010). Maggot debridement therapy for laminitis. *Vet. Clin. Equine* 26: 447–450.

51 Lepage, O.M., Doumbia, A., Perron-Lepage, M.F., and Gangl, M. (2012). The use of maggot debridement therapy in 41 equids. *Equine Vet. J. Suppl.* 44 (43): 120–125.

52 Sherman, R.A., Stevens, H., Ng, D. et al. (2007). Maggot debridement therapy for serious horse wounds – a survey of practitioners. *Vet. J.* 173: 86–91.

53 Andersen, A.S., Joergensen, B., Bjarnsholt, T. et al. (2010). Quorum sensing-regulated virulence factors in *Pseudomonas aeruginosa* are toxic to *Lucilia sericata* maggots. *Microbiology* 156: 400–407.

54 Michelle, L.M., Mark, T.H., Karen, M.S. et al. (2011). Maggot debridement therapy in the treatment of complex diabetic wounds. *Hawaii Med. J.* 70 (6): 121–124.

55 Sherman, R.A. (1997). A new dressing design for treating pressure ulcers with maggot therapy. *Plast. Reconstr. Surg.* 100: 451–456.

56 Dumville, J.C., Worthy, G., Bland, J.M. et al. (2009). Larval therapy for leg ulcers (VenUS II): randomized controlled trial. *BMJ* 338: b773.

57 Mumcuoglu, K.Y., Davidson, E., Avidan, A., and Gilead, L. (2012). Pain related to maggot debridement therapy. *J. Wound Care* 21 (8): 400–405.

58 Courtenay, M., Church, J.C., and Ran, T.J. (2000). Larva therapy in wound management. *J. R. Soc. Med.* 93: 72–74.

59 Zubir, M.Z.M., Holloway, S., and Noor, N.M. (2020). Maggot therapy in wound healing: a systematic review. *Int. J. Environ. Res. Public Health* 17: 6103. https://doi.org/10.3390/ijerph17176103.

60 Campbell, N. and Campbell, D. (2014). A retrospective, quality improvement review of maggot debridement therapy outcomes in a foot and leg ulcer clinic. *Ostomy Wound Manage.* 60 (7): 16–25.

61 Sun, X., Chen, J., Zhang, J. et al. (2016). Maggot debridement therapy promotes diabetic foot wound healing by up-regulating endothelial cell activity. *J. Diabetes Complicat.* 30 (2): 318–322.

62 Opletalova, K., Blaizot, X., Mourgeon, B. et al. (2012). Maggot therapy for wound debridement: a randomized multicenter trial. *Arch. Dermatol.* 148 (4): 432–438.

63 Tian, X., Liang, X.M., Song, G.M. et al. (2013). Maggot debridement therapy for the treatment of diabetic foot ulcers: a meta-analysis. *J. Wound Care* 22 (9): 462–469.

64 Polat, E., Kutlubay, Z., Sirekbasan, S. et al. (2017). Treatment of pressure ulcers with larvae of *Lucilia sericata*. *Turk. J. Phys. Med. Rehabil.* 63 (4): 307–312.

65 Wilasrusmee, C., Margareonrungrung, M., Earnkong, S. et al. (2014). Maggot therapy for chronic ulcer: a retrospective cohort and a meta-analysis. *Asian J. Surg.* 37 (3): 138–157.

66 Sun, X., Jiang, K., Chen, J. et al. (2014). A systematic review of maggot debridement therapy for chronically infected wounds and ulcers. *Int. J. Infect. Dis.* 25: 32–37.

67 Cangel, U., Sirekbasan, S., and Polat, E. (2022). Comparison of larval therapy and vacuum-assisted closure therapy after revascularization in peripheral artery disease patients with ischemic wounds. *Evid. Based Complement. Alternat. Med.* 2022: 8148298. https://doi.org/10.1155/2022/8148298.

68 Malekian, A., Esmaeeli Djavid, G., Akbarzadeh, K. et al. (2019). Efficacy of maggot therapy on *Staphylococcus aureus* and *Pseudomonas aeruginosa* in diabetic foot ulcers: a randomized controlled trial. *J. Wound Ostomy Continence Nurs.* 46 (1): 25–29.

69 Zarchi, K. and Jemec, G.B.E. (2012). The efficacy of maggot debridement therapy-a review of comparative clinical trials. *Int. Wound J.* 9 (55): 469–477.

70 Shi, E. and Shofler, D. (2014). Maggot debridement therapy: a systematic review. *Br. J. Commun. Nurs. Suppl. Wound Care* S6–S13.

71 Wayman, J., Nirojogi, V., Walker, A. et al. (2000). The cost effectiveness of larval therapy in venous ulcers. *J. Tissue Viability* 10: 91–94.

72 Soares, M.O., Iglesias, C.P., Bland, J.M. et al. (2009). Cost effectiveness analysis of larval therapy for leg ulcers. *BMJ* 338: b825.

73 Nigam, Y., Williams, S., Humphreys, L. et al. (2022). An exploration of public perceptions and attitudes towards maggot therapy. *J. Wound Care* 31 (9): 756–770.

74 Hopkins, R.C.N., Williams, S., Brown, A. et al. (2022). *J. Wound Care* 31 (10): 846–863.

12

Bandages

Kristin A. Coleman[1] and Nicole J. Buote[2]

[1] *Gulf Coast Veterinary Specialists, Houston, TX, USA*
[2] *Department of Clinical Sciences, Cornell University, Ithaca, NY, USA*

Introduction

Bandages are one of the most commonly used tools for wound care in veterinary medicine [1]. Bandages commonly consist of four layers whether you are stabilizing a fracture or covering a wound (Figure 12.1). The innermost layer is in direct contact with the wound and is known as the "contact" or "primary" layer. The "secondary" or "absorbent" layer is next and then the "support" layers finish the bandage structure (consists of two layers). The contact layer for a wound bandage comprises a topical application and or a dressing (see Chapters 7 and 8). These dressings may be adherent (e.g., wet-to-dry gauze) or non-adherent (e.g., calcium alginate) and may be employed to debride and clean a wound or to cover and protect a wound. The absorbent layer is usually multiple layers of roll cotton or cast padding. It is important to note that this layer cannot be tightened to a deleterious degree as the cotton will tear. This layer can be added upon as needed to absorb and wick away exudate from wounds. A layer of nonelastic conforming roll gauze is then placed around the absorbent layer to support this layer in position, but care should be taken to avoid over-tightening this layer as constriction of the underlying tissue can occur. The outermost layer most commonly consists of an elastic wrap to secure the bandage materials and provide a water-resistant covering. Some clinicians prefer to place a strong flexible elastic tape at the edges of limb bandages: proximally to help keep bandages from slipping and distally around the edges to discourage absorption of substances on the ground.

Many different bandages can be applied for veterinary patients, but the following bandages are most relevant to wound management. Orthopedic bandages such as Ehmer slings, 90–90, Spica, and casting are discussed in other references [2, 3].

Light or Modified Robert Jones Bandage

Indications:
A light bandage is the most common type used to cover a wound. This can be considered any bandage covering limbs or the trunk (Cross-Your-Heart bandage) (Figure 12.2a and b). A true Robert Jones bandage is usually used to immobilize fractures and decrease swelling. The difference between a light bandage and a "modified" Robert Jones is subjective but typically indicates the addition of more padding (secondary layer).

Description of Technique (Figure 12.3):
Most commonly the patient is placed in lateral recumbency if a limb is to be bandaged. If the chest or abdomen is bandaged, it is easiest to do this in awake patients as they can stand and support their weight. For a wound bandage of the limb, it is helpful to place tape stirrups first. These are made from elastic tape, placed on opposite sides of the limb (lateral-medial or dorso-plantar/palmar). The author prefers non-waterproof tape as she has seen skin removed when the adhesive in waterproof tape melts to the skin if these bandages are left in place for more than a few days. The free ends can be stuck together or to a tongue depressor while the contact and support layers are created. After the tape is applied, the contact layer of choice

Techniques in Small Animal Wound Management, First Edition. Edited by Nicole J. Buote.
© 2024 John Wiley & Sons, Inc. Published 2024 by John Wiley & Sons, Inc.
Companion website: www.wiley.com/go/buote/wounds

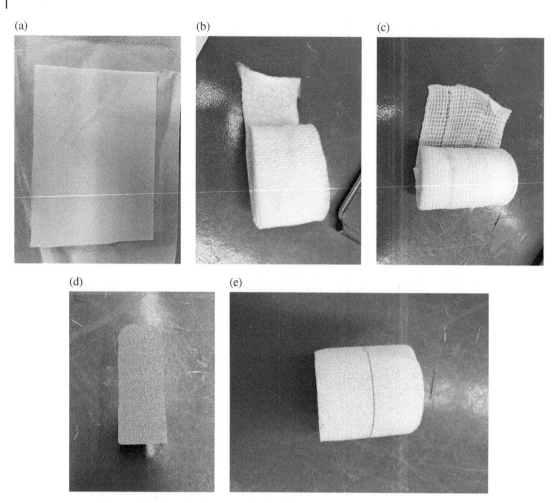

Figure 12.1 Photographs of common bandage material. (a) non-adherent dressing; (b) roll cotton; (c) conforming roll gauze; (d) elastic wrap bandage; (e) elastic tape. *Source:* Courtesy of Nicole Buote, DVM, DACVS.

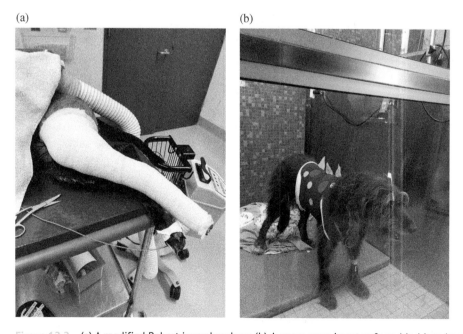

Figure 12.2 (a) A modified Robert jones bandage; (b) A cross-your-heart soft padded bandage. *Source:* Courtesy of Nicole Buote, DVM, DACVS.

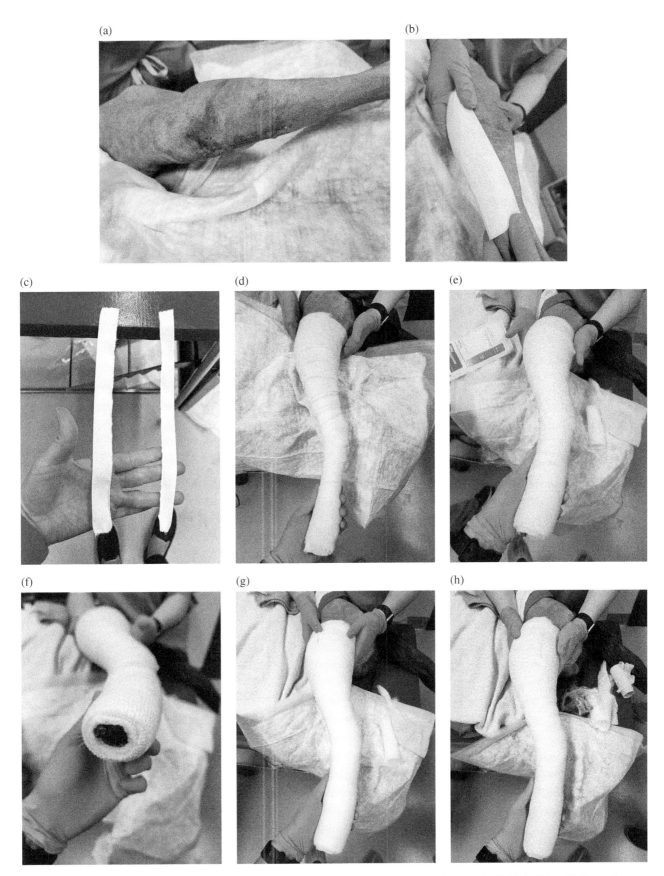

Figure 12.3 Photographs of a modified Robert Jones bandage being placed over a stifle incision. (a) Stifle incision. (b) Non-adherent dressing placed over stifle incision. (c) Stirrups made from white non-waterproof tape can be added before cast padding is applied to help keep the bandage in place. Adequate length is important to ensure enough surface area grips both the patient's skin and the bandage material. (d) First layer of cast padding roll cotton. Always start at the toes and work proximally. (e) Bandage after three layers of cast padding roll cotton applied. Note the distal aspect of the bandage is nearly as thick in diameter as the proximal aspect. This will help to keep the bandage from slipping down. (f) Note the bandage does not cover the toes completely. It is very important to see the distal aspect of digits 3 and 4 so that owners can check for swelling, pain, color change, temperature change or discharge. (g) Bandage after conforming roll gauze applied. (h) Bandage after elastic wrap applied. *Source:* Courtesy of Colin Chik, DVM.

is applied over the wound. The secondary absorbent layer affixed by overlapping 50% of the diameter of the cotton roll as used. An important tip is to try to create a tube rather than a funnel with this layer. Build up the bottom (distal aspect) of the bandage so that it is close to the diameter of the proximal aspect. This lessens the chance of the bandage slipping distally. This is especially helpful in short-legged animals (chondrodystrophic breeds). If a thicker modified Robert Jones is to be placed, cotton roll or cast padding is added until the absorptive capacity is appropriate, usually two to three layers of cotton.

The conforming gauze is then applied. If the wound is on a limb, the gauze is applied from toes upward and then back down with a 50% overlap. If the wound is on the chest, application begins at the caudal aspect and proceeds cranially. As this layer can be over-tightened, it is important to provide even tension while applying this layer to avoid constricting venous and lymphatic flow. For limb bandages, once the conforming gauze is placed, the stirrups are separated and applied vertically to limb to help hold the bandage in place.

Postoperative Care:
Postoperative care of bandages depends on the location and wound being treated. Specific printed instructions should always be provided to the owner so there is no miscommunication of care required (Table 12.1, Box 12.1). In general, bandages need to be kept clean and dry. This means keeping pets' mouths from them and keeping them from wetting or soiling them in water, urine, feces, etc. An E-collar should always be provided. There are many commercial protective booties to protect bandages but recycled IV fluid bags are also very effective (Figure 12.4). It is extremely important to explain to owners that if bandages become wet, bacteria can proliferate, or tissue maceration can occur therefore the pet needs to be brought in for a bandage evaluation as soon as possible. Another important postoperative recommendation is to ensure decreased activity because excessive pressure or movement could lead to slipping or twisting of the materials leading to pain and potential venous congestion and/or tissue damage (Figure 12.5). The author commonly asks owners to monitor how the patient is using the limb, noting a dramatic change for the worse (was weight-bearing and now is not) could indicate a problem with the bandage that is not visible on the outside.

Outcome/Complications:
Bandage complications are common and usually consist of skin irritation (especially at the site of any tape application) and dermatitis (between the toes) which can be managed with timely bandage changes and addition of new/different topicals or dressings. If bandages need to be changed more frequently, owners may become frustrated at the time commitment and cost but wound management is a marathon, not a sprint. Unfortunately, these minor complications can quickly evolve into more severe issues including full-thickness skin loss and the need for digit or limb amputation (Figure 12.5) [4, 5]. Close monitoring of bandages at home must be performed by caretakers to decrease the chance of minor complications becoming more serious.

Wet-to-Dry or Dry-to-Dry Bandages

Indications:
As discussed in Chapters 7 and 8, there is an increasing number of available topical treatments and dressings for wounds. The historic indication for wet-to-dry (WTD) and dry-to-dry (DTD) bandages is debridement of a contaminated wound. Their use for debridement is currently discouraged for a number of reasons, most importantly due to the non-selective manner in which they remove exudate and debris (Table 12.2) [1, 6]. They are effective at removal of not only surface exudate and debris through the *physical action* of drying to the surface and then pulling that debris away during contact layer removal. This can be highly effective but also removes healthy fibroblasts, epithelial cells, and granulation tissue. As their use requires the primary contact layer to "dry" to the external layer of the wound, these bandages can be uncomfortable for the patient and when removed, sedation should be provided.

Description of Technique:
These bandages can be employed under soft padded bandages or tie-over bandages. A WTD utilizes gauze or lap pad materials moistened with sterile saline (lactated Ringer or Plasmalyte solutions also appropriate) as the contact layer. The gauze/lap pads should not be soaking wet, merely moist, to aid in diluting the exudate created by the wound. As the contact layer dries, the bandage material sticks to the wound. DTD bandages are employed when wounds are considered highly exudative therefore no additional moisture is required. If the contact layer never dries, the physical debridement of the surface of the wound will not be effective therefore more frequent bandage changes are required. With the strong evidence that wounds heal best in a warm moist environment, the use of WTD and DRD bandages is declining.

Table 12.1 Home care instructions.

Keep bandage dry	• do not wash pet while bandage in place • cover bandage when walking outside
Keep bandage clean	• do not allow pet to play in dirt • do not allow pet to lick or chew bandage - USE the provided E-collar
Exercise restriction	• NO running, jumping, or rough-housing (this may cause the bandage to slip or twist/tighten) • Monitor for any slipping of the bandage
Monitor pet's behavior	• If the bandage is on a limb, pay close attention to the use of that limb. If the patient stops using the limb suddenly, bring him/her in for evaluation. • Touching the bandage gently should NOT hurt. If you notice discomfort on gentle manipulation of the bandage bring him/her in for evaluation.
Monitor for odor and fluid (strike-through)	• There should be NO foul smell coming from the bandage • There should be NO fluid soaking through the bandage
Check toes daily	• Check your pets toes daily to ensure they are not swelling or becoming bruised of painful

---

Box 12.1 Bandage Care Instructions

Medical Record #

[Insert Name] **has been discharged with a soft bandage.**

The following instructions apply to casts, splints and bandages:

It is essential that the bandage stay clean and dry. You may place a plastic bag over the bandage when your pet goes outside but remove the plastic bag when you bring him or her back inside. Keeping a plastic bag over the bandage for extended periods of time will trap moisture inside the bandage, which may cause skin problems underneath.

If the bandage becomes wet or extremely dirty, please call the hospital to make an appointment for a bandage change. This includes the bandage becoming wet from your pet licking or chewing on it. If you notice your pet licking or chewing on his or her bandage, please place an Elizabethan Collar on your pet. These are available from a pet store or we can provide you with one. However, if your pet's behavior toward the bandage changes suddenly or the bandage seems extremely uncomfortable to him or her, please call the hospital as there may be a problem with the bandage. (For example, he or she has had the bandage for a week and has not bothered it at all then begins chewing at it excessively)

If the bandage is being cared for properly, there should not be any kind of odor associated with the bandage. If you notice any type of foul odor coming from your pet's bandage, there may be a problem such as an infection. Please call the hospital for a bandage change if this were to occur.

Check the toes every day. If you notice that your pet's toes are red or swollen, please call the hospital, as there may be a problem with your pet's bandage.

If you notice that your pet's bandage has slipped from its original position, please call the hospital for a bandage change.

No matter what the reason for your pet's bandage, his or her activity should be restricted to short leash walks for dogs and limited activity for cats including no jumping or running.

If you have any concerns regarding your pet's bandage, please do not hesitate to call the hospital.

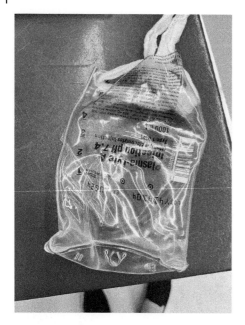

Figure 12.4 Photograph of an IV bag that can be used for bandage protection. Note holes have been cut at the top to weave roll gauze to allow the bag to be tightened to the bandage. *Source:* Courtesy of Nicole Buote, DVM, DACVS.

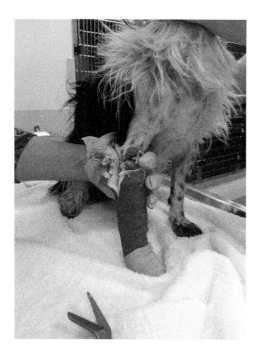

Figure 12.5 Photograph of a bandage-associated wound with full-thickness disruption of skin and underlying muscle due to a tight bandage with tape at the proximal aspect. *Source:* Courtesy of Nicole Buote, DVM, DACVS.

Postoperative care, Outcomes, Complications:

The frequency of changes for WTD and DRD bandages depends on the stage of wound healing and the amount of exudate being produced. The balance between a moist wound environment and maceration to the tissues can be difficult to achieve so frequent bandage evaluations are required while establishing a healthy wound bed. These bandages should not be placed on wounds with granulation tissue therefore their use is only during the beginning phase when physical debridement might be employed. Complications seen with these bandages include delayed wound healing, peri-wound tissue maceration, and patient discomfort.

Tie-Over Bandages

Indications:

The tie-over bandage is arguably the most versatile of bandages that may be created to be any size, may incorporate any primary contact layer, and may applied almost anywhere on the body. While this bandage is ideal for areas that are difficult to reach with other bandages, such as on the proximal limbs, thorax, abdomen, or neck, it is not always the bandage of choice for wounds spanning joints. A tie-over bandage has a variety of uses, from addressing wounds requiring a bandage or covering to providing tension relief over a tight surgical incision. It may also be used in combination with other types of bandages, such as a distal limb bandage being wrapped over a proximal limb tie-over bandage to assist in securing the distal limb bandage and preventing slipping.

Description of technique:

Minimal equipment is required for placement of a tie-over bandage. Needle-holders, thumb forceps, suture scissors, umbilical tape (sterile or non-sterile), and one or more packs of large non-absorbable suture (e.g., 0-Prolene or 2-0 nylon) (Figure 12.6) are needed for the most important and unique aspect of this bandage: stay suture placement, which is preferably performed circumferentially around the wound or area to be covered by the bandage. The bandage itself should contain a primary contact layer and a secondary layer, with the most commonly utilized by the author being laparotomy sponges for their absorbency or a stack of soft gauze if laparotomy sponges would be too bulky in certain areas, and if desired, a piece of water-impermeable drape for covering the final product.

After clipping, prepping, and quarter-draping the area of interest, the stay sutures are placed. Non-absorbable stay sutures should be placed at least 1 cm from the wound or incision and should be a wide bite of at least 1 cm at a depth into the subcutaneous layer, and in the case of wounds with crushing injury and bruising, the stay sutures should be placed outside of the bruised tissue (Figure 12.7). Stay sutures are ideally placed in even numbers with each pair directly across from each other (Figure 12.8) to allow for a stable bandage with individual knots between each pair of stay sutures using the tensioned umbilical tape. After placing the primary contact layer (Figure 12.9) with sterile gloves, the secondary layer of gauze or laparotomy sponges is put on top of the

Table 12.2 Disadvantage of wet-to-dry and dry-to-dry bandages.

Disadvantages to WTD/DTD bandages

Nonselective debridement- both healthy and unhealthy tissue is removed

Dry environment not ideal for wound healing

Remove helpful growth factors and cytokines found in wound fluid

Bacteria can proliferate in wet gauze/lap pads

Dry gauze may disperse bacteria into the air during bandage changes

Fibers from material may become embedded

Painful to wear and remove

Figure 12.6 These sutures (0-Prolene for dogs, 2-0 nylon for cats) are examples of non-absorbable suture types acceptable for tie-over bandage stay suture placement. *Source:* Courtesy of Kristin Coleman, DVM, MS, DACVS.

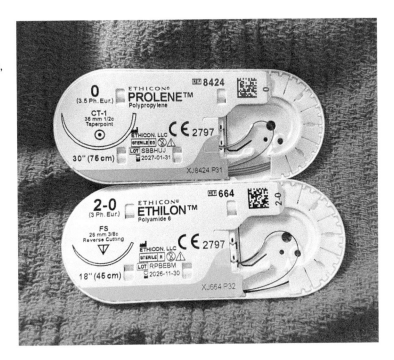

Figure 12.7 Stay sutures should be placed at least 1 cm from the wound or incision and should be a wide bite of at least 1 cm at a depth into the subcutaneous layer (a and b). Enough of a gap should be created in the suture to allow for ease of threading umbilical tape (b). *Source:* Courtesy of Kristin Coleman, DVM, MS, DACVS.

(a)

(b)

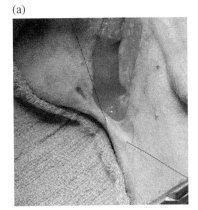
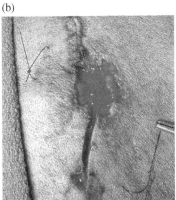

(a)

(b)

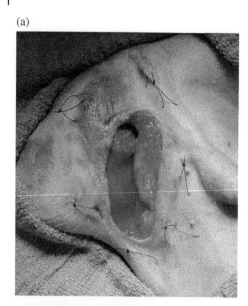

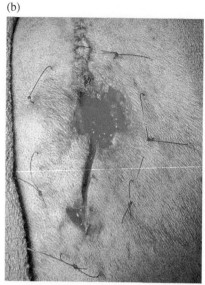

Figure 12.8 Stay sutures are ideally placed in even numbers with each pair directly across from each other (a and b). *Source:* Courtesy of Kristin Coleman, DVM, MS, DACVS.

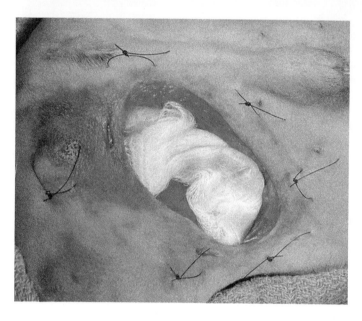

Figure 12.9 The primary contact layer is placed into the wound. In this case, a single loosely woven gauze barely dampened with hypertonic saline is positioned to contact all surfaces of the wound bed. *Source:* Courtesy of Kristin Coleman, DVM, MS, DACVS.

primary contact layer. Usually, a water-resistant layer of blue drape material is placed over the secondary layer before the umbilical tape is tied (Figures 12.10b and 12.12b). The umbilical tape is threaded through 2 stay sutures across from each other, and it is pulled until the ends are even (Figure 12.10a). A single throw is made for half of a square knot and pulled to the desired tension across the wound, and an assistant's finger is helpful in maintaining tension before the second throw is made to complete the square knot (Figure 12.11). The next two stay sutures across from each other have umbilical tape threaded through them, and the process is repeated until a flower or wagon wheel appearance results with tension controlled between each pair of stay sutures (Figure 12.12).

Postoperative care:

As with any bandage, tie-over bandages should be protected from the patient's mouth with application of a hard Elizabethan collar until a day or so after bandage removal. While the bandage is somewhat protected by the impermeable drape from a light drizzle when a canine patient is taken outside for eliminations, it should be changed immediately if soaked. In cases when the client is advised to return if soaking through of the secondary bandage layer is noted, no impermeable drape is applied. Frequency of bandage changes is dictated by the nature of the wound and primary contact layer being used, and need for sedation is determined by the temperament of the patient and possible need for replacing stay sutures, especially those applied for chronic wounds in high-motion areas of the body.

(a) (b)

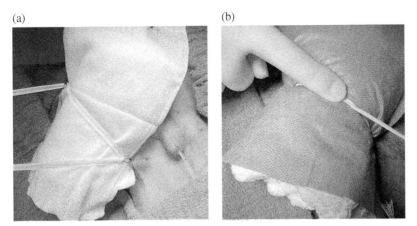

Figure 12.10   The umbilical tape is threaded through the 2 stay sutures across from each other, and it is pulled until the ends are even (a and b). In (a), the umbilical tape is being placed directly over the laparotomy sponges. In (b), an impermeable drape is included on top of the laparotomy sponges. *Source:* Courtesy of Kristin Coleman, DVM, MS, DACVS.

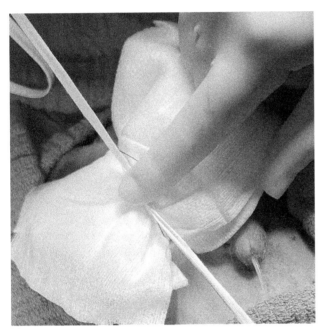

Figure 12.11   After creating half of a square knot with a single throw and analyzing the appropriate tension needed across the wound and put onto both stay sutures, an assistant's finger is placed on top of the throw to maintain tension while the second throw is made to complete the square knot. *Source:* Courtesy of Kristin Coleman, DVM, MS, DACVS.

(a) (b)

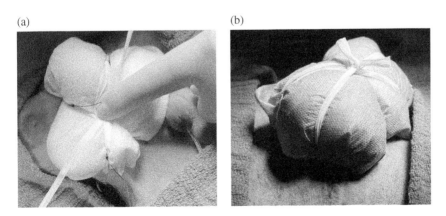

Figure 12.12   The next two stay sutures across from each other have umbilical tape threaded through them (a), and the process is repeated until a flower or wagon wheel appearance results (b). *Source:* Courtesy of Kristin Coleman, DVM, MS, DACVS.

Outcomes/complications:

When the tie-over bandage is no longer needed, the stay sutures and bandage are removed. There will often be small punctures with crusting where the stay sutures were removed, and this should be gently cleansed at the time of bandage removal. Potential complications with tie-over bandages include the need to add or replace stay sutures if any sutures are noted to be attached by only a thin section of skin; this complication may be mitigated by wide bites with the suture when initially placing the stay sutures and by using a large gauge of suture.

References

1 Campbell, B.G. (2006). Dressings, bandages, and splints for wound management in dogs and cats. *Vet. Clin. North Am. Small Anim. Pract.* 36 (4): 759–791.

2 Campbell, B.G. (2018). Bandages and drains. In: *Veterinary Surgery: Small Animal Expert Consult*, 2e (ed. S. Johnston and T. DAK), 246–255. St. Louis, MO: Elsevier Health Sciences.

3 Simpson, A.M., Radlinsky, M., and Beale, B.S. (2001). Bandaging in dogs and cats: external coaptation. *Compendium* 23 (2): 157–164.

4 Anderson, D.M. and White, R.A. (2000). Ischemic bandage injuries: a case series and review of the literature. *Vet. Surg.* 29: 488–498.

5 Buote, N.J. (2014). The use of medical leeches for venous congestion. A review and case report. *Vet. Comp. Orthop. Traumatol.* 27 (3): 173–178.

6 Hosgood, G. (2018). Open wounds. In: *Veterinary Surgery: Small Animal Expert Consult*, 2e (ed. S. Johnston and T. DAK), 1410–1421. St. Louis, MO: Elsevier Health Sciences.

13

Hyperbaric Oxygen Therapy

Cheryl Braswell

Spring City, TN, USA

Introduction

Hyperbaric oxygen therapy (HBOT) has a long history, having been investigated since 1960 [1]. Research has been conducted validating the use of HBOT in multiple conditions. In human medicine, there are now 14 conditions for which HBOT is reimbursable from insurance companies and Medicare. Included on this list are disease states such as refractory osteomyelitis, diabetic foot ulcers, crush injury and other traumatic ischemias, necrotizing soft tissue infections, compromised flaps and grafts, and clostridial infections. Human research and prospective clinical trials form the basis for translational HBOT use in veterinary patients with commiserate conditions [2]. In treating difficult wounds, HBOT is currently recognized as one of the more promising adjuvant treatments in this field [3].

Physiology

There are two primary effects of HBOT: decreased gas bubble size and hyperoxygenation. Decreasing gas bubble size is the physiology by which decompression sickness (the bends) is effectively treated. This can also be utilized to mitigate air embolism. This application has not been reported in any veterinary clinical cases to date. Hyperoxygenation initiates a cascade of events (secondary effects) that benefit our patients with respect to wound care. Hyperoxygenation is achieved when the patient breaths 100% oxygen under pressure. When a patient breaths 100% oxygen at 2ATA, (atmospheres absolute) the amount of oxygen (O_2) pressure is nine times that compared to breathing ambient air at sea level [1]. This increase in O_2 pressure in the alveoli creates a gradient resulting in an increased number of oxygen molecules diffusing across the alveoli and into the plasma. The increased dissolved oxygen in the plasma creates a gradient increasing oxygen diffusion into the tissues. The enhanced diffusion of oxygen molecules out of the plasma also improves offloading of oxygen from hemoglobin forming what has been termed an "oxygen bridge."

Normal wound healing is divided into different stages (see Chapter 2). For this discussion, we will use the following terms: hemostasis/inflammation, proliferation, and maturation [2]. HBOT has effects in each of the stages of healing (Table 13.1) and these actions overlap in the healing process. Failure to progress through these stages results in abnormal wound healing (chronic wound) most often characterized by hypoxia and prolonged inflammation.

Acute Wounds

Briefly, during the initial phase, vessels supplying the wounded tissue undergo vasoconstriction, platelets are activated and the coagulation cascade is induced. Disruption of blood vessels, lymphatics, and cell membranes occurs along with vasodilation resulting in fluid migration into the tissues with subsequent swelling (vasogenic and cytotoxic edema). HBOT causes arteriolar vasoconstriction of normal blood vessels leading to decreased tissue edema and therefore increased comfort. Due to the hyperoxygenation of the plasma and the enhanced diffusion gradient to tissues, hypoxia is alleviated and cellular integrity is maintained [1].

Techniques in Small Animal Wound Management, First Edition. Edited by Nicole J. Buote.
© 2024 John Wiley & Sons, Inc. Published 2024 by John Wiley & Sons, Inc.
Companion website: www.wiley.com/go/buote/wounds

Table 13.1 HBOT action during phases of healing.

1) Hemostasis and inflammation	– Arteriolar vasoconstriction
	– Decreased tissue edema
	– Eliminates hypoxia
	– Maintains cellular integrity
	– Reduced monocyte-macrophage pro-inflammatory cytokine levels
	– Decreased endothelial adhesion molecules
	– Increased production of heat shock proteins which stabilize hypoxia-inducible factor which in turn increases VEG-F, SDF, and PDGF
2) Proliferation	– Induces fibroblast growth factor
	– Increased fibroblast migration and proliferation
	– Increased collagen production
	– Decreased matrix degradation
3) Maturation	– Increases collagen cross-linking improving tensile strength

The acute inflammatory response is characterized by cytokine activation of neutrophils, monocytes, and macrophages. After successive HBOT treatments, patients with a prolonged or elevated proinflammatory states will have reduced monocyte–macrophage proinflammatory cytokine levels. This has been documented in both humans and animals *in vitro* and *in vivo* studies [1]. HBOT has also been shown to decrease endothelial adhesion molecules, reducing cellular wall adhesions.

The proliferation phase involves neovascularization and recruitment of endothelial progenitor cells from bone marrow. Fibroblasts provide collagen deposition and during the maturation stage, there is wound retraction and remodeling [2]. Hyperoxygenation increases production of reactive oxygen species (ROS) and reactive nitrogen species (RNS). Both ROS and RNS stimulate wound healing factors such as vascular endothelial growth factor (VEGF), transforming growth factor β1 (TGFβ1), and angiopoetin [1]. Endothelial cells exposed to HBOT exhibit enhanced capillary formation due to these growth factors. Hyperoxygenation also has multiple positive effects on fibroblasts. Hyperoxia induces fibroblast growth factor (FGF) improving fibroblast migration and proliferation. Hyperoxia has also been reported to increase collagen production by fibroblasts and improve collagen crosslinking, thereby enhancing tissue tensile strength [1, 4].

Chronic Wounds

Tissue loss due to excessive matrix degradation is a common characteristic of chronic wounds. Upregulation of proteolytic enzymes, matrix metalloproteinases (MMPs), are responsible for this condition. MMPs have natural antagonists that regulate the activity of MMPs called tissue inhibitors of matrix metalloproteinases (TIMP). HBOT stimulates the production of TIMP therefore decreasing matrix degradation [5].

Another area under investigation centers on the affect HBOT has on heat shock proteins (HSP). HBOT is thought to increase production of HSP's which are responsible for the cell's response to stress (not exclusively thermal stress). By increasing HSP production, a stabilizing effect on another factor, hypoxia-inducible factor 1 (HIF-1) is seen. HIF-1 is a cytokine expressed under conditions of hypoxia with a very short half-life (minutes) in normal environments. In chronic wounds, HIF-1 supports keratinocyte migration and epithelial regeneration. HIF-1 stimulates production of vascular endothelial growth factor (VEGF), platelet-derived growth factor (PDGF), and stromal cell-derived factor (SDF). By stabilizing HIF-1, HBOT may ultimately enhances secretion of VEGF, PDGF, and SDF. This premise needs further study and validation [4].

Contaminated Wounds

A hyperoxygenated environment is toxic for bacteria and fungi due to the production of increased superoxide levels. Elevated superoxide leads to increased hydrogen peroxide and other toxic oxygen radicals that damage microbial DNA and interfere with metabolic functions. This is particularly true with Clostridial species. HBOT also promotes phagocytosis of organisms by leukocytes. In the hyperoxic environment, there is increased oxidative burst from neutrophil-like cells enhancing infection control. Hyperoxygenation can also enhance effectiveness of antibiotics that require oxygen to transport across cell membranes. Antibiotic classes in this category include aminoglycosides, fluoroquinolones, Amphotericin B, and the antimetabolites/sulfonamides trimethoprim, sulfamethoxazole, and sulfasoxazole. HBOT may also be an effective adjunct in antibiotic-resistant infections [1].

In a preliminary study by Gouveia et al., HBOT was shown to be helpful in severe wounds classified according to the Modified Vancouver Scale (MVS) [3]. This study evaluated wounds in 41 patients before and after HBOT. Results reported a decrease in the MVS classification over time with HBOT in difficult-to-heal wounds. This study also concluded that HBOT was a safe therapy as no major side effects were seen after 289 sessions of HBOT [3].

Indications

HBOT has shown beneficial effects in a wide range of veterinary and human conditions. The conditions currently approved for third-party reimbursement in human medicine include:

air or gas embolism
carbon monoxide poisoning
clostridial myositis and myonecrosis (gas gangrene)
crush injury, compartment syndrome, and other traumatic ischemia
decompression sickness
arterial insufficiencies
several anemia
intracranial abscess
necrotizing soft tissue infections
osteomyelitis (refractory)
delayed radiation injury (soft tissue and bony necrosis)
compromised grafts and flaps
acute thermal burn injury
idiopathic sudden sensorineural hearing loss

There is a plethora of scientific investigations of HBOT in human medicine, but comprehensive studies are lacking in veterinary medicine [5–10]. Due to this lack of research on veterinary patients, the indications for and treatment protocols used have mostly been translated from human data and anecdotal experience. Indications for use of HBOT in veterinary medicine can be classified into seven categories.

1) Wound Healing: HBOT stimulates angiogenesis, enhances collagen synthesis, and improves immune function, leading to accelerated wound healing. It is particularly useful in cases of non-healing wounds, infected wounds, and compromised tissue perfusion.
2) Traumatic Injuries: Animals suffering from traumatic injuries such as fractures, crush injuries, and spinal cord injuries can benefit from HBOT. The increased oxygen availability promotes tissue repair and reduces inflammation, helping to mitigate secondary damage.
3) Postsurgical Recovery: HBOT can aid in the recovery process after surgical procedures by improving tissue oxygenation, reducing swelling, and promoting faster healing. It is especially useful in cases involving compromised blood supply or tissue viability.
4) Neurological Disorders: Conditions like spinal cord injuries, intervertebral disc disease, and brain trauma can benefit from HBOT due to its ability to reduce edema, modulate inflammation, and enhance tissue repair mechanisms.
5) Infection Management: Hyperbaric oxygen has antimicrobial properties and can enhance the effectiveness of certain antibiotics. It is beneficial in managing infections that are resistant to conventional therapies, such as anaerobic bacteria and certain fungal infections.
6) Carbon Monoxide Poisoning: HBOT facilitates the removal of carbon monoxide from the bloodstream, preventing further tissue damage and promoting a faster recovery.
7) Other Applications: HBOT has also been used in conditions such as smoke inhalation, near-drowning, snakebites, heatstroke, and immune-mediated diseases.

HBOT has been successfully used in veterinary medicine for envenomation, CNS injury, and ischemia reperfusion injury in addition to those listed above (Figures 13.1–13.4) [5, 6, 11, 12].

(a)

(c)

(b)

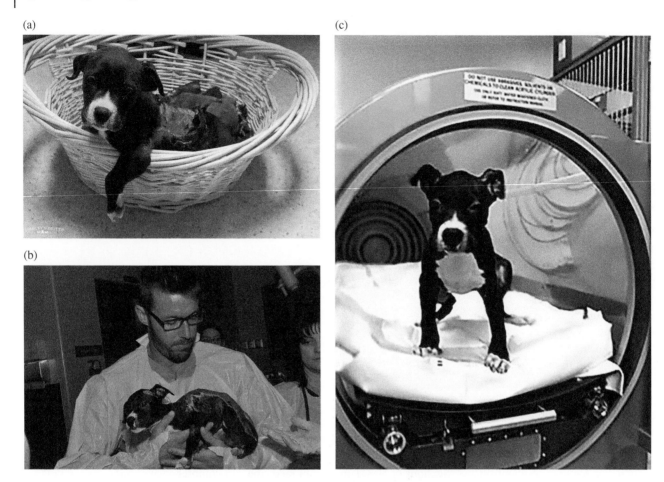

Figure 13.1   (a,b) Photographs of two 8-week-old puppies presented one week post structure fire with thermal injury and Pseudomonas infection. (a) Patient had full-thickness burns to the midbody almost 360° around the circumference. (b) Patient had full-thickness burns along entire dorsum from shoulders to base of tail. (c) Patient in A within the hyperbaric chamber. Adjunctive HBOT was employed with their ongoing critical care. Survival was initially thought questionable. HBOT daily for two weeks produced a healthy bed of granulation tissue. Both puppies survived. *Source:* Courtesy of Cheryl Braswell, DACVECC, CHT-C, CVPP, CHPV.

Patient Considerations and Description of Technique

By far, the most important consideration when delivering HBOT to humans or animals is safety. Oxygen, and particularly oxygen under pressure, can have catastrophic consequences if not safely administered. Since there is a potential risk for fire in the hyperbaric oxygen environment, patient preparation includes removing any metal items from the patient, for example, collars and harnesses (even if the only metal is the buckle). This author typically covers post-op staples with a cotton bandage material. The patient's coat can be wiped down with a wet towel and/or a pan of water placed in the chamber to help humidify the environment decreasing the chance of sparking. It is also advisable to only use cotton material for blankets and bedding. Any bandages on the patient or bedding in the chamber should be only cotton material. The patient should be evaluated for the potential of containment anxiety. It is perfectly acceptable to pretreat with a sedative if deemed necessary. Often, once the patient has undergone the treatment a few times, sedation is no longer necessary. Smaller patients are generally confined in a suitable plastic crate (with no metal parts). This will also allow more than one patient to be treated at a time if necessary (multiple burn victims for example).

The specific treatment protocol for HBOT will vary depending on the patient's condition and the equipment available. The provider determines a treatment plan that consists of pressure, time, and frequency (Table 13.2). In the author's practice, the pressure within the chamber is typically set at 1.3–2.8 times atmospheric pressure, and treatment sessions can range from 60 to 90 minutes. The length of treatment includes time to pressurize, time at pressure, and time to decompress. The frequency and duration of the treatment will be determined based on the individual patient's response

Figure 13.2 Photographs of an eight-year-old MN German Shepherd who underwent pelvic fracture surgery three years prior to presentation for chronic draining tract presumed to be associated with an orthopedic wire. The wire was removed, cultures taken (negative), and biopsies taken (nondiagnostic). (a) After eight weeks of treatment, the patient presented for adjunctive HBOT with a wound flushing system in place. (b) The flushing system was removed and HBOT applied three times per week for four weeks. (c) The fistula completely healed with no other treatments. *Source:* Courtesy of Cheryl Braswell, DACVECC, CHT-C, CVPP, CHPV.

(a)
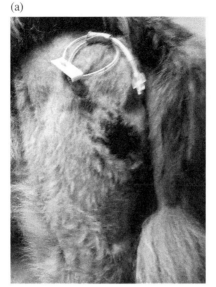

(c)
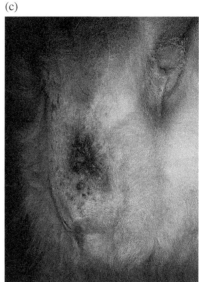

(b)
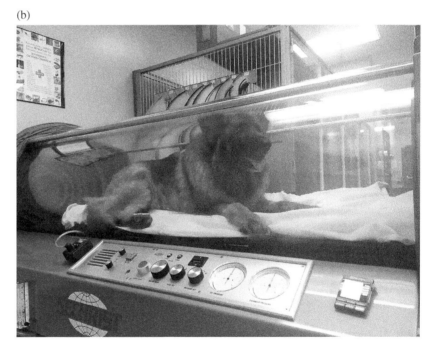

and the severity of the condition being treated. Frequency is usually one to two times per day; however, this is often modified depending on client finances and scheduling availability.

Equipment and Costs

Hyperbaric chambers come in two basic constructs, a soft-sided and a hard shell. The soft-sided chambers are much less expensive however they are restricted to 1.3 ATA maximum pressure and generally provide only 24–32% oxygen concentration.

Hard-shell units require a dedicated liquid oxygen system with reserve, pipping, and an alarm that meets National Fire Protection Association codes. These systems cost between $15 and 20,000 and are not included in the cost of the chamber itself. In the United States, there are only a few veterinary-specific hard-shell chambers manufactured. One company that has been producing human equipment for 50 years, Sechrist Industries, produces chambers that cost approximately $100,000.00. Hyperbaric Veterinary Medicine (HVM) produces chambers that run $45,000–$75,000 depending on whether

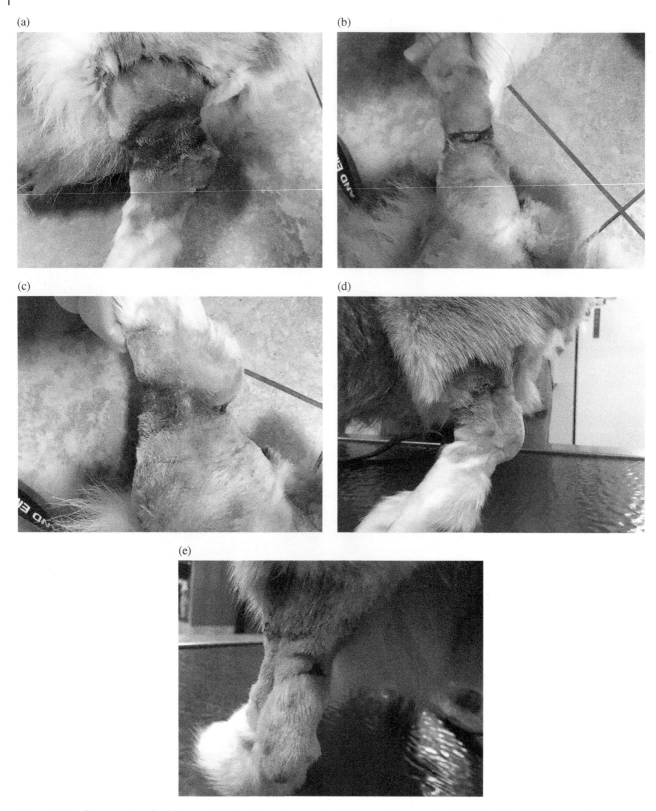

Figure 13.3 Photographs of a 10-year-old MN mix breed presented for traumatic wound to the left pelvic limb from cord wrapped around limb. No oral or topical antibiotics were administered. Routine daily cleaning and hydrotherapy plus adjunctive HBOT three times per week. (a–c) Wounds at presentation (a-lateral aspect, b-caudal aspect, c-medial aspect). (d,e) Healed wounds 10 days post-HBOT (c-lateral aspect, d-caudal aspect). *Source:* Courtesy of Cheryl Braswell, DACVECC, CHT-C, CVPP, CHPV.

Figure 13.4 Photographs of a one-year-old MI Labrador presented after having been at the trainers for 10 days. The owners were told he developed a wound on the medial aspect of his left pelvic limb that had progressed to necrotic tissue that had been debrided by the trainer's veterinarian. Two multidrug-resistant bacteria were cultured. In addition to medical care, HBOT was initiated twice daily for three days, then a negative pressure wound therapy bandage was applied for three days then the defect was grafted. HBOT was continued once daily for two weeks post-grafting. (a) original presentation, (b) condition on the day of grafting, (c) two weeks post grafting, (d) two months post-procedure. *Source:* Courtesy of Cheryl Braswell, DACVECC, CHT-C, CVPP, CHPV.

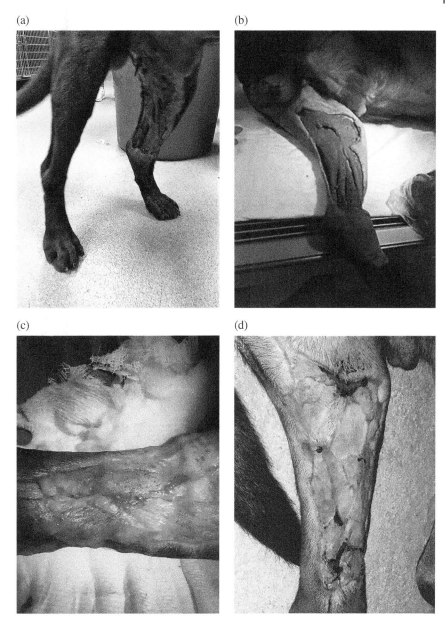

Table 13.2 Author's recommendations.

Condition	Pressure	Time	Frequency
Envenomation	2 ATA	60 min	Every 12 h
Severe MDR infections	2 ATA	60 min	Every 8 h
Inflammatory diseases	2 ATA	60 min	Every 12 h or every 24 h if outpatient
IVDD medical management	1.5 ATA	90 min	Every 12 h or every 24 h if outpatient
Post hemilaminectomy	1.5 ATA	90 min	Every 12 h
CNS injury in general	1.5 ATA	90 min	Every 12 h
Wounds of various etiology	2.0 ATA	60 min	Every 8–24 h pending severity and chronicity

Note: Time listed is actual treatment time. Usually 15 min allowed before and after treatment to compress and decompress.

Table 13.3 Daily and weekly checklist.

DAILY-prior to beginning treatments for the day, the following inspections should be performed.

1) Assure that the supply pressure is between 50.0 and 70.0 psig (3.5 and 4.9 kg/cm², 344.8 and 482.7 kPa).
2) Visually inspect the acrylic cylinder for any discoloration, scratches, blisters, cracks, pits, and crazing.
3) Visually inspect the chamber interior and exterior for clean lines dust, lint, fluff, and hair are fire hazards.
4) Visually inspect the door gasket for damage and cleanliness. Replace or clean as required.
5) Ensure patient grounding mat (and ground cords if needed) is in place.
6) Check the chamber ground and patient ground by utilizing the methods described in Section 4 – Safety Features and Procedures. Ensure patient grounding mat (and cord if needed) is in place and ready for use.
7) Inspect chamber supply and vent hoses for kinks and loose connections. Insure proper function before use.
8) Ensure over-pressure relief valve is in the open position. Do not use chamber with the valve in the closed position.
9) Ensure ventilation control is set to 240 LPM for SV250, 400 LPM for SV500.
10) Perform a visual inspection of the complete chamber for damage, loose knobs, etc. The chamber must be in optimum working condition before use.
11) When at pressure, make sure the readings on electronic display panel are at an acceptable range per your facility requirements (i.e., O_2 values). These values should be in conjunction with your facility's policies and procedures.

WEEKLY PERFORMANCE VERIFICATION
To ensure proper operation of the Chamber the following systems should be checked on a weekly basis: the Ventilation Flow, Emergency Vent System, Safety Lock Pin Device System, and Intercommunication System.

they are new or refurbished. Another popular option is to purchase a used human monoplace chamber. Class C chambers, are the type designated for veterinary use, and are the equivalent of Class B human monoplace chamber. Most chambers use transparent acrylic walls to permit constant patient monitoring and visualization. Some systems have intercoms to allow for communication with the patient and most chambers have digital displays providing data on chamber gas content (percent of O_2 and CO_2), humidity, and temperature inside the chamber. Chambers may also allow for CO_2 level adjustment. Daily and monthly checklists based on manufacturer recommendations to ensure safety and proper function (Table 13.3).

Complications

While HBOT is generally considered safe, there are some precautions and potential risks to be aware of. The presence of a pneumothorax is a strict contraindication with devastating consequences to the patient if overlooked. Patients with pulmonary bullae are also at significant risk of creation of a fatal tension pneumothorax therefore thoracic radiographs should be performed before any HBOT. Previous treatment with bleomycin is a contraindication for HBOT due to the potential risk of developing pulmonary toxicity. Bleomycin is an antineoplastic medication not commonly used in veterinary medicine but it is known to cause lung damage as a side effect, particularly when administered in high doses or over a prolonged period. The combination of bleomycin-induced lung injury and the increased oxidative stress caused by HBOT can increase the risk of severe lung complications, including pulmonary fibrosis.

Patients with certain conditions, such as uncontrolled seizures, or preexisting severe respiratory disease, may not be suitable candidates for HBOT. Veterinary patients should also be evaluated for otitis media and/or sinus infections as these conditions can precipitate extreme discomfort to the patient in the pressurized environment. Additionally, there is a risk of barotrauma and oxygen toxicity. Proper training, adherence to safety protocols, and close monitoring of patients during treatment are essential to minimize these risks. It is important to remember that even in the absence of otitis or sinusitis, patients can be uncomfortable during the pressurization phase which is manifested by head shaking or ear scratching [3]. If this is observed, the rate of pressurization should be slowed.

Patients who are prone to hypoglycemia (diabetics/sepsis/liver disease etc.) should be evaluated on a case-by-case basis. Hyperoxygenation increases metabolism and therefore glucose utilization. In susceptible patients, this creates a potential for hypoglycemia severe enough to result in seizures. This author typically treats patients in this category at a lower pressure (1.5 ATA). Any CNS injury (traumatic brain injury, spinal cord injury, etc.) is also typically treated at a lower pressure to minimize ROS formation and CNS oxygen toxicity. CNS oxygen toxicity can manifest as a seizure. It is noteworthy that in human medicine, excessive production of ROS has resulted in oxygen toxicity in other organ systems. To date, only CNS toxicity has been documented in veterinary medicine.

Clinical outcomes of HBOT in veterinary patients have been promising, with many reported cases showing improved healing, reduced infection rates, and enhanced recovery. A rat study in 2016 evaluated wound healing in the face of ischemia and hyperglycemia as a model for diabetic wounds which are notoriously difficult to treat [7]. This study included a control group that only received treatment with a semiocclusive wound dressing. In both hyperbaric oxygen groups (those with ischemia and hyperglycemia), the authors found increased blood flow, accelerated wound healing, contraction, and reepithelialization. There was also increased collagen deposition in early time points in the ischemic wounds leading authors to postulate that HBOT applied early in wound healing may be beneficial [7].

In a retrospective analysis of 2792 HBOTs, it was found that the occurrence of major adverse events (CNS toxicity) was 0.7%. These treatments were provided across multiple species including dogs, cats, macaw parrots, capuchin monkeys, opossum, bat, gray squirrel, skunk, iguana, and goat. The primary indication for therapy was external wounds or abscesses [13]. Another smaller study of 78 dogs and 12 cats reported results after treatment for a variety of conditions including intracranial disease, immune-mediated disease, postoperative skin flaps, and gastrointestinal disease [14]. The treatment protocol was 2 ATA for 45–60 minutes and there was a total of 230 treatments provided. No major adverse events, defined as those contributing to mortality or persistent patient morbidity, causing significant distress, or requiring emergency decompression, were noted [14]. The authors concluded that HBOT was well-tolerated and safe when performed appropriately but objective assessment of therapeutic benefit is still lacking.

In a study of HBOT effects on patients with two or more criteria consistent with SIRS, the patients were divided into traumatic and nontraumatic etiologies [15]. There was a total of 624 treatments at 2.4–2.8 ATA for 60–90 minutes. The authors reported that 73.5% of patients improved after treatment, 24.5% died or were euthanized and 2% showed no change to their clinical status. No difference was seen between traumatic and nontraumatic etiologies and outcomes after HBOT but the number of days between diagnosis and the beginning of HBOT resulted in a significant difference leading authors to recommend early treatment. It is important to note this study did not have a control and was not blinded or randomized [15].

A 2021 study on the molecular mechanisms of hyperbaric oxygen in tissue repair documented changes in factors/biomarkers of inflammation and healing [6].

Factors up-regulated included:

* enzymes enhancing growth or differentiation
* factors with cytoprotective and anti-apoptotic effects
* mechanisms facilitating reduction of oxidative stress
* cell-to-cell contacts, especially tight junctions

Factors downregulated included:

* enzymes involved in pro-inflammatory cascades
* enzymes enhancing production of reactive oxygen species (ROS)
* functions involved in adhesion to endothelium and migration
* pro-inflammatory mechanisms inducing or effectuating apoptosis or cell cycle arrest

To date, there are mixed results in the few veterinary studies evaluating the use of HBOT to improve wound healing with planned surgical incisions [4, 16, 17]. One recent study evaluating the use of HBOT after hemimastectomy found improved subjective healing parameters (decreased swelling, discharge, and less visible scar) in patients treated with low-pressure HBOT [16]. The authors removed skin sutures earlier in the HBOT-treated group. This was a non-blinded study of only 12 dogs and no objective criteria were utilized to warrant the added cost to owners [16]. A second study by Gautier et al., investigating the use of HBOT after routine ovariohysterectomy evaluated multiple objective variables including C-reactive protein, circulating cytokines, and serum oxidant status [17]. Subjective data such as pain scores and incision scores were also collected. The authors found no significant differences between the control and treatment groups in any of the variables but also reported no adverse effects with HBOT [17].

Further research is needed to establish standardized treatment protocols, determine optimal conditions for different indications, and evaluate short-term and long-term outcomes in veterinary patients. Additionally, the cost of equipment and limited availability of hyperbaric chambers pose challenges to its widespread adoption in veterinary practice. In conclusion, HBOT may be a valuable adjunctive therapy for numerous conditions in veterinary patients. With proper patient selection, treatment protocols, and safety precautions, this modality can significantly contribute to improving outcomes and quality of life for veterinary patients, especially in the sphere of wound care. Continued research and collaboration among veterinary professionals will further advance our understanding and utilization of HBOT in the years to come.

References

1 Levitan, D.M., Hitt, M., Geisler, D.R., and Lyman, R. (2021). Rationale for hyperbaric oxygen therapy in traumatic injury and wound care in small animal veterinary practice. *J. Small Anim. Pract.* 62 (9): 719–729. https://doi.org/10.1111/jsap.13356.

2 Lam, G., Fontaine, R., Ross, F.L., and Chiu, E.S. (2017). Hyperbaric oxygen therapy: exploring the clinical evidence. *Adv. Skin Wound Care* 30 (4): 181–190. https://doi.org/10.1097/01.ASW.0000513098.75457.22.

3 Gouveia, D., Bimbara, S., Carvalho, C. et al. (2021). Effect of hyperbaric oxygen on wound healing in veterinary medicine: a pilot study. *Open Vet. J.* 11 (4): 544–554.

4 Ruzicka, J., Dejmek, J., Bolek, L. et al. (2021). Hyperbaric oxygen influences chronic wound healing -a cellular level review. *Physiol. Res.* 70 (S3): 261–273. https://doi.org/10.33549/physiolres.934822.

5 Lindermann, J., Smolle, C., Kamolz, L.P. et al. (2021). Survey of molecular mechanism of hyperbaric oxygen in tissue repair. *Int. J. Mol. Sci.* 11754. https://doi.org/10.3390/ijms22211754.

6 Teguh, D.N., Bol Raap, R., Koole, A. et al. (2021). Hyperbaric oxygen therapy for non healing wounds: treatment results of a single center. *Wound Repair Regen.* 29 (2): 254–260. https://doi.org/10.1111/wrr.12884.

7 Andre-Levigne, D., Modarressi, A., Pignel, R. et al. (2016). Hyperbaric oxygen therapy promotes wound repair in ischemic and hyperglycemic conditions, increasing tissue perfusion and collagen deposition. *Wound Repair Regen.* 24: 954–965.

8 Smolle, C., Lindermann, J., Kamolz, L. et al. (2021). The history and developement of hyperbaric oxygenation (HBO) in thermal burn injury. *Medicina* 57: 49. https://doi.org/10.3390/medicina57010049.

9 Lansdorp, C.A., Buskens, C.J., Gecse, K.B. et al. (2022). Hyperbaric oxygen therapy for the treatment of perianal fistulas in 20 patients with Crohn's disease: results of the HOT-TOPIC trail after 1-year follow-up. *United Euro. Gastroenterol. J.* 10 (2): 160–168. https://doi.org/10.1002/ueg2.12189.

10 Coxene, B., Sadanandan, N., Gonzolez-Portillo, B. et al. (2020). An extra breath of fresh air: hyperbaric oxygenation as a stroke therapeutic. *Biomolecules* 10 (9): 1279. https://doi.org/10.3390/biom10091279.

11 Tian, C., Yang, Q., Bi, S. et al. (2022). Application of whole-body hyperbaric oxygen therapy in the treatment of grade III exposed dog bite wounds. *Emerg. Med. Int.* 2022: 2570883. https://doi.org/10.1155/2022/2570883.

12 Cooper, N.A., Unsworth, I.P., Turner, D.M. et al. (1976). Hyperbaric oxygen used in the treatment of gas gangrene in a dog. *J. Small Anim. Pract.* 17 (11): 759–764. https://doi.org/10.1111/j.1748-5827.1976.tb06940.x.

13 Montalbano, E., Kiorpes, C., Elaml, L. et al. (2021). Common uses and adverse effects of hyperbaric oxygen therapy in a cohort of small animal patients: a retrospective analysis of 2,792 treatment sessions. *Front. Vet. Sci.* 8: 764002. https://doi.org/10.3389/fvcts.2021.764002.

14 Birnie, G.L., Fry, D.R., and Best, M.P. (2018). Safety and tolerability of hyperbaric oxygen therapy in dogs and cats. *J. Am. Anim. Hosp. Assoc.* 54 (4): 188–194. https://doi.org/10.5326/JAAHA-MS-6548.

15 Gouvela, D., Chichorro, M., Cardos, A. et al. (2022). Hyperbaric oxygen therapy in systemic inflammatory response syndrome. *Vet. Sci.* 9 (2): 33. https://doi.org/10.3390/vetsci9020033.

16 Tunkiewicz, W., Kielbowicz, Z., Kallsiak, K. et al. (2020). Effect of hyperbaric oxygen on the healing of postoperative wounds in bitches after hemimastectomy. *Pol. J. Vet. Sci.* 23 (4): 495–499. https://doi.org/10.24425/pjvs.2020.134698.

17 Gautier, A., Graff, E.C., Backe, L. et al. (2020). Effects of ovariohysterectomy and hyperbaric oxygen therapy on systemic inflammation and oxidation in dogs. *Front. Vet. Sci.* 6: 506. https://doi.org/10.3389/fvets.2019.00506.

14

Low Level Laser, Photobiomodulation and Electromagnetics for Wound Therapy

Nicole J. Buote

Department of Clinical Sciences, Cornell University, Ithaca, NY, USA

Low Level Laser Therapy

Physiology

Low level laser therapy (LLT) also known as cold laser is defined as any device which emits <10 W of power when applied to the skin or other tissue. Much is still unknown regarding the exact mechanism of action these devices have on healing wounds, but some studies have shown encouraging results [1–3]. One theory posited involves photon activation of cytochrome oxidase creating energy production and synthesis of proteins implicated in cellular repair. Other authors theorize possible effects of radiation on cellular differentiation and prostaglandin synthesis [3–5].

Indications

Reported indications for LLLT are acute or chronic wounds, closed incisions as well as various musculoskeletal injuries [3, 6, 7].

Technique

There are many different types of commercial devices available in laser classes I–IV that produce different wavelengths and varied energy density. A recent review indicated that daily laser exposure at a wavelength within the 600 or 800 nm range was the most beneficial across the rodent studies reviewed but more studies were required in rabbit, canine, and equine models to determine the correct treatment parameters for these species [8]. The most commonly used wavelength in studies of LLLT in wound healing is 635 nm (Helium-Neon) (Figure 14.1) but other studies looking at 980 nm lasers have also been performed [1, 9]. Recommended treatment times and number of treatments per week will vary according to the wound being treated and the device. In most studies, the laser is applied three times per week for five minutes at a time. The authors recommend consulting with the manufacturer before embarking on LLT to determine the safest protocol for your patient. Appropriate eye protection for the clinician using LLLT must be worn.

Post-Treatment Care/Complications

No specific posttreatment care is required. No clinically adverse side effects or complications have been observed in any patient treated with LLLT.

Techniques in Small Animal Wound Management, First Edition. Edited by Nicole J. Buote.
© 2024 John Wiley & Sons, Inc. Published 2024 by John Wiley & Sons, Inc.
Companion website: www.wiley.com/go/buote/wounds

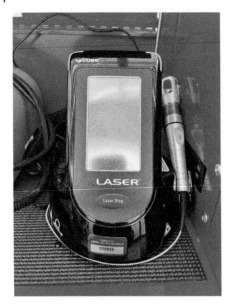

As with many new wound therapies, there are inconsistencies in the literature regarding the effects of LLLT for wound healing. This is most likely due to the use of different machines, treatment dosages, and outcome measures. *In vitro* studies have shown effects on cellular migration and proliferation of cultured canine keratinocytes [10, 11]. A veterinary experimental randomized study using a class II He–Ne laser (635 nm) three times a week failed to show a benefit in an acute canine wound model over a 21 day period but the authors did encourage ongoing studies as different protocols may yield altered results [1]. Another experimental prospective study in dogs with created open dermal punch wounds and closed ovariectomy incisions reported that wound treated with a class IV laser (980 nm) once daily for five days did not show any subjective effect on wound healing or wound measurements [9]. A recent prospective, randomized, blinded, placebo-controlled pilot study investigating the use of LLLT in infected traumatic wounds in dogs treated wounds with two different dosages (2 or 6 J/cm^2 with four wavelengths used simultaneously: 660, 800, 905, and 970 nm) [12]. A significant decrease in the bacterial count and improved wound scores were reported in the 2 J/cm^2 group when compared to controls.

Figure 14.1 Photograph of a K laser®, a class 4 therapeutic laser. *Source:* Courtesy of Nicole Buote, DVM, DACVS.

The lack of standardization of wavelength, energy density, and treatment schedules hamper conclusive recommendations regarding this modality of wound therapy. Future research is required to justify the use of LLLT in a clinical veterinary setting.

Photobiomodulation

Physiology

Photobiomodulation therapy (PBMT) is a broad term that incorporates LLLT and other devices consist of light-emitting devices (LED) proposed to stimulate cellular transduction pathways. Research into the uses of these devices for many diseases including orthopedic and neurologic has shown some promise in this non-invasive modality [13]. PBM may be beneficial in chronic and infected wounds [12, 14]. The biological processes affected by PMBT are promoted through activation of photoacceptors or chromophores present in cells and tissue. A full understanding of the mechanisms of action of PMBT is not known and some proposed processes have only been studied *in vitro* [15–17]. The three main mechanisms focus on interactions with adenosine triphosphate (ATP), nitric oxide (NO), and reactive oxygen species (ROS). When specific chromophores are excited by the appropriate wavelength of light (500–1100 nm – red and infrared spectrum) a chain reaction occurs whereby ATP production is increased, circulating nitric oxide increases, and ROS are released [13]. Many consequences can be seen due to these effects (Table 14.1) leading to the proposed benefits to wound healing [13].

A study using PBMT (BTL 5800 SL Combi, 830 nm) on chronic wounds in client-owned dogs found a significant decrease in wound area in treated dogs compared to controls [14]. A different type of PBMT called fluorescence photobiomodulation (FPBM) has been studied in veterinary medicine [18–20]. With FPBM, light-absorbing molecules convert the light emitted by the device to broader wavelengths and lower energy which penetrates the skin and encourages healing [21, 22]. When the chromophores in the topical photoconverter (carbopol-based amorphous hydrogel) are activated by the LED light source, they release photons at varying wavelengths in the form of fluorescence. The Phovia device (KT-V lamp; Klox Technologies, Laval, Quebec, Canada) is a commercially available device which delivers a blue light with wavelengths between 440 and 460 nm and a power density ranging between 55 and 129 mW/cm^2 (Figure 14.2). This device has been researched and found to have positive effects on epithelialization and collagen production as well as decrease bacterial counts and inflammation [12, 18].

Table 14.1   Proposed mechanisms of action of PMBT.

ATP production increased	
	Increased available energy for reparative tasks
	Increased cellular signaling and intracellular calcium
	± Neurotransmitter
Increased NO circulation	
	Increased metabolic turnover
	Vasodilatory effects via relaxation of endothelial cells
	Increased angiogenesis
	Alteration of inflammation and immune responses
Release of ROS	
	Activation of antioxidant enzymes
	Stimulation of cellular growth
	Augment stem cell differentiation

ATP, adenosine triphosphate; NO, nitric oxide; ROS, reactive oxygen species.

Figure 14.2   (a,b) Photographs of the commercially available Phovia device (KT-V lamp; Klox Technologies, Laval, Quebec, Canada) which delivers a blue light with wavelengths between 440 and 460 nm. *Source:* Courtesy of Nicole Buote, DVM, DACVS.

(a)
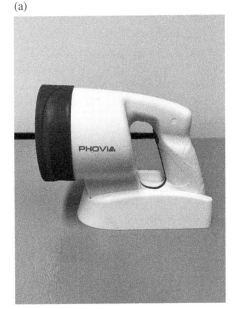

(b)
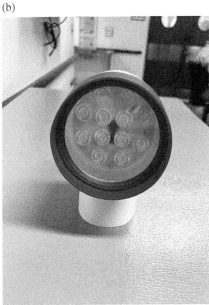

Indications

Distinct recommendations for PBMT for wound healing are difficult to ascertain. A recent systematic review highlighted the paucity of high-quality reproducible studies in veterinary medicine [3]. Indications based on available existing literature include chronic and infected wounds. PBMT for incisional healing could also be considered as there are no known side effects if incisional healing is precarious.

Technique

For healing surgical incisions, a published treatment recommendation consisted of 2 mm of photoconverter gel applied to the closed incision and use of the Phovia device for two minutes at a wavelength between 440 and 460 nm and a power density of between 55 and 129 mW/cm^2. The first treatment was on day 1 postoperative with follow-up treatments of two minutes every three days until day 13 [18].

The treatment protocol for burn wounds stated by the manufacturer is two treatments a week, of two minutes per 10 × 10 cm region after application of the photoconverter gel. An alternative treatment regimen performed with good success (see Figure 14.3) is a once-a-week application of the light using two treatments per region. This double treatment regimen can be performed every five to seven days. Because the gel has hydrogen peroxide in it, the wound should be flushed when the treatment is done.

For chronic wounds, recommended treatment dosages depend on the device used (Table 14.2). Treatments were performed in one study every other day for two weeks [14]:

Specific treatment times and number of treatments per week will vary according to the wound being treated and the device (Figure 14.3). The authors recommend consulting with the manufacturer to determine the safest protocol for your patient. Appropriate eye protection for the clinician using LED devices must be utilized.

Post-Treatment Care/Complications

No specific posttreatment care is required. No clinically adverse side effects have been observed in any patient treated with LED treatments and no adverse reactions have been reported associated with the photoconverter gel. No known complications have occurred during or after PBMT in veterinary patients.

Outcomes

Outcomes for wounds treated with LED therapies have been positive in the few veterinary studies published to date. In the study by Salvaggio et al., looking at the effects on closed clean wounds, the LED-treated (Phovia) tissue achieved lower histologic inflammation scores, and greater deposition of collagen. The authors concluded that Phovia therapy improved reepithelialization and matrix formation in closed clean surgical incisions [18]. A study investigating chronic wounds in canine patients assessed the use of multiple wavelength doses (single wavelength of 830 nm or superpulsed multi-wavelength – 660, 875, and 905 nm) on client-owned patients [14]. These investigators found a significant difference in the percentage of wound area reduction for both PBMT groups compared to the control leading them to conclude that either uni- or multi-wavelength dosages can improve wound healing for chronic wounds in dogs. Another study evaluating surgical incisions (hemilaminectomies) in canine patients created a novel scar scale to compare treated and controlled incisions [23]. Patients received 8 J/cm^2 of laser therapy once a day for seven days in the treatment group and incisions were scored over 21 days based on digital photographs. The authors concluded that laser therapy improved the cosmetic healing by day 7 in the treatment group and this effect continued after cessation of daily laser therapy [23]. While this study is promising, objective histologic data was not performed, and this scar score has not been independently validated.

Pulsed Electromagnetic Field Therapy

Physiology

Pulsed electromagnetic field (PEMF) therapy utilizes electromagnetic fields in tissue to encourage healing through noninvasive nonthermal devices. Faraday's Law is the main physical mechanism underlying PEMF devices. This law states that the induced electromotive force in any closed circuit is equal to the rate of change of the magnetic flux enclosed by the circuit [24]. The known characteristics of the electromagnetic pulse (i.e., frequency, duration, amplitude) determine the magnitude of the magnetic and electrical fields provided to the tissues; this information to use to compare efficacy of treatment and safety. Specific proposed mechanisms include the effect of PEMF on calcium ion signaling, nitric oxide signaling, heat shock proteins, and adenosine receptor expression [24]. It is important to note that different PEMF devices exist (targeted versus non-targeted) and the results of investigations show varying usefulness depending on the device characteristics.

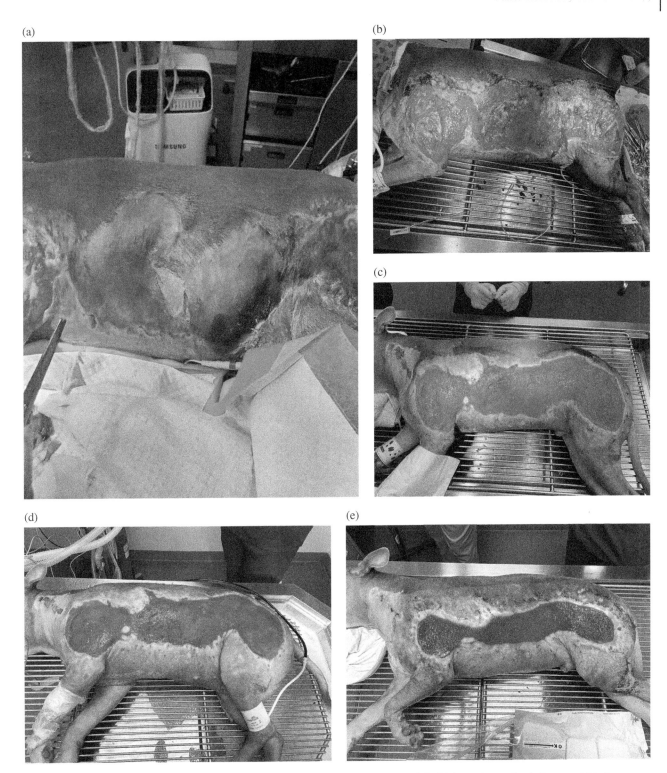

Figure 14.3 Photographs of a four-year-old male neutered Pitt bull with a severe full-thickness burn after being caught below a fallen roof in a mobile home fire. The burn was treated with Phovia light treatments every five-days. The treatment protocol: 1–2 mm of photoconverter gel was applied, the light was applied for two minutes, the gel was removed and a new covering of gel reapplied and light applied again. An area of 10 cm × 10 cm can be treated by the laser therefore this large wound required the laser to be moved to sequentially cover the tissue (two treatments per each area treated). (a) Initial eschar, (b) After initial debridement, (c) 12 days after initial debridement – weekly treatments had been performed, (d) 14 days after initial debridement, (e) 24 days after initial debridement, (f) 31 days after initial debridement, (g) 38 days after initial debridement, (h) Photoconverter gel by Vetoquinol (a part of the Phovia system) being applied before a treatment – the gel is mixed with an activator and applied about 1–2 mm thick for each treatment, (i,j) Phovia laser in action during treatment. *Source:* Courtesy of Katie Barry, DVM, DACVS.

(f) (g)

(h) (i) (j)

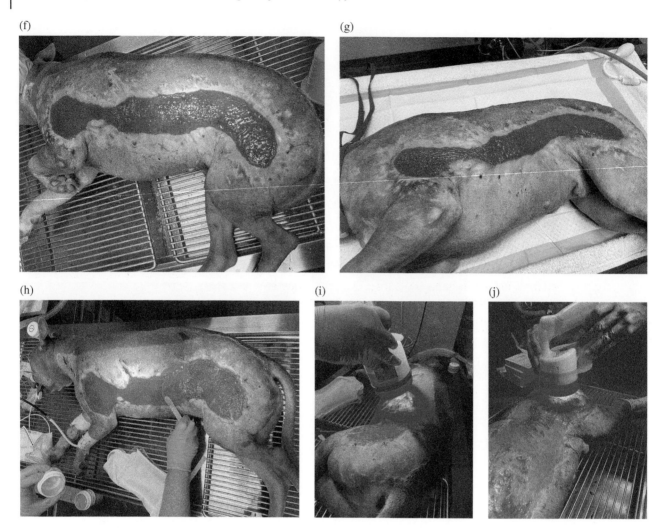

Figure 14.3   (Continued)

Table 14.2   Treatment regimens for chronic wounds [14].

1) Device: BTL-5800 SL Combi, BTL Industries Ltd., UK
   Dose: 830 nm wavelength with fluence of 4 J/cm^2
         Power of 200 mW, and frequency of 50 Hz
         Time of treatment was calculated from the wound area which is between 3.45 and 41.40 min
2) Device: MR4 ActiVet Pro, Multi Radiance Medical®, USA
   Dose: Synchronous use of light power of SPMW (100 mW of 660 nm; 250 mW of 875 nm)
         Peak pulse power 50 W (pulse duration of 110 ± 20 s) of 905 nm
         Time of treatment used was 1 min/4 cm^2 of wound area which is between 1 and 5 min

Indications

While PEMF devices have been awarded FDA clearance for orthopedic indications (bone healing, osteoarthritis, fasciitis) in human medicine, these devices have also been studied in inflammatory, postsurgical, and chronic wound models as well as in neurologic and psychiatric trials [24]. In veterinary medicine, PEMF has been studied in bone healing models [25] (Inoue), clinical osteoarthritis [26] (Sullivan), a postoperative surgical discomfort (OVH) model [27] (Shafford), and more recently in dogs with intervertebral disk disease [28, 29] (Alvarez, Zidan). No effect was seen in the ovariohysterectomy model with regards to postoperative discomfort and no clinical studies have been performed studying wound healing in veterinary patients.

Technique

Only one clinical veterinary study to date discusses the use of PEMF and its subjective effects on healing hemilaminectomy incisions [28]. In this study, an Assisi Loop (Assisi Animal Health, Northvale, New Jersey, Figure 14.4) was utilized every 6 hours for 15 minutes during hospitalization (number of days not specified), followed by every 12 hours for 7 days.

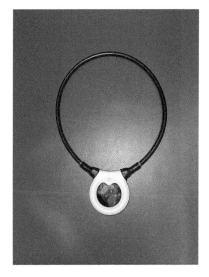

Figure 14.4 Photograph of the Assisi Loop (Assisi Animal Health, Northvale, New Jersey, USA). *Source:* Courtesy of Pamela Schwartz, DVM, DACVS.

Post-Treatment Care/Complications

No specific posttreatment care is required. While the dangers of non-ionizing electromagnetic fields are due to thermal effects, non-thermal PEMF devices have reports of clinically adverse side effects or adverse reactions in any patient treated with this technology [30]. (Guo)

Outcomes

As discussed above, these devices have been used to treat multiple orthopedic diseases in human medicine but to date, very few rigorous veterinary studies have been performed [24]. As with all of the therapies in this chapter, there are many different devices commercially available, all providing varied dosages. A discussion of outcomes unrelated to wounds can be found in other resources [24] but the one veterinary study mentioning incisional effects of PEMF reported subjective wound healing (as evaluated by visual analog scores and wound evaluation scales), was significantly improved at the six week recheck [28]. This study examined hemilaminectomy incisions and no histologic comparisons between the control and treated groups were performed. Subjective wound scores can be inaccurate and more rigorously tested, data-driven studies should be performed before recommendations can be made. No studies to date have investigated PEMF with chronic or infected wounds.

References

1 Kurach, L.M., Stanley, B.J., Gazzola, K.M. et al. (2015). The effect of low-level laser therapy on the healing of open wounds in dogs. *Vet. Surg.* 44: 988–996.

2 Kim, H., Choi, K., Kweon, O.-K., and Kim, W.H. (2012). Enhanced wound healing effect of canine adipose-derived mesenchymal stem cells with low-level laser therapy in athymic mice. *J. Dermatol. Sci.* 68 (3): 149–156.

3 Millis, D.L. and Bergh, A. (2023). A systematic literature review of complementary and alternative veterinary medicine: laser therapy. *Animals* 13 (4): 667.

4 da Silva, J.P., da Silva, M.A., Almeida, A.P. et al. (2010). Laser therapy in the tissue repair process: a literature review. *Photomed. Laser Surg.* 28: 17–21.

5 Kushibiki, T., Hirasawa, T., Okawa, S. et al. (2013). Regulation of miRNA expression by low-level laser therapy (LLLT) and photodynamic therapy (PDT). *Int. J. Mol. Sci.* 14: 13542–13558.

6 Enwemeka, C.S., Parker, J.C., Dowdy, D.S. et al. (2004). The efficacy of low power lasers in tissue repair and pain control: a meta-analysis study. *Photomed. Laser Surg.* 22: 323–329.

7 Leal Junior, E.C., Lopes-Martins, R.A., Frigo, L. et al. (2010). Effects of low level laser therapy (LLLT) in the development of exercise induced skeletal muscle fatigue and changes in biochemical markers related to post exercise recovery. *J. Orthop. Sports Phys. Ther.* 40: 524–532.

8 Lopez, A. and Brundage, C. (2019). Wound photobiomodulation treatment outcomes in animal models. *J. Vet. Med.* https://doi.org/10.1155/2019/6320515.

9 Gammel, J.E., Biskup, J.J., Drum, M.G. et al. (2018). Effects of low-level laser therapy on the healing of surgically closed incisions and surgically created open wounds in dogs. *Vet. Surg.* 47: 499–506.

10 Gagnon, D., Gibson, T.W.G., Singh, A. et al. (2016). An in vitro method to test the safety and efficacy of low-level laser therapy (LLLT) in the healing of a canine skin model. *BMC Vet. Res.* 12: 73.

11 Peplow, P.V., Chung, T.Y., and Baxter, G.D. (2010). Laser photobiomodulation of wound healing: a review of experimental studies in mouse and rat animal models. *Photomed. Laser Surg.* 28: 291–325.

12 Rico-Holgado, S., Ortiz-Dı́ez, G., Martı́n-Espada, M.C. et al. (2021). Effect of low-level laser therapy on bacterial counts of contaminated traumatic wounds in dogs. *J. Lasers Med. Sci.* 12 (1): e78. https://doi.org/10.34172/jlms.2021.78.

13 Bunch, J. (2023). Photobiomodulation (therapeutic lasers): an update and review of current literature. *Vet. Clin. North Am. Small Anim. Pract.* 53 (4): 783–799.

14 Hoisang, S., Kampa, N., Seesupa, S., and Jitpean, S. (2021). Assessment of wound area reduction on chronic wounds in dogs with photobiomodulation therapy: a randomized controlled clinical trial. *Vet. World* 14 (8): 2251–2259.

15 Hochman, L. (2018). Photobiomodulation therapy in veterinary medicine: a review. *Top. Companion Anim. Med.* 33 (3): 83–88.

16 Anders, J.J., Ketz, A.K., and Wu, X. (2017). Basic principles of photobiomodulation and its effects at the cellular, tissue, and system levels. In: *Laser Therapy in Veterinary Medicine* (ed. R.J. Riegel and J.C. Godbold Jr.), 36–51. Wiley.

17 Hamblin, M.R. (2017). Mechanisms and applications of the anti-inflammatory effects of photobiomodulation. *AIMS Biophys.* 4 (3): 337–361.

18 Salvaggio, A., Magi, G.E., Rossi, G. et al. (2020). Effect of the topical Klox fluorescence biomodulation system on the healing of canine surgical wounds. *Vet. Surg.* 49: 719–727.

19 Marchegiani, A., Spaterna, A., Cerquetella, M. et al. (2019). Fluorescence biomodulation in the management of canine interdigital pyoderma cases: a prospective, single-blinded, randomized and controlled clinical study. *Vet. Dermatol.* 30 (5): 371–e109. https://doi.org/10.1111/vde.12785.

20 Tambella, A.M., Cerquetella, M., Attili, A.R. et al. (2017). Klox biophotonic system, a promising innovative approach to canine chronic oti tis externa: preliminary report of a randomized controlled clinical trial. *Vet. Surg.* 46 (6): E50–E51.

21 Nikolis, A., Grimard, D., Pesant, Y. et al. (2016). A prospective case series evaluating the safety and efficacy of the Klox BioPhotonic system in venous leg ulcers. *Chron. Wound Care Manag. Res.* 3: 101–111.

22 Romanelli, M., Piaggesi, A., Scapagnini, G. et al. (2017). EUREKA study—the evaluation of real-life use of a biophotonic system in chronic wound management: an interim analysis. *Drug Des. Devel. Ther.* 11: 3551–3558.

23 Wardlaw, J.L., Gazzola, K.M., Wagoner, A. et al. (2018). Laser therapy for incision healing in 9 dogs. *Front. Vet. Sci.* 5: 349.

24 Gaynor, J.A., Hagberg, S., and Gurfein, B.L. (2018). Veterinary applications of pulsed electromagnetic field therapy. *Res. Vet. Sci.* 119: 1–8.

25 Inoue, N., Ohnishi, I., Chen, D. et al. (2002). Effect of pulsed electromagnetic fields (PEMF) on late-phase osteotomy gap healing in a canine tibial mode. *J. Orthop. Res.* 20 (5): 1106–1114.

26 Sullivan, M.O., Gordon-Evans, W.J., Knap, K.E., and Evans, R.B. (2013). Randomized, controlled clinical trial evaluating the efficacy of pulsed signal therapy in dogs with osteoarthritis. *Vet. Surg.* 42 (3): 250–254.

27 Shafford, H.L., Hellyer, P.W., Crump, K.T. et al. (2002). Use of a pulsed electromagnetic field for treatment of post-operative pain in dogs: a pilot study. *Vet. Anaesth. Analg.* 29 (1): 43–48.

28 Alvarez, L.X., McCue, J., Lam, N.K. et al. (2019). Effect of targeted pulsed electromagnetic field therapy on canine postoperative hemilaminectomy: a double-blind, randomized, placebo-controlled clinical trial. *J. Am. Anim. Hosp. Assoc.* 55 (2): 83–91.

29 Zidan, N., Fenn, J., Griffith, E. et al. (2018). The effect of electromagnetic fields on post-operative pain and locomotor recovery in dogs with acute, severe thoracolumbar intervertebral disc extrusion: a randomized placebo-controlled, prospective clinical trial. *J. Neurotrauma* 35 (15): 1726–1736.

30 Guo, L., Kubat, N.J., Nelson, T.R., and Isenberg, R.A. (2012). Meta-analysis of clinical efficacy of pulsed radio frequency energy treatment. *Ann. Surg.* 255: 457–467.

15

Platelet Rich Plasma and Stem Cell Therapy

Aarthi Rajesh, Rebecca M. Harman, and Gerlinde R. Van de Walle

Department of Microbiology and Immunology, Baker Institute for Animal Health, Cornell University, Ithaca, NY, USA

Platelet Rich Plasma (PRP) Therapy

Physiology and Indications

Platelet Rich Plasma (PRP) is defined as a volume of plasma with a platelet concentration higher than that of peripheral blood [1]. PRP therapy differs from stem cell therapy in that it uses the therapeutic factors found in blood plasma to heal acute or degenerative damage. It can be prepared and administrated as an autologous therapy for a multitude of clinical conditions in small companion animals, including osteoarthritis [2], muscle damage, burns [3], ulcers [4], and even hair restoration [5]. The therapeutic properties of PRP rely on the fact that platelets under physiological conditions secrete a wide variety of growth factors such as epidermal growth factor (EGF), fibroblast growth factor (FGF), transforming growth factor beta (TGF-β), platelet-derived growth factor (PDGF), vascular endothelial growth factor (VEGF), and insulin-like growth factor 1 (IGF-1). During injury, when platelets come in contact with collagen, they release alpha granules and growth factors. Concentrating platelets results in concentrated growth factors that can be used as a treatment to assist in healing.

The use of PRP as a treatment for the healing of cutaneous wounds in small companion animals has been reported in both clinical and experimental studies. The clinical outcomes of PRP treatments of large skin defects have been generally positive [6–8]. Large and contaminated natural skin defects in cats and dogs that previously showed no improvement with conventional therapies, such as antibacterial medications and saline washes, showed promising reduction in wound size after treatment with PRP (Table 15.1).

Experimentally-induced wounds in dogs and rabbits treated with PRP generally exhibit both macroscopically and microscopically faster healing phenotypes with no abnormal tissue formation, keloids, or pathologic scarring, when compared to the control group (Table 15.2).

PRP Promotes Wound Contraction

Most small companion animals have loose skin, so they rely on effective wound contraction to shorten healing time [15]. Wound contraction is a healing response that functions to reduce the size of the wound margins, through movement of fibroblasts in the granulation tissue. PRP treatment of experimentally-induced wounds in dogs and rabbits significantly promoted wound contraction, as demonstrated by increased fibroblast migration and collagen deposition [16, 17, 23]. Specifically, greater fibroblast migration was noted [14, 16, 17], as well as increased collagen deposition and a more orderly arrangement of collagen fibers in the wounds, thus reducing the possibility of hypertrophic or keloid scarring [9] (Table 15.2).

PRP Enhances Reepithelialization

The enriched growth factors in PRP act on the epidermal and dermal layers of the skin. PRP treatment accelerated reepithelialization and epidermal differentiation [12, 14, 17, 21, 23–26] (Tables 15.1 and 15.2). Reepithelialization results from the proliferation and differentiation of epidermal cells, in which multiple growth factors [27], including EGF, FGF,

Techniques in Small Animal Wound Management, First Edition. Edited by Nicole J. Buote.
© 2024 John Wiley & Sons, Inc. Published 2024 by John Wiley & Sons, Inc.
Companion website: www.wiley.com/go/buote/wounds

Table 15.1   Platelet-rich plasma (PRP) applications for healing of naturally occurring wounds in cats and dogs.

PRP formulation	Number of animals	Nature of natural lesion	Outcome	References
Cats				
2 ml injection, 2 doses, autologous	1	Post-operative wound	• Increased granulation tissue formation, gradual reduction of necrotic tissue	[4]
2 ml topical PRP formulation, heterologous (canine origin)	1	Large skin defect	• No signs of inflammation, necrosis, or infection • Increased reepithelialization, and wound contraction • Slight scar formation	[9]
Dogs				
0.1 ml topical gel, autologous	1	Large skin defect	• Complete healing with reduced edema • Complete hair regrowth observed	[2]
0.1 ml topical gel, allogeneic	1	Large skin defect	• Reduced inflammation • Increased reepithelialization and granulation tissue formation • Complete hair regrowth observed	[3]
3–6 ml (depending on wound size) topical, autologous	6	Various skin defects	• Increased reepithelialization, wound contraction, and angiogenesis. • Hair growth restored • No abnormal scarring present	[6]

Table 15.2   Platelet-rich plasma (PRP) applications for healing of experimentally-induced wounds in dogs and rabbits.

PRP formulation	Number of animals	Treatment of control group	Size and nature of wounds	Outcome	References
Dogs					
1.5 ml topical gel, autologous	5	Untreated	2×2 cm excisional wounds	• No significant difference in wound contraction, reepithelialization	[10]
1.5 ml topical gel, autologous	5	Untreated	2×2 cm excisional wounds	• No significant difference between the two groups	[11]
Unknown volume of topical gel, autologous	15	Untreated	10 cm long incisional wounds.	• Accelerated reepithelialization, increased neo-vascularization • No difference in collagen deposition	[12]
3 ml injection dose, autologous	6	Untreated	2×2 cm excisional wounds	• Rate of healing did not differ significantly with PRP treatment. • Increased collagen production and better collagen orientation with PRP treatment	[13]
0.5 ml injection dose, autologous	3	Saline	6 mm diameter excisional wounds	• No significant difference in wound closure rate. • Increased angiogenesis, granulation tissue, collagen deposition, and reepithelialization	[14]

Table 15.2   (Continued)

PRP formulation	Number of animals	Treatment of control group	Size and nature of wounds	Outcome	References
3 ml injection dose, autologous	5	Untreated	3 mm diameter excisional wounds	• Reduced wound size • Increased wound contraction, reepithelialization, migration of fibroblasts, and MMP-9 activity • Organized collagen deposition with parallel orientation • Reduced polymorphonuclear cells and scar formation	[15]
5 ml injection dose, autologous	10	Saline	2×2 cm excisional wounds	• Increased wound contraction, reepithelialization, granulation tissue, and skin appendages • Increased macrophages and fibroblasts through TGF beta production.	[7]
Rabbits					
0.3, 0.6, and 0.9 ml topical PRP formulation, autologous	15	Untreated	2.5×2.5 cm excisional wounds	• Increased reepithelialization, reduced contraction, and fibroblast recruitment in the 0.6- and 0.9-ml dose • No difference in neutrophil, macrophage numbers, and angiogenesis	[16]
Unknown volume of topical gel, autologous	20	Untreated	6 mm diameter excisional wounds	• Reduced inflammation • Increased granulation tissue formation and reepithelialization	[17]
0.5 ml injection dose, autologous	20	Saline solution + Tegaderm™ dressing	2×2 cm excisional wounds	• PRP-treated rabbits healed faster. • Delayed healing was seen in 1 out of 20 showed in the PRP-treated group and 6 out 20 in the control group	[18]
0.5 ml topical gel, heterologous (canine origin)	6	Untreated	8 mm diameter excisional wounds	• No difference in size of the wound, contraction. • Mild-to-moderate inflammatory infiltrate observed in 90% of PRP-treated wounds	[19]
0.5 ml topical gel, autologous, allogenic, and heterologous (canine origin)	24	Saline	8 mm diameter excisional wounds	• Wound treated with PRP showed complete and enhanced reepithelialization and angiogenesis when compared to controls. • Similar levels of wound contraction, migration of fibroblasts between the treatments • Potential analgesic effect • Increased neutrophil recruitment in heterologous PRP	[8]
0.5 ml topical gel + Rosuvastin, autologous	8	Saline	8 mm diameter excisional wounds	• PRP treatment alone showed no difference in wound contraction or wound closure • Combined treatment showed increased reepithelialization, neovascularization, and collagen production more than individual treatments	[20]
0.5 ml topical study ointment, heterologous (equine origin)	24	Study ointment	3 cm diameter excisional wounds	• Increased immune response • Decreased edema • Early formation of scabs and granulation tissue • Increased neovascularization and fibrosis • No difference in wound size with control	[21]
0.4 ml of topical PRP formulation, allogeneic and heterologous (human origin)	21	Platelet poor plasma	2×2 cm excisional wounds	• Larger scar retraction observed with heterologous PRP • No significant difference between healing	[22]

TGF-beta, PDGF, and IGF-1, all secreted by platelets, play critical roles. Furthermore, a significant increase in matrix metalloproteinase 9 (MMP-9) in PRP-treated wounds has been reported, which may aid in reepithelialization [14]. MMP-9 is essential for degrading the basement membrane to allow for efficient keratinocyte migration during reepithelialization [9], although an overexpression may also result in delayed wound healing and chronic wounds [28].

PRP Enhances Granulation Tissue Formation and Angiogenesis

Most studies report enhanced granulation tissue formation and angiogenesis in PRP-treated wounds in cats, dogs, and rabbits [7, 8, 12, 16, 17, 21, 23, 26, 29]. Granulation tissue is essential for effective wound healing as it provides a conducive environment for wound repair by increasing vascularization that provides nutrients and oxygen. The quality and quantity of neovascularization thus determines the quality of wound healing. *In vitro* and *in vivo* studies using human and mouse models have demonstrated PRP's strong angiogenic potential through enhanced production of VEGF [30]. The ability of PRP to promote angiogenesis makes it a highly suitable treatment for chronic wounds, which are commonly characterized by poor vascularization.

PRP Improves Regrowth of Appendages

The regeneration of skin appendages, which include hair, nails, sweat glands, and sebaceous glands, is still one of the most significant challenges in regenerative medicine. Poor regrowth of skin appendages has been associated with delayed wound healing and excessive scarring. The growth of hair and sebaceous glands showed improvement in PRP-treated experimentally-induced canine wounds when compared to the control group [6, 17, 23]. Epidermal stem cells play a key role in the regeneration of hair follicles and skin appendages in the skin [31], and PRP treatment was found to increase survival and activation of mouse epidermal stem cells *in vitro* [32].

PRP Provides Analgesic Effects

Pain is a frequently experienced, yet often overlooked factor in wound care, that can reduce a patient's quality of life [33]. One study showed that rabbits treated with PRP had reduced signs of pain [16]. Similarly, human studies suggest that PRP treatment can reduce pain at the lesion site and provide potential analgesic effects by producing endocannabinoids [11, 20, 34]. PRP used for the treatment of carpal tunnel syndrome in humans revealed a long-term analgesic effect after a single PRP injection in mild-to-moderate cases [22]. PRP treatment has been shown to result in significant pain reduction in dogs [10] and cats [13] suffering from osteoarthritis. Further investigation into the analgesic effects of different PRP formulations in small companion wound healing is warranted.

Description of Technique

PRP formulations can be classified into four types based on their leukocyte content and fibrin architecture [19] (Table 15.3). The type of PRP prepared depends on the type of collecting tube and centrifugation speed, which both play a role in the final concentration of platelets and leukocytes in the PRP preparation [18].

Various protocols are being used to prepare PRP (Tables 15.4 and 15.5). In general, the process begins with obtaining whole blood from a patient at volumes ranging from 3 ml [41] to 120 ml [21]. Needle size used to draw blood is not standardized across published studies in small companion animals (Tables 15.4 and 15.5). For reference, human PRP studies recommend using a needle size of 21 gauge or larger as smaller needle sizes may prematurely activate platelets [42].

Centrifugation, at relative centrifugal forces (RCF) ranging between 400 and 900, is done to separate plasma and leukocytes from red blood cells (Figures 15.1 and 15.2). This process usually results in a 2-3-fold increase of platelets when compared to the original blood sample. An additional faster centrifugation step (<1000 RCF) may be included to further concentrate the platelets [42]. Although the resulting platelet concentrations can be three to eight times higher than the baseline, leukocytes remain in the preparation [42].

Multiple commercial PRP systems have been developed for small companion animal use, particularly for dogs. A study comparing the efficacy of five different commercial systems (i.e., SmartPrep 2 ACP+, Arthrex ACP, CRT Pure PRP, ProTec PRP, C-PET Canine Platelet Enhancement Therapy) for the preparation of canine PRP showed that PRP concentration results varied among these systems [43]. Limitations of this study were that different dogs were used for each PRP system and thus, the authors acknowledge that the observed variations could be attributed to inherent patient factors as well. Three of the systems (i.e., Arthrex ACP, Protec PRP, and C-PET) were tested in another study using canine blood and revealed similar platelet concentrations [44]. However, there were slight variations in initial blood volumes and protocols

Table 15.3 Classification of platelet-rich plasma formulations.

Preparation	Leukocyte count	Fibrin density
Pure platelet-rich plasma (P-PRP)	Poor	Low
Leukocyte- and platelet-rich plasma (L-PRP)	Rich	Low
Pure platelet-rich fibrin (P-PRF)	Poor	High
Leukocyte- and platelet-rich fibrin (L-PRF)	Rich	High

Table 15.4 Summary of platelet-rich plasma (PRP) protocols used in wound healing studies of naturally occurring wounds in cats and dogs.

Blood volume (ml)	Needle size (gauge)	Centrifuge speed	Centrifuge time (min)	Activator	References
Cats					
16	22	2800 RPM	20	NI	[8]
		1300 RPM	15		
16	18	Unknown	Unknown	NI	[25]
Dogs					
8	Unknown	629 RCF	10	10% Calcium chloride	[6]
		1233 RCF	15		
8	Unknown	629 RCF	10	10% Calcium chloride	[7]
		1233 RCF	14		
15–25	Unknown	2800 RPM	20	NI	[23]
		1300 RPM	15		

RPM, rotations per minute; RCF, relative centrifugal force; NI, Not Included

used between the two studies [44]. Currently, only one study reports the use of a commercial system, namely the PRO-PRP kit, for a wound healing study in dogs [21] (Table 15.5). In this system, 18 ml of blood is injected into the PRP-separation containers and centrifuged at 290 RCF for six minutes, which separates the blood into three fractions – red blood cells, platelet-poor plasma, and platelet-rich plasma with leukocytes [21].

In many PRP preparations, activators are added to stimulate the platelets and help release alpha granules. Use of exogenous activators can be used to control the timing of growth-factor release [45]. Bovine thrombin [24] and calcium chloride [6, 7, 14] are most commonly used for PRP preparations from companion animal studies (Tables 15.4 and 15.5). These activators catalyze the fibrinogen-to-fibrin reaction that begins to congeal the plasma [45]. However, the use of activators is not necessary, as improved healing of wounds from small companion animals has been reported without their use [8, 21, 25].

Considerations for PRP Therapy

One of the major challenges in evaluating the success of PRP treatments is the lack of standardization in preparation and dosage of PRP. While a majority of the studies indicate a positive healing effect with PRP, several experimental studies in dogs and rabbits found no effect on wound healing after PRP treatment when compared to control wounds [35–37, 39–41] (Table 15.2). In addition, a study in rabbits showed an evident clinical deterioration in one of the 20 wounds treated with PRP, although this number was lower compared to the six out of the 20 wounds that showed delayed healing in the control

Table 15.5 Summary of platelet-rich plasma (PRP) protocols used in wound healing studies of experimentally-induced wounds in dogs and rabbits.

Blood volume (ml)	Needle size (gauge)	Centrifuge speed	Centrifuge time (min)	Activator	References
Dogs					
40	Unknown	120 RCF	5	NI	[35]
		280 RCF	5		
Unknown	Unknown	120 RCF	5	Unknown % Calcium chloride	[36]
		280 RCF	5		
20	Unknown	3000 RPM	10	NI	[26]
53	Unknown	4000 RPM		NI	[37]
120	19	209 RCF	6	NI	[21]
Unknown	Unknown	250 RCF	10	10% Calcium chloride	[14]
		2000 RCF	10		
		3000 RCF	20		
52	19 g	209 RCF	6	NI	[17]
Rabbits					
20	Unknown	Unknown	Unknown	Bovine thrombin	[24]
10	Unknown	460 RCF	8	10% Calcium Chloride	[12]
24.5	22	Unknown	11	NI	[38]
4	Unknown	200 RCF	10	NI	[39]
		400 RCF	10		
4	25	200 RCF	10	NI	[16]
		400 RCF	10		
8	25	Unknown	10	NI	[40]
		400 RCF	10		
40	24	400 RCF	20	5% Calcium chloride	[29]
		400 RCF	10		
3	Unknown	800 RCF	8	NI	[41]
		3000 RCF	15		

RPM, rotation per minute; RCF, relative centrifugal force; NI, Not included

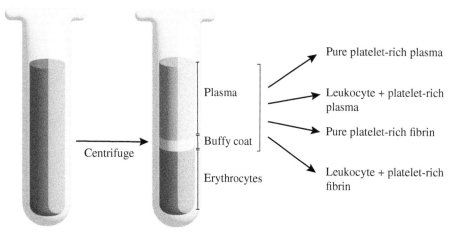

Figure 15.1 General methodology for the preparation of platelet rich plasma (PRP) formulations.

group [38] (Table 15.2). Discrepancies in these results could be attributed to variations in the PRP preparation and techniques, including number of spins, application of PRP activation procedures such as calcium chloride or bovine thrombin, dosage, and route of administration [46].

Platelet Concentration

One of the major drawbacks of using autologous PRP is that the final product of the composition of platelets can be highly variable among patients. While it is suggested that PRP should contain at least a three to fivefold increase in platelet concentration in order to ensure a therapeutic effect [47], a sixfold increase in final platelet count compared to the patient's

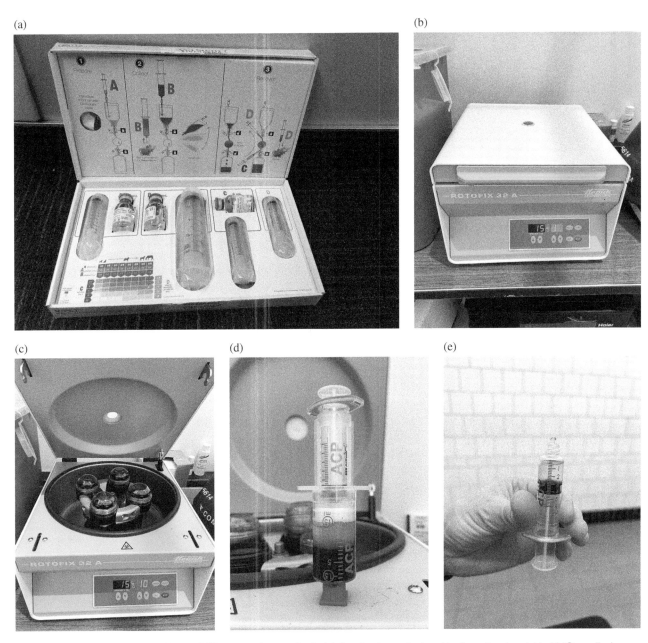

(a)

(b)

(c)

(d)

(e)

Figure 15.2 Photographs of different PRP preparation methods. (a) Gravity-dependent method previously sold by VetStem. (b,c) Arthrex the centrifugation unit for ACP separation. *Source:* Photographs courtesy of Nicole Buote, DVM, DACVS. (d) Arthrex double syringe post centrifugation of blood with separate platelet concentrate sitting above red blood cell concentrate. (e) Syringe of platelet concentrate. Courtesy of Allison Miller, DVM, CVA, CCRP-Regenerative Medicine Center and Tissue Culture Laboratory Cornell College of Veterinary Medicine. (f, g) Injection of PRP into a tendon via ultrasound guidance. *Source:* Courtesy of Nicole Buote DVM, DACVS.

(f)

(g)

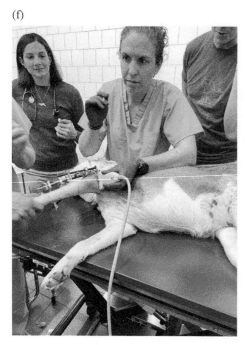
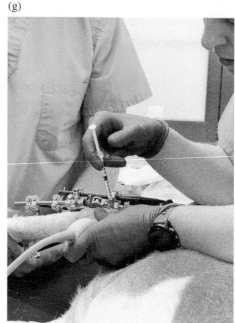

Figure 15.2   (Continued)

baseline platelet count showed more consistent and histologically apparent beneficial effects in humans [48]. In contrast, higher concentrations of platelets could result in decreased angiogenic potential, which could negatively affect healing [49]. Further studies are thus required to establish the ideal concentration of platelets required to generate positive effect during healing.

Dosage

Studies have shown that a single application of PRP does not always lead to improvement in the healing process [35–37] (Table 15.2). Based on the biological half-life of platelets being ten days, the application of two or more PRP doses, given at a 10-day interval based on the half-life of platelets, was found to have a superior improvement in healing [8, 23, 50, 51] (Table 15.2).

Similarly, using an increased volume of topical PRP based on the size of the lesion suggests a positive effect on healing [23]. In rabbits, higher volumes but with the same PRP concentration (i.e., 0.6 and 0.9 ml) exhibited a higher reepithelialization rate compared to the 0.3 ml PRP dose and no treatment controls [24] (Table 15.2). The reduction in the amount of growth factors released when using a smaller volume, combined with an incomplete coverage of the entire wound area, could explain the differences in healing.

Administration Routes

The administration route might also influence the efficacy of PRP treatment. Topical PRP gels, typically made by adding calcium gluconate or calcium chloride at various ratios depending on the study, were found to stimulate the production of excessive inflammatory exudates that provide a moist wound environment which may negatively impact wound contraction [52]. Intralesional injections of PRP (Figure 15.3) might be more efficient, as they provide selective distribution in target regions of the wound that require more aid in healing and allow for regular dressing changes to be performed without loss of PRP from the wound [38]. A study in humans that directly compared the efficacy on wound healing of a PRP gel versus a PRP injection showed no major differences in efficacy [53]. The PRP gel was prepared by adding 0.1 ml of calcium chloride to 1 ml of PRP and was left in a petri dish until a gel was formed and then applied to the wounds. In parallel, two-thirds of 1 ml of PRP with 0.1 ml of calcium chloride was injected into the perilesional site and the remaining one-third into the wound bed. Despite seeing no difference, the authors still proposed that the increased penetration of PRP via injection might be beneficial for the treatment of chronic ulcers [53].

Figure 15.3 Photographs of PRP-treated wounds. (a) Linear wound on the palmar surface of the thoracic limb seven days after wounding on a hike. 2 ml of PRP was injected in 0.2 ml aliquots around the periphery of the wound. (b) The same wound at next bandage change (5 days after PRP injection), significant contraction has occurred. *Source:* Courtesy of Nicole Buote DVM, DACVS.

(a) 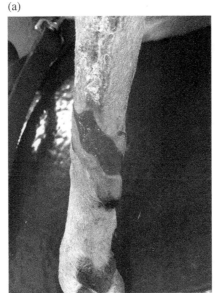 (b)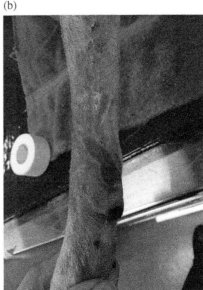

Xenogenic PRP

Since a large volume of blood is required for the preparation of PRP, it can be challenging to obtain enough blood to generate autologous PRP from small companion animals. Similarly, the hematologic status of the patient can affect the final preparation of PRP, which can prevent it from being used in those patients [54]. In these cases, heterologous PRP can be used as it has been shown to behave similarly to autologous PRP to promote skin healing, [16, 25, 29] (Tables 15.1 and 15.2). No signs of infection or higher leukocyte concentration have been found in heterologous PRP-treated wounds in small companion animals, which could be associated with the increased antimicrobial activity by the PRP [29, 39] (Table 15.2). However, concerns have been raised of the increased, but not statistically significant, recruitment of neutrophils in the wound when compared to autologous PRP in rabbits [16]. Neutrophil depletion studies in mice suggest that increased numbers of neutrophils in the wound may contribute to slower healing [55, 56]. However, since no significant impact on the healing process was observed between autologous and heterologous PRP treatments in a wound healing study in rabbits [16]. Heterologous PRP appears to be a safe option in circumstances where a patient's blood cannot be used.

Conclusions

Both clinical and experimental *in vivo* studies with PRP have provided encouraging results for cutaneous wounds. The powerful regenerative capabilities of growth factors in PRP may have synergistic and composite action on wound healing. However, further studies are needed to elucidate the exact underlying mechanisms. PRP therapy is well tolerated, rarely leads to complications, and is easy to prepare and administer. Despite the widespread and frequent usage of PRP, the therapy still warrants standardization to ensure direct comparison between studies and demonstrate reproducibility. There is also a lack of information on long-term outcomes of cutaneous wound healing after PRP treatment. Finally, additional well-controlled clinical studies in small companion animals including more variables in a larger cohort are required to confirm and further improve the clinical efficacy of PRP products.

Stem Cell Therapy

Physiology

Stem cells are undifferentiated cells that can self-renew to maintain the stem cell pool and can differentiate into mature cell types. They are classified based on potency as follows: (i) totipotent stem cells in the zygote, which can differentiate into all cell types; (ii) pluripotent embryonic stem cells (ESCs) and induced pluripotent stem cells (iPSCs), which can develop into

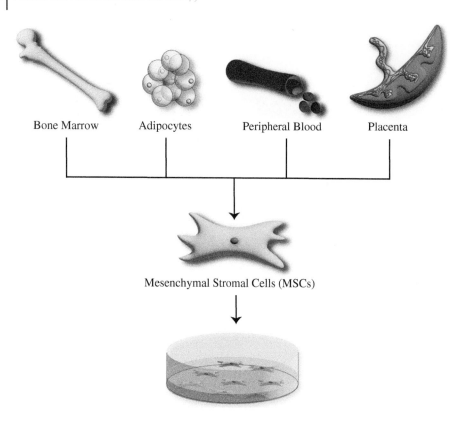

Figure 15.4 Overview of the isolation and culture of mesenchymal stromal cells (MSCs).

Bone Marrow   Adipocytes   Peripheral Blood   Placenta

Mesenchymal Stromal Cells (MSCs)

all cells except placental cells; and (iii) multipotent, tissue-specific, adult stem cells, which can produce limited sets of cells characteristic of a certain tissue [57]. Tissue-specific adult stem cells, more specifically mesenchymal stromal cells (MSCs), have thus far been the most explored as a therapy for small companion animal wound management. MSCs can be isolated from many tissues including, but not limited to, bone marrow, adipose tissue, peripheral blood, and placental tissues (Figure 15.4). They have been isolated from many species and can be readily expanded in culture. Another cell source for therapeutic use is the stromal vascular fraction (SVF) which is isolated from adipose tissue. SVF consists of a heterogeneous population of cells including MSCs, endothelial precursors and mature endothelial cells, immune cells, smooth muscle cells pericytes, and pre-adipocytes. Proposed benefits of SVF cells over MSCs are based on the facts that (i) the diversity of cell types comprising the SVF secrete a wider range of regenerative factors than MSCs and (ii) SVF is generally administered immediately after isolation, and not maintained in culture like MSCs [58]. SVF cells have been studied in the context of wound healing in humans [59, 60], whereas the therapeutic benefits of SVF in small companion animals have primarily been examined in the context of orthopedic diseases [61–63].

There is evidence that cultured MSCs delivered as therapy can migrate through blood vessels, homing to damaged tissues through injury/inflammation/hypoxia signals [64, 65] (Figure 15.5).

MSCs interact with target cells and tissues via direct cell–cell contact and paracrine signaling, including the secretion of soluble factors and the release of extracellular vesicles [66–68] (Figure 15.6a). The most studied therapeutic outcomes of the application of MSCs and MSC-secreted factors are the regulatory effects they have on immune cells (Figure 15.6b) and the reparative effects on dysregulated cells and tissues. In companion animal medicine, MSCs and MSC products have been tested *in vivo* as treatments for musculoskeletal, cardiovascular, neurologic, renal, and gastrointestinal diseases, as well as neoplasia [69–73], and more recently, they have been used to treat skin wounds, primarily in dogs.

Description of Technique

MSCs can be successfully isolated from various sources of small companion animals [74–79] (Figure 15.4). The regions of adipose tissue harvested for MSC isolation from small companion animals have traditionally been caudal the scapula, inguinal fat pad, or falciform [80]. However, since tissue yields from these locations may be low and post-operative

Figure 15.5 Overview of the molecular mechanisms facilitating each step of MSC homing. (a) MSCs express CD44 receptors that "catches" onto the selectins expressed by endothelial cells, (b) resulting in rolling of MSCs along the vascular wall. (c) MSCs secrete matrix metalloproteinases (MMPs) and tissue inhibitors of metalloproteinases (TIMPs) that break down the basement membrane and enable transmigration of MSCs through the endothelial cell layer. (d) Chemotactic signals in response to the tissue damage triggers the MSCs to migrate toward the inflamed site.

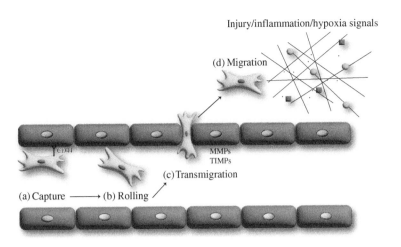

Figure 15.6 MSC mechanism of action and immunomodulatory capabilities. (a). MSCs exert their functions on their target cells by cell-to-cell contact and secretion of paracrine factors. (b). MSCs dynamically express different receptors affecting the pro- or anti- inflammatory properties of immune cells according to the microenvironment. MSCs can block the differentiation and maturation of dendritic cells (DCs) and are strong inhibitors of natural killer (NK) cell proliferation and toxicity. MSCs can suppress both T- and B-lymphocyte proliferation and polarize the cells toward an immunosuppressive phenotype. MSCs dampen pro-inflammatory M1 macrophages and promote the induction of an anti-inflammatory M2 phenotype.

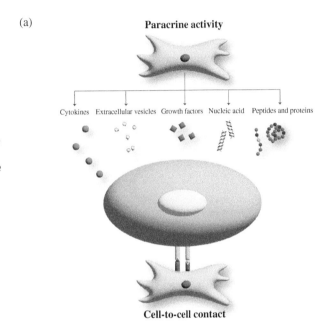

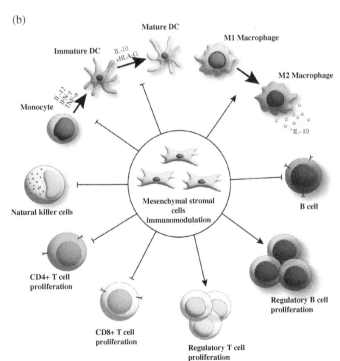

complications are common, a recent study explored a laparoscopic collection of canine adipose tissue for MSC isolation using a bipolar sealing device [81]. The authors demonstrated that the technique is feasible, productive, and not associated with any complications. In dogs, bone marrow for MSC collection is generally obtained from the humerus [82] and placental MSCs are derived from term placentas [83, 84]. In contrast to horses, peripheral blood as a source for MSCs is not well-described for small companion animals.

For MSC isolation, irrespective of the tissue source, initial cells are seeded in flasks with primary MSC culture media [85, 86]. Non-adherent cells are removed by regularly changing the media, while the adherent cells that remain are mostly spindle-shaped, fibroblast-like cells that form discrete, dense colonies. MSCs typically proliferate rapidly and can be expanded to obtain high numbers of cells (Figures 15.7 and 15.8).

indications

Acute and Chronic Wounds

In one of the few clinical studies with control groups, 24 dogs of various breeds ranging 1–10 years of age with acute or chronic wounds were treated with one or two doses (depending on wound area) of 3×10^7 allogeneic adipose-derived MSCs that were injected intradermally around the wound perimeter [87]. Animals were divided into four groups: (i) six dogs with acute wounds received conventional treatment, (ii) 10 dogs with acute wounds were treated with MSCs, (iii) four dogs suffering from chronic wounds were treated conventionally, and (iv) four dogs with chronic wounds received MSCs. The regenerative area in patients with acute and chronic wounds treated with MSCs was significantly greater than in patients in the control groups at each study time point, strongly suggesting that MSC therapy has beneficial effects on the healing of acute and chronic wounds. Although acute wounds appeared to respond to treatment more quickly than chronic wounds, all MSC-treated wounds were nearly closed by day 90. In addition to measuring wound closure, a panel of serum cytokines were evaluated to determine safety, and the only difference between control and treatment groups was an increase in IL-8 in the serum of MSC-treated dogs. Because the increased values of IL-8 fell within the median range of IL-8 levels in healthy dogs, it was concluded that MSC therapy is clinically safe based on the absence of a negative systemic inflammatory immune response. Wound biopsies were collected for analysis of *GM-CSF, VEGF-A, MMP-2,* and *IL-10,* genes relevant to wound healing, and elevated *GM-CSF* expression levels in biopsy tissues from MSC-treated wounds led the authors to speculate that MSCs do not only act directly to improve wound healing, but also induce resident cells to secrete secondary factors involved in wound healing.

Experimentally-Induced Full-Thickness Skin Wounds

In a well-controlled *in vivo* study, treatment with canine allogeneic adipose-derived MSCs was compared to treatment with canine allogeneic adipose-derived MSCs overexpressing platelet-derived growth factor (PDGF), a protein regulating wound healing processes [88, 89]. Six $1.5\,cm^2$ wounds/animal were created on the back of twelve 2–3-year old beagles, with each wound receiving a different treatment: (i) MSCs, (ii) PDGF-MSCs, (iii) cell sheets comprised of MSCs, (iv) cell sheets comprised of PDGF-MSCs, (v) PBS (vehicle control), and (vi) no treatment (control). At day 10 post-wounding, all treated wounds exhibited significantly more epithelialization, contraction, and total wound healing, compared to the control wounds that received PBS or no treatment. Treated wounds also had more total granulation tissue, higher histological scores, greater vascular density, more abundant and well-organized collagen, thicker epidermal layers, and more cells positive for the proliferation marker Ki67. When comparing the four different treatments, MSCs overexpressing PDGF, both in cell sheets or as individual cells, were more effective when compared to regular MSCs.

Xenotransplantation of MSCs

MSCs are typically considered to be non-immunogenic due to low expression levels of MHCII [64, 65]. This allows not only for the use of allogeneic MSCs from the same species, but also for xenotransplantation of MSCs from a different species. A clinical report described the use of human MSCs isolated from Wharton's jelly to treat non-healing large skin lesions in two dogs [90]. MSCs were applied in conjunction with a polyvinyl alcohol hydrogel (PVA) membrane, to prevent wound dehydration, at a concentration of 1×10^5 cells/cm² wound area. Wounds on both animals demonstrated skin repair with little ulceration. Although no controls were included in this report, the authors concluded that Wharton's jelly MSCs associated with a PVA membrane showed promising results. A second study in dogs with surgically created wounds and a novel Wharton's jelly matrix reported earlier epithelialization in treated dogs compared to control wounds (Figure 15.9) [91]. A larger laboratory study with controls evaluated the therapeutic potential of 1×10^6 canine bone marrow-derived MSCs

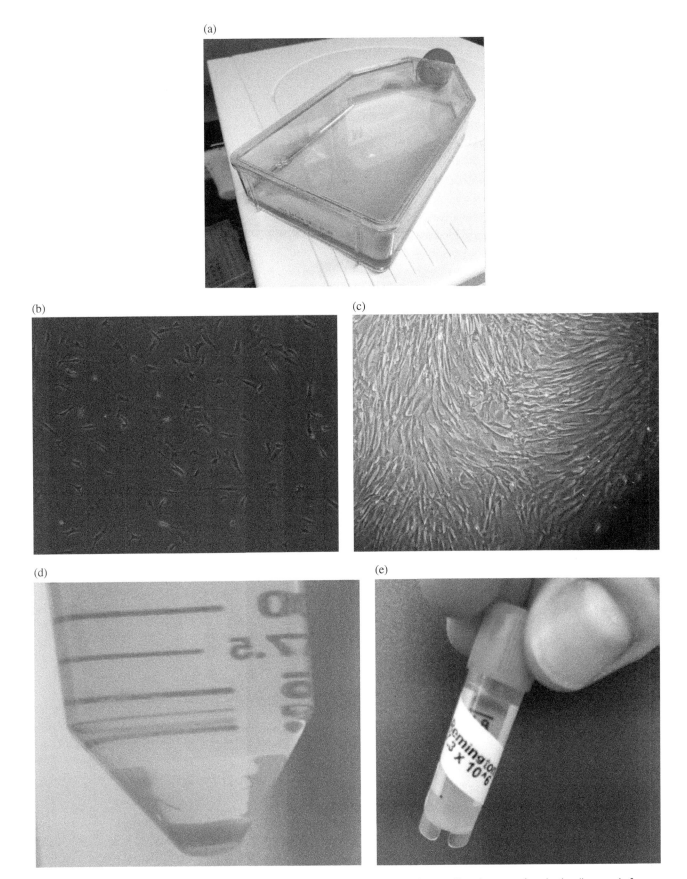

Figure 15.7 (a) Canine mesenchymal stem cells in cell culture; (b) Canine mesenchymal stem cells – demonstrating plastic adherence before reaching confluence; (c) Canine mesenchymal stem cells – demonstrating confluence for passage; (d) Tripsinized, washed, and centrifuged canine mesenchymal stem cell pellet; (e) Canine mesenchymal stem cells resuspended in autologous serum for therapeutic delivery. *Source:* Courtesy of Christopher Frye DVM, DACVSMR-Regenerative Medicine Center and Tissue Culture Laboratory Cornell College of Veterinary Medicine.

(a)   (b)

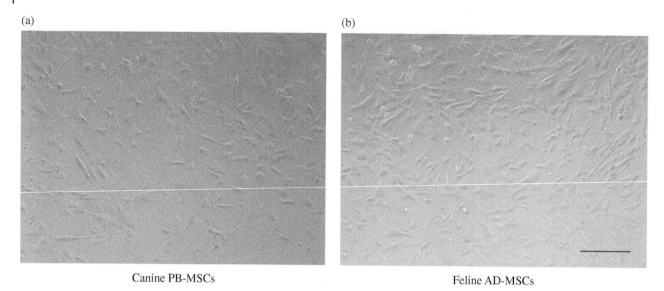

Canine PB-MSCs   Feline AD-MSCs

Figure 15.8 Peripheral blood-derived MSCs from dogs (a) and adipose-derived MSCs from cats (b). Scale bar represents 200 μm.

embedded in a mesh scaffold in experimentally-induced 2 cm^2 full-thickness skin wounds in guinea pigs [92]. Treatments included (i) systemic antibiotic and inflammatory drugs only, (ii) PVA mesh only, (iii) fresh MSCs only, (iv) PVA mesh with fresh MSCs, and (v) PVA mesh with cryopreserved MSCs. The meshes were removed from the wounds 48 hours after wound creation/treatment. Fourteen days post-wounding, MSC-treated wounds not only showed more contraction and closed faster, but also exhibited better histological scores for epithelialization, neovascularization, collagen density, and collagen thickness, when compared to control wounds that received PVA mesh or antibiotics/inflammatory drugs only. The authors concluded that canine bone marrow-derived MSCs induce quality wound healing, that meshes can be used to deliver MSCs, and that cryopreserved MSCs are as effective as fresh.

Conclusions

Based on currently published case reports and experimental studies, stem cell therapy for companion animal skin wounds is promising. Specifically, MSC application and injection in dogs appear safe and may be effective. More well-controlled studies in dogs and other small companion animals need to be conducted to define the benefits of MSC therapy, determine what types of skin wounds respond best to MSCs, and refine treatment protocols.

Combinational Therapy Using PRP and Stem Cell Therapy

A combined PRP and stem cell therapy has been shown to have an added advantage. PRP offers a suitable microenvironment for MSCs to promote proliferation and differentiation. A case report described the use of autologous adipose-derived MSCs in combination with PRP to treat a large skin wound on a one-year-old Labrador, after the dog was struck by a train [93]. PRP was applied by dripping or spraying over the wound surface every 48–72 hours, as well as by injection along the wound edge every 4–6 days, for 56 days. In addition, MSCs were applied topically by spraying the cells over the wound surface on days 11, 17, 23, 31, and 41 for a total of five treatments. Granulation tissue was visible four days after the first PRP application and the wound was fully closed after three months. The wound did not show any signs of infection or necrosis following PRP/MSC therapy, and it was concluded that PRP and MSCs are an effective option to manage large wounds with substantial soft tissue removed. Studies using mouse wound models support that PRP can be used as an adjuvant to boost the wound healing efficacy of MSC by improving their proangiogenic potential [94]. Similarly, PRP was found to enhance the survival and repair potential of MSCs following their administration into acute wounds in pigs [95] and rat diabetic wound models [96, 97]. However, whether the therapeutic effect of combined treatment of PRP and MSCs results from the sum of separate effects of the two biological compounds or rather from a synergistic action has not yet been formally addressed.

(a)

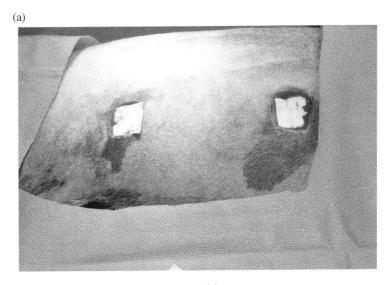

(b)   (c)

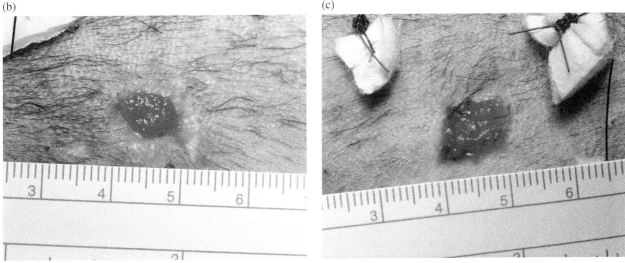

Figure 15.9 (a) Photograph of a Wharton's jelly novel matrix in place in surgically created wounds in a dog. (b,c) Photographs of wounds at day 14 after treatment with novel Wharton's jelly matrix (b) or control treatment (c) of hydrogel and non-adherent dressing. Marked difference in epithelialization from the edges is visible. *Source:* Courtesy of Nicole Buote DVM, DACVS.

References

1 Marx, R.E. (2001). Platelet-rich plasma (PRP): what is PRP and what is not PRP? *Implant Dent.* 10 (4): 225–228.
2 Alves, J.C., Santos, A., and Jorge, P. (2021). Platelet-rich plasma therapy in dogs with bilateral hip osteoarthritis. *BMC Vet. Res.* 17 (1): 207.
3 Lee, S., Cheong, J., and Lee, J.-M. (2018). Clinical application of autologous platelet-rich plasma (PRP) on delayed wound healing of a dog with burns. *J. Vet. Clin.* 35 (5): 229–232.
4 Farghali, H.A., AbdElKader, N.A., AbuBakr, H.O. et al. (2021). Corneal ulcer in dogs and cats: novel clinical application of regenerative therapy using subconjunctival injection of autologous platelet-rich plasma. *Front. Vet. Sci.* 8: 641265.
5 Diamond, J.C., Schick, R.O., Savage, M.Y., and Fadok, V.A. (2020). A small scale study to evaluate the efficacy of microneedling in the presence or absence of platelet-rich plasma in the treatment of post-clipping alopecia in dogs. *Vet. Dermatol.* 31 (3): 214. -e45.
6 Kim, J.H., Park, C., and Park, H.M. (2009). Curative effect of autologous platelet-rich plasma on a large cutaneous lesion in a dog. *Vet. Dermatol.* 20 (2): 123–126.

7 Chung, T.H., Baek, D.S., Kim, N. et al. (2015). Topical allogeneic platelet-rich plasma treatment for a massive cutaneous lesion induced by disseminated intravascular coagulation in a toy breed dog. *Ir. Vet. J.* 68 (1): 4.

8 Aminkov, K., Aminkov, B., Zlateva-Panayotova, N., and Botev, C. (2016). Application of platelet-rich plasma (PRP) in treating of a complicated postoperative wound in cat: a clinical case. *Tradition Modern. Vet. Med.* 1: 33–37.

9 Xue, M. and Jackson, C.J. (2008). Autocrine actions of matrix metalloproteinase (MMP)-2 counter the effects of MMP-9 to promote survival and prevent terminal differentiation of cultured human keratinocytes. *J. Invest. Dermatol.* 128 (11): 2676–2685.

10 Catarino, J., Carvalho, P., Santos, S. et al. (2020). Treatment of canine osteoarthritis with allogeneic platelet-rich plasma: review of five cases. *Open Vet. J.* 10 (2): 226–231.

11 Descalzi, F., Ulivi, V., Cancedda, R. et al. (2013). Platelet-rich plasma exerts antinociceptive activity by a peripheral endocannabinoid-related mechanism. *Tissue Eng. Part A* 19 (19–20): 2120–2129.

12 Molina-Minano, F., Lopez-Jornet, P., Camacho-Alonso, F., and Vicente-Ortega, V. (2009). The use of plasma rich in growth factors on wound healing in the skin: experimental study in rabbits. *Int. Wound J.* 6 (2): 145–148.

13 Chun, N., Canapp, S., Carr, B.J. et al. (2020). Validation and characterization of platelet-rich plasma in the feline: a prospective analysis. *Front. Vet. Sci.* 7: 512.

14 Farghali, H.A., AbdElKader, N.A., Khattab, M.S., and AbuBakr, H.O. (2017). Evaluation of subcutaneous infiltration of autologous platelet-rich plasma on skin-wound healing in dogs. *Biosci. Rep.* 37 (2): BSR20160503.

15 Bohling, M.W., Henderson, R.A., Swaim, S.F. et al. (2004). Cutaneous wound healing in the cat: a macroscopic description and comparison with cutaneous wound healing in the dog. *Vet. Surg.* 33 (6): 579–587.

16 Barrionuevo, D.V., Laposy, C.B., Abegao, K.G. et al. (2015). Comparison of experimentally-induced wounds in rabbits treated with different sources of platelet-rich plasma. *Lab. Anim.* 49 (3): 209–214.

17 Hussein, S.M. (2018). Effects of autologous platelet-rich plasma on skin healing in dogs. *Iraqi J. Vet. Sci.* 32: 275–283.

18 Mazzocca, A.D., McCarthy, M.B., Chowaniec, D.M. et al. (2012). Platelet-rich plasma differs according to preparation method and human variability. *J. Bone Joint Surg. Am.* 94 (4): 308–316.

19 Dohan Ehrenfest, D.M., Rasmusson, L., and Albrektsson, T. (2009). Classification of platelet concentrates: from pure platelet-rich plasma (P-PRP) to leucocyte- and platelet-rich fibrin (L-PRF). *Trends Biotechnol.* 27 (3): 158–167.

20 Carter, M.J., Fylling, C.P., and Parnell, L.K. (2011). Use of platelet rich plasma gel on wound healing: a systematic review and meta-analysis. *Eplasty* 11: e38.

21 Jee, C.H., Eom, N.Y., Jang, H.M. et al. (2016). Effect of autologous platelet-rich plasma application on cutaneous wound healing in dogs. *J. Vet. Sci.* 17 (1): 79–87.

22 Lai, C.Y., Li, T.Y., Lam, K.H.S. et al. (2022). The long-term analgesic effectiveness of platelet-rich plasma injection for carpal tunnel syndrome: a cross-sectional cohort study. *Pain Med.* 23 (7): 1249–1258.

23 Iacopetti, I., Patruno, M., Melotti, L. et al. (2020). Autologous platelet-rich plasma enhances the healing of large cutaneous wounds in dogs. *Front. Vet. Sci.* 7: 575449.

24 Lee, H.W., Reddy, M.S., Geurs, N. et al. (2008). Efficacy of platelet-rich plasma on wound healing in rabbits. *J. Periodontol.* 79 (4): 691–696.

25 Gemignani, F., Perazzi, A., and Iacopetti, I. (2017). Use of canine sourced platelet-rich plasma in a feline contaminated cutaneous wound. *Can. Vet. J.* 58 (2): 141–144.

26 Alishahi, M.K., Kazemi, D., Mohajeri, D. et al. (2013). Histopathological evaluation of the effect of platelet-rich fibrin on canine cutaneous incisional wound healing. *Iran. J. Vet. Sci. Technol.* 5 (2): 19–32.

27 Yamakawa, S. and Hayashida, K. (2019). Advances in surgical applications of growth factors for wound healing. *Burns Trauma* 7: 10.

28 Reiss, M.J., Han, Y.P., Garcia, E. et al. (2010). Matrix metalloproteinase-9 delays wound healing in a murine wound model. *Surgery* 147 (2): 295–302.

29 Rezende, R.S., Eurides, D., Alves, E.G.L. et al. (2020). Co-treatment of wounds in rabbit skin with equine platelet-rich plasma and a commercial ointment accelerates healing. *Med. Vet.* 21: e-56274.

30 Kakudo, N., Morimoto, N., Kushida, S. et al. (2014). Platelet-rich plasma releasate promotes angiogenesis in vitro and in vivo. *Med. Mol. Morphol.* 47 (2): 83–89.

31 Yang, R., Liu, F., Wang, J. et al. (2019). Epidermal stem cells in wound healing and their clinical applications. *Stem Cell Res. Ther.* 10 (1): 229.

32 Xu, P., Wu, Y., Zhou, L. et al. (2020). Platelet-rich plasma accelerates skin wound healing by promoting re-epithelialization. *Burns Trauma* 8: tkaa028.

33 Bechert, K. and Abraham, S.E. (2009). Pain management and wound care. *J. Am. Col. Certif. Wound Spec.* 1 (2): 65–71.

34 Gardner, M.J., Demetrakopoulos, D., Klepchick, P.R., and Mooar, P.A. (2007). The efficacy of autologous platelet gel in pain control and blood loss in total knee arthroplasty. An analysis of the haemoglobin, narcotic requirement and range of motion. *Int. Orthop.* 31 (3): 309–313.

35 Kazemi Mehrjerdi, H., Sardari, K., Emami, M.R. et al. (2008). Efficacy of autologous platelet-rich plasma (PRP) activated by thromboplastin-D on the repair and regeneration of wounds in dogs. *Iran J. Vet. Surg.* 3 (4): 19–30.

36 Sardari, K., Reza Emami, M., Kazemi, H. et al. (2011). Effects of platelet-rich plasma (PRP) on cutaneous regeneration and wound healing in dogs treated with dexamethasone. *Compar. Clin. Path* 20 (2): 155–162.

37 Karayannopoulou, M., Psalla, D., Kazakos, G. et al. (2015). Effect of locally injected autologous platelet-rich plasma on second intention wound healing of acute full-thickness skin defects in dogs. *Vet. Comp. Orthop. Traumatol.* 28 (3): 172–178.

38 Dionyssiou, D., Demiri, E., Foroglou, P. et al. (2013). The effectiveness of intralesional injection of platelet-rich plasma in accelerating the healing of chronic ulcers: an experimental and clinical study. *Int. Wound J.* 10 (4): 397–406.

39 Abegao, K.G., Bracale, B.N., Delfim, I.G. et al. (2015). Effects of heterologous platelet-rich plasma gel on standardized dermal wound healing in rabbits. *Acta Cir. Bras.* 30 (3): 209–215.

40 Tetila, A.F., Breda, M.R.S., Nogueira, R.M.B. et al. (2019). The use of platelet-rich plasma and rosuvastatin in wound healing in rabbits: a longitudinal study. *Adv. Skin Wound Care* 32 (9): 1–5.

41 Meira, R.O., Braga, D.N.M., Pinheiro, L.S.G. et al. (2020). Effects of homologous and heterologous rich platelets plasma, compared to poor platelets plasma, on cutaneous healing of rabbits. *Acta Cir. Bras.* 35 (10): e202001006.

42 Lansdown, D.A. and Fortier, L.A. (2017). Platelet-rich plasma: formulations, preparations, constituents, and their effects. *Oper. Tech. Sports Med.* 25 (1): 7–12.

43 Carr, B.J., Canapp, S.O. Jr., Mason, D.R. et al. (2015). Canine platelet-rich plasma systems: a prospective analysis. *Front. Vet. Sci.* 2: 73.

44 Franklin, S.P., Garner, B.C., and Cook, J.L. (2015). Characteristics of canine platelet-rich plasma prepared with five commercially available systems. *Am. J. Vet. Res.* 76 (9): 822–827.

45 Arnoczky, S.P. and Shebani-Rad, S. (2013). The basic science of platelet-rich plasma (PRP): what clinicians need to know. *Sports Med. Arthrosc. Rev.* 21 (4): 180–185.

46 Tambella, A.M., Attili, A.R., Dupre, G. et al. (2018). Platelet-rich plasma to treat experimentally-induced skin wounds in animals: a systematic review and meta-analysis. *PLoS One* 13 (1): e0191093.

47 Monteiro, S.O., Lepage, O.M., and Theoret, C.L. (2009). Effects of platelet-rich plasma on the repair of wounds on the distal aspect of the forelimb in horses. *Am. J. Vet. Res.* 70 (2): 277–282.

48 Hom, D.B., Linzie, B.M., and Huang, T.C. (2007). The healing effects of autologous platelet gel on acute human skin wounds. *Arch. Facial Plast. Surg.* 9 (3): 174–183.

49 Giusti, I., Rughetti, A., D'Ascenzo, S. et al. (2009). Identification of an optimal concentration of platelet gel for promoting angiogenesis in human endothelial cells. *Transfusion* 49 (4): 771–778.

50 Yurtbay, A., Say, F., Cinka, H., and Ersoy, A. (2021). Multiple platelet-rich plasma injections are superior to single PRP injections or saline in osteoarthritis of the knee: the 2-year results of a randomized, double-blind, placebo-controlled clinical trial. *Arch. Orthop. Trauma Surg.* 142 (10): 2755–2768.

51 Tavassoli, M., Janmohammadi, N., Hosseini, A. et al. (2019). Single- and double-dose of platelet-rich plasma versus hyaluronic acid for treatment of knee osteoarthritis: a randomized controlled trial. *World J. Orthop.* 10 (9): 310–326.

52 Choate, C.S. (1994). Wound dressings. A comparison of classes and their principles of use. *J. Am. Podiatr. Med. Assoc.* 84 (9): 463–469.

53 Elgarhy, L.H., El-Ashmawy, A.A., Bedeer, A.E., and Al-Bahnasy, A.M. (2020). Evaluation of safety and efficacy of autologous topical platelet gel vs platelet rich plasma injection in the treatment of venous leg ulcers: a randomized case control study. *Dermatol. Ther.* 33 (6): e13897.

54 Jain, N.K. and Gulati, M. (2016). Platelet-rich plasma: a healing virtuoso. *Blood Res.* 51 (1): 3–5.

55 Zhu, S., Yu, Y., Ren, Y. et al. (2021). The emerging roles of neutrophil extracellular traps in wound healing. *Cell Death Dis.* 12 (11): 984.

56 Dovi, J.V., He, L.K., and DiPietro, L.A. (2003). Accelerated wound closure in neutrophil-depleted mice. *J. Leukocyte Biol.* 73 (4): 448–455.

57 Harman, R.M., Theoret, C.L., and Van de Walle, G.R. (2019). The horse as a model for the study of cutaneous wound healing. *Adv. Wound Care* 10 (7): 381–399.

58 Bora, P. and Majumdar, A.S. (2017). Adipose tissue-derived stromal vascular fraction in regenerative medicine: a brief review on biology and translation. *Stem Cell Res. Ther.* 8 (1): 145.

59 Zhao, X.S., Guo, J.M., Zhang, F.F. et al. (2020). Therapeutic application of adipose-derived stromal vascular fraction in diabetic foot. *Stem Cell Res. Ther.* 11 (1): 1–8.

60 Bi, H.S., Li, H., Zhang, C. et al. (2019). Stromal vascular fraction promotes migration of fibroblasts and angiogenesis through regulation of extracellular matrix in the skin wound healing process. *Stem Cell Res. Ther.* 10 (1): 1–21.

61 Upchurch, D.A., Renberg, W.C., Roush, J.K. et al. (2016). Effects of administration of adipose-derived stromal vascular fraction and platelet-rich plasma to dogs with osteoarthritis of the hip joints. *Am. J. Vet. Res.* 77 (9): 940–951.

62 Kemilew, J., Sobczyska-Rak, A., Zyliska, B. et al. (2019). The use of allogenic stromal vascular fraction (SVF) cells in degenerative joint disease of the spine in dogs. *In Vivo* 33 (4): 1109–1117.

63 Franklin, S.P., Stoker, A.M., Bozynski, C.C. et al. (2018). Comparison of platelet-rich plasma, stromal vascular fraction (SVF), or SVF with an injectable PLGA nanofiber scaffold for the treatment of osteochondral injury in dogs. *J. Knee Surg.* 31 (7): 686–697.

64 Naji, A., Eitoku, M., Favier, B. et al. (2019). Biological functions of mesenchymal stem cells and clinical implications. *Cell. Mol. Life Sci.* 76 (17): 3323–3348.

65 Markov, A., Thangavelu, L., Aravindhan, S. et al. (2021). Mesenchymal stem/stromal cells as a valuable source for the treatment of immune-mediated disorders. *Stem Cell Res. Ther.* 12 (1): 192.

66 Elahi, F.M., Farwell, D.G., Nolta, J.A., and Anderson, J.D. (2020). Preclinical translation of exosomes derived from mesenchymal stem/stromal cells. *Stem Cells* 38 (1): 15–21.

67 de Windt, T.S., Saris, D.B.F., Slaper-Cortenbach, I.C.M. et al. (2015). Direct cell–cell contact with chondrocytes is a key mechanism in multipotent mesenchymal stromal cell-mediated chondrogenesis. *Tissue Eng. Part A* 21 (19–20): 2536–2547.

68 Bogatcheva, N.V. and Coleman, M.E. (2019). Conditioned medium of mesenchymal stromal cells: a new class of therapeutics. *Biochemistry* 84 (11): 1375–1389.

69 Thomson, A.L., Berent, A.C., Weisse, C., and Langston, C.E. (2019). Intra-arterial renal infusion of autologous mesenchymal stem cells for treatment of chronic kidney disease in cats: phase I clinical trial. *J. Vet. Intern. Med.* 33 (3): 1353–1361.

70 Webb, T.L. (2020). Stem cell therapy and cats: what do we know at this time. *Vet. Clin. N. Am. Small Anim. Pract.* 50 (5): 955–971.

71 Kang, M.H. and Park, H.M. (2020). Challenges of stem cell therapies in companion animal practice. *J. Vet. Sci.* 21 (3): e42.

72 Gugjoo, M.B., Fazili, M.R., Gayas, M.A. et al. (2019). Animal mesenchymal stem cell research in cartilage regenerative medicine - a review. *Vet. Q.* 39 (1): 95–120.

73 Ganiev, I., Alexandrova, N., Aimaletdinov, A. et al. (2021). The treatment of articular cartilage injuries with mesenchymal stem cells in different animal species. *Open Vet. J.* 11 (1): 128–134.

74 Zhang, W., Zhang, F., Shi, H. et al. (2014). Comparisons of rabbit bone marrow mesenchymal stem cell isolation and culture methods in vitro. *PLoS One* 9 (2): e88794.

75 Sato, K., Yamawaki-Ogata, A., Kanemoto, I. et al. (2016). Isolation and characterisation of peripheral blood-derived feline mesenchymal stem cells. *Vet. J.* 216: 183–188.

76 Rashid, U., Yousaf, A., Yaqoob, M. et al. (2021). Characterization and differentiation potential of mesenchymal stem cells isolated from multiple canine adipose tissue sources. *BMC Vet. Res.* 17 (1): 388.

77 Park, S.G., An, J.H., Li, Q. et al. (2021). Feline adipose tissue-derived mesenchymal stem cells pretreated with IFN-gamma enhance immunomodulatory effects through the PGE(2) pathway. *J. Vet. Sci.* 22 (2): e16.

78 Munoz, J.L., Greco, S.J., Patel, S.A. et al. (2012). Feline bone marrow-derived mesenchymal stromal cells (MSCs) show similar phenotype and functions with regards to neuronal differentiation as human MSCs. *Differentiation* 84 (2): 214–222.

79 Li, X., Lu, X., Sun, D. et al. (2016). Adipose-derived mesenchymal stem cells reduce lymphocytic infiltration in a rabbit model of induced autoimmune dacryoadenitis. *Invest. Ophthalmol. Visual Sci.* 57 (13): 5161–5170.

80 Black, L.L., Gaynor, J., Gahring, D. et al. (2007). Effect of adipose-derived mesenchymal stem and regenerative cells on lameness in dogs with chronic osteoarthritis of the coxofemoral joints: a randomized, double-blinded, multicenter, controlled trial. *Vet. Ther.* 8 (4): 272–284.

81 Buote, N.J. (2022). Laparoscopic adipose-derived stem cell harvest technique with bipolar sealing device: outcome in 12 dogs. *Vet. Med. Sci.* 8 (4): 1421–1428.

82 Benavides, F.P., Pinto, G.B.A., Heckler, M.C.T. et al. (2021). Intrathecal transplantation of autologous and allogeneic bone marrow-derived mesenchymal stem cells in dogs. *Cell Transplant.* 30: 09636897211034464.

83 Zhan, X.-S., El-Ashram, S., Luo, D.-Z. et al. (2019). A comparative study of biological characteristics and transcriptome profiles of mesenchymal stem cells from different canine tissues. *Int. J. Mol. Sci.* 20 (6): 1485.

84 Long, C., Lankford, L., Kumar, P. et al. (2018). Isolation and characterization of canine placenta-derived mesenchymal stromal cells for the treatment of neurological disorders in dogs. *Cytometry A* 93 (1): 82–92.

85 Soleimani, M. and Nadri, S. (2009). A protocol for isolation and culture of mesenchymal stem cells from mouse bone marrow. *Nat. Protoc.* 4 (1): 102–106.

86 Huang, S., Xu, L., Sun, Y. et al. (2015). An improved protocol for isolation and culture of mesenchymal stem cells from mouse bone marrow. *J. Orthop. Translat.* 3 (1): 26–33.

87 Enciso, N., Avedillo, L., Fermin, M.L. et al. (2020). Cutaneous wound healing: canine allogeneic ASC therapy. *Stem Cell Res. Ther.* 11 (1): 261.

88 Pierce, G.F., Mustoe, T.A., Altrock, B.W. et al. (1991). Role of platelet-derived growth factor in wound healing. *J. Cell. Biochem.* 45 (4): 319–326.

89 Kim, N., Choi, K.U., Lee, E. et al. (2020). Therapeutic effects of platelet derived growth factor overexpressed-mesenchymal stromal cells and sheets in canine skin wound healing model. *Histol. Histopathol.* 35 (7): 751–767.

90 Ribeiro, J., Pereira, T., Amorim, I. et al. (2014). Cell therapy with human MSCs isolated from the umbilical cord Wharton jelly associated to a PVA membrane in the treatment of chronic skin wounds. *Int. J. Med. Sci.* 11 (10): 979–987.

91 Kierski, K., Buote, N.J., Rishniw, M. et al. (2023). Novel extracellular matrix wound dressing shows increased epithelialization of full thickness skin wounds in dogs. *Am. J. Vet. Res.* 84: https://doi.org/10.2460/ajvr.23.05.0105.

92 Bharti, M.K., Bhat, I.A., Pandey, S. et al. (2020). Effect of cryopreservation on therapeutic potential of canine bone marrow derived mesenchymal stem cells augmented mesh scaffold for wound healing in guinea pig. *Biomed. Pharmacother.* 121: 109573.

93 Zubin, E., Conti, V., Leonardi, F. et al. (2015). Regenerative therapy for the management of a large skin wound in a dog. *Clin. Case Rep.* 3 (7): 598–603.

94 Hersant, B., Sid-Ahmed, M., Braud, L. et al. (2019). Platelet-rich plasma improves the wound healing potential of mesenchymal stem cells through paracrine and metabolism alterations. *Stem Cells Int.* 2019: 1234263.

95 Blanton, M.W., Hadad, I., Johnstone, B.H. et al. (2009). Adipose stromal cells and platelet-rich plasma therapies synergistically increase revascularization during wound healing. *Plast. Reconstr. Surg.* 123 (2 Suppl): 56S–64S.

96 Samberg, M., Stone, R. 2nd, Natesan, S. et al. (2019). Platelet rich plasma hydrogels promote in vitro and in vivo angiogenic potential of adipose-derived stem cells. *Acta Biomater.* 87: 76–87.

97 Lian, Z., Yin, X., Li, H. et al. (2014). Synergistic effect of bone marrow-derived mesenchymal stem cells and platelet-rich plasma in streptozotocin-induced diabetic rats. *Ann. Dermatol.* 26 (1): 1–10.

16

Reconstructive Techniques for Wounds

Jill K. Luther[1] and Nicole J. Buote[2]

[1] *Heartland Veterinary Surgery, LLC, Columbia, MO, USA*
[2] *Department of Clinical Sciences, Cornell University, Ithaca, NY, USA*

Equipment

Multiple resources detail numerous procedures for varied wounds or resections and this chapter does not plan to recreate the wheel but instead will feature some of the most important aspects and methods for wound reconstruction [1–4]. Reconstructive surgery is often quite delicate therefore the instrumentation used is of the highest importance. Using damaged or dull instruments can be both frustrating to the surgeon and detrimental to the tissues. Surgical instruments are designed for a specific purpose, and it is important to use them only for the purpose intended to maximize their usefulness.

A basic instrument set used for reconstructive surgery should include needle holders, gentle forceps such as Brown-Adson thumb forceps or DeBakey vascular tissue forceps, hemostatic forceps, Metzenbaum scissors, Mayo scissors, a Bard-Parker blade handle, towel clamps, and scissors for cutting drape material and suture. (Figure 16.1) Forceps used in reconstructive surgery should be non-crushing (Adsons, Brown-Adson, etc.). Any instrument used for cutting should be sharp and precise. For more delicate procedures, ophthalmic instruments such as Castroviejo needle holders and iris scissors may be useful (see Chapter 17).

Skin incisions are most commonly performed using a blade handle and #10 or #15 blades. However, there are other cutting instruments that are useful for providing precise incisions. If scissors are to be used, a high-quality scissor should be reserved only for this purpose and not used to cut or dissect any other tissue or material. Scissors appropriate for skin use are often designated as "supercut" with a ceramic or tungsten carbide coating. One such example is the Freeman-Kaye Facelift Scissors used in plastic reconstruction of humans. The addition of cartilage scissors to a reconstructive pack is useful as they transect skin smoothly with the least amount of crushing (Figure 16.2).

Electrosurgery may be used both to cut and coagulate tissue. The most commonly used tip for monopolar electrosurgery is a flat blade which allows for painting a bleeding surface, transecting tissue, and spot cauterization (Figure 16.3). Electrosurgery creates heat by passing a current through the tissue between two points of contact (the ground plate and handpiece for monopolar or the two tips of the pencil for bipolar). An advantage of monopolar electrosurgery is the ability to move through vascular tissues such as subcutaneous tissue and muscle efficiently without having to stop to tie ligatures while keeping visualization maximized. However, the thermal damage to surrounding tissues has been documented [5]. Additionally, it has been noted that electrosurgery incisions have increased healing times and increased complications within the first week following surgery compared with scalpel incisions [6].

The CO_2 laser has also been used to create a bloodless incision as the laser coagulates vessels 0.6 mm or smaller. CO_2 lasers also come with a variety of tips with straight and right-angle being the most commonly used (Figure 16.4). Heat is generated resulting in tissue ablation and vaporization as the light energy from the CO_2 laser is absorbed by intracellular and extracellular water molecules. Lymphatics and nerve endings are also sealed by the laser, which may decrease

Techniques in Small Animal Wound Management, First Edition. Edited by Nicole J. Buote.
© 2024 John Wiley & Sons, Inc. Published 2024 by John Wiley & Sons, Inc.
Companion website: www.wiley.com/go/buote/wounds

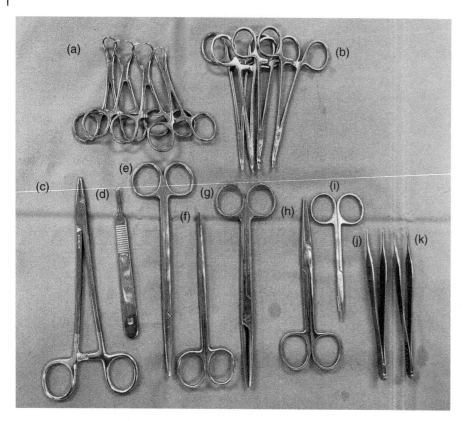

Figure 16.1 A standard instrument set used for soft tissue surgery. (a) Penetrating towel clamps, (b) mosquito hemostats, (c) needle holders, (d) Bard-Parker blade handle, (e) long Metzenbaum scissors, (f) short curved Metzenbaum scissors, (g) Mayo scissors, (h) suture scissors, (i) Tenotomy scissors, (j) Adson forceps, (k) Brown-Adson forceps. *Source:* Courtesy of Nicole Buote, DVM, DACVS.

(a)

(b)

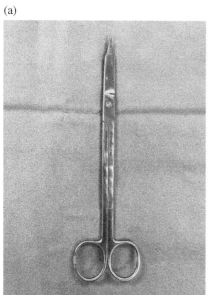
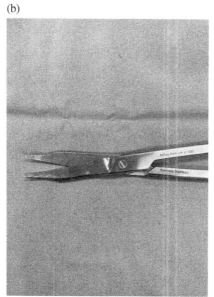

Figure 16.2 (a) Martin cartilage scissors are very sharp and cut skin smoothly without crushing. (b) Close-up view of tips of Martin cartilage scissors. *Source:* Courtesy of Nicole Buote, DVM, DACVS.

postoperative edema and pain sensation. One study comparing the CO_2 laser and conventional surgical techniques found delayed healing in skin flaps created by the CO_2 laser [7]. The authors concluded that in areas of increased skin mobility or tension, skin flaps created with the CO_2 laser may be more susceptible to dehiscence. Another study in a dog model found decreased bursting strength and histologic collagen content in skin flaps created with a CO_2 laser or electrosurgery compared with sharp dissection [8]. While simultaneous coagulation and cutting may be considered ideal in patients with

(a)

(b)

(c)

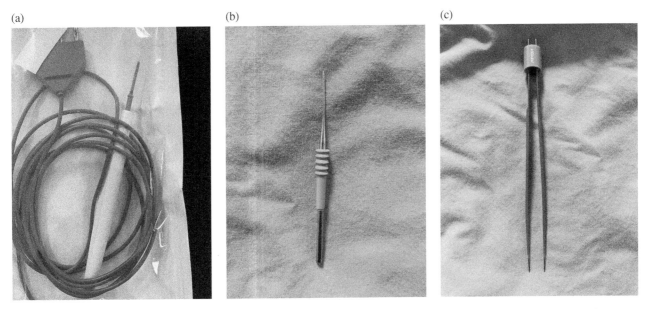

Figure 16.3   (a) Photograph of a monopolar electrosurgery pen with a flat tip. (b) Needle tip for monopolar cautery. (c) Bipolar electrosurgery forceps. *Source:* Courtesy of Nicole Buote, DVM, DACVS.

coagulopathies or other comorbidities, judicious use of these modalities should be considered in reconstructive procedures due to the potential for delayed healing.

Retraction is an important part of reconstructive surgery. Once a segment of skin has been surgically isolated for use in a local or distant location, gentle handling of the tissue is imperative. Forceps come in a variety of forms and the appropriate type is based on the tissue being handled. When possible, avoiding "thumb" forceps to grasp the skin is recommended as this type of forceps has small grooves along the inside edge but no teeth on the tips and the amount of crushing varies with pressure and can be difficult to control. Atraumatic tissue forceps (Adsons or Brown-Adsons) may be used on the deeper hypodermis or subcutaneous tissue to avoid crushing the skin. Skin hooks may be purchased or made using hypodermic needles (Figure 16.5) [9]. Alternatively, stay sutures using 3-0 or 4-0 suture with a small swaged-on needle may be placed in the skin and manipulated using hemostatic forceps to provide gentle retraction that uses gravity in place of an assistant (Figure 16.6). In the instance that an incision must be retracted in an open position, self-retaining retractors such as the Gelpi, Weitlaner, or ring-retractor may be useful (Figure 16.7).

Having a designated room or area for management of open wounds is ideal to prevent cross-contamination between patients, especially in hospitals in which orthopedic implants are used. The area should have easy access to supplies and dressings needed for wound management as well as standard operating procedures for routine daily cleaning and sanitizing between uses. A wet table is invaluable, as

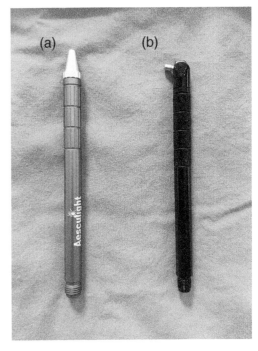

(a)   (b)

Figure 16.4   Photograph of CO_2 laser handles with straight (a) and right-angle (b) tips. Some laser handles require a ceramic tip to be inserted while others are "tip-less." *Source:* Courtesy of Nicole Buote, DVM, DACVS.

lavage is typically involved in contaminated wound management. If ventilation and cleaning protocols are appropriate the risk of cross-contamination between patients and across areas of the hospital is decreased.

(a)

(b)

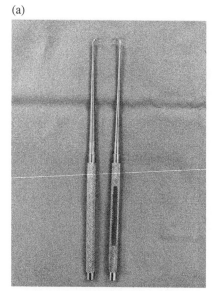

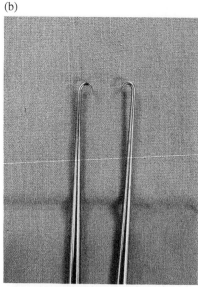

Figure 16.5 (a) Skin hooks, (b) close-up of hooks – note they have rounded edges similar to taper point needles. *Source:* Courtesy of Nicole Buote, DVM, DACVS.

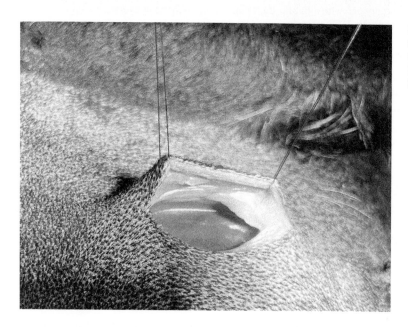

Figure 16.6 Skin sutures being used for elevation and manipulation. 3-0 PDS suture with a cutting needle placed through the skin and clamped with hemostatic forceps to provide gentle retraction. *Source:* Courtesy of Nicole Buote, DVM, DACVS.

Basic Tissue Handling Tenants

Tenants of tissue handling that remain valuable today were described by Dr. William Halstead in the late 1800's. These include gentle handling of tissue, meticulous hemostasis, preservation of blood supply, strict aseptic technique, minimum tension on tissues, accurate tissue apposition, and obliteration of dead space. These principles are used to guide every aspect of wound management from how one holds and uses instruments to how skin is chosen for reconstruction of the wound. Additional tenants that may be added to Halstead's include optimizing wound exposure, attention to moist wound healing, and planning for wound closure.

It is frequent that a surgeon must increase wound bed exposure in order to optimize the treatment plan. In wounds created by traumatic means, the open area of the skin may not approximate that of the deeper tissues. For example, bite wounds may only leave punctures in the skin, while larger defects in the subcutaneous and muscle layers may be present. It is important to have adequate exposure to these deeper tissues to evaluate for viability, ensure hemostasis, and to resect necrotic tissue. Additionally, dead space may be present deep in the skin and ultimately closing that dead space necessitates first increasing the exposure by lengthening the wound or skin incision. A surgeon must not be hesitant to open a wound

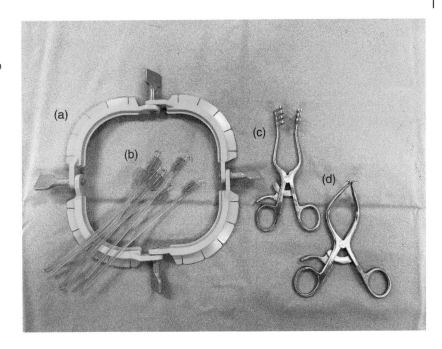

Figure 16.7 Self-retaining retractors. (a) Ring-retractor (Lonestar retractor), (b) flexible skin hooks that attach to the ring-retractor. These hooks come with sharp points (pictured) or blunt points. (c) Blunt-tipped Weitlaner retractor. (d) Sharp-tipped Gelpi retractor. *Source:* Courtesy of Nicole Buote, DVM, DACVS.

further to increase exposure. Once the wound is thoroughly evaluated, the decision can be made if a portion of the wound or the entire wound is healthy enough for closure.

Tissues that are dry become unhealthy and are unlikely to survive. However, tissues that are bathed in exudates can cause tissue layer separation and delayed healing [10]. Therefore, care must be taken to maintain an open wound with absorptive dressings appropriate for the amount of exudate present while preventing desiccation (see Chapters 8 and 9). In surgically created wounds, during a skin flap procedure, for example, the donor tissues should be covered with moistened sponges or periodically bathed in sterile saline to prevent desiccation while the recipient bed is prepared.

Having multiple plans in place for wound closure is imperative to minimize complications and maximize a successful outcome. This is true whether the wound is surgically created, in cases of tumor resection, or an open traumatic wound. Additionally, part of the plan may be continued open wound management or second intention healing if there is not a feasible closure option at the time of assessment. From one of the leading human plastic and reconstructive surgeons of the twentieth century, Sir Harold Gillies, "Never do today what can best be done tomorrow" [11].

Skin Tension

Histologic evaluation of skin has shown that it is a matrix of collagen tissue fibers that become oriented based on the tensile forces acting on them such as gravity and muscle pull [12]. Understanding the lines of tension on any anatomic region helps to plan for a tension-free closure, as tension on any closed skin incision can be devastating to the healing of the incision. Relying on sutures alone to hold an incision together where there is tension leads to ischemic necrosis of the skin edges. Additionally, if the wound is on a distal extremity the tension can lead to lymphatic and vascular compromise distal to the wound, creating a biological tourniquet effect [13]. Dehiscence and secondary bacterial infection are common sequela when there is tension on an incision.

Lines of tension of the dog are illustrated in multiple reference texts [1, 3] based on a terminal study of six dogs in 1966 [12] but most times real-time palpation of the skin is used to determine individual reconstructive plans. In a study by Baker, it was noted that a skin incision made *across a line of tension* creates a larger gap which takes longer to heal, requires more sutures, and results in a wider scar. A skin incision made *parallel to the tension lines* requires fewer sutures and heals quicker with minimum scarring [14]. Therefore, wounds are best closed *parallel* to the lines of tension, rather than perpendicular or diagonal.

In veterinary medicine, there is dramatic variation in elasticity and amount of skin between species and breeds. Feline skin, for example, is more pliable than that of the dog. Obese patients lose skin elasticity from heavy fat

(a) (b)

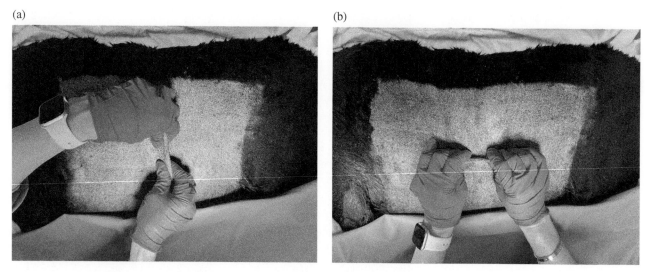

Figure 16.8 Photographs of subjective "pinch testing" of patient's skin elasticity. Patient's head is to the left. (a) In this photograph the skin overlying the chest is being pinched in a cranio-caudal direction (along tension lines). (b) In this photograph, the skin overlying the chest is being pinched in a dorsoventral direction (perpendicular to tension lines). The surgeon is able to grasp less tissue in photograph B when pinching perpendicular to the tension lines. *Source:* Courtesy of Nicole Buote, DVM, DACVS.

deposits in the subcutis [15]. Additionally, there are differences in the same animal in the pliability of skin in different anatomic regions. The most pliable skin is located in the axilla, flank, and dorsum of the neck and has more loosely woven dermal collagen bundles and greater numbers of elastic fibers. The least pliable is located in the tail, ear, and digital pads and has wider, more closely packed collagen bundles with less elastic fibers [15]. Extreme geriatric age has been found to affect cellular content of the skin in dogs as well, leading to thinner skin, although how this affected pliability was not examined [14]. A device capable of measuring directionality of forces on the skin (Reviscometer®) has been developed for use in people. While the dog has been used as a validated model for this objective measure of tension lines [16], it is not being used currently in clinical veterinary practice. Subjective "pinch testing" of the individual patient's skin elasticity is still the primary assessment tool used by veterinary surgeons prior to determining wound closure (Figure 16.8, Video 16.1 ☉). The direction in which skin is most easily moved is called the line of maximum distensibility and is perpendicular to the line of maximum tension [11]. A method of assessment of tension has also been adopted when removing a tumor with a circular incision. Following removal, the tensile forces tend to turn a round incision into a mild ellipse naturally, allowing for real time determination of the patient's lines of tension.

Tension-Relieving Techniques

Some of the most common tension-relieving techniques used in veterinary medicine include undermining, tension-relieving suture patterns, and releasing incisions. It is common to use a variety of techniques in concert to enable a tension-free closure.

Undermining

Undermining is one of the most basic, and therefore useful, techniques to close a wound without tension. Undermining allows the surgeon to draw upon the full elastic potential of the skin in the portion that has been undermined. The skin is anchored to deeper tissues such as fascia through subcutaneous attachments [17]. In order to allow use of the elasticity of the skin to advance over a wound, these connections must be gently broken down with a combination of blunt and sharp dissection. There is generally a distinct layer that guides where to perform the dissection – when there is a panniculus muscle present such as the platysma or cutaneous trunci, this should be included with the skin. Pay close attention to preserve the blood supply as much as possible, especially direct cutaneous vessels and the subdermal plexus.

Undermining can be performed using electrosurgery. However, to limit thermal damage a "pure cut" setting rather than "blend" should be used. Additionally, using a needle tip may provide a more controlled dissection plane [18]. Blunt undermining involves advancing closed scissor tips, such as Mayo scissors, into the wound edge and opening them to push and shear fibrous bands and loose connective tissue (Figure 16.9, Video 16.2). Sharp undermining can be performed with either scissors or a surgical blade. Oftentimes when contraction and epithelialization has begun, a blade must be employed to create a separation of the skin from the granulation tissue bed. However, care must be taken not to penetrate too deeply and to stop the incision when the proper plane of dissection has been reached. Sharp dissection with scissors involves advancing the instrument with open tips and closing at the level of tissue to be severed. This technique should never be performed blindly, and care must be taken to avoid inadvertent cutting of neurovascular structures. Incremental undermining is recommended to determine the lateral extent required for a tension-free closure. Intermittently, the surgeon should test the elasticity of the skin segment undermined for ability to stretch over the wound to meet the corresponding skin edge. Excessive undermining can lead to vascular compromise of a segment and increased dead space, increasing the risks of poor flap viability or seroma, respectively (see Chapter 3). For larger wounds undermining may be needed in combination with other tension-relieving techniques [18–20].

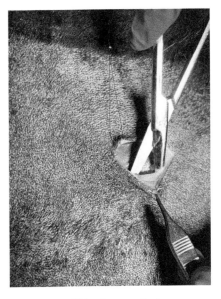

Figure 16.9 This photograph shows blunt dissection by advancing closed Mayo scissor tips into the wound edge and opening them to push and shear fibrous bands and loose connective tissue. *Source:* Courtesy of Nicole Buote, DVM, DACVS.

Tension-Relieving Sutures

Tension-relieving sutures can provide aid to achieve a tension-free closure. One such technique is an intradermal layer closure (sometimes called subdermal). Sutures should be placed in the *fibrous subdermal layer*, also known as the subcutaneous fascia or "white line," rather than the looser subcutaneous layer to bring the skin edges closer together (Figure 16.10) [19]. Using a subdermal layer in the closure will substantially reduce stress on the skin sutures. This layer may be performed using either a simple interrupted or continuous technique. But in areas of higher tension, a cruciate pattern or a far-near-near-far or far-far-near-near may be preferred in the subdermal tissue [20]. Absorbable swaged-on suture material should be used for this suture layer and size 3-0 or 4-0 material should be sufficient in holding ability without creating knots that are excessively large. Polydioxanone is recommended because it is present for more than 20 days, approximately the time it will take for collagen fibers to be produced in the healing process [19].

Walking sutures are also placed in the fibrous subdermal layer and then *walked* toward the incision by tacking to the underlying muscular fascia. This aids in obliterating dead space and spreading the tension out along the skin rather than concentrating it on the skin edges. Polydioxanone in size 2-0 or 3-0 is generally preferred for these sutures. To place walking sutures, a bite is first taken in the subdermis, then a bite in the wound bed fascia such that when pulled tight, the free skin edge advances toward the opposite wound edge by 1–3 cm. When the suture has been appropriately placed in the subdermis, a dimple can be seen in the epidermis when tension is placed on the suture (Figure 16.11, Video 16.3). An assistant is useful to aid in retraction to maximize the advancement of each suture placed. Multiple rows of walking sutures may be placed advancing both free skin edges toward the center of the wound. Excessive numbers of sutures should be avoided as they could lead to vascular compromise of the tissue [15].

External tension-relieving suture patterns may be placed in the skin to further decrease the tension on the incision. Vertical mattress sutures or far-near-near-far or far-far-near-near patterns will distribute tension away from the incision and will cause very minimal circulatory compromise because they are perpendicular to the incision (Figure 16.12) [15]. Horizontal mattress sutures have a greater tendency for impairing blood flow and should be avoided as a tension-relieving pattern unless used with a stent or bolster. Vertical suture patterns should be placed with the near suture at least 0.5 cm and the far suture at least 1 cm from the wound edge. They should be in a straight line and are perpendicular to the wound edge. They are quite useful where there may be cyclic increases and decreases in tension during motion such as on the foot pad, over a joint, or near an orifice [20]. Ideally, non-reactive suture material is used such as a non-absorbable monofilament

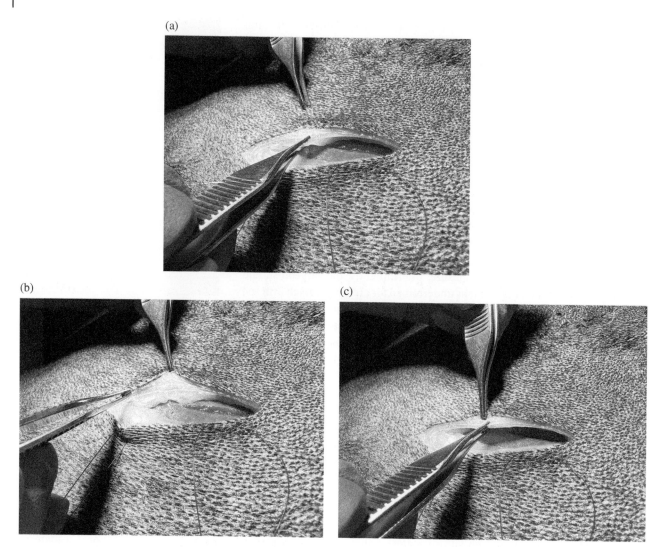

Figure 16.10 (a) Looser subcutaneous layer being grasped by Brown-Adson forceps, this would be considered the subcutaneous layer. (b) Skin being retracted slightly to highlight the "white line" where the dermis meets the subcutaneous layer, (c) Adson forceps resting on the white line/subdermal fascia. *Source:* Courtesy of Nicole Buote, DVM, DACVS.

(nylon or polypropylene) and these sutures may be alternated with simple interrupted in an incision. They must not be overtightened to prevent suture line inversion and knots should not be placed overlying the incision (Figure 16.13).

Stents and bolsters can also be used to spread tension out over a wider area and prevent the stent sutures from cutting through the skin. Penrose drains work well as stents and rolled gauze or laparotomy sponges work very well as bolsters (Figure 16.14). Buttons are not ideal, as they do not spread the tension out nearly enough and pressure necrosis can occur under the button. Before the skin is closed, the bolster sutures should be placed with a larger non-absorbable monofilament material such as nylon or polypropylene but not yet tied. Following skin closure the bolster is added and sutures are tied over it. If using a Penrose drain as a stent, the sutures must be placed through the drain and left in place to tie following skin closure. The bolsters and stent sutures should be removed within three to four days, as skin relaxation will have occurred.

Skin Stretching

When there is time to plan a closure in advance, skin stretching can be a very useful technique for closure of moderately sized wounds with local tissues. By applying a stretching force to skin, tissue fluid is slowly displaced from around the randomly arranged dermal collagen filaments as they progressively align and compact longitudinally in the direction of the

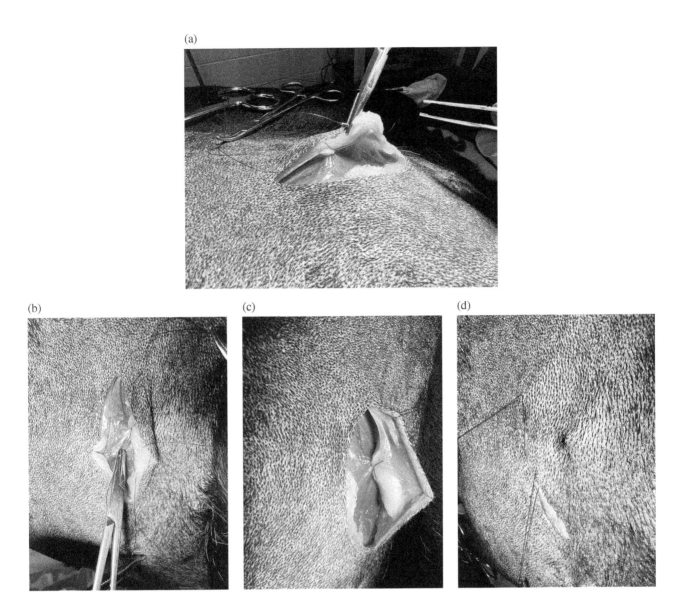

Figure 16.11   Walking sutures. (a) Grasping deep subcutaneous tissue under the skin flap. (b) Taking a bite of deep muscle at the incision center. (c) Tied suture bringing together deep subcutaneous tissue to the center of the incision. (d) Visible skin "dimple" from suture grabbing the dermis. *Source:* Courtesy of Nicole Buote, DVM, DACVS.

Figure 16.12   Far-far-near-near patterns. (a) Line drawing, (b) photograph of a far-far-near-near suture being pre-placed. *Source:* Courtesy of Nicole Buote, DVM, DACVS.

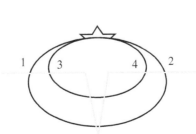

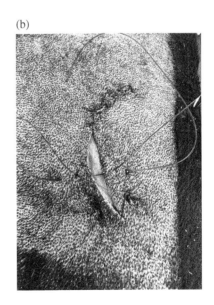

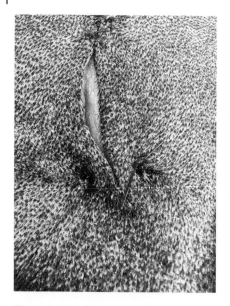

Figure 16.13 Photograph of a far-far-near near suture with the knot to the side of the incision. Note the slight eversion of the skin edges. *Source:* Courtesy of Nicole Buote, DVM, DACVS.

stretching force (aka mechanical creep). Stress relaxation is the phenomenon in which there is a progressive reduction in the force required to keep the stretched collagen fibers at a given length, i.e., the stretched fibers do not recoil when the load is removed [20, 21]. These biomechanical mechanisms allow skin to stretch beyond the conventional suturing limits of its inherent extensibility and is made possible by alteration of its basic structural components. Under external tension, the interrelated networks of collagen, elastin, and ground substance in the extracellular matrix of the tissue deform, inflicting tissue elongation, allowing skin stretching to occur [22]. Patients that develop very large masses or pregnant bitches or queens have this natural phenomenon of skin stretching over time (Figure 16.15).

Presuturing

The simplest method of skin stretching involves stretching before the extra skin is needed. Prior to a planned excision, skin may be *presutured*, using mattress sutures or Lembert sutures to stretch the skin adjacent to a proposed wound. This method is most useful in areas of very little extra skin such as the distal extremities. Ample stretching can reportedly occur within 2.5 hours to 3 days, but 24 hours of stretching is average [15, 20, 21]. Large (2-0 or 0) non-absorbable monofilament suture material is recommended and can be used alone or with tubing placed to aid in spreading out the tension and prevention of suture cutting through tissue (Figure 16.16).

Pretensioning

In an existing wound, the edges can be *pretensioned*, using one of several possible methods. Pretensioning is similar to presuturing in principle but is used after the formation of an open wound. Pretensioning can be done through placement of sutures at the wound edges or through an externally placed stretching device. For the suture method, 0 or 2-0 non-absorbable monofilament (multifilament may be seen through the tissue if placed in tension) is placed through the skin and fibrous hypodermis to pull the wound edges closer together. This can be done using reusable split shot fishing sinkers (tin rather than lead-based) in order to continue to adjust the tension daily, as stress-relaxation occurs (Figure 16.17) [23]. Alternatively,

(a)

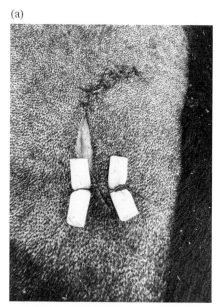

(b)

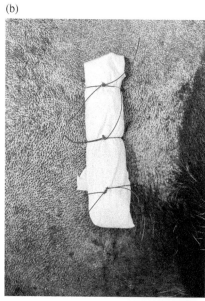

Figure 16.14 (a) Penrose drains as stents under tension-relieving vertical mattress sutures. (b) Rolled gauze placed as a bolster over an incision. *Source:* Courtesy of Nicole Buote, DVM, DACVS.

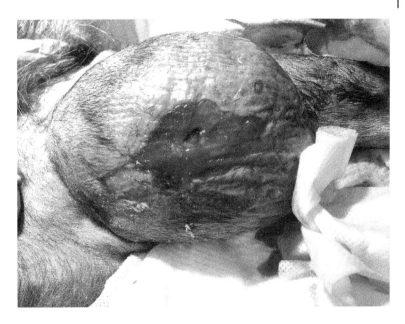

Figure 16.15 Photograph of a very large mammary mass on a canine patient. The skin has been stretched to the point of necrosis over the center and cranial aspects. *Source:* Courtesy of Nicole Buote, DVM, DACVS.

two methods are described using sutures held to the wound edge using staples or hypodermic needles in the distal extremities [24]. The hypodermic needle method may spread the tension out over a larger surface area along the wound edge.

Another method of pretensioning skin was described by Pavletic and involves a bit more planning but is very effective. Skin glue may be used to secure Velcro on opposing sides of the wound [25]. Then Velcro strips are used to gradually tighten, thereby stretching the skin adjacent to the wound. Successful use of the device requires a reasonable source of donor skin that can be recruited for wound closure and one study found that this method was ineffective for distal extremities corroborating the need for recruitable skin [24]. This method can also be used following wound closure to decrease tension on the incision.

Commercial tissue expanders are available that are implanted under the skin and gradually inflated with saline. These are expensive and require multiple surgeries, making these less practical for veterinary patients. One big advantage is that the expanders can be used acutely in plastic surgery. Expanders are not to be placed in damaged skin.

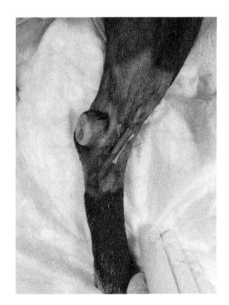

Figure 16.16 Photograph of an 11-year-old MC Boston terrier with a MCT on tarsus. Owners chose a marginal resection with primary closure. Pre-tensioning was performed to stretch his skin. *Source:* Courtesy of Jill Luther, DVM, MS, DACVS.

Relaxing/Releasing Incisions

Relaxing incisions (also known as releasing incisions) can either be one or two simple incisions on either side of the wound or many small incisions (aka mesh expansion). This is a technique most commonly used on the distal extremities but can be used anywhere to pull wound edges together with less tension. Special attention must be paid to incise through the dermis with these incision in order to get relaxation. The incisions should "open" and look like an ellipse if done appropriately. This technique does require new incisions to be created in healthy adjacent skin so owners should be prepared preoperatively. The relaxing incisions are usually left to heal by second intention and depending on their number, location, and the patient this may lead to increased home care (keeping the incisions clean, keeping the housing area clean, applying ointment to them, etc.) and scarring (especially in short-haired animals). Fortunately, these incisions usually heal with a scab within five to seven days so the added care is short-lived. Care must be taken to stagger the rows of these small 1–2 cm incisions enough to avoid vascular compromise (Figure 16.18).

(a)

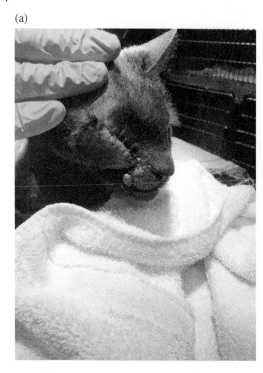

(b)

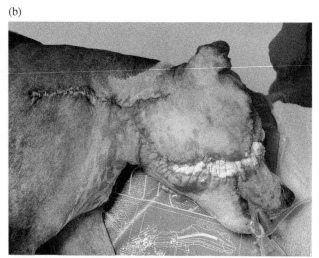

Figure 16.17 (a) Photograph of a feline patient after a large facial sarcoma removal. A fishing weight or split shot is placed at the end of the continuous line. The weight is loosened and then pushed down the suture (tightening it) daily to gradually bring the skin edges together. (b) Photograph of open wound management in a canine patient after a previous reconstruction for a large maxillary tumor failed. Multiple running sutures with split shots were used to gradually tension the skin edges to facilitate primary closure. *Source:* Courtesy of Nicole Buote, DVM, DACVS.

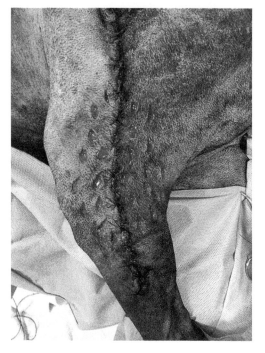

Figure 16.18 Photograph of extensive releasing incisions on the thoracic limb of a canine patient. *Source:* Courtesy of Nicole Buote, DVM, DACVS.

Triangular, Square, Rectangle Wounds

Triangular

Triangular wounds present a challenge due to the wide area that must be covered at the base of the triangle. The triangular wound is closed by undermining each side and bringing the sides toward each other in a centripetal closure (Figure 16.19, Video 16.4 ⊙). This closure is a "Y" shape. The closure point where more than two edges meet must be handled with care and with the knowledge that at least partial dehiscence in this area is common. The other common method of triangular wound closure is to use one or more rotational flaps. The advantage with this type of closure is the avoidance of the three-point closure. Rotational flaps allow recruitment of more skin than the Y closure in areas such as the face or perineum (Figure 16.20).

Square or Rectangular Defects

Square or rectangular defects can be closed using a variety of methods, and largely depends on wound location and amount of local skin available for recruitment. A centripetal movement of skin is possible with this wound configuration similar to the triangle with the resultant shape of an "X" when closed (Figure 16.21). Additional closure options for these defects include advancement (Figure 16.22) or transpositional flaps.

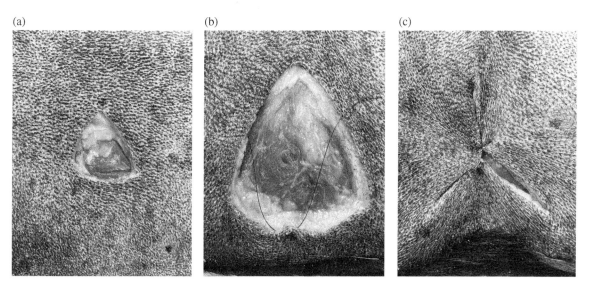

Figure 16.19 Photographs of a triangular wound being closed with a three-sided suture bringing the sides toward each other (centripetal closure). (a) Triangular wound, (b) suture placement, (c) appearance after suture tied. *Source:* Courtesy of Nicole Buote, DVM, DACVS.

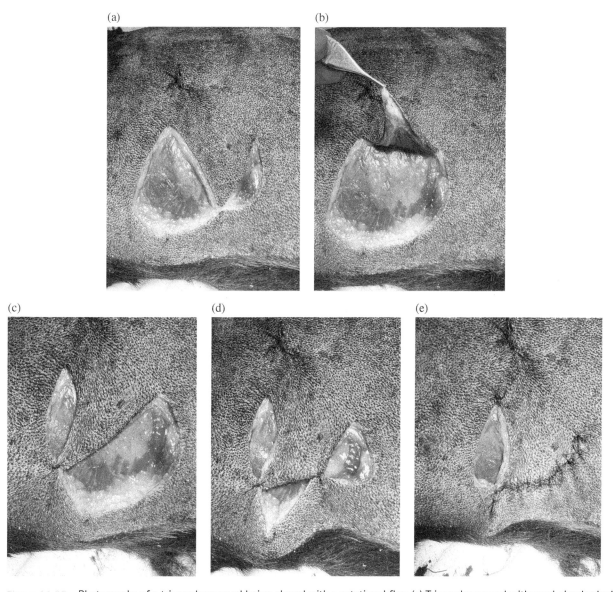

Figure 16.20 Photographs of a triangular wound being closed with a rotational flap. (a) Triangular wound with semi-circular incision made from one edge, (b) undermining flap, (c) placement of first suture to bring tip of flap to edge of original triangle, (d) second suture at halfway point of flap and the incision created by the original triangle + the flap incision, (e) closure of one side of the incision. This type of closure will make a "V" instead of a "Y." *Source:* Courtesy of Nicole Buote, DVM, DACVS.

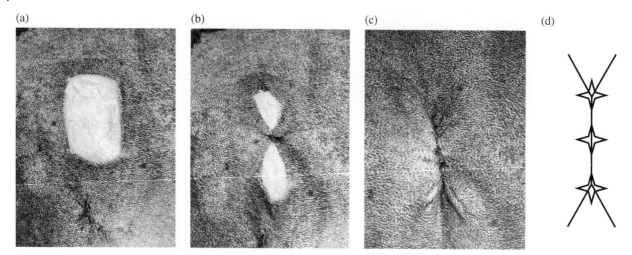

Figure 16.21 Square or rectangular defects can be closed using a variety of methods, and largely depends on wound location and amount of local skin available for recruitment. A centripetal movement of skin is possible with this wound configuration similar to the triangle with the resultant shape of an "X" when closed. (a) Rectangular wound, (b) first suture is placed from side to side, (c) second and third sutures are placed in the same manner as closing a triangular wound (Figure 16.19b) to create to "Y" incisions meeting at the center, (d) line drawing of closure. Stars signify suture knots. *Source:* Courtesy of Nicole Buote, DVM, DACVS.

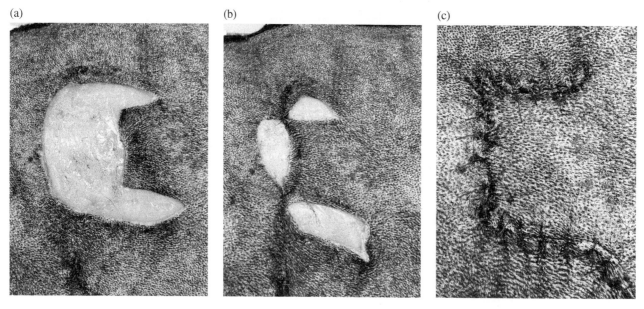

Figure 16.22 Closure of a rectangular wound by advancement flap. (a) H-plasty flap created along one of the wound edges, (b) initial sutures to advance the flap into the wound bed, (c) Final appearance. *Source:* Courtesy of Nicole Buote, DVM, DACVS.

Circular and Crescentic Wounds

Circular Defects

Circular defects can be some of the most difficult to heal by second intention as epithelial cells at the edges can contact each other more readily halting centripetal movement. Chronic or acute open circular wounds should be closed primarily whenever possible for this reason. As circular incisions are recommended over ellipsoid ones for tumor resections, understanding the many available techniques for closure is essential. Circular incisions allow for accurate assessment of the tension lines in a given region leading to a simpler closure on the one hand, but additional adjacent tissue is usually removed so incisions may appear quite extensive to owners. The most straightforward method for closure of a circular wound is to create a linear

(a)	(b)	(c)

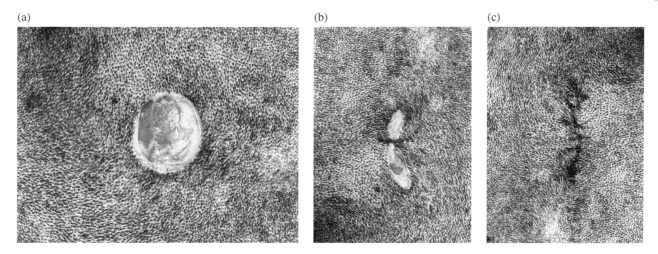

Figure 16.23	Photographs of a linear closure for a circular wound. (a) Circular wound, (b) initial suture placement in the mid-point of the wound, (c) final appearance. *Source:* Courtesy of Nicole Buote, DVM, DACVS.

incision. It is important to test for tension before closure as in the author's experience, many times this incision is best closed at an angle as opposed to strictly dorsoventral or craniocaudal. Start by placing a simple buried interrupted suture at the midpoint of the diameter and then begin filling in interrupted sutures on either side (Figure 16.23). Depending on the size of the wound, "dog ears" will be present with this technique and can be surgically excised or left in place. Many dog ears will flatten over time. An additional technique for circular wound closure is the "Bow tie" technique [3]. This technique is useful for larger wounds that would create large dog ears if closed in a linear fashion. Equilateral triangles removed from opposite sides of the defect, spaced approximately 30° from the long axis of the wounds tension line are removed (Figure 16.24). The resulting triangular flaps are then rotated into new positions to create a wavy line.

Crescentic Defects

Crescentic defects occur when one side of a wound or incision is longer than the other. This is quite common in bite wounds or lacerations and the closure technique useful for planned resections as well. The recommended technique is to start closure in the middle with a simple interrupted suture to decrease tension across the wound/incision. When placing additional sutures, on either side, it is critical to place suture bites closer together on the shorter arc (or concave side) compared to the longer arc (convex side) (Figure 16.25).

Incisional Plasties

Incisional plasties help redistribute tensile forces to close wounds with challenging anatomy. A "V-Y" plasty is most commonly used to counteract the functional consequences of wound contraction on normal structures adjacent to the wound such as the eyelid (see Chapter 17) but can be used in any location with high tension if tissue is available nearby. The vertex of the V should be pointed opposite to the direction of movement and undermining is usually required between the initial defect and the new "V" incision to allow for skin to move (Figure 16.26). A Z-plasty is used for redistribution of tension in opposing directions. This plasty provides length. The central arm is made in the direction that is needed for lengthening and can be the primary incision or wound or be a separate incision nearby. The other two arms are created at 30–90° (60° ideal) from the central arm and are the same length as the central arm. The triangular flaps are then undermined and reversed (Figure 16.27).

Skin Flaps

A skin flap is a portion of skin and subcutaneous tissue with or without a specific vascular supply that is moved from one area of the body to another. Flaps can be described in numerous ways depending on their blood supply (axillary pattern), location (flank fold) and tissue type (myocutaneous). Multiple resources exist which describe in detail the

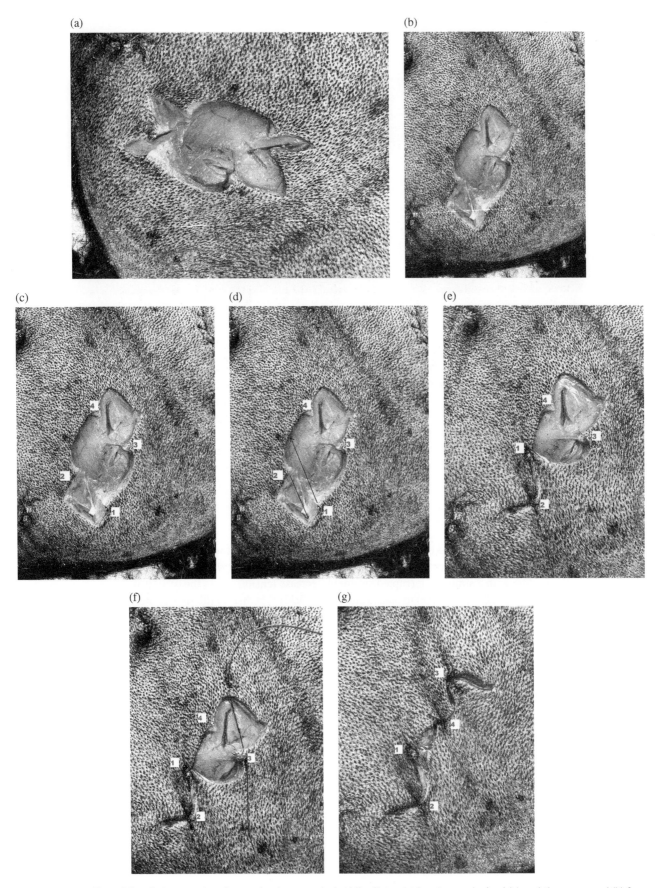

Figure 16.24 "Bow tie" technique to close larger circular wounds. (a,b) Equilateral triangles are incised (a) and then removed (b) from opposite sides of the defect, (c) the corners of the triangles are number 1–4, (d,e) corner 2 is rotated down into the triangles base and corner 1 is rotated toward the center of the circle opposite it (d), resulting in a "zig-zag" incision (e), (f,g) the same process is performed for corners 3 and 4. *Source:* Courtesy of Nicole Buote, DVM, DACVS.

(a)

(b)

(c)

(d)

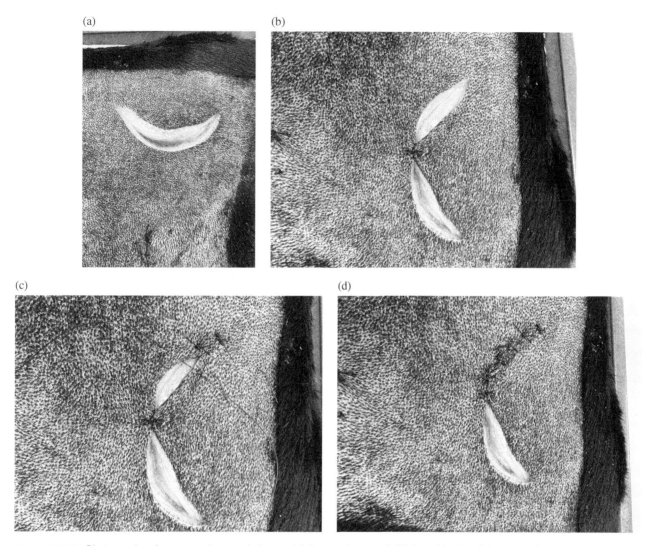

Figure 16.25 Photographs of a crescentic wound closure. (a) Crescentic wound, (b) the midpoint of the wound is closed first, (c) sutures can be placed from one edge, or by splitting the difference again, (d) closure of half of the incision – sutures are placed farther apart on the convex side and closer together on the concave side to bring the edges together. *Source:* Courtesy of Nicole Buote, DVM, DACVS.

various flaps that can be employed but a brief overview of the most common flaps will be presented (1–4). The blood flow is maintained or immediately reestablished when skin segment is moved to new position. Indications for a skin flap include large defects (tumor resections or trauma), defects with poor vascularity, areas difficult to immobilize with a bandage (face, perineum, over joints), defects overlying cavities (orbit), and areas where padding and durability are essential. The blood supply to local (advancement or transpositional) skin flaps comes from the subdermal plexus, which are the terminal branches of a directly penetrating cutaneous artery. Common types of subdermal plexus flaps include rotational, advancement, and transposition (skin fold) flaps. The survival rate of this type of flap is reported to be close to 90%.

Advancement Flaps

Advancement flaps are considered any subdermal plexus flap that "advances" skin to an adjacent area. Examples include single-pedicle, bipedicle flap (a single incision parallel to the wound or incision), H-plasty, and V-Y plasty (Figures 16.20, 16.22, and 16.26). The flaps must be created along lines of tension and require undermining of adjacent tissue but for small wounds in areas with available adjacent skin, they are quite helpful.

(a)   (b)

(c)   (d)

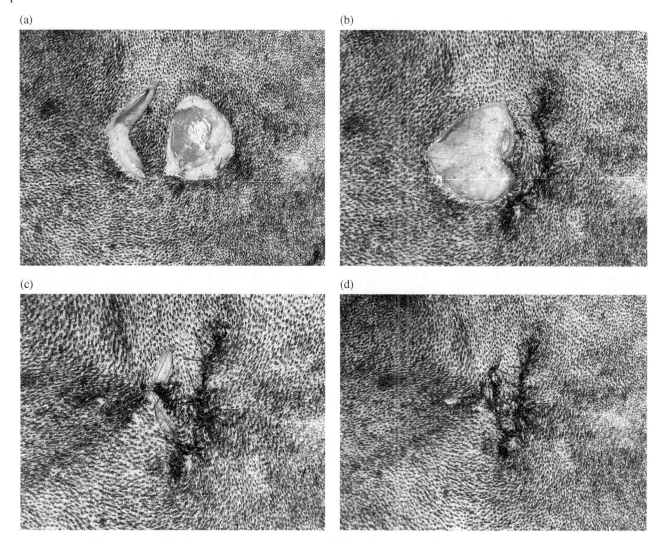

Figure 16.26   Photographs of "V-Y" plasty for a circular wound. (a) "V" incision created adjacent to wound, (b) tissue undermined and advanced to close original wound, (c) remaining wound closed in a "Y" configuration (red lines) with first suture placed at the center, (d) final appearance. *Source:* Courtesy of Nicole Buote, DVM, DACVS

Rotational Flaps

Rotational flaps include any subdermal (but axial pattern flaps [APF] can be included) flap that uses skin that is rotated into a defect or wound that includes a common border. A curved incision is used to harvest the donor tissue, and these can be used to close irregular shaped wounds and triangular wounds. If a subdermal plexus flap is used as a rotational flap, care must be taken to ensure excessive tension is not created and the length of the skin is not too great (Figure 16.20)

Transposition Flaps

Transposition or rotational flaps are rectangular or crescentic skin flaps that are also rotated into a nearby wound or incision (Figure 16.28). The most commonly used transposition flaps are the elbow fold and flank fold flaps (also considered axial pattern flaps). Usually, the flap is harvested parallel to the tension lines to allow for simple closure of the donor site and the length and width of the flap are determined by the defect size and the arc of rotation. Elbow and flank fold flaps can be harvested bilaterally to close large wounds in the sternal and inguinal regions, but they have also been reported for defects affecting the thorax, abdomen, hip, stifle, and elbow (Figure 16.28) [3]. These flaps are harvested by creating

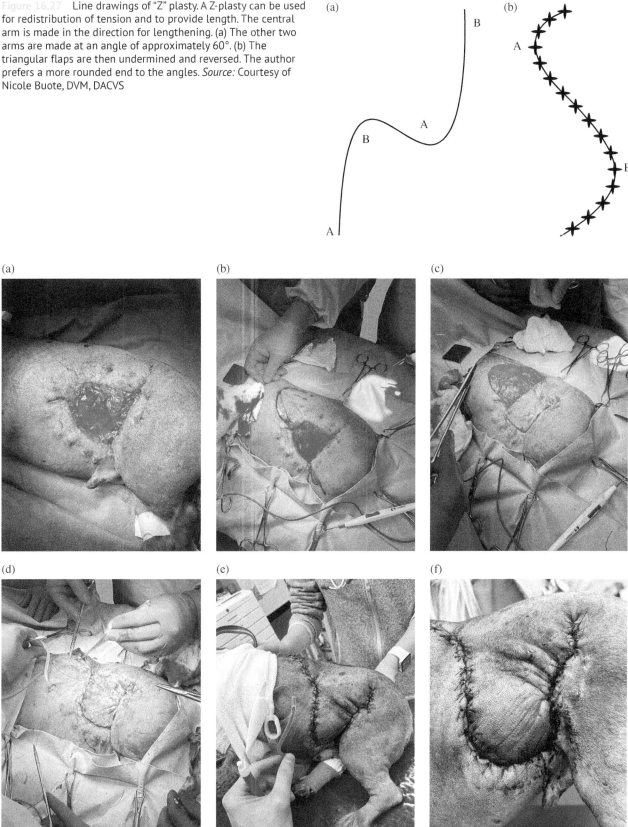

Figure 16.27 Line drawings of "Z" plasty. A Z-plasty can be used for redistribution of tension and to provide length. The central arm is made in the direction for lengthening. (a) The other two arms are made at an angle of approximately 60°. (b) The triangular flaps are then undermined and reversed. The author prefers a more rounded end to the angles. *Source:* Courtesy of Nicole Buote, DVM, DACVS

Figure 16.28 Photographs of a transposition/rotation flap to close a large flank wound. (a) Large wound on lateral abdomen of canine patient. This wound had been managed with a tie-over bandage until the wound bed was healthy enough for primary closure. (b) The rotational flap is incised. One of the edges of the flap is shared with the wound. (c) The flap has been rotated into the wound bed. (d) Subcutaneous sutures have been placed to secure the flap and close the donor site. Note a closed suction drain has been placed under the flap. (e) One-day postoperatively mild edema is present, but no congestion is noted. (f) Three-days postoperatively continued edema and mild reddish bruising present distally. A thin rim of scabbing or partial thickness necrosis is present along the incision line ventrally – the author does not recommend debriding these scabs as many time the flap will heal uneventfully under them. *Source:* Courtesy of Nicole Buote, DVM, DACVS.

Table 16.1   Useful axial pattern flaps for wound reconstruction.^a

Name (artery supply)	Anatomic landmarks	Indications
Caudal auricular	Wing of the atlas and spine of the scapula	Dorsal and lateral facial region, pinna, and chin
Superficial temporal	Caudal zygomatic arch and lateral border of the orbit	Dorsal and lateral facial area, and bridge of nose
Angularis oris	Lip commissure	Palate, lateral face, neck, chin
Thoracodorsal	Spine of the scapula and caudal edge of the scapula	Lateral thorax, lateral forelimb, and axilla
Caudal superficial epigastric	Midline of abdomen and lateral to mammary teats	Lateral flank, abdomen, inguinal, perineum, lateral hindlimb
Elbow fold (lateral thoracic artery)	Elbow skin fold (pinchable skin)	Medial and lateral elbow, axilla, sternum
Genicular	Patella, tibial tuberosity, and Greater trochanter	Lateral and medial distal hindlimb (from stifle to hock)
Flank fold (deep circumflex iliac artery)	Flank fold skin (pinchable skin)	Medial and lateral proximal hindlimb (thigh), inguinal, and flank

^a Breed and body conformation will determine the extent to which many of these flaps can be harvested and rotated.

symmetric incisions on the lateral and medial aspects of the elbow/flank fold once the determination of the extent of tissue that can be resected is made. The skin is elevated from underlying fascial attachments and rotated into the recipient bed. Special attention should be given to the donor sites when using these flaps as excessive tension in these high-motion areas (axilla and inguinal) can lead to seroma formation and dehiscence.

Axial Pattern Flaps

APF are considered any skin flap that is supplied by a direct cutaneous artery and vein position at the pedicle base. These flaps can be rotated directly into a wound or defect that shares a common border or bridging incision can be created to produce a path for the flap to reach the defect. Most APF's are considered robust because they do not rely on circulation from the subdermal plexus and therefore perfusion is considered superior. Descriptions of every APF is not possible as new options are constantly evolving and other references exist with detailed images of these reconstructive techniques [1–4]. An abbreviated discussion of the most commonly used APFs in the authors' experience is below (Table 16.1). The major disadvantages of APFs include the invasiveness of the donor dissection leading to increased discomfort and the potential for complications (infection, dehiscence, necrosis).

Axial pattern flaps require meticulous planning to minimize surgical misjudgments, but the authors admit that many decisions must be made once the patient is anesthetized to gain full insight into the best flap option. Once the ideal flap is determined, care must be paid to appropriate positioning on the surgical table to decrease tension and improve harvest and closure. The cosmetic results for APFs are better than those for second intention healing or mesh skin grafts as the skin is of normal thickness and durability. While most clinicians anecdotally feel that APF's result in good outcomes, it is important to choose these procedures wisely. To date, the only broad retrospective on outcomes of APF's in 73 dogs reported good to excellent outcomes in only 64% of patients, with complications occurring in 89% [26].

Specific Axial Pattern Flaps

Caudal Auricular Flap

This flap can be used for defects of the dorsal and lateral head, neck, chin, and pinna [27–29]. The main arterial blood supply is positioned between the base of the pinna and the wing of the atlas and the width of the flap is approximately 1/3 of the lateral neck circumference of the patient in lateral recumbency. The length of the flap is dependent on the patient's conformation but can reach the scapular spine (Figure 16.29). The authors have had good success with this flap for a variety

Figure 16.29 Postoperative photograph of an axillary (elbow) fold flap used to help close a large lateral thoracic incision after sarcoma removal. Note-releasing incisions were also used to ease tension for this closure. *Source:* Courtesy of Nicole Buote, DVM, DACVS.

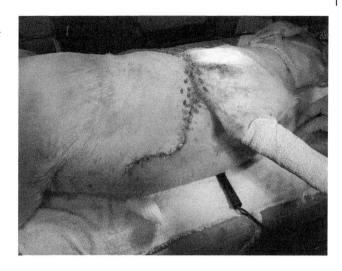

(a)

(b)

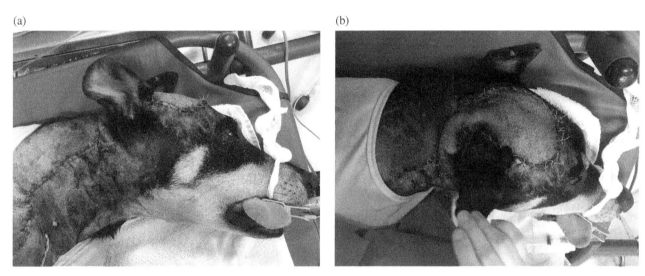

Figure 16.30 Postoperative photographs of a caudal auricular flap. (a) Lateral aspect (note an active suction drain is exiting ventrally), (b) dorsal aspect. *Source:* Courtesy of Nicole Buote, DVM, DACVS.

of wound closures, but a 2019 study reported partial flap necrosis and dehiscence in 63% of dogs [28]. About 42% of patients also required a revision surgery (50% of dogs and 25% of cats) [28]. This flap has also been used successfully to recreate the dorsal pinna in a brachycephalic dog after a traumatic bite wound when pinnectomy was declined [27].

Superficial Temporal

This flap is based on a cutaneous branch of the superficial temporal artery and is best used for defects involving the dorsal and lateral head. The arterial supply is positioned at the base of the zygomatic arch and extends rostrally along the zygomatic arch. The caudal aspect of the flap is considered to be the caudal aspect of the zygomatic arch and the rostral aspect is the lateral orbital rim. Two parallel lines extending from these points dorsally and laterally to the middle of the dorsal orbital rim of the contralateral eye complete the flap (Figure 16.30). The width of the flap should be limited to the width of the orbit. This flap should be elevated with the underlying frontalis muscle (thin muscle over the temporalis muscle). In one study, investigating this flap postoperative complications occurred in 42% of patients but only 5% consisted of a major complication of full-thickness necrosis of the flap when the flap length exceeded the recommended guidelines [30]. Minor complications occurred in 21–26% of patients and included partial flap necrosis, wound discharge, mild ectropion or exposure of the eye, and reduced ability to blink [30].

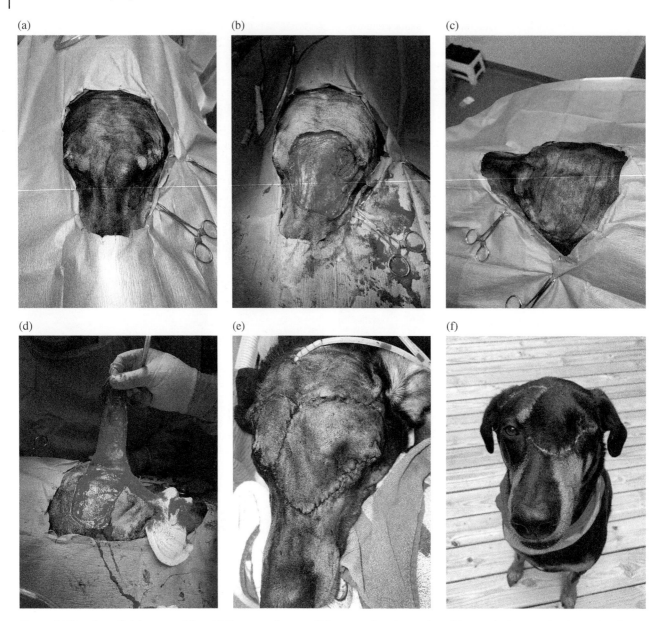

Figure 16.31 Superficial temporal flap. (a) Tumor on dorsomedial aspect of canine patient, (b) wound after enucleation and wide resection of tumor, (c) margins of superficial temporal flap, (d) flap raised, (e) appearance of flap sutured in place, (f) two-week recheck showing healed flap. *Source:* Courtesy of Justin Ganjei, DVM, DACVS.

Angularis Oris

This flap is useful for a variety of facial defects including the lateral aspect of the head and neck, oral cavity, and chin. This flap is based on the cutaneous branch of the facial artery and the base is positioned at the caudal commissure of the lips. The dorsal border of the flap consists of the ventral aspect of the zygomatic arch and a parallel line at the level of the ventral mandible forms the ventral border (Figure 16.31). The recommended caudal boundary is the wing of the atlas. Meticulous dissection in this region is required to avoid the auriculopalpebral branches of the facial nerve, branches of the auriculotemporal nerve, and the parotid duct. The division of the linguofacial and maxillary vein will also be prominent in some patients (especially cats). This flap has the added advantage of availability for palate and oral mucosa closures. In these cases, skin does not need to be resected along with the buccal mucosa. A single incision through the skin caudal to the lip commissure can be made and retracted and the underlying subcutaneous tissue and buccal mucosa harvested and rotated

Figure 16.32 Postoperative photograph of an angularis oris flap for closure of a small tumor resection wound bed. *Source:* Courtesy of Nicole Buote, DVM, DACVS.

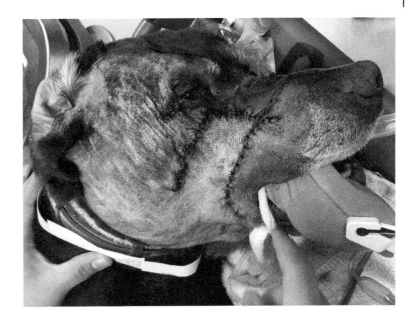

into place [31]. As with all flaps, distal flap necrosis and dehiscence have been reported with this flap but functional and cosmetic outcomes have been reported in both cats and dogs [32–34].

Thoracodorsal

The thoracodorsal flap is a robust APF that can be rotated to cover defects involving the shoulder, forelimb (elbow down to carpus depending on conformation), axilla, and craniolateral thorax. This flap is based on an arterial supply positioned at the caudal shoulder depression at the level of the acromion. The flaps cranial border is a line overlying the scapular spine and the caudal incision is parallel to this with a width twice the distance from the acromion to the caudal shoulder depression. The dorsal border is created by connecting these two lines at the dorsal midline of the patient (Figure 16.32). An "L" flap can be created to extend the size of the flap by extending the flap along the dorsum. When creating this flap, it is important to undermine deep to the cutaneous trunci muscle to improve uptake of the donor flap. While this flap is more robust than the omocervical flap and has more versatility and rotational length than the axillary fold flap, it does require a large donor site and moderate patient morbidity. Distal flap necrosis is common with this flap therefore owners should be prepared for this complication [31]. In the author's practice, this flap has not been used as frequently recently as local rotational flaps have been shown to have good outcomes and create less discomfort. In cats, this flap can be used with omental pedicle grafts to close chronic nonhealing axillary wounds with good success [35].

Caudal Superficial Epigastric

The caudal superficial epigastric flap is one of the most widely used APF's in the author's oncologic reconstructive practice. This flap can be used to cover defects of the caudal abdomen, perineum, prepuce, thigh, and lateral hindlimb [36–38]. In cats, due to their highly elastic skin, this flap can extend as far down the limb to the metatarsal joint, whereas in most dogs, it will not reach past the stifle. The flap is based on the caudal superficial epigastric artery which exits the abdomen near the inguinal ring. The ventral midline of the patient acts as the medial border. The width of the flap is determined by using the distance between the nipples and the ventral midline as the same distance between the nipples and the lateral most aspect. The cranial border (length of the flap) is determined by the size of the defect or the distance the flap will need to travel. This flap is dissected superficial to the external abdominal oblique fascia but does include the supramammarius muscle (Figure 16.33).

Genicular

The genicular axial pattern flap is most commonly used to cover defects of the lateral and medial tibia [39–41]. This flap is based on the short genicular artery off the saphenous artery and the base is positioned slightly proximal to patella and ~2cm distal to tibial tuberosity on lateral aspect of the limb. The cranial and caudal incisions are parallel to the femoral

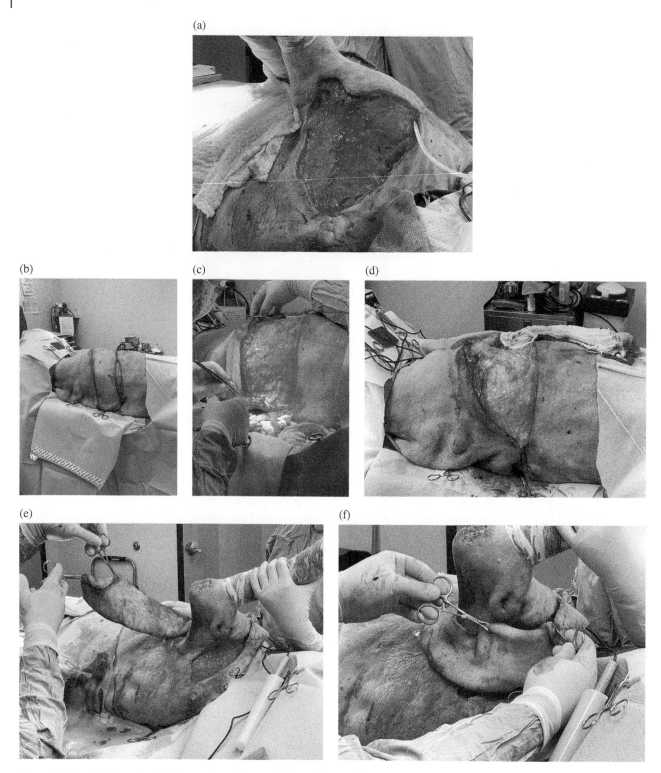

Figure 16.33 Photographs of a thoracodorsal flap used in a golden retriever which had a grade I soft tissue sarcoma in the cranial axillary region. Initially, an omocervical artery APF was used to close the resection site, but it became infected and dehisced. The resulting wound was revised using this thoracodorsal flap, which healed uneventfully. (a) Wound after dehiscence of omocervical flap, (b) thoracodorsal flap incision on dorsolateral aspect, (c) donor site wound, (d) initial closure of donor site (note flap is in far-field wrapped in saline soaked lap sponge), (e) sternal view with flap elevated, (f) placement of flap into wound, (g) a bridge has been made to allow the flap to reach this axillary/sternal wound and the subcutaneous sutures have started to be placed, (h) final closure, (i,j) day 2 postoperatively, (k,l) day 14 postoperatively – note very minor dehiscence cranially, (k) and evidence of minor second intention healing at the rotation point (l). *Source:* Courtesy of Rodrigo Rosa, MV, CVPP, MANZCVS (SA Surgery), DABVP (canine/feline).

(g)

(h)

(i)

(j)

(k)

(l)

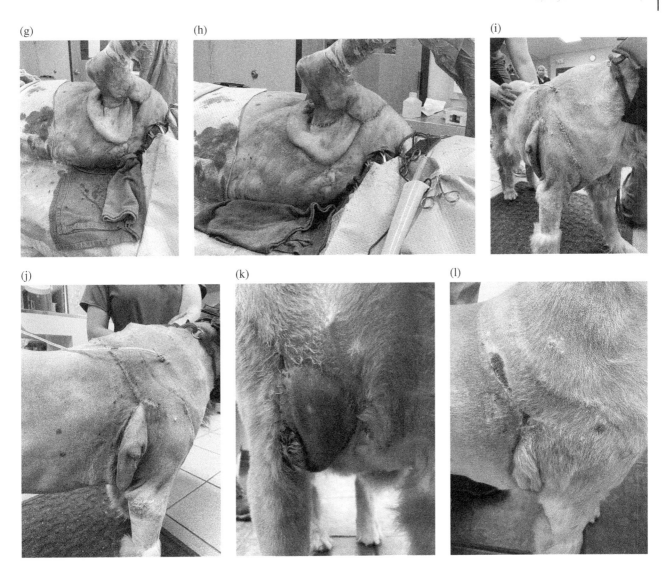

Figure 16.33 (Continued)

shaft from the stifle and the dorsal border is distal to the greater trochanter (Figure 16.34). While originally thought to be a more tenuous flap, a study by Emmerson et al., in 2019, concluded that average flap survival was 99% with major complications requiring a second surgery in less than 15% of patients [41]. Proper case selection, for small to medium defects of the tibia region are the best candidates for this flap.

Elbow/Axillary Flank Fold Flaps

While the elbow/axillary flank fold flaps can be considered subdermal plexus flaps [42], they both can be based on arterial vessels as well (lateral thoracic artery for the elbow fold, and deep circumflex iliac artery for the flank fold) therefore they can function as APFs too [43–45]. The skin in these areas is incised to create a "U"-shaped flap which is attached to the chest [44] or inguinal region (Figures 16.35 and 16.36). For the axillary and flank flaps, the skin can then be rotated into wounds overlying the lateral chest or sternum and inguinal region, ventral abdomen, or lateral thigh, respectively. In most cases, closure of medium-large skin defects can be attained without undue tension or limitation of range of motion to the adjacent limb.

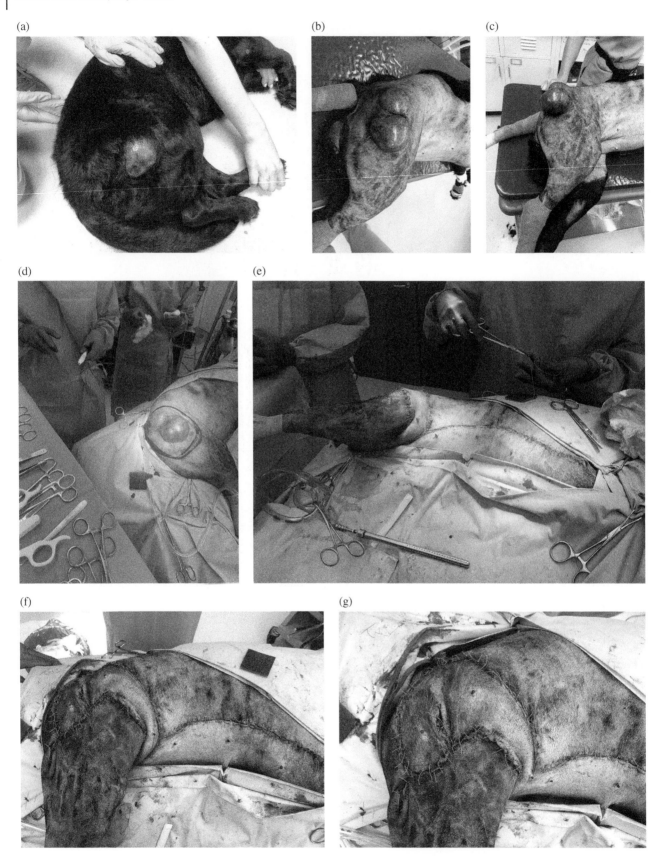

Figure 16.34   Photographs of a Caudal Superficial Epigastric flap used in a Labrador retriever after resection of a grade 2 soft tissue sarcoma from the lateral aspect of the right pelvic limb. (a) Preoperative view during initial consult, (b,c) after clipping the full extent of the mass is visible, (d) wide margins are incised around the primary tumor, (e) abdominal closure, (f) view of caudal rotation of flap – a bridge incision was made to connect the resection site and the flap to allow the edge to be sutured, (g) the flap has been folded in a gentle arc caudally to fill the circular resection site, (h,i) two weeks postoperatively, healed incisions. *Source:* Courtesy of Nicole Buote, DVM, DACVS.

(h)   (i)

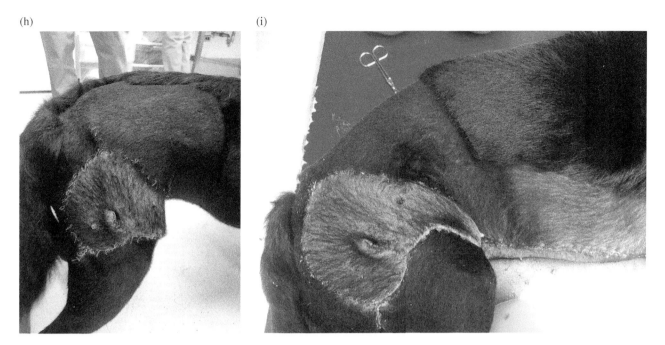

Figure 16.34   (Continued)

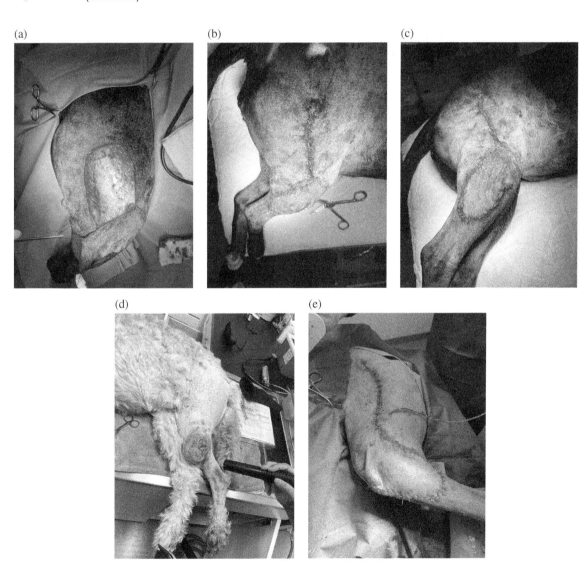

Figure 16.35   Photographs of genicular flaps. (a) Flap raised in patient after tumor resection on proximal lateral tibia region, (b) closure of donor site, (c) final appearance of flap rotated distally into wound bed. (d) Preoperative photograph of patient with large tumor over the lateral aspect of left pelvic limb distal to stifle, (e) postoperative appearance. *Source:* Courtesy of Dan Linden, DVM, DACVS, ACVS Fellow Surgical Oncology.

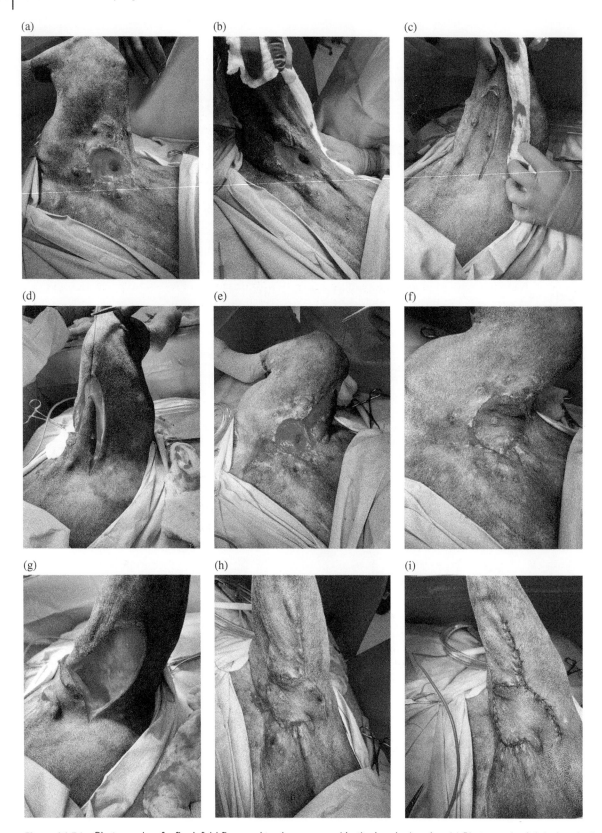

Figure 16.36 Photographs of a flank fold flap used to close a wound in the inguinal region. (a) Photograph of right inguinal wound, (b) medial incision along flank fold, (c) lateral incision along flank fold, (d) flap raised, a suture is used to manipulate the flap during dissection, (e) the tissue between the flap and the wound is incised to allow the flap to be rotated medially, (f) flap rotated into place, (g) view of donor site after flap rotation, (h) subcutaneous closure complete, (i) final closure. *Source:* Courtesy of Nicole Buote, DVM, DACVS.

Skin grafting techniques employ the relocation of a free segment of skin (full or partial thickness) to a distant location. These techniques are an especially useful option for wounds on distal extremities as many flaps do not easily reach those locations. Full-thickness free grafts include epidermis and dermis and have the advantage of including hair follicles. Partial thickness free grafts include epidermis but not the entire dermis which makes them excellent options for larger reconstructions (thorax, abdomen), and the donor site does not require closure. Skin grafts can be categorized as autografts (from the same animal), allografts (from the same species), and xenografts (from different species). Allografts and xenografts act as a primary contact layer and are not incorporated into the wound. Allografts are not used in clinical practice and xenografts are discussed in Chapter 8; therefore, autografts will be the focus of the following discussion.

Skin Graft Survival

Graft survival depends on multiple factors including recipient bed characteristics and free graft harvest technique and postoperative care (i.e., ingrowth of blood supply, fluid absorption/drainage, stability of the graft). In order for a graft to "take" or be incorporated into the recipient bed, revascularization must occur by the seventh to eighth day [3, 46]. Stages of graft healing are: (i) Fibrin adherence, (ii) Plasmatic imbibition, (iii) Inosculation, (iv) Revascularization.

Stages of Healing

Fibrin Adherence
The graft originally adheres to the recipient bed by fibrin contraction. Fibrous tissue is formed by invasion of fibroblasts and white blood cells. Over the first 10 days, as more fibrous tissue is created, a strong adhesion forms. It is during this time frame that graft-recipient bed contact is crucial. If any irregularities in the recipient bed are present (divits, holes, irregular surfaces), techniques such as a negative pressure wound bandage (NPWB) should be considered. In the author's practice, a NPWB is placed over every free skin graft for a minimum of four days without being changed to increase the chance of graft uptake. The use of soft padded bandages with or without splints to immobilize a limb is commonly used but special attention must be paid that these bandages are cared for properly. If bandages slip, are too tight, or become wet, the underlying graft can become irrevocably damaged.

Plasmatic Imbibition
Plasmatic Imbibition describes the capillary action that pulls a serum-like fluid and cells from the recipient bed into the dilated vessels of the free graft. This is the first type of nutrition the graft receives from the wound bed. This fluid is free of fibrinogen but contains hemoglobin which gives the free graft its typical blue–purple color during this phase. The fluid absorption can lead to edema of the tissue for the first 72 hours until venous and lymphatic drainage begins to improve. As this process is easily arrested if the graft is manipulated off the recipient bed, the author does not change the bandage overlying a graft for the first four days regardless of bandage type.

Inosculation
The next phase includes anastomosis of the free graft vessels and vessels of the same size in the wound bed (inosculation). This begins shortly after graft placement (day 1 postoperatively) but it is a slow process requiring anastomoses to form between previously severed vessels over the course of a week. Initially, blood flow is slow but this normalizes by the sixth day.

Revascularization
New vessels from endothelial sprouting from the recipient bed may also revascularize the free graft starting within 48–72 hours after graft placement. Over time, vessels differentiate into venules, arterioles, and lymphatics and by day 5 lymphatic drainage begins.

Recipient Bed Factors

The recipient bed must be appropriate for skin grafts to become incorporated. They must be free of debris or infection and have an adequate blood supply. Healthy granulation tissue, muscle, periosteum, or peritenon can support free skin grafts. Bone, cartilage and avascular fat, and infected or damaged tissue cannot support free skin grafts. Even chronic or hypertrophic (proud) granulation tissue cannot incorporate free skin grafts and should be excised. Regardless of the recipient site tissue type, gentle debridement immediately before graft placement should be performed by rubbing gauze or a #10 blade over the surface to encourage a mild amount of bleeding and freshen the edges of the wound.

Free Graft Harvest Techniques

Free grafts can be divided into full-thickness grafts and split-thickness grafts. Full-thickness grafts have the benefit of including hair follicles therefore cosmesis is improved. Hair growth is not guaranteed as the hair follicles may be damaged during graft preparation but, when possible, usually is seen within three weeks of grafting. The healed skin is more durable as it is inherently thicker. The disadvantage to full-thickness grafts lies in the necessity to create a new wound (donor site) which needs to be closed, increasing morbidity. Split-thickness wounds can be taken over a wide area but are less durable and still create morbidity at the donor sites. Hair growth at split-thickness donor sites is also variable depending on the depth of the removed graft [47]. While either type of graft can be placed as a sheet or a mesh graft, mesh grafts are more commonly employed. Mesh grafts allow for improved drainage, conformability to the wound bed and can expand over the wound site.

Full-Thickness Mesh Graft Technique

Creating a template of the wound bed to be covered is recommended and can be achieved with sterile glove packaging or drape material. Once the margins of donor tissue are marked, the skin is harvested removing as little subcutaneous fat as possible. This sheet graft can be meshed with a specific meshing tool or more commonly by hand. The degree of expansion is directly related to the length of the slits created but the graft will shorten in the plane perpendicular to the slits. Freehand meshing is easily performed by attaching the harvested sheet graft to a piece of sterile cardboard, pack of lap pads, or a roll of adhesive bandage material with skin staples or needles (Figure 16.37). Subcutaneous tissue is meticulously removed with fine scissors or a blade until hair follicles can be seen. Slits are then created in the sheet graft with a #15 blade approximately 5–15 mm long and 4–6 mm apart oriented in staggered rows [46].

The cosmetic appearance can be good with full-thickness mesh grafts depending on survival. Some references report a survival of up to 80–100% when grafts are applied appropriately and managed correctly [46, 48, 49] but in the authors' experience graft survival of 60–70% is more commonly appreciated.

Split-Thickness Skin Grafts

Split-thickness grafts require the use of a dermatome in most cases. Thin-skinned patients, especially cats, are not good candidates for split-thickness grafts. Certain areas of the body are more amenable to split-thickness harvesting because there are wide flat donor sites (chest, dorsum, lateral thigh) but the elasticity of the skin can make harvesting more difficult in certain regions (chest, abdomen). If using a dermatome, the skin can be lubricated with sterile water-soluble gel applied directly to the surface. Sterile saline can also be injected under the donor skin site to help elevate the skin to make harvesting easier. A #10 blade is used to make a partial thickness incision perpendicular to the skin surface. The skin is pulled taut and then fed into the modified razor of the dermatome. Stay sutures can be placed at the edge of the graft to apply constant traction while pushing the dermatome forward.

Split-thickness grafts have been extensively researched in humans and equine patients, but no prospective comparative studies exist on their use in small animal clinical patients. Concerns in human patients include chronic pain at the donor and recipient site, itch and dryness at the donor site, dysregulation of sensation and scarring [47, 50]. While cosmesis is not a concern to our animal patients, pain and sensory issues should be considered when contemplating these grafts.

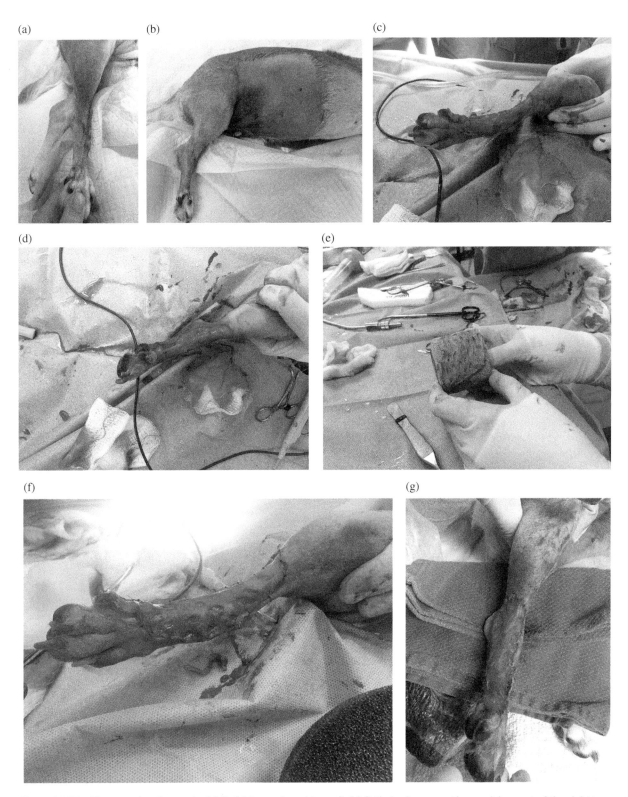

Figure 16.37 Photographs of a meshed full-thickness free skin graft. (a) Pathologic scar on the cranial aspect of the right tarsus after a wound was allowed to heal by second intention. The patient was lame on this limb and had decreased range of motion to the tarsal joint. (b) Preoperative preparation of the limb and the donor site on the right lateral abdomen. (c,d) Dorsal and lateral views after resection of the scar tissue. (e) The graft has been placed on a roll of adhesive wrap with staples and the subcutaneous tissue removed. Incisions have been made in a staggered orientation. (f) Meshed graft sutured in place. (g) Five days postoperatively – note black discoloration to a small portion of the distomedial aspect of the graft, the rest of the graft looks adhered and well-incorporated. *Source:* Courtesy of Nicole Buote, DVM, DACVS.

Graft Placement and Donor Site Management

Once the graft is harvested, and meshed if applicable, it should be placed in the recipient bed with the hair growth oriented in the same direction as the adjacent skin. It is also recommended that the slits in meshed grafts are placed parallel to the lines of tension in the recipient bed. It is typical to overlap the wound edges with graft by ~2 mm and to anchor the graft with simple interrupted monofilament absorbable sutures. The author will place a non-adherent dressing (Adaptic™) with an additional thin layer of triple antibiotic ointment applied to the dressing over the graft as the contact layer. The secondary layer is either a NPWB (preferred) or an absorbent hydrophilic foam or dry gauze to soak up any exudate produced during the healing process. A tie-over or soft padded bandage is then applied to aid in immobilization of the skin graft. The donor site of a full-thickness graft must be primarily closed or treated as an open wound to heal by second intention. The donor site of a split-thickness graft should be covered with hydrogel and a hydrocolloid dressing to encourage healing.

Postoperative Care

While some texts recommend performing the first bandage change 24–48 hours after surgery, the author usually waits four to five days to decrease the chance of iatrogenic damage to the fragile graft-wound bed ecosystem. With the advent of NPWB, the chances of a seroma or hematoma under the graft are much lower due to the effective suction of this bandage therefore the need to check grafts earlier is decreased (Figure 16.38) [51]. If a traditional soft padded bandage or tie-over is applied and fluid is seen under the graft, an incision should be made to allow drainage or aspiration so that the graft can sit flush against the recipient bed.

While grafts are usually pale initially, they will change color over time as they become vascularized. It should be expected that the graft will appear blue–purple if checked at the three to four day period due to revascularization process – this is not detrimental congestion or necrosis (Figure 16.39). By the end of the first week, a reddish hue should be appreciated if the graft is integrating appropriately. Areas that remain white or gray or black are avascular and will eventually slough. It is not usually necessary to sharply debride this tissue as it is removed during bandage changes by gentle cleaning. Any overlapping tissue will necrose and scab but this can be gently cleaned away once the graft is healed (Figure 16.38). Bandages should be changed as infrequently as possible (usually once per week for three to four weeks) because every bandage change can create trauma to the underlying graft [52].

(a) (b) (c)

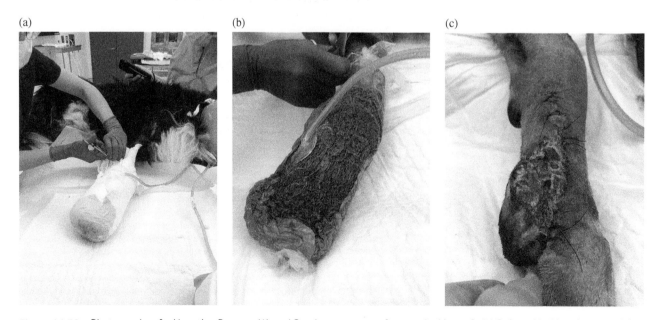

Figure 16.38   Photographs of a Negative Pressure Wound Bandage on a paw-free mesh skin graft. (a) Soft padded bandage overlying the vacuum bandage to help with immobilization, (b) NPWB, (c) appearance of graft four days post-placement – note the purplish color to the majority of the central graft with a white rim of tissue at the very edge where the graft overlapped the wound bed. *Source:* Courtesy of Nicole Buote, DVM, DACVS.

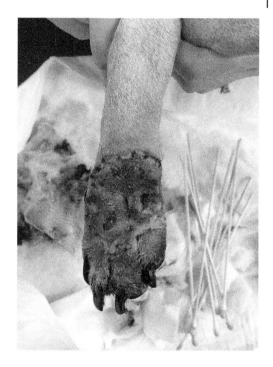

Figure 16.39 Photograph of full thickness free mesh graft six days post-placement. Note the congestion in the center of the graft as revascularization slowly begins – this can be normal for this point in graft healing. Distally there is evidence of necrosis of the overlapped tissue. *Source:* Courtesy of Nicole Buote, DVM, DACVS.

Complications and Considerations

Complications with skin graft uptake occur due to one or more of the following causes: fluid accumulation under the graft, movement of the graft, tension on the graft, and infection. Fluid accumulation under the graft prevents inosculation and revascularization and is one of the most common reasons for graft failure. Meshed grafts allow for fluid drainage but the benefit of a NPWB cannot be overstated with regards to this specific graft consideration [51]. Movement of the graft also disrupts adherence, nutritional transport, inosculation, and revascularization. Movement can also create trauma leading to hematoma or seroma formation. Movement of the graft is most commonly caused by a slipping bandage and an overly active patient. NPWB is also highly effective at adhering the graft to the underlying recipient site therefore movement of the graft is unlikely. Tension on the graft is created if the graft becomes adhered to overlying bandage material. This would lead to inadvertent removal of the graft when the bandage is changed. This can be avoided by placing non-adherent dressings over the graft and meticulous care during bandage changes. While infection is not common if appropriate recipient site preparation is performed, it does happen occasionally. Bacteria may interfere with the fibrin adherence of the graft (via plasminogen activators and proteolytic enzymes) as well as produce wound exudate that separates the graft from the wound bed. Pseudomonas infections can be especially damaging as those bacteria also produce elastase which breaks down elastin which is necessary for graft adherence [3, 46].

A long-term consideration of skin grafts is sensory dysregulation at the recipient site. Reinnervation of skin grafts depends on many factors including the type of graft (full-thickness versus split-thickness), amount of graft uptake, and the innervation of the recipient site. Sensation is greater in full-thickness grafts compared to split-thickness grafts but homogeneity of sensation across a graft is not guaranteed. It is important to remember that reinnervation starts at the margins of the wound bed/graft and that pain is the first sensation to return to the grafted tissue. Following pain, the next sensation to return is touch and then temperature perception [3, 46]. The author has unfortunately seen patients with chronic sensory dysregulation at graft recipient sites manifesting as chronic self-harm (licking or biting). These patients required topical treatments (lidocaine cream), oral pain medications (gabapentin, amantadine), or in one case surgical denervation.

References

1 Pavletic, M.M. (2018). *Atlas of Small Animal Wound Management and Reconstructive Surgery*, 4e. Hoboken, NJ: Wiley.

2 Kirpensteijn, J. and ter Haar, G. (2013). *Reconstructive Surgery and Wound Management of the Dog and Cat*. London: Mason Publishing.

3 Fossum, T.W. (2019). Surgery of the integumentary. In: *Small Animal Surgery*, 5e (ed. T.W. Fossum), 179–265. Philadelphia, PA: Elsevier.

4 Johnston, S.A. and Tobias, K.M. (2018). *Veterinary Surgery: Small Animal Expert Consult*, 2e. St. Louis, MO: Elsevier.

5 Silverman, E.B., Read, R.W., Boyle, C.R. et al. (2007). Histologic comparison of canine skin biopsies collected using monopolar electrosurgery, CO_2 laser, radiowave radiosurgery, skin biopsy punch, and scalpel. *Vet. Surg.* 36 (1): 50–56.

6 Scott, J.E., Swanson, E.A., Cooley, J. et al. (2017). Healing of canine skin incisions made with monopolar electrosurgery versus scalpel blade. *Vet. Surg.* 46 (4): 520–529.

7 Mison, M.B., Steficek, B., Lavagnino, M. et al. (2003). Comparison of the effects of the CO_2 surgical laser and conventional surgical techniques on healing and wound tensile strength of skin flaps in the dog. *Vet. Surg.* 32 (2): 153–160.

8 Gelman, C.L., Barroso, E.G., Britton, C.T. et al. (1994). The effect of lasers, electrocautery, and sharp dissection on cutaneous flaps. *Plast. Reconstr. Surg.* 94 (6): 829–833.

9 Gupta, S., Mohapatra, D.P., Chittoria, R.K. et al. (2018). Innovative skin hook. *J. Cutan. Aesthet. Surg.* 11 (3): 148–149.

10 Hedlund, C. (2007). Surgery of the integumentary system. In: *Small Animal Surgery*, 3e (ed. T.W. Fossum), 159–259. St Louis, MO: Elsevier.

11 Williams, J.M. and Fowler, D. (1999). Preface. In: *Manual of Canine and Feline Wound Management and Reconstruction* (ed. D. Fowler and J.M. Williams), 3. London: British Small Animal Veterinary Association.

12 Irwin, D.H. (1966). Tension lines in the skin of the dog. *J. Small Anim. Pract.* 7 (9): 593–598.

13 Boothe, H.W. (2018). Instrument and tissue handling techniques. In: *Veterinary Surgery: Small Animal Expert Consult*, 2e (ed. S.A. Johnston and K.M. Tobias), 225–238. St. Louis, MO: Elsevier.

14 Baker, K.P. (1967). Senile changes of dog skin. *J. Small Anim. Pract.* 8 (1): 49–54.

15 Pavletic, M.M. (2018). The skin. In: *Atlas of Small Animal Wound Management and Reconstructive Surgery*, 4e (ed. M.M. Pavletic), 1–15. Hoboken, NJ: Wiley.

16 Deroy, C., Destrade, M., Mc Alinden, A., and Ní, A.A. (2017). Non-invasive evaluation of skin tension lines with elastic waves. *Skin Res. Technol.* 23 (3): 326–335.

17 de Lahunta, A. and Evans, H.E. (2013). The integument. In: *Miller's Anatomy of the Dog*, 4e (ed. H.E. Evans and A. de Lahunta), 61–80. St. Louis, MO: Saunders/Elsevier.

18 Chen, D.L., Carlson, E.O., Fathi, R., and Brown, M.R. (2015). Undermining and hemostasis. *Dermatol. Surg.* 41 (Suppl 10): S201–S215. https://doi.org/10.1097/DSS.0000000000000489.

19 Johnston, D.E. (1990). Tension-relieving techniques. *Vet. Clin. North Am. Small Anim. Pract.* 20 (1): 67–80.

20 Stanley, B.J. (2018). Tension relieving techniques. In: *Veterinary Surgery: Small Animal Expert Consult*, 2e (ed. S.A. Johnston and K.M. Tobias), 1422–1446. Louis, MO: Elsevier.

21 Pavletic, M.M. (2018). Tension-relieving techniques. In: *Atlas of Small Animal Wound Management and Reconstructive Surgery*, 4e (ed. M.M. Pavletic), 265–322. Hoboken, NJ: Wiley.

22 Topaz, M., Carmel, N.N., Topaz, G. et al. (2014). Stress-relaxation and tension relief system for immediate primary closure of large and huge soft tissue defects: an old-new concept: new concept for direct closure of large defects. *Medicine* 93 (28): e234. https://doi.org/10.1097/MD.0000000000000234.

23 Song, A.H. and Tobias, K.M. (2017). Tensioning suture for open wounds. *Clinician's Brief* 33–38.

24 Tsioli, V., Papazoglou, L.G., Papaioannou, N. et al. (2015). Comparison of three skin-stretching devices for closing skin defects on the limbs of dogs. *J. Vet. Sci.* 16 (1): 99–106.

25 Pavletic, M.M. (2000). Use of an external skin-stretching device for wound closure in dogs and cats. *J. Am. Vet. Med. Assoc.* 217 (3): 350–354, 339.

26 Field, E.J., Kelly, G., Pleuvry, D. et al. (2015). Indications, outcome and complications with axial pattern skin flaps in dogs and cats: 73 cases. *J. Small Anim. Pract.* 56 (12): 698–706.

27 Katarwala, K.R. and Buote, N.J. (2022). The use of a caudal auricular axial pattern flap for repair of a degloving pinna wound in a dog. *Can. Vet. J.* 63 (3): 275–280.

28 Proot, J.L.J., Jeffery, N., Culp, W.T.N. et al. (2019). Is the caudal auricular axial pattern flap robust? A multi-centre cohort study of 16 dogs and 12 cats (2005 to 2016). *J. Small Anim. Pract.* 60 (2): 102–106.

29 Del Magno, S., Giuseppe, P., Pisani, G. et al. (2020). Caudal auricular axial pattern flap for the reconstruction of the upper eyelid in three cats. *J. Am. Anim. Hosp. Assoc.* 56 (4): 236–241.

30 de la Puerta, B., Buracco, P., Ladlow, J. et al. (2021). Superficial temporal axial pattern flap for facial reconstruction of skin defects in dogs and cats. *J. Small Anim. Pract.* 62 (11): 984–991.

31 Warlaw, J.L. and Lanz, O.I. (2018). Axial pattern and myocutaneous flap. In: *Veterinary Surgery: Small Animal Expert Consult*, 2e (ed. S.A. Johnston and K.M. Tobias), 1457–1473. St. Louis, MO: Elsevier.

32 Albernaz, V.G.P., Oblak, M.L., and Quitzan, J.G. (2021). Angularis oris axial pattern flap as a reliable and versatile option for rostral facial reconstruction in cats. *Vet. Surg.* 50 (8): 1688–1695.

33 Guzu, M., Rossetti, D., and Hennet, P.R. (2021). Locoregional flap reconstruction following oromaxillofacial oncologic surgery in dogs and cats: a review and decisional algorithm. *Front. Vet. Sci.* 21 (8): 685036. https://doi.org/10.3389/fvets.2021.685036.

34 Nakahara, N., Mitchell, K., Straw, R., and Kung, M. (2020). Hard palate defect repair by using haired angularis oris axial pattern flaps in dogs. *Vet. Surg.* 49 (6): 1195–1202.

35 Lascelles, B.D. and White, R.A. (2001). Combined omental pedicle grafts and thoracodorsal axial pattern flaps for the reconstruction of chronic, nonhealing axillary wounds in cats. *Vet. Surg.* 30 (4): 380–385.

36 Forster, K., Cutando, L.S., Ladlow, J. et al. (2022). Outcome of caudal superficial epigastric axial pattern flaps in dogs and cats: 70 cases (2007-2020). *J. Small Anim. Pract.* 63 (2): 128–135.

37 Remedios, A.M., Bauer, M.S., and Bowen, C.V. (1989). Thoracodorsal and caudal superficial epigastric axial pattern skin flaps in cats. *Vet. Surg.* 18 (5): 380–385.

38 Aper, R.L. and Smeak, D.D. (2005). Clinical evaluation of caudal superficial epigastric axial pattern flap reconstruction of skin defects in 10 dogs (1989-2001). *J. Am. Anim. Hosp. Assoc.* 41 (3): 185–192.

39 Murdoch, A.P., Greenaway, S.N., Owen, L.J., and Danielski, A. (2016). Murdoch evaluation of an axial pattern flap based on the cranial cutaneous branch of the saphenous artery: a cadaveric perfusion study. *Vet. Surg.* 45 (7): 922–928.

40 Ober, C., Milgram, J., McCartney, W. et al. (2019). Ober evaluation of a genicular axial pattern flap to repair large cutaneous tibial defects in two dogs. *BMC Vet. Res.* 15 (1): 158.

41 Emmerson, T., de la Puerta, B., and Polton, G. (2019). Genicular artery axial pattern flap for reconstruction of skin defects in 22 dogs. *J. Small Anim. Pract.* 60 (9): 529–533.

42 Jones, C.A. and Lipscomb, V.J. (2019). Indications, complications, and outcomes associated with subdermal plexus skin flap procedures in dogs and cats: 92 cases (2000-2017). *J. Am. Vet. Med. Assoc.* 255 (8): 933–938.

43 Hunt, G.B. (1995). Skin fold advancement flaps for closing large sternal and inguinal wounds in cats and dogs. *Vet. Surg.* 24 (2): 172–175.

44 Brinkley, C.H. (2007). Successful closure of feline axillary wounds by reconstruction of the elbow skin fold. *J. Small Anim. Pract.* 48 (2): 111–115.

45 Nevill, B.G. (2010). Bilateral axillary skin fold flaps used for dorsal thoracic skin wound closure in a dog. *J. S. Afr. Vet. Assoc.* 81 (1): 58–61.

46 Bohling, M.W. and Swaim, S.F. (2018). Skin Grafts. In: *Veterinary Surgery: Small Animal Expert Consult*, 2e (ed. S.A. Johnston and K.M. Tobias), 1473–1494. St. Louis, MO: Elsevier.

47 Burnett, L.N., Carr, E., Tapp, D. et al. (2014). Patient experiences living with split thickness skin grafts. *Burns* 40 (6): 1097–1105.

48 Bonaventura, N.C. and Ganjei, J.B. (2021). Comparison of outcomes for single-session and delayed full-thickness applications of meshed skin grafts used to close skin defects after excision of tumors on the distal aspects of the limbs in dogs. *J. Am. Vet. Med. Assoc.* 258 (4): 387–394.

49 Brown, Y., Cinti, F., Mattioli, V., and Pisani, G. (2021). Single, large, meshed full-thickness free skin graft for reconstruction of a dorsal lumbosacral wound defect in a dog. *J. Am. Vet. Med. Assoc.* 259 (12): 1441–1445.

50 Sinha, S., Schreiner, A.J., Biernaskie, J. et al. (2017). Treating pain on skin graft donor sites: review and clinical recommendations. *J. Trauma Acute Care Surg.* 83 (5): 954–964.

51 Stanley, B.J., Pitt, K.A., Weder, C.D. et al. (2013). Effects of negative pressure wound therapy on healing of free full-thickness skin grafts in dogs. *Vet. Surg.* 42 (5): 511–522.

52 Pavletic, M.M. (2014). Skin grafting techniques. In: *Current Techniques in Small Animal Surgery*, 5e (ed. M.J. Bojrab, D.R. Waldron, and T.P. Toombs), 595–614. Jackson, WY: Teton New Media.

17

Specific Wounds

Subsection A: Bite Wounds – A Case Study

Nicole J. Buote

Department of Clinical Sciences, Cornell University, Ithaca, NY, USA

Presenting Signs

A 14-year-old female spayed beagle was presented after a housemate attacked her in her home earlier in the day. The owner had recently adopted the other dog and had left them alone for multiple hours only to come home and find the patient bleeding. The patient was deaf and had poor eyesight but had no other major medical concerns and was not on any medications.

Examination and Initial Wound Characteristics

Physical exam was unremarkable except for age-related changes (nuclear sclerosis OU, moderate dental disease) and multiple bite wounds to the right caudal thigh and dorsum. The wounds were actively oozing and ranged in size from 0.5 to 2 cm in length. There was significant pocketing and communication between the largest dorsum wound and the caudal thigh wound.

Diagnostics

Point of care blood work (venous blood gas) was unremarkable. An AFAST and TFAST revealed not free fluid or abnormalities and pulse oximetry was 94% on room air. Other diagnostics:

Lactate = 2.3
PCV = 38
TP = 5.4
Azo = 5–15
urine specific gravity = 1.028
creatinine = 0.8 mg/dl.

Initial Therapy and Procedure

The patient was provided a methadone injection (0.2 mg/kg IV), Plasmalyte IV fluid bolus at 10 ml/kg over 30 minutes, and then began on a continuous rate of 60 ml/kg/day. The patient was induced with ketamine (2 mg/kg IV) and Propofol to effect IV and the wounds were clipped and cleaned with chlorhexidine scrub and saline. A laceration repair was performed

Techniques in Small Animal Wound Management, First Edition. Edited by Nicole J. Buote.
© 2024 John Wiley & Sons, Inc. Published 2024 by John Wiley & Sons, Inc.
Companion website: www.wiley.com/go/buote/wounds

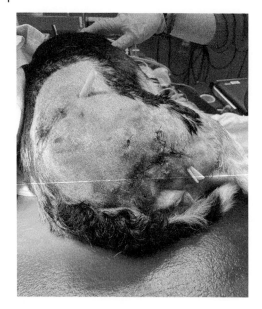

Figure 17.A.1 Photograph of patient on the night of presentation after wounds to the dorsum and right thigh have been clipped, cleaned, and primarily sutured with Penrose drains placed. *Source:* Courtesy of Nicole Buote, DVM, DACVS.

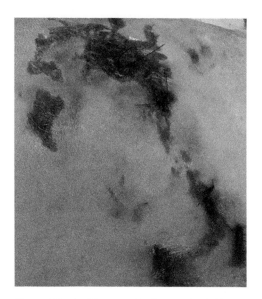

Figure 17.A.2 Photograph of necrosis of skin at previous wound sites when patient represented three days after initial closure for drain removal. *Source:* Courtesy of Nicole Buote, DVM, DACVS.

after copious lavage with sterile saline. The edges of the wound were apposed in one layer with 2-0 Nylon cruciate and Penrose drains were placed (Figure 17.A.1). The patient was given an injection of Convenia (8 mg/kg SQ) and sent home the same day on Carprofen (2.2 mg/kg PO BID), Gabapentin (15 mg/kg PO TID), and Trazodone (6 mg/kg PO TID).

Follow-up Bandage Care

The patient returned for drain removal and evaluation three days later and necrosis of the skin and purulent material was visible at all the previous closure sites (Figure 17.A.2). The patient was booked into the hospital and transferred to the surgery service for debridement and wound management. The patient was placed under general anesthesia and all necrotic skin was sharply debrided. A deep tissue sample was taken for aerobic and anaerobic culture. Tie-over bandages with honey as the primary contact layer and lap sponges were applied. Ampicillin/sulbactam was initiated at this time. Daily bandage changes occurred over the following two days. At each bandage change, any necrotic tissue visualized within the wounds was sharply dissected but wound edges were not freshened or resected unless black/gray (Figure 17.A.3). On the third hospitalized day, the granulation present appeared pale pink and the decision was made to switch to a calcium alginate dressing (Figures 17.A.4, 17.A.5, 17.A.6). The wounds were highly exudative, and the patient required sedation for daily bandage changes. It was also noted that moderate to severe pitting edema was present in the right hind leg so massage with warm-packing was instituted every six hours. The patient was eating small amounts, so a liquid protein diet (Royal Canin Recovery) was added to her daily meals.

The recommendation was to apply a negative pressure wound bandage (NPWB) due to the size of the wounds, the amount of exudate produced, and the slow progress of granulation tissue formation and contraction (see Chapter 10 for more information). On day 5 of hospitalization, a NPWB was placed. The patient was placed on general anesthesia and the wounds were flushed copiously with sterile saline. Any discolored or necrotic tissue was debrided. Sterile sliver-impregnated open-cell foam was cut to size for both wounds and sutured to the wound edges with 2-0 Nylon (simple interrupted sutures). The dorsal piece of foam was placed into the deep connecting defect between the two wounds to ensure suction of exudate would occur. Stoma paste was placed around the circumference of the wound to help create a seal when the clear the occlusive dressing was placed over the foam (Figures 17.A.7, 17.A.8). A "Y" connector was used to connect two individual suction pads (one placed over each wound) to the same suction unit (KCI V.A.C. Freedom™, 3M Medical). The NPWB was programmed for continuous suction at a pressure of 125 mmHg and was left in place for 48 hours. The plan was to reevaluate the wounds in two days and determine whether reapplication of a NPWB or closure was indicated. Due to the size of the defects and the patient's lack of skin elasticity, reconstructive techniques such as rotation flaps were considered highly likely. On Day 6, the initial culture results revealed a methicillin-resistant *Staphylococcus intermedius, Enterococcus gallinarum,* and *Klebsiella pneumoniae* infection. The only appropriate antibiotic was chloramphenicol which was initiated.

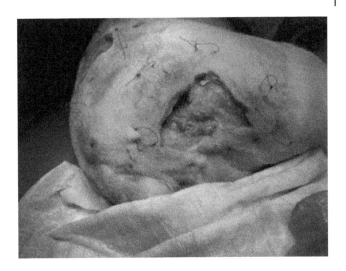

Figure 17.A.3   Photograph of caudal thigh wound after two days of honey-impregnated bandages. The granulation tissue is pale and there is no evidence of contraction or epithelialization of the wound edges. *Source:* Courtesy of Nicole Buote, DVM, DACVS.

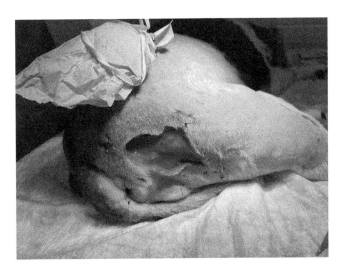

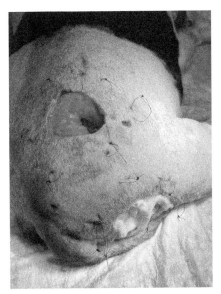

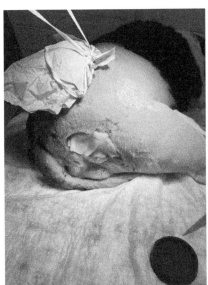

Figures 17.A.4, 17.A.5, 17.A.6   Photographs of the wounds after one day of calcium alginate dressing. The granulation tissue in both the perineal (17.A.4) and the dorsum wound (17.A.5) is a healthier dark pink/red color, and the edges are starting to adhere to the underlying tissue. The calcium alginate dressing seen in Figures 17.A.5 and 17.A.6 is similar to a felt pad which will absorb wound exudate to create a gel. Tie-over bandages with sterile lap sponges were placed over each wound. *Source:* Courtesy of Nicole Buote, DVM, DACVS.

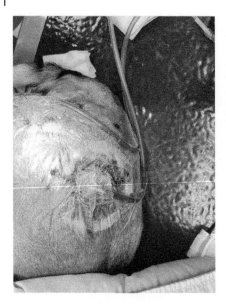

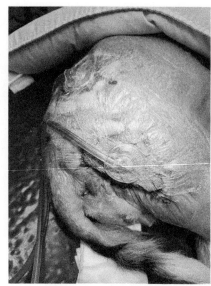

Figures 17.A.7, 17.A.8 Photographs of the negative pressure wound bandage (NPWB) placed over the dorsum (17.A.7) and perineal wound (17.A.8). Yellow stoma paste can be seen on the skin around the edges of the wound to help seal the occlusive dressing. It is extremely important that the vacuum maintain pressure in order to reap the benefits of these bandages so liberal application of stoma paste should be considered especially in hard-to-bandage regions. *Source:* Courtesy of Nicole Buote, DVM, DACVS.

Surgical Procedure

On day 7 of hospitalization, the NPWB was removed under general anesthesia and the wounds were assessed. No ongoing tissue necrosis was identified, and the underlying granulation tissue was a deep healthy red (Figure 17.A.9). The patient was moved to an operating suite and the wounds were both primarily closed with rotational flaps (Figures 17.A.10, 17.A.11). The right thigh wound was closed using a flank fold flap rotated caudally into the wound (Figure 17.A.10, 17.A.11). An active suction (Jackson Pratt) drain was placed in the deep defect to remove wound fluid and aid in apposition of the skin to the underlying tissues.

Outcome

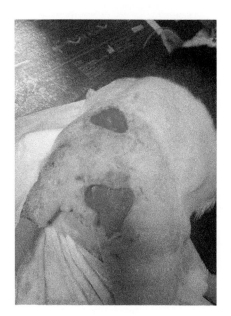

The patient recovered from surgery uneventfully and remained hospitalized for four more days until the drain was removed. On day 1, postoperatively distal necrosis of the flank fold flap began to show signs of venous congestion and mild dehiscence (Figure 17.A.12). The incision was cleaned and covered, and medicinal leech therapy was instituted for two days. Approximately 3 cm of the incision remained open to heal by second intention. The patient was sent home 12 days after hospitalization for bite wound complications. A recheck exam performed at the local veterinarian 14 days postoperatively revealed healed incisions.

Figure 17.A.9 Photograph of wounds on Day 7 of hospitalization. The granulation tissue is bright red and bled when the foam was removed. After only two days of the NPWB, the tissue was considered healthy enough for primary closure with rotation flaps. *Source:* Courtesy of Nicole Buote, DVM, DACVS.

Prognosis

The long-term prognosis for this patient is excellent once the skin is healed even with prolonged wound management.

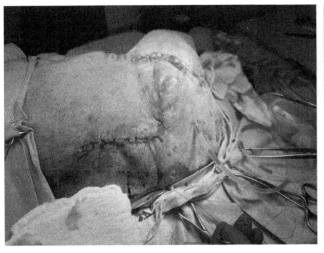
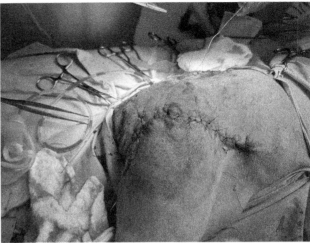

Figures 17.A.10, 17.A.11   Photographs of primary closure over a Jackson Pratt drain. Figure 17.A.10 – dorsal wound; Figure 17.A.11 – right caudal thigh wound. *Source:* Courtesy of Nicole Buote, DVM, DACVS.

Clinical Lessons

Many important lessons can be learned from this case as it highlights the complexity of bite wound management.

1. The initial closure was done outside of the "Golden Period" of six hours post-wounding therefor primary closure carries a higher risk of sealing in infection but

2. Many times, the full extent of the injuries is not visible on initial presentation ("tip of the mountain" analogy) therefore owners must be advised that bite wounds may require multiple evaluations and visits. The better the communication with the owner in the beginning, the smoother ongoing care for the patient will be.

3. Honey bandages have many advantages but in the face of a considerable exudate these attributes are diluted, and healing progress can stall. Pay attention to the color and texture of the granulation tissue and change the contact layer dressing based on the phase of healing and wound characteristics.

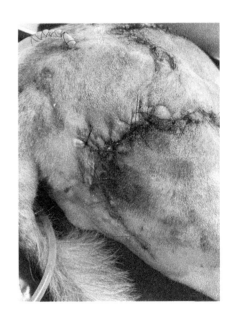

Figure 17.A.12   Photograph of minor dehiscence and venous congestion at the distal aspect of the flank fold flap used to close the right caudal thigh wound. *Source:* Courtesy of Nicole Buote, DVM, DACVS.

4. Negative pressure bandages are excellent for highly exudative wounds, wounds on difficult-to-bandage areas and wounds will unhealthy granulation tissue as they have effective suction, preserve a moist wound environment, and encourage angiogenesis.

5. Outcome references:

   a. Shamir, M.H., Leisner, S., Klement. E. et al. (2002). Dog bite wounds in dogs and cats: a retrospective study of 196 cases. *J. Vet. Med. A Physiol. Pathol. Clin. Med.* 49 (2):107–112.

   b. Klainbart, S., Shipov, A., Madhala, O. et al. (2022). Dog bite wounds in cats: a retrospective study of 72 cases. *J. Feline Med. Surg.* 24 (2):107–115. https://doi.org/10.1177/1098612X211010735. Epub 2021 May 13.

   c. Davros, A.M., Gregory, C.W., Cockrell, D.M., and Hall, K.E. (2023). Comparison of clinical outcomes in cases of blunt, penetrating, and combination trauma in dogs: A VetCOT registry study. *J. Vet. Emerg. Crit. Care (San Antonio).* 33 (1):74–80.

17

Specific Wounds

Subsection B: Penetrating Wounds
Galina Hayes

Department of Clinical Sciences, Cornell University, Ithaca, NY, USA

Clinical Presentation

Penetrating wounds represent a diverse population of clinical presentations sharing the common origin of an object piercing the tissue and causing injury to deeper underlying structures. Short-term morbidity is due to the immediate tissue disruption and damage with common sequela including hemorrhage, pneumothorax, or septic peritonitis when vasculature or internal organs are injured. Long-term morbidity can result if object fragments and debris such as hair or dirt are left behind in the wound tract. Thus, the surgical focus is not only on repairing the immediate injury but also on ensuring the complete removal of the penetrating object, or if this is no longer present then decontaminating the wound tract. Specific wound scenarios are discussed below.

Bite Wounds

Bite wounds after dog-on-dog attacks are a common clinical presentation. The external skin wounds can appear relatively minor and typically belie the severity of the deeper injury (Figure 17.B.1). Dogs can apply a bite force of over 3000N at the carnassial teeth [1], with a combination of both severe crush and shear. For dog-on-dog bite wounds over the thoracic cavity, 20% were found to have penetrated the thorax necessitating exploratory thoracotomy [2], while in dog-on-cat bites 36% of thoracic wounds penetrated the thoracic cavity [3]. Bite wounds positioned over a body cavity should be assumed to have entered that cavity with risk of damage to internal organs until proven otherwise. For penetrating bite wounds to the limbs, neck or dorsal musculature, the severe crush injury can result in devitalization of soft tissues that may take several days to fully manifest clinically (Figure 17.B.2) and require serial debridement before definitive repair and closure (Figure 17.B.3). Bite wounds in the cervical area can cause secondary laryngeal paralysis following injury to the recurrent laryngeal nerves.

Oropharyngeal Stick Injury

Oropharyngeal/esophageal stick injuries are frequently self-inflicted during play. Self-impalement via the mouth can occur while attempting to capture a stick at speed that has one end embedded in the ground, while injury can also occur during apparently routine chewing or carrying. The injury event may not be observed by owners. Clinical presentation can include gagging, ptyalism, the presence of blood within the saliva, pain around the oral cavity or neck, reluctance to eat, and in some cases cervical emphysema. Perforation can occur at the level of the oropharynx (66%) or esophagus (34%) [4]. Wood fragments are commonly retained in the wound tract and were found at surgery in 32% of dogs presenting with stick injury and radiographic cervical emphysema [4]. Morbidity and mortality are substantially higher when esophageal perforation occurs [4].

Techniques in Small Animal Wound Management, First Edition. Edited by Nicole J. Buote.
© 2024 John Wiley & Sons, Inc. Published 2024 by John Wiley & Sons, Inc.
Companion website: www.wiley.com/go/buote/wounds

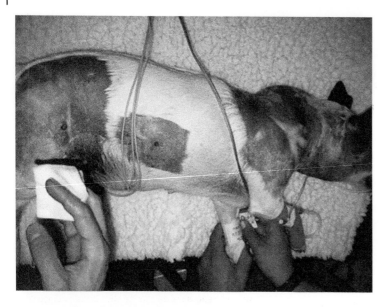

Figure 17.B.1 Bite wounds following a dog-on-dog attack- despite the relatively minor skin wounds, this dog had multiple rib fractures, a thoracic wall defect, and a lung perforation requiring lung lobectomy. *Source:* Courtesy of Galina Hayes, BVSc, DVSc, PhD, DACVECC, DACVS.

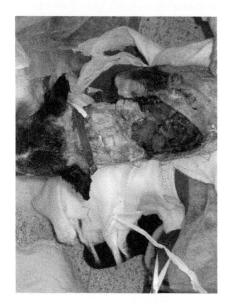

Figure 17.B.2 Progressive necrosis requiring serial debridement and open management of a dog-on-dog bite wound to the cervical area. *Source:* Courtesy of Galina Hayes, BVSc, DVSc, PhD, DACVECC, DACVS.

Gunshot Wounds

Penetrating gunshot wounds are relatively unusual in veterinary medicine but can be misdiagnosed as vehicular or bite trauma when the projectile is not retained in the wound tract. Gunshot wounds are over-represented in young, intact male dogs and hunting dogs (Figure 17.B.4) [5]. Injury severity is related to projectile velocity. High-velocity gunshot wounds to the thorax are frequently associated with tension pneumothorax [6]. In cats, 80% of projectile injuries result from airguns [7].

Porcupine Quills

Quill injuries frequently initiate around the muzzle and forelimbs (Figure 17.B.5). The quill structure consists of backward-pointing barbs that result in the migration of any embedded quills into deeper tissues. Quill injuries are more common in the spring and fall and are more likely to occur in large-breed dogs, with >20 quills typically embedded during a single incident [8]. In one study, 10.8% of dogs that received urgent treatment for a quilling incident went on to experience a complication [8]. Complications included abscess or cellulitis at the previous quilling site (68.8%), lameness due to periarticular or intra-articular migration (18.8%), and ocular injury (12.5%). Numerous other negative sequelae have been reported, including migration into the lung lobes with pneumothorax, cardiac migration with pericardial tamponade and valvular injury, intracranial migration, and migration through the organs of the abdominal cavity. As the migration is progressive and deep quills are challenging to detect and can be numerous, negative sequelae can take several months to fully manifest [9].

Impalement Injuries

The injury from impalement by arrows, stakes, knives, etc. depends on the site of entry, trajectory, and force of penetration as well as the shape and material of the object. Perforated vascular structures or viscus organs may be temporarily sealed by the continued presence of the penetrating object. Impalement wounds in dogs most commonly involve the head, neck, or cranial thorax as a result of running onto a stationary pointed object but can also occur from deer antlers or miscellaneous other objects [10]. As the entry wound can sometimes be small and hidden in fur, if the animal breaks off the penetrating object the owner may be unaware of the original injury (Figure 17.B.6). This can result in delayed presentation, in some cases for months. Reverse impalement injuries can also occur, in which an ingested foreign object, often a barbecue skewer, perforates the gastric or intestinal wall followed by the abdominal wall after traversing the abdominal cavity (Figure 17.B.7). Migration retrograde through the diaphragm with pulmonary or cardiac injury can also occur [11].

Triage and Imaging

In general terms, animals with penetrating wounds benefit from expeditious stabilization in the ER with early multidisciplinary consultation and a low threshold for urgent surgical intervention.

Bite Wounds

For penetrating bite wounds located over a body cavity radiographs and/or focused ultrasound should be performed, and findings assessed in the context of the physical exam and direct wound palpation. CT scan has higher sensitivity than radiographs for body wall penetration and internal organ injury. While imaging findings can assist with the decision-making regarding the need for abdominal or thoracic exploratory surgery, it should be recognized that negative thoracic radiographs are not always predictive of absence of thoracic penetration.

Oropharyngeal/Esophageal Stick Injury

Identification of the site of perforation requires careful examination under general anesthesia using a combination of direct visualization and endoscopy. CT scan is insensitive for identifying the perforation site in this context, although retained stick fragments may be detected with a sensitivity of 79% and specificity of 93% [12]. Ultrasound is unhelpful in the presence of cervical emphysema. Radiographs of the thoracic cavity are performed prior to endoscopy to assess for pneumothorax and/or pneumomediastinum. If either are present care should be taken with insufflation during subsequent esophagoscopy, with equipment and expertise available for rapid placement of a chest tube if necessary. A flexible gastroscope is used to assess the esophagus. If the soft or hard palate has been penetrated, then rhinoscopy using a rigid endoscope and irrigation will be useful to evaluate for retained stick fragments. The airway should be protected at all times due to the risk of aspiration of saliva/hemorrhage/esophageal or gastric contents. In the authors' experience, it is not uncommon to find oropharyngeal perforations dorsal or lateral to the upper esophageal sphincter, and these can be easily missed. Firm retraction of the larynx ventrally using a long-bladed laryngoscope may be necessary for visualization/ direct repair.

Gunshot Wounds

In the author's experience, in the urban setting dogs presenting emergently with gunshot wounds may be accompanied by emotionally volatile individuals with handguns – thus it may be prudent to prepare staff appropriately and notify local law enforcement early in the course of triage.

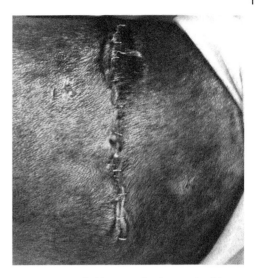

Figure 17.B.3 Dehiscence of a dog-on-dog bite wound treated six days prior with primary closure following thorough debridement and closed suction drain placement. Re-exploration of the wound found a substantial burden of additional necrotic tissue that had not yet declared non-viabilit at the initial surgery. *Source:* Courtesy of Galina Hayes, BVSc, DVSc, PhD, DACVECC, DACVS.

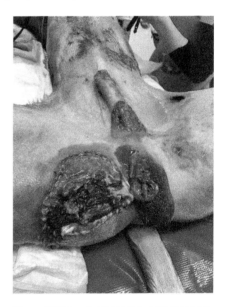

Figure 17.B.4 Accidental gunshot wound from a hunting rifle in a 3-year-old intact male large breed dog that was mistaken for a deer. The bullet entered the left flank fold with a through and through wound before grazing the ventral prepuce and hitting the right testicle with severance of the right testicular artery and exiting the right thigh. The arterial bleeding required prompt ligation on ER admission. Note the relatively small entry wound and large exit wound typical of hunting ammunition with a "mushrooming" projectile. *Source:* Courtesy of Galina Hayes, BVSc, DVSc, PhD, DACVECC, DACVS.

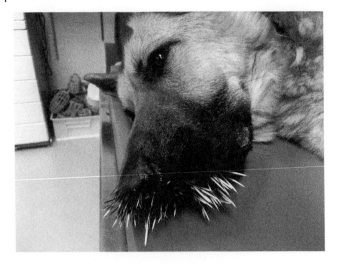

Figure 17.B.5 Image of a patient shortly after a quilling. This German shepherd attacked the porcupine and sustained hundreds of quills to the muzzle. The patient was sedated for meticulous quill removal. *Source:* Courtesy of Nathan Peterson, DVM, MS, DACVECC.

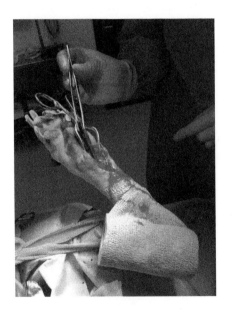

Figure 17.B.6 This substantial wood fragment was removed from a dog with a six-month history of recurrent interdigital ulceration and infection that was referred for fusion podoplasty. Ultrasound successfully identified the fragment deep to the flexor tendons. *Source:* Courtesy of Galina Hayes, BVSc, DVSc, PhD, DACVECC, DACVS.

Porcupine Quills

Early presentation for quill removal is associated with a reduced incidence of complications [8]. Radiographs are insensitive to detection of a migrating quill, although the consequences such as a pneumothorax or gas tract may be observed. Quills can be identified on CT scan, MRI scan, and ultrasound, although the relative sensitivity of each modality is unknown. If surgery is planned, the advanced imaging should be performed contemporaneously due to the potential for rapid migration.

Impalement Injuries

Where possible, it is preferable to leave the intra-corporeal component of the penetrating object in situ prior to definitive treatment (Figure 17.B.8). If the impaling object is too large to be moved or is unwieldy, it can be cut to either free the animal from it (wooden stakes) or shorten it for safer transport (arrows). Again, wherever possible the object should be stabilized relative to the patient. Maintaining the object in situ reduces the risk of widespread leakage of GI contents where intra-abdominal penetrations have occurred as well as reducing the risk of exsanguination for vascular penetrations. This approach also facilitates accurate identification and decontamination of the wound tract. Computed tomography (CT) scan can facilitate assessment of the trajectory of penetration. CT angiogram may be helpful for surgical planning if major vessels are implicated. In cases where it is unclear whether foreign material remains in the wound tract, CT scan is most accurate compared with magnetic resonance imaging (MRI) and ultrasound for detecting wooden foreign bodies in the canine manus [13], while ultrasound has greater sensitivity than CT or MRI for the detection of subcutaneous foreign bodies associated with chronic abscesses or draining tracts [14]. However, in the context of acutely retained wooden material the strong possibility of a false negative result based on CT scan should be considered – in a case series of acute trunk impalement by wooden objects, pre-operative CT failed to identify wood material that was subsequently found on surgical exploration in 4 of 11 cases [10].

Management Plans

General principles of penetrating wound management include systemic stabilization combined with expeditious administration of broad-spectrum antibiotics and surgical exploration of the wound tract where appropriate. Surgical goals include decontamination, debridement, and source control where necessary. Primary repair of injuries may be acute or delayed depending on context. Provision may be made for ongoing drainage or decompression of the injury site. In common with other traumatic wounds, penetrating wounds are considered contaminated at the point of injury – negative cultures likely reflect incomplete sensitivity of the test rather than wound sterility. Approximately 20% of traumatic wounds subsequently became infected despite appropriate antibiotic selection based on admission cultures in one study, and acute cultures were not predictive of the bacterial species in subsequent infections [15].

Bite Wounds

Bite wounds over the thoracic cavity require surgical exploration. When the thoracic cavity is penetrated, various surgical interventions may prove necessary, including placement of a chest tube, lung lobectomy, and restoration of thoracic wall integrity. For this reason, when exploration of a penetrating wound over the thoracic cavity is planned, there should be provision of equipment and expertise to convert quickly to positive pressure ventilation and exploratory thoracotomy if needed. This is typically performed via the wound site. Similarly for bite wounds over the abdomen, abdominal cavity penetration with injury to the internal organs may occur. This is typically accompanied by an increase in the volume of peritoneal fluid. When a high index of suspicion for abdominal cavity penetration is present, exploratory laparotomy is indicated. Due to the relative mobility of the abdominal

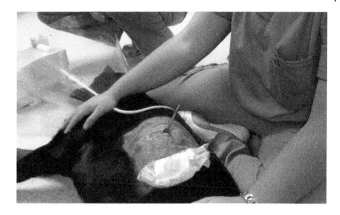

Figure 17.B.7 Dog presenting with an intra-gastric barbecue skewer which subsequently perforated the gastric wall, diaphragm, caudal mediastinum, and thoracic wall. The lung was not injured, although a pneumothorax was present secondary to the exit wound. *Source:* Courtesy of Galina Hayes, BVSc, DVSc, PhD, DACVECC, DACVS.

organs within the cavity, this is typically performed via midline approach. This allows both a full exploration to be performed and simplifies repair of the abdominal wall defect from the peritoneal surface. When contamination of the cavity with GI contents has occurred, a closed suction drain is placed following primary repair of the defects. Bite wounds by their nature are contaminated at the point of injury and merit coverage with broad-spectrum antibiotics. Clinical outcome was not improved by the addition of enrofloxacin to a single agent amoxicillin-clavulanic acid protocol [16].

Figure 17.B.8 (a and b) This dog impaled itself on a branch while running in the woods. The referring veterinarian attended to the patient at the scene to provide IV access, fluids, analgesia, and sedation as well as broad-spectrum antibiotic coverage which allowed the branch to be cut and the dog safely transported. Note the entry point in the right axilla and the exit site in the left perineum. *Source:* Courtesy of Tom Gibson, DVM, DACVS.

(a)

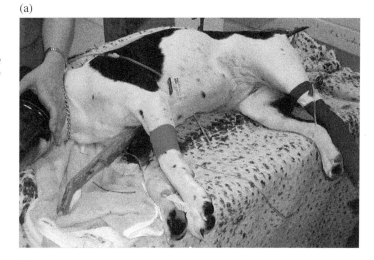

(b)

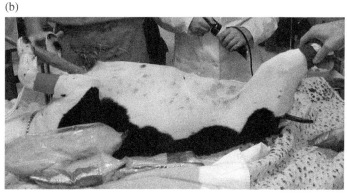

Oropharyngeal/Esophageal Stick Injury

For oropharyngeal penetrations, the defect is repaired at the level of the mucosa. When the soft palate is perforated, the oral surface of the defect can be enlarged if necessary to allow identification and primary closure of the nasopharyngeal mucosa. For hard palate penetrations, reconstruction options include buccal mucosal flaps, sliding palatal flaps, or angularis oris flaps depending on size and location. For wounds deep in the pharynx or at the level of the upper esophageal sphincter, the use of 4/0 V-loc suture on a small needle can be useful as it avoids the technical challenges associated with knotting suture in a small working space. As long as mucosal apposition can be achieved then oral feeding can be recommended.

Esophageal perforations are challenging to manage with a high complication rate, and a strong evidence base to guide treatment direction is lacking in companion animals. Based on the human patient experience, non-operative management can be considered for perforations characterized by the presence of a pneumomediastinum with no fluid accumulations combined with a swallow study using an iodine-based oral contrast medium (Gastrografin) that shows no contrast extravasation on CT or esophagogram. In this situation, all food and drink by mouth is avoided for five to seven days, and a gastrostomy tube is placed [17, 18]. For larger defects, rapid operative intervention is required to reduce the risk of progressive inflammation and tissue necrosis. Both endoscopic and open-surgical treatment options are available, with the choice of therapy largely dictated by the relative accessibility of the perforation site and the availability of local expertise and equipment. Endoscopic options include the placement of endoscopic clips when the mucosa appears healthy, or placement of temporary covered self-expanding metallic stents for two to four weeks combined with mediastinal and/or pleural decontamination and drainage and bypass feeding [17, 19]. There is a risk of premature stent migration, and the placement of suture anchors can be considered. If an open surgical procedure is performed, primary repair relies on the absence of diffuse necrosis. The mucosal defect is frequently longer than the defect in the overlying muscle layers, and myotomy cranial and caudal to the defect may be required to allow complete identification of the mucosal margin and closure. The esophageal defect is closed in two layers. A transoral bougie such as an orogastric tube may be useful to ensure that adequate esophageal diameter can be achieved if debridement has been necessary. The repair can be augmented with a vascularized tissue flap taken from the longus colli m., latissimus dorsi m., or diaphragm as dictated by location [4, 20].

Gunshot Wounds

In general, gunshot wounds should be approached and managed like any other penetrating wound, with judicious debridement of the wound tract and evaluation for injury to internal organs. As the metal fragments from projectile injuries can remain clinically silent for years after injury, the necessity for removal reflects a balance between location, clinical signs, and the surgical trauma involved.

Porcupine Quills

To avoid late and potentially serious complications due to deep quill migration, every effort should be made to remove all quills at the time of initial presentation. This may require the use of ultrasound to detect subcutaneous quills combined with surgical extraction. For animals with a delayed presentation indicating deep quill migration, whole-body advanced imaging may be prudent to evaluate for multiple quills causing both manifest and occult injury. Quills may be very difficult to locate by palpation alone or by advanced imaging. Locating quills during surgery may be aided by the use of intra-operative ultrasound and the author recommends its use in any case where deep tissues may be penetrated.

Impalement Injuries

Removal of the penetrating object is preferably performed under general anesthesia in the operating room under direct vision. For body cavity penetration, a median sternotomy or midline celiotomy or both are performed as needed (Figure 17.B.9). Endoscopic assistance may also be useful and facilitate a more focused surgical approach. The goals of surgery include the removal of the penetrating object without causing further injury followed by local debridement and decontamination, primary repair of injuries where necessary and provision for ongoing decompression or drainage particularly when the brain or spinal cord is involved. For large penetrating objects, segmental removal may be less traumatic, and provision should be made for appropriate cutting equipment to achieve this. When the object is no longer *in situ*, CT and if necessary, CT fistulograms, can assist with surgical planning.

Figure 17.B.9   (a and b) Images from a patient with a known penetrating injury. (a) Preoperative image after surgical preparatory clip. (b) Intraoperative image of retained wood fragment removed at surgical explore. The wood fragment was not identified on CT scan.

(a)
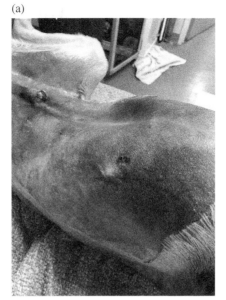

(b)
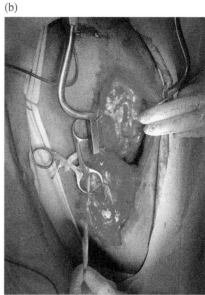

Prognosis

In general, the prognosis for penetrating wounds is good to excellent, although specific morbidity, mortality, and complication rates can be dependent on the type and the severity of the initial injury together with time since wounding. For 10,816 dogs presenting for penetrating trauma and recorded in the VetCOT registry between 2017 and 2019, a 96.5% survival rate was recorded [21]. For 54 dogs managed for truncal impalement, long-term survival was 90%, although major complications occurred in 11% [10]. In the context of oropharyngeal/esophageal stick injuries, the prognosis following esophageal perforation is relatively poor with a mortality of close to 50% reported, in contrast to 100% survival with oropharyngeal injuries [4].

References

1 Ellis, J.L., Thomason, J.J., Kebreab, E. et al. (2008). Calibration of estimated biting forces in domestic canids: comparison of post-mortem and in vivo measurements. *J. Anat.* 212: 769–780.

2 Von Hekkel, A., Pegram, C., and Halfacree, Z. (2020). Thoracic dog bite wounds in dogs: a retrospective study of 123 cases. *Vet. Surg.* 49 (4): 694–703.

3 Von Hekkel, A. and Halfacree, Z. (2020). Thoracic dog bite wounds in cats: a retrospective study of 22 cases. *J. Feline Med. Surg.* 22 (2): 146–152.

4 Doran, I., Wright, C., and Hotston Moore, A. (2008). Acute oropharyngeal and esophageal stick injury in forty-one dogs. *Vet. Surg.* 38 (8): 781–785.

5 Capak, H., Bottegaro, N., and Manojlovic, A. (2016). Review of 166 gunshot injury cases in dogs. *Top. Companion Anim. Med.* 31: 146–151.

6 Baker, J.L., Havas, K.A., and Miller, L.A. (2013). Gunshot wounds in military working dogs in Operation Enduring Freedom and Operation Iraqi Freedom: 29 cases (2003–2009). *J. Vet. Emerg. Crit. Care* 23 (1): 47–52.

7 Vnuk, D., Capak, H., and Gusak, V. (2016). Metal projectile injuries in cats: review of 65 cases (2012–2014). *J. Feline Med. Surg.* 18: 626–631.

8 Johnson, M., Magnusson, K., and Shmon, C. (2006). Porcupine quill injuries in dogs: a retrospective of 296 cases (1998–2002). *Can. Vet. J.* 47 (7): 677–682.

9 Flesher, K., Lam, N., and Donovan, T. (2017). Diagnosis and treatment of massive porcupine quill migration in a dog. *Can. Vet. J.* 58 (3): 280–284.

10 Matiasovic, M., Halfacree, Z., and Moores, A. (2017). Surgical management of impalement injuries to the trunk of dogs: a multicentre retrospective study. *J. Small Anim. Pract.* 59 (3): 139–146.

11 Garcia-Pertierra, S., Das, D., and Burton, C. (2022). Surgical management of intra-thoracic wooden skewers migrating from the stomach and duodenum in dogs: 11 cases (2014–2020). *J. Small Anim. Pract.* 63 (5): 403–411.

12 Lamb, C.R., Pope, E.H., and Lee, K.C. (2017). Results of computed tomography in dogs with suspected wooden foreign bodies. *Vet. Radiol. Ultrasound* 58 (2): 144–150.

13 Ober, C., Jones, J., and Larson, M. (2008). Comparison of ultrasound, CT and MRI imaging in the detection of acute wooden foreign bodies in the canine manus. *Vet. Radiol. Ultrasound* 49 (5): 411–418.

14 Blondel, M., Sonet, J., and Cachon, T. (2021). Comparison of imaging techniques to detect migrating foreign bodies. Relevance of pre-operative and intra-operative ultrasonography for diagnosis and surgical removal. *Vet. Surg.* 50 (4): 833–842.

15 Hamil, L., Smeak, D., and Johnson, V. (2020). Pretreatment aerobic bacterial swab cultures to predict infection in acute open traumatic wounds – a prospective clinical study in 64 dogs. *Vet. Surg.* 49 (5): 914–922.

16 Kalnins, N.J., Haworth, M., and Croton, C. (2021). Treatment of moderate grade dog bite wounds using amoxicillin-clavulanic acid with and without enrofloxacin: a randomized non-inferiority trial. *Aust. Vet. J.* 99 (9): 369–377.

17 Khaitan, P., Famiglietti, A., and Watson, J. (2022). The etiology, diagnosis and management of esophageal perforation. *J. Gastrointest. Surg.* 2606–2615.

18 Teh, H., Winters, L., and James, F. (2018). Medical management of esophageal perforation secondary to esophageal foreign bodies in 5 dogs. *J. Vet. Emerg. Crit. Care* 28 (5): 464–468.

19 Gurwara, S. and Clayton, S. (2019). Esophageal perforations: an endoscopic approach to management. *Curr. Gastroent. Rep.* 57: 1–6.

20 Bouayad, H., Caywood, D., and Alykine, H. (1992). Surgical reconstruction of partial circumferential esophageal defect in the dog. *J. Invest. Surg.* 5 (4): 327–342.

21 Davros, A., Gregory, C., and Cockrell, D. (2023). Comparison of clinical outcomes in cases of blunt, penetrating and combination trauma in dogs: a VetCOT registry study. *J. Vet. Emerg. Crit. Care* 33 (1): 74–80.

17

Specific Wounds

Subsection C: Abscess Case Study
James D. Crowley and Julia P. Sumner

Small Animal Specialist Hospital, Sydney, Australia

Presenting Signs

A 12-year-old male neutered Australian Cattle Dog presented for assessment of a persistent draining tract on the medial aspect of the proximomedial tibia. Tibial plateau leveling osteotomy had been previously performed 11 months prior due to cranial cruciate ligament rupture. The dog made a complete recovery from surgery prior to development of soft tissue swelling over the surgical site eight months postoperatively. The swelling was recurrent despite multiple antimicrobial medications and wound exploration. The dog had good clinical function of the limb, with low-grade lameness at the walk at the time of referral.

Examination and Wound Characteristics

On physical examination, the dog was bright, alert, and responsive with normal vital signs. At the walk, there was mild weight-bearing right pelvic limb lameness. The right stifle was stable in tibial thrust. On the proximomedial aspect of the tibia, there was a 1 cm open wound with serosanguinous discharge (Figure 17.C.1). There was moderate-poorly demarcated alopecia at this location, and it was noted to be uncomfortable for the dog.

Diagnostics (Part 1)

Orthogonal mediolateral and craniocaudal radiographic projections of the right stifle revealed a Kirschner wire that remained *in situ*, consistent with an anti-rotational pin (Figure 17.C.2). There was no obvious peri-implant osteolysis. Screw holes were present following recent implant removal. The radiographic appearance of the proximal tibia was otherwise within normal limits. There was no stifle effusion. There were mild osteoarthritic changes, including osteophyte formation on the tibial plateau and patella apex.

Treatment (Part 1)

A second draining tract was noted following clipping of the limb (Figure 17.C.3a,b), and communication between these draining tracts confirmed by saline flushing with a 25 ml syringe and 18 g catheter (Figure 17.C.4). The draining sinus was surgically explored and the remnant orthopedic implant removed (Figure 17.C.5a,b). Next, the draining tract on the proximomedial right tibial region was excised *en bloc* in an elliptical fashion (Figure 17.C.6). Purulent material was noted beneath, excised, and collected for microbial culture and sensitivity testing (Figure 17.C.7). The surgical wound was closed routinely, with a small opening at the distal extent to facilitate ongoing drainage. A light growth of methicillin-resistant *Staphylococcus pseudintermedius* was cultured, with sensitivity to Clindamycin amongst others. The dog was discharged

Techniques in Small Animal Wound Management, First Edition. Edited by Nicole J. Buote.
© 2024 John Wiley & Sons, Inc. Published 2024 by John Wiley & Sons, Inc.
Companion website: www.wiley.com/go/buote/wounds

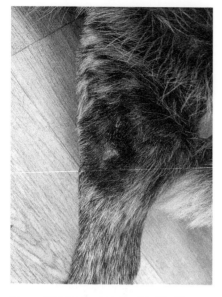

Figure 17.C.1 Open wound (~10 × 10 mm) with serosanguinous discharge on the proximomedial aspect of the right tibia, with moderate-poorly demarcated alopecia. *Source:* Courtesy of Jieming Cheng.

with a 14-day course of Meloxicam (0.1 mg/kg PO q 24 hours) and 4-week course of Clindamycin (300 mg PO q 12 hours). The owner was instructed to topically clean the wound daily using dilute chlorhexidine solution until the wound had closed.

Diagnostics (Part 2)

Four weeks post-implant removal and deep tissue exploration, the dog represented for discharging sinuses (serosanguinous consistency), again over the proximomedial aspect of the tibia and immediately caudal to the stifle joint in the popliteal region (Figure 17.C.8a–c). We recommended and proceeded with a computed tomography scan and focused ultrasound of the region that was consistent with abscess formation (Figure 17.C.9). No obvious foreign material could be visualized though there was roughly linear hyperechoic material visible on ultrasound in the popliteal region.

An ultrasound-guided exploratory approach was made to the proximomedial and caudomedial aspect of the tibia, and caudomedial to the right stifle. All three draining sinus tracts were explored with a combination of sharp, blunt, and electrosurgical dissection. Communication of all three tracts was achieved through this dissection, culminating in a surgical swab being found immediately caudal to the proximal tibia, cranial to the popliteus muscle (Figure 17.C.10a–c).

Treatment (Part 2)

The swab was moderately adhered to the caudal aspect of the tibia though able to be removed with periosteal elevator dissection. An in-dwelling 7 mm Jackson-Pratt drain was placed and secured externally. The surgical wounds were closed routinely. The draining tracts at the skin surface were excised *en bloc* and included in the primary closure. The dog was managed postoperatively with opioid analgesia (Methadone 0.2 mg/kg IV q 4 hours, transitioned to Buprenorphine 0.02 mg/kg slow IV q 8 hours), non-steroidal anti-inflammatories (Meloxicam 0.1 mg/kg PO q 24 hours) and Clindamycin (300 mg PO q 12 hours). Deep tissue collected from adjacent to the swab reported a light growth of *S. pseudintermedius*.

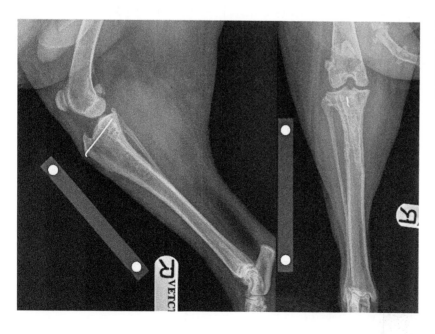

Figure 17.C.2 Orthogonal mediolateral and craniocaudal radiographic projections of the right stifle demonstrating the Kirschner wire (anti-rotational pin) left *in situ*, empty screw holes and osteoarthritic changes. *Source:* Courtesy of Jieming Cheng.

Figure 17.C.3 (a) Persistent draining tracts on the medial aspect of the proximomedial tibia. (b) Persistent draining tracts on the medial aspect of the proximomedial tibia. *Source:* Courtesy of Jieming Cheng.

(a)

(b)

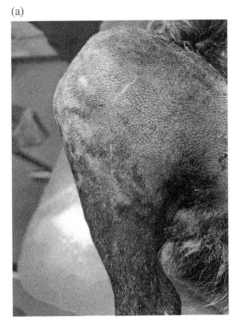
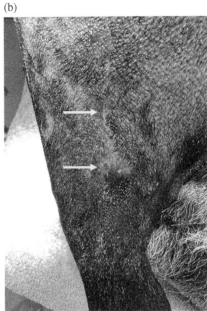

Figure 17.C.4 Communication between the draining tracts was confirmed by instilling saline using a 25 ml syringe and 18 g catheter. *Source:* Courtesy of Jieming Cheng.

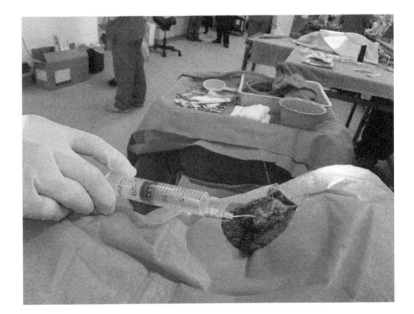

Outcome

Two weeks postoperatively, the surgical wounds were well healed, and the dog was clinically sound on the limb. At most recent follow-up eight weeks post-operatively, no draining sinus has recurred, and the dog continues to be clinically well.

Prognosis

This dog's long-term prognosis is excellent given appropriate source control has been performed with the identification of and removal of surgical swab foreign material. Draining tracts secondary to foreign bodies typically have an excellent prognosis once the foreign body is removed.

(a)

(b)

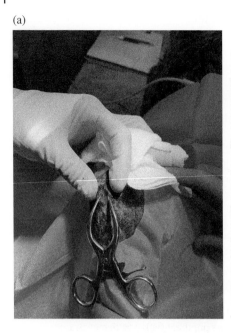

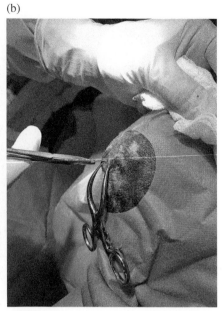

Figure 17.C.5 (a) Targeted surgical approach to the Kirschner wire (anti-rotational pin) in the tibial tuberosity left *in situ*. The wire can be visualized in the center of the wound. (b) The Kirschner wire was removed from the tibial tuberosity using needle holders. *Source:* Courtesy of Jieming Cheng.

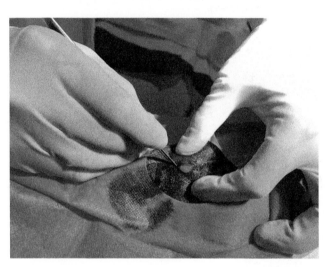

Figure 17.C.6 Surgical approach to the proxomedial right tibial region for wound exploration and deep tissue culture. *Source:* Courtesy of Jieming Cheng.

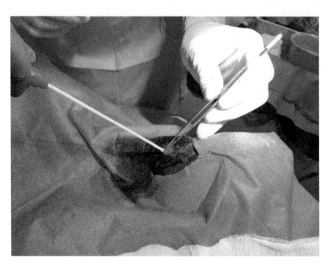

Figure 17.C.7 Swab used to collect sample of deep tissue within the explored wound for microbial culture and sensitivity testing. *Source:* Courtesy of Jieming Cheng.

(a)

(b)

(c)

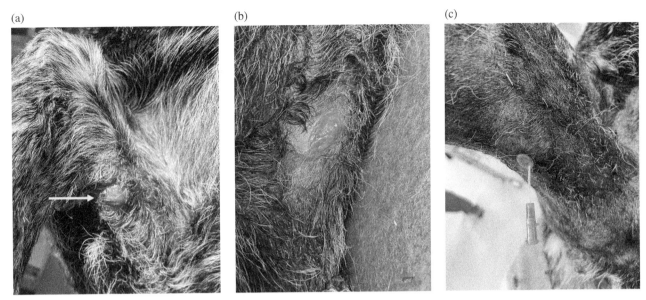

Figure 17.C.8 (a) Draining sinus tract in the popliteal region of the right pelvic limb. (b) Draining sinus tract in the popliteal region of the right pelvic limb. (c) 22 g intravenous cannula placed within the draining sinus in the popliteal region to demonstrate communication between the skin and deeper structures. *Source:* Courtesy of Jieming Cheng.

Figure 17.C.9 Intravenous contrast computed tomography images in the dorsal (a) and transverse (b) planes that identified a moderately well-demarcated region of soft tissue attenuation, hyperattenuating relative to local musculature, with peripheral contrast rim enhancement, consistent with abscess formation. *Source:* Courtesy of Jieming Cheng.

(a)

(b)

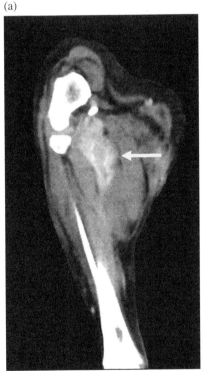

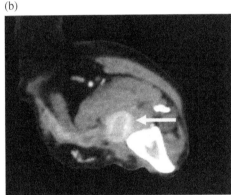

Abscesses may form secondary to the presence of foreign material within the body. For similar cases, identification of and removal of foreign material is critical to successful case management. This is in combination with appropriate "source control," including evacuation of purulent material and devitalized tissue, in-dwelling active suction drain placement if indicated, and appropriate systemic and local antimicrobial therapy directed by deep tissue culture.

(a)   (b)   (c)

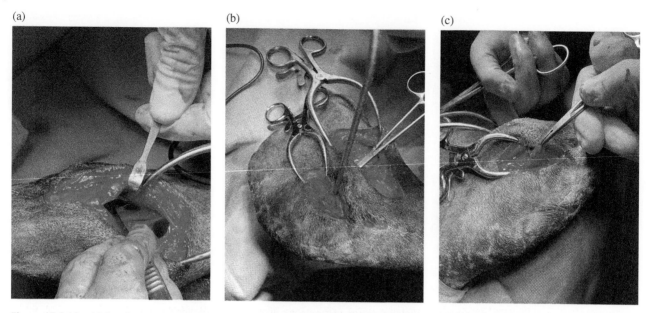

Figure 17.C.10 (a) Surgical swab identified and retrieved in the popliteal region, immediately caudal to the proximal right tibia, cranial to the popliteus muscle. (b) Surgical swab identified and retrieved in the popliteal region, immediately caudal to the proximal right tibia, cranial to the popliteus muscle. (c) Surgical swab being retrieved from the popliteal region, immediately caudal to the proximal right tibia, cranial to the popliteus muscle. *Source:* Courtesy of Jieming Cheng.

17

Specific Wounds

Subsection D: Burns

Galina Hayes

Department of Clinical Sciences, Cornell University, Ithaca, NY, USA

Clinical Presentation

Burns can theoretically present anywhere on the animal, but in small animal practice, some locations represent commoner patterns of injury than others. Electrical burns most commonly affect the oral cavity. Splash burns from hot liquids are often located on the dorsum [1], as are car exhaust burns, while burns from electrical heating pads may affect the flank or dorsum. The full extent of any burn may take several days to declare, and it is common in veterinary practice for burned animals to be presented relatively late, with symptoms that include lethargy or anorexia. The burn may only become evident to the owner when the eschar and associated hair start to lift away from the underlying wound.

Anatomy and Physiology of Burns

Burns can be broadly categorized as superficial partial, deep partial, and full thickness. Superficial partial thickness burns do not include the dermis or hair follicles and heal rapidly (within a few days) by reepithelialization. Due to the insulative and protective hair coat, these injuries are relatively rare in cats and dogs. Deep partial-thickness burns leave part of the dermis and a small number of hair follicles unaffected, and can also heal by reepithelialization although the process may be slower. Full-thickness burns include the entire dermis and go on to develop an eschar. The eschar represents denatured collagen and devitalized dermis. As the eschar develops, the skin appears thickened, hard, brown, and leathery and infection may develop beneath the eschar as it gradually lifts away from the viable tissue beneath. Full-thickness burn wounds heal by second intention (contraction and epithelialization from the wound margin) or are surgically closed. However, despite this (and other) classification schemes it is important to note that:

- Typically, multiple burn depths co-exist within the same heterogenous wound (Figure 17.D.1)
- It is very challenging to differentiate between a deep partial thickness and full thickness burn in the acute phase. The full extent and depth of a burn may take several days to fully clinically manifest.

Comparative Aspects of Burn Physiology

Much of the literature regarding the systemic effects of burns has been extrapolated from human patients; however, human and small animal skin differs fundamentally in anatomy – small animals typically have a much denser hair coat, which may be protective, and lack the rich superficial dermal plexus of blood vessels found in human skin. Extensive burns in humans result in a diffuse but transient capillary leak that leads to the extravasation of fluids, electrolytes, and colloids into both burned and unburned soft tissues. This systemic capillary leak may be profound and manifest clinically as severe

Techniques in Small Animal Wound Management, First Edition. Edited by Nicole J. Buote.
© 2024 John Wiley & Sons, Inc. Published 2024 by John Wiley & Sons, Inc.
Companion website: www.wiley.com/go/buote/wounds

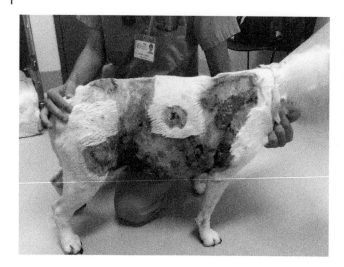

Figure 17.D.1 Patient with declaring wounds following a heating pad burn sustained 10 days prior. The eschar has peeled away over the right shoulder, while the area in the right flank fold has not fully declared. The patient is febrile and anorexic with purulent drainage from beneath the eschars. *Source:* Courtesy of Galina Hayes, BVSc, DVSc, PhD, DACVECC, DACVS.

generalized tissue edema affecting all parts of the body combined with hypovolemic shock. This phase lasts until 24 hours post-injury, when it is superseded by a hypermetabolic state. This early global systemic capillary leak, tissue edema, and resulting high demand for IV fluid support has not been well documented in small animals, with the burn literature limited mostly to isolated case reports [2, 3], and it is unclear if the same syndrome exists and to what degree.

Acute Management Plan

Patient Presenting with a History of a Known Recent Burn

Thoroughly assess for presence of oral (electrical cord) injury or smoke inhalation injury including carbon monoxide toxicity and treat accordingly. Clip and palpate the suspected burn area carefully. If the injury has occurred within the preceding hour, then cool the area with cold running tap water 12–18 °C (55–64 °F) for 20 minutes. Do not apply freezing water or ice to burns as studies have shown their application produces results similar to no treatment. If injury is focal with no systemic signs, then cover with an alginate/hydrocolloid semi-occlusive dressing, provide analgesic coverage, and schedule frequent re-checks (Q-24–48 hours) until the full extent of injury has been defined. If the burned area is very small or in a hard-to-bandage area, silver sulfadiazine cream can be applied twice daily. If the burned area is large or suspected to be large, and/or systemic signs are present, then the patient will likely require admission for a customized IV fluid plan based on hemodynamic parameters, IV analgesic support (opioids, ketamine), nutritional support and urine output and electrolyte monitoring. Unfortunately, for large burns, while the initial evaluation and resuscitation period may be completed in 72 hours, serial wound debridements may be necessary up to seven days post-injury (Figure 17.D.2) while the extent and depth of wounding fully declares, and definitive wound closure can take substantially longer. During the early phases of management of large wounds, the wound bed can be highly exudative following sharp debridement, with resulting need for frequent bandage changes and relatively high protein and fluid losses. This component of systemic loss should be factored into the supportive plan. Use of a vacuum-assisted closure device (VAC) during this phase can make these losses more quantifiable, reduce the need for frequent deep sedation for bandage changes, and may improve the perfusion gradient to questionably viable tissue. Early enteral nutritional support, often by means of a nasogastric tube, can reduce the severity of systemic hypoproteinemia (Figure 17.D.3). Large burns can be very painful. For patients who are systemically affected and requiring IV fluid support, non-steroidal anti-inflammatories should be avoided due to the risk of acute kidney injury. Use of constant rate infusions of opioids, with the addition of ketamine or dexmedetomidine as needed should be considered. However, these medications need to be carefully titrated to ensure the patient is not over-sedated to the point of complete immobility or the loss of a normal swallowing reflex, as this will increase the risk of aspiration pneumonia substantially. Due to financial burden associated with the protracted duration of therapy and the resulting high incidence of financial euthanasia, measures directed at reducing costs where possible and expediting the time to definitive wound closure should be considered.

(a)

(b)

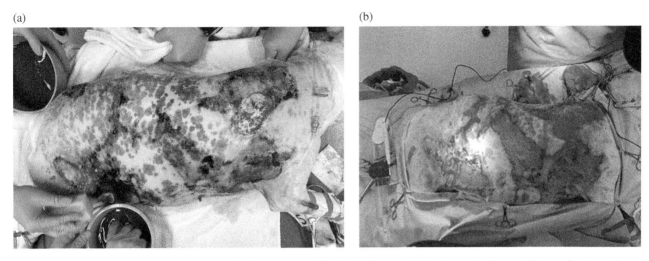

Figure 17.D.2 (a and b) Large area burn over the dorsum and right flank before and after sharp debridement. *Source:* Courtesy of Galina Hayes, BVSc, DVSc, PhD, DACVECC, DACVS.

Figure 17.D.3 Patient with VAC and NG tubes in place over a large burn wound. *Source:* Courtesy of Galina Hayes, BVSc, DVSc, PhD, DACVECC, DACVS.

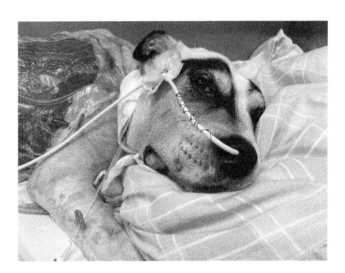

Patient Presenting with Dermal Injuries and a History of Possible Burn Exposure within the Last 14 days

In the case of unobserved or unknown burns, patients may not present until several days after injury. They may be presented for the presence of wounds or draining tracts, but also for anorexia/lethargy/pain with the presence of the wound or eschar only revealed by a thorough physical exam, particularly when hair coats are thick. The eschar that develops over a full-thickness burn wound is a rigid, leather-like scab that is composed of dead tissue and dried secretions. While this material may be initially mechanically protective of the viable tissue beneath, the secretions beneath the eschar become readily colonized by dermal flora and abscessation develops, often with systemic effects. The presence of the eschar also ultimately inhibits myofibroblast contraction and delays wound contraction and second-intention healing. Thus, early debridement of well-demarcated eschars is recommended. This involves sharp excision of the eschar under general anesthesia to the point that only viable tissue remains. Following eschar removal, extensive wounds without mature granulation coverage tissue coverage may be revealed, with resulting free drainage of protein-rich exudate. This then requires diligent bandage management, analgesic, fluid, and nutritional support. Early surgical reconstruction of the wound reduces pain, ongoing fluid and protein losses and the catabolic state associated with prolonged trauma and cytokine release. Surgical reconstruction can be accomplished through primary closure, axial pattern flaps, or split thickness-free grafting when wound areas are large [4].

Bandage Management

In the early phases of debridement while some necrotic tissue is still present alginate dressings work well and are highly absorbent. In this phase of management, dressing changes occur every 12–24 hours. Honey can also be used [5]. Once granulation tissue starts to establish, a foam semiocclusive dressing maintains an appropriately moist wound bed and appears comfortable, with dressing changes reducing to every 48–72 hours. For a wound with a healthy granulation bed that is healing by secondary intention, or for partial thickness burns, a commercially prepared (chemical sterilization, glycerolization, and irradiation) xenograft such as tilapia skin may be an option to reduce the need for frequent bandage changes; however, this should not be applied until the wound appears healthy and is becoming less exudative (see Chapter 8) [6, 7].

Split Thickness Grafts

While full-thickness autografts can be very successful on smaller extremity wounds (Figure 17.D.4), when wound areas are very large, split-thickness autografts may be the only good option to achieve wound closure in a timely manner. While second-intention healing of a full thickness wound can ultimately be successful even over very large areas, the process may be very lengthy and labor intensive. Split-thickness grafts are best harvested using a powered dermatome – this is a device that shaves skin off a donor site to a predetermined depth and width (Figure 17.D.5). As an intact dermis is retained at the donor site, healing occurs within a few days by reepithelialization, predominantly with epidermal stem cell migration from the hair follicle buds (Figure 17.D.6). Another advantage is that the thinness of the graft typically ensures reliable inosculation and revascularization, making graft "take" more certain. To harvest the graft, the donor skin is clipped and lubricated with sterile mineral oil before being tensioned using stay sutures or penetrating towel clamps. The dermatome is run at full speed before applying to the skin to be harvested, and then applied with a firm "scooping" motion at a depth setting of 0.015 in. The graft is retrieved and meshed (Figure 17.D.7). Meshers designed for human skin may be variably effective on canine or feline skin; however, the Padgett skin graft expander (a rolling pin with a staggered blade "table") is effective. The graft is secured in the wound bed using suture/bandaging as required to ensure immobilization (Figure 17.D.8). The donor site is covered with a semi-occlusive foam or gel-type dressing while it reepithelializes.

(a)

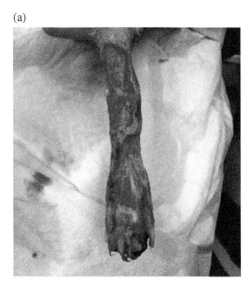

(b)

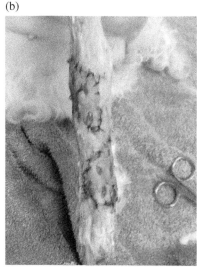

Figure 17.D.4 (a and b) Patient with an extremity wound following a chemical burn. A good granulation bed was challenging to establish initially, requiring derail sharp debridement, but ultimately responded well to a full-thickness autograft. *Source:* Courtesy of Galina Hayes, BVSc, DVSc, PhD, DACVECC, DACVS.

Possible Complications

Deep burns can result in severe local tissue injury which may make establishing a healthy granulation bed more challenging than usual. If this is the case, points to consider include whether additional debridement is needed due to a residual burden of tissue necrosis, use of a VAC to promote rapid granulation, or use of a topical antibacterial such as unpasteurized honey if the wound has become over-colonized with a multidrug resistant bacteria.

Burns can extend through the dermis and subcutaneous fat to injure the underlying musculature. When such wounds are adjacent to a limb and subsequently heal by secondary intention, the resulting pronounced fibrosis and contracture can inhibit limb motion to a degree that requires excision and reconstruction.

Future Directions

Autologous skin cell suspension is a proven technology where $1\,cm^2$ of donor skin can be expanded to treat a much larger area on a 1 : 80 ratio using a commercial kit (ReCell). An autologous split-thickness graft is harvested from a small area and treated with enzymatic denaturation. The cells are then mechanically disaggregated from the skin, filtered, and "sprayed" into the wound bed. Cultured epidermal autografts are also available commercially (Epicel). In this process, a small biopsy of donor skin is expanded in culture with the aid of irradiated 3T3 mouse cells to generate sheets of skin cells for wound coverage ranging from 2 to 8 cell layers thick. Unfortunately, financial limitations currently prohibit the widespread use of these technologies in animal patients.

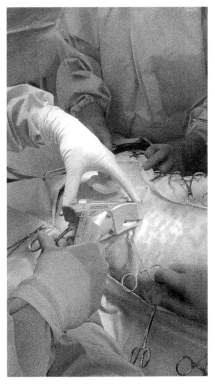

Figure 17.D.5 Dermatome in use with appropriate width plate and depth set. An assistant is tensioning the skin ahead of the blade, while the operator applies firm downward pressure at the leading edge using the non-dominant hand. *Source:* Courtesy of Galina Hayes, BVSc, DVSc, PhD, DACVECC, DACVS.

Prognosis

The prognosis for burns, as for most wounds, is excellent as long as systemic complications can be managed or avoided and the financial burden of care can be tolerated.

Figure 17.D.6 Donor sites immediately following split graft harvest. Sites over the ribs or bony prominences are best avoided, as they make harvest of an intact graft challenging. *Source:* Courtesy of Galina Hayes, BVSc, DVSc, PhD, DACVECC, DACVS.

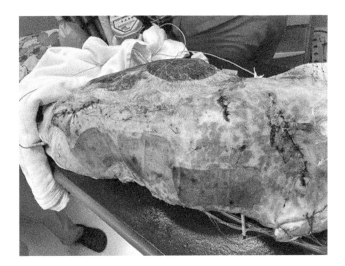

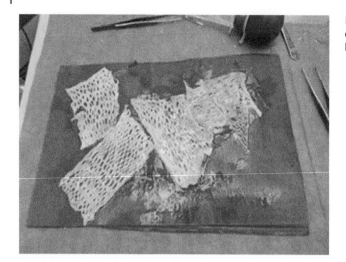

Figure 17.D.7   Meshing of a split-thickness graft using a graft expander. Courtesy of Galina Hayes, BVSc, DVSc, PhD, DACVECC, DACVS.

(a)   (b)

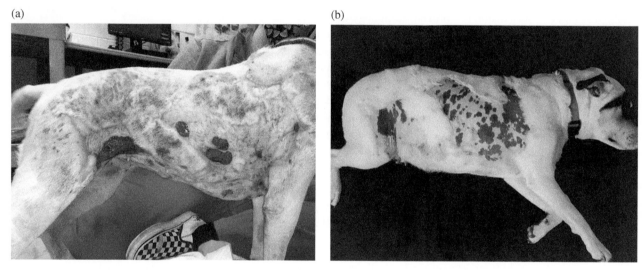

Figure 17.D.8   (a) Burn wounds seven days after grafting with partial loss of graft in flank fold wound. (b) Six months following injury. *Source:* Courtesy of Galina Hayes, BVSc, DVSc, PhD, DACVECC, DACVS.

References

1 Quist, E., Tanabe, M., and Mansell, J. (2012). A case series of thermal scald injuries in dogs exposed to hot water from garden hoses (garden hose scalding syndrome). *Vet. Dermatol.* 23 (2): 162–166.

2 Dawson, K., Mickelson, M., and Blong, A. Management of severe burn injuries with novel treatment techniques including maggot debridement and applications of acellular fish skin grafts and autologous skin suspension in a dog. *J. Am. Vet. Med. Assoc.* 202 (260): 428–435.

3 Zingel, M.M. and Sakals, S.A. (2017). Use of skin stretching techniques before bilateral caudal superficial epigastric axial flaps in a dog with severe burns. *Can. Vet. J.* 58: 835–838.

4 Pavletic, M.M. and Trout, N.J. (2006). Bullet, bite and burn wounds in dogs and cats. *Vet. Clinic. Small Anim.* 36: 873–893.

5 Moustafa, A. and Atiba, A. The effectiveness of a mixture of honey, beeswax and olive oil in the treatment of canine deep second degree burn. *Glob. Vet.* 14 (2): 244–250.

6 Lima Júnior, E.M., de Moraes Filho, M.O., Costa, B.A. et al. (2020). Innovative burn treatment using tilapia skin as a Xenograft: a phase II randomized controlled trial. *J. Burn Care Res.* 41: 585–592.

7 Buote, N.J. (2022). Updates in wound management and dressings. *Vet. Clin. North Am. Small Anim. Pract.* 52 (2): 289–315.

17

Specific Wounds

Subsection E: Wounds Over Joints

Galina Hayes

Department of Clinical Sciences, Cornell University, Ithaca, NY, USA

Clinical Presentation

Wounds over joints can occur for all the usual traumatic reasons including bites, degloving injuries, lacerations, and burns. Similar to wounds over body cavities, determining whether the joint has been penetrated and identifying concurrent intra-articular injuries such as fractures or luxations is a key step that may change the surgical plan and alter the prognosis. Radiographs of the area are performed to evaluate underlying bony structures and evaluate for evidence of intra-articular penetration. Depending on the visible soft tissue damage, stressed radiographs combined with manipulation of the joint under sedation should be performed to evaluate for concurrent ligamentous injury and joint instability. Intra-articular fractures or luxations are prioritized for early definitive treatment with open reduction and internal fixation. Fortunately, joint instability due to collateral ligament injury occurring as a component of major open or degloving wounds may not always require specific intervention despite substantial instability noted at the time of injury. Typically, the joint will self-stabilize with the peri-articular fibrosis that occurs during second intention healing over a period of several weeks with external coaptation alone. If there is a concern for traumatic joint penetration antibiotic coverage should be provided. If clinical presentation has been delayed and there is concern for an established septic arthropathy, arthrocentesis for culture and cytology should be performed followed by through-and-through lavage. Wounds over joints can also occur following oncologic resections where the size of the tumor or need for lateral margins results in lack of available skin to achieve primary closure. Prolonged bandaging or casting of the limb can also result in wounds developing over bony prominences close to the elbow and hock joints which may be challenging to resolve. Ehmer slings in particular are associated with a high incidence of iatrogenic wounds over the tarsus, which may be strangulating and necessitate amputation [1].

Specific Challenges

Challenges unique to wounds over joints include the high mobility of the area, the lack of available skin and soft tissue for joints located in the distal extremities, and the pressure points that may be associated with certain joints. If the joint is fully exposed but the wound can be categorized as clean or clean contaminated, the joint capsule can and should be primarily closed with 3-0 monofilament delayed absorbable suture. If the wound is contaminated or infected, open management with healing by second intention will be necessary. Commonly, clinicians are concerned about joint fluid leaking from an open joint creating swelling or edema, but the joint capsule will heal by second intention and the amount of joint fluid produced daily is minimal. The tensile forces placed on the skin during flexion and extension of the underlying joint can create a relatively hostile environment to wound healing and place additional stress on healing surgical incisions. For wounds undergoing second intention healing, normal myofibroblast contraction may be inhibited, and epithelialization delayed. Repetitive motion against any overlying bandage can also delay healing. Lack of soft tissue structures in the wound bed, when a wound bed is composed of areas of bone or tendon, can make it difficult to establish a suitable environment for transfer of a graft

Techniques in Small Animal Wound Management, First Edition. Edited by Nicole J. Buote.
© 2024 John Wiley & Sons, Inc. Published 2024 by John Wiley & Sons, Inc.
Companion website: www.wiley.com/go/buote/wounds

or flap. When the wound exposes a pressure point such as the caudal aspect of the olecranon, the weight of the animal in recumbency can both compromise perfusion to the wound bed and place high mechanical forces on the area.

Management Plans

External Coaption

Temporary partial or complete immobilization of the underlying joint combined with a bandage that redistributes pressure away from the wound area can go some way to address some of the challenges discussed above. Specific bandaging approaches have been described [2], but in general, the goal is to heavily pad the areas of healthy skin adjacent to the wound with relatively minimal padding over the wound itself, causing redistribution of the weight-bearing load away from the wound. Custom braces can also be constructed to achieve this, which may have the added benefit of allowing progressive increases in range of motion in the area (Figure 17.E.1a–c). Transarticular fixators or the use of the Rudy external fixator boot may be helpful in certain situations as they will provide complete immobilization of the joint while allowing access to the wound for bandage management. Placement of external fixators requires specific care and the principles of fixator application need to be carefully adhered to, particularly the diameter and number of pins used. Complications including proximal fracture due to the long lever arm generated and distal devascularization of the pes as well as pin breakage and loosening have been reported [3]. Once immobilization is achieved and pressure redistributed away from the wound, second intention healing can be accelerated. Other criteria common to good husbandry of all wounds healing by second intention also need to be met, including maintaining a clean, moist, and healthy wound environment with appropriately timed dressing changes, lavage, and appropriate contact layer selection. Finally, counterintuitively, for wounds that have been caused by splints or casts applied for orthopedic disease, the wound may only ultimately fully heal when the splint or cast is removed together with the bandage. This appears to be particularly true for pressure ulcers over the point of the elbow (Figure 17.E.2). Following bandage removal, twice daily hydrotherapy performed by the owners together with clean, soft bedding may be sufficient to allow the wound to progress positively.

(a)   (b)   (c)

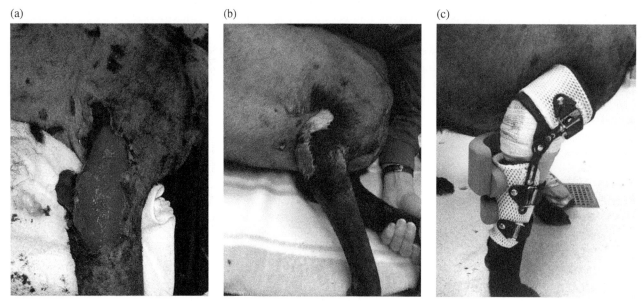

Figure 17.E.1   (a–c) This challenging wound in a 6 yo FS Labrador developed following a large peri-articular abscess suspected to be secondary to a cat bite. The wound shown in (a) developed subsequent to necrosis of the overlying skin. At this point, the wound had been debrided and managed for several days with a debridement dressing consisting of unpasteurized honey-soaked laparotomy sponges. The wound was then closed using a flank fold flap which partially dehisced (not shown) and was further managed with a medial and cranial releasing incision which also partially necrosed over the caudal aspect of the olecranon (b). At this stage, the articulated brace (Jim Alaimo, mypetsbrace.com) shown in (c) was constructed to redistribute weight in recumbency away from the wound area. This allowed rapid progression of second intention healing to close the remaining defect. *Source:* Courtesy of Galina Hayes, BVSc, DVSc, PhD, DACVECC, DACVS.

Releasing Incisions

This technique, discussed in detail in Chapter 16, can be a useful method (Figure 17.E.3) in select situations where the wound is mostly confined to an aspect of the joint that acts as a load-bearing surface during recumbency. While highly conforming bedding can be tried as a first-line approach, some animals are surprisingly resistant to resting on anything other than hard surfaces. If the wound is proving frustrating to manage, a releasing incision made over an aspect of the joint that is not load bearing and has excellent soft tissue coverage may be performed to allow sufficient mobilization of skin to surgically close the original wound. Because the created wound is in a less hostile environment, second intention healing of this wound may be much more rapid.

Axial Pattern Flaps

Depending somewhat on the patient's individual conformation, thoracodorsal flaps [4] can be very useful for managing elbow wounds while caudal superficial epigastric flaps [4] can be helpful for wounds around the stifle (Figure 17.E.4). While reverse saphenous flaps have been described for tarsal wounds, in the authors hands these have not proven consistently reliable, and an autograft may provide an alternative option. The author avoids bandaging or splinting the limb after flap closure in an attempt to optimize perfusion to the flap; however, there is currently sparse evidence in the literature to support or disprove this approach. Keys to success may include ensuring that the flap is not sutured under excessive tension when the limb is in the fully extended position, and backlighting the flap as it is raised from the tip towards the axial vessel to ensure the axial vessel is identified early and the flap raised in such a way that it is both centralized and not inadvertently injured. The author uses the light cable from a laparoscopic tower for this purpose, but any high-intensity light source will serve the purpose (see Chapter 16 for more detailed information on reconstructive techniques).

Autografts

The biggest challenge with the use of autografts on a wound over a joint is maintaining the necessary immobility of the graft relative to the underlying wound bed over the first few days following grafting (Figure 17.E.5a,b). For distal joints, this may be achieved with external coaptation. For more proximal joints, the necessary immobilization can be very challenging, and an axillary pattern flap may be a better choice. Subjectively, the larger the animal the more challenging distal immobilization seems to be, and in this setting punch or seed grafts [5] may be a good solution. Because these grafts are recessed into a pocket of granulation tissue and function as islands independent of each other, motion appears to be better tolerated without disrupting the process of individual graft inosculation and graft failure is rare (Figure 17.E.6). However, they can be time-consuming to harvest, prepare and place over a large area.

Prognosis

Prognosis for joint wounds is typically excellent as long as the clinician is prepared to be both creative and persistent.

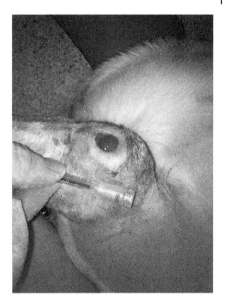

Figure 17.E.2   Chronic ulcer over the caudal aspect of the olecranon resulting from prolonged casting. This healed rapidly once all bandages were removed. *Source:* Courtesy of Galina Hayes, BVSc, DVSc, PhD, DACVECC, DACVS.

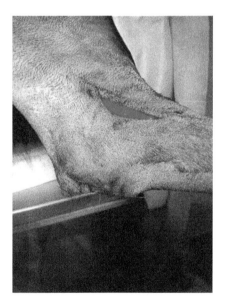

Figure 17.E.3   Releasing incision placed over the medial aspect of the elbow to allow closure of the caudal wound over the point of the olecranon. The limb was then placed in a soft padded bandage with a foam buttress to minimize pressure over the point of the elbow. The caudal wound healed routinely with suture removal at two weeks, while the created wound healed over that same two-week period. *Source:* Courtesy of Galina Hayes, BVSc, DVSc, PhD, DACVECC, DACVS.

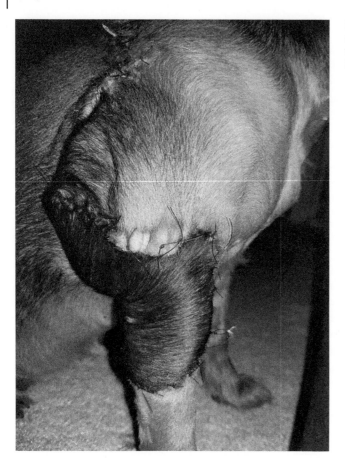

Figure 17.E.4 Thoracodorsal flap used to close a large wound over the elbow and proximal antebrachium, image taken two weeks following surgery. *Source:* Courtesy of Galina Hayes, BVSc, DVSc, PhD, DACVECC, DACVS.

(b)

(a)

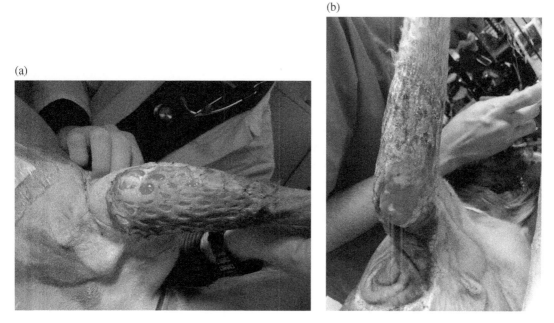

Figure 17.E.5 (a and b) Full-thickness meshed autograft used to close a large defect over the elbow and antebrachium. Failure of the graft over the point of the olecranon can be seen (a) and should have been anticipated. Closure was then attempted with a flank fold flap which initially partially failed (b) but was subsequently remobilized to achieve closure. *Source:* Courtesy of Galina Hayes, BVSc, DVSc, PhD, DACVECC, DACVS.

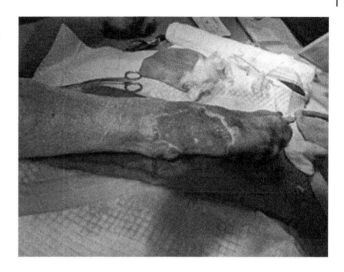

Figure 17.E.6 A carpal wound on a 60 kg mastiff. The dog tolerated bandaging poorly, becoming non-ambulatory with any form of forelimb splint. Punch grafts were used in combination with a soft padded bandage – this image was taken five days after grafting, with excellent take of the grafts evident. *Source:* Courtesy of Galina Hayes, BVSc, DVSc, PhD, DACVECC, DACVS.

References

1 Schlag, A., Hayes, G., Taylor, A. et al. (2019). Analysis of outcomes following treatment of craniodorsal hip luxation with closed reduction and Ehmer sling application in dogs. *J. Am. Vet. Med. Assoc.* 254 (12): 1436–1440.

2 Pavletic, M. (2011). Use of commercially available foam pipe insulation as a protective device for wounds over the elbow joint area in 5 dogs. *J. Am. Vet. Med. Assoc.* 239 (9): 1225–1231.

3 Toombs, J.P. (1992). Transarticular application of external skeletal fixation. *Vet. Clin. North Am. Small Anim. Pract.* 22: 181–194.

4 Pavletic, M.M. (1990). Axial pattern flaps in small animal practice. *Vet. Clin. North Am. Small Anim. Pract.* 20: 105–125.

5 Crowley, J.D., Hosgood, G., and Appelgrein, C. (2020). Seed skin grafts for reconstruction of distal limb defects in 15 dogs. *J. Small Anim. Pract.* 61 (9): 561–567.

17

Specific Wounds

Subsection F: Shearing Wounds – Case Study

James D. Crowley

Small Animal Specialist Hospital, Sydney, Australia

Presenting Signs

A 1-year-old male neutered Bengal presented for assessment of a traumatic, full-thickness shearing wound on the dorsal aspect of the right pes following road traffic trauma.

Examination and Wound Characteristics

On physical examination, the cat was quiet, alert, and responsive with appropriate mentation. The cat was non-weight bearing on the right pelvic limb. Neurological function was within normal limits. There was a full-thickness shearing injury to the dorsal aspect of the right metatarsus, with exposure of all extensor tendons over the entire dorsal surface of the metatarsus (Figure 17.F.1). There was obvious fracture and dislocation of P1 of the 5th digit. The metatarsus and tarsus were stable on palpation. The wound was heavily contaminated with grit and road debris.

Diagnostics

Point of care thoracic and abdominal ultrasound excluded serious systemic injuries. Orthogonal mediolateral and cranio-caudal radiographic projections of the right pes demonstrated a complete, short oblique proximal diaphyseal fracture of P1 with metatarsophalangeal dislocation. No other orthopedic injuries were identified.

Treatment

Under general anesthesia, the wound was assessed, and decontamination was performed. Sterile lubricant was placed within the wound prior to clipping of fur. The wound was copiously flushed with sterile saline to remove as much gross contamination as possible. Any devitalized skin was sharply excised using a no. 10 scalpel blade. The wound was dressed with a hypertonic saline primary dressing (Mesalt, Molnlycke Healthcare), polyurethane foam secondary dressing (Allevyn, Smith, and Nephew), followed by secondary and tertiary dressing supportive dressings. The cat was hospitalized for seven days for daily bandage changes under general anesthesia. At each change, any tissue that had "declared itself" as nonviable was sharply excised, the wound cleaned with sterile saline, and dressings applied based on the clinical appearance of the wound (Figure 17.F.2). Once granulation tissue was present, the primary wound dressing was polyurethane foam (Allevyn, Smith, and Nephew) followed by supportive dressings. During this hospitalization period, the cat was managed on opioid analgesia (Methadone 0.2 mg/kg IV q 4 hours transitioned to Buprenorphine 0.02 mg/kg transmucosal q 8 hours), Meloxicam 0.05 mg/kg Po q 24 hours, Gabapentin 75 mg PO q 8 hours, Amoxicillin–clavulanic acid 20 mg/kg PO q 12 hours.

Techniques in Small Animal Wound Management, First Edition. Edited by Nicole J. Buote.
© 2024 John Wiley & Sons, Inc. Published 2024 by John Wiley & Sons, Inc.
Companion website: www.wiley.com/go/buote/wounds

(a)   (b)   (c)

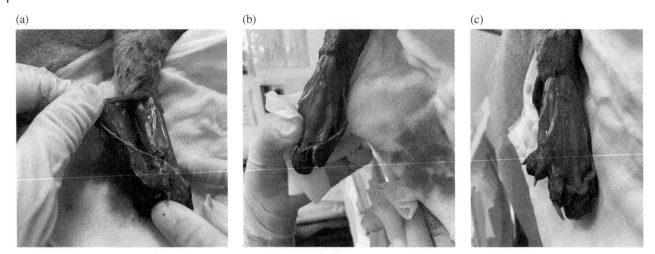

Figure 17.F.1 (a–c) Day 0 – Full thickness shearing wound over the dorsal aspect of the right metatarsus with exposure of the extensor tendons in a 1-year-old male neutered Bengal. (a) Lateral aspect; (b) Dorsal aspect; (c) Medial aspect. *Source:* Courtesy of James D. Crowley, BVSc (Hons), MANZCVS (Small Animal Surgery).

(a)   (b)

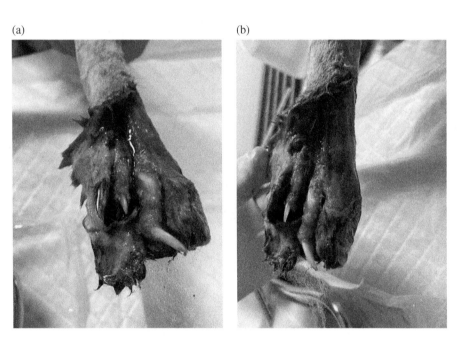

Figure 17.F.2 (a and b) Day 4 – Appearance of the dorsal metatarsal wound following open wound management. (a) Lateral aspect; (b) Dorsal aspect. *Source:* Courtesy of James D. Crowley, BVSc (Hons), MANZCVS (Small Animal Surgery).

Day 7 post-trauma, amputation of the 5th digit of the right pes was performed using an oscillating bone saw at the level of the distal diaphyseal region of the 5th metatarsal bone. A modified phalangeal fillet technique was performed to close a portion of the wound on the lateral aspect of the dorsal metatarsus. The remainder of the dorsal surface of the pes was covered in early granulation tissue. Once recovered, the cat was discharged and returned for bandage changed every four to five days.

Day 16 post-trauma, the entire dorsal surface of the metatarsus was covered in a healthy, hyperemic layer of granulation tissue (Figure 17.F.3) and deemed an appropriate recipient bed for a full thickness, meshed-free skin graft. An estimation of skin required to cover the defect was done by placing a sterile piece of paper over the metatarsal skin defect (Figure 17.F.4) and the template traced using a marker pen on the donor site on the right lateral thorax (Figure 17.F.5). A traumatic technique was used during graft harvest aided by the placement of stay sutures (4-0 PDS). Care was taken to avoid handling of the graft. The graft was stretched over a roll of bandaging material to facilitate the dissection of subcutaneous and adipose tissue from the graft. The grafted was then tacked to a roll of bandaging material (Figure 17.F.6a) and "meshed" by making full-thickness staggered fenestrations using a #11 scalpel blade (Figure 17.F.6b). The skin graft was placed into defect with the direction of hair growth appropriately aligned and to ensure complete wound coverage. The edges of graft were secured in a simple interrupted pattern using 4/0 Nylon suture (Figure 17.F.7). The donor site was routinely closed. An antibiotic topical ointment (Tricin, Jurox) was placed at the margins of the graft/recipient wound bed. The graft site was covered with one to two layers of non-adherent petrolatum-impregnated gauze (Jelonet, Smith and Nephew), followed by polyurethane foam (Allevyn, Smith and Nephew), an absorbent layer, (Soffban, BSN medical) and a tertiary cohesive layer (Fun-Flex Pet Bandage, Kruuse). A plantar splint was incorporated into the dressing to assist with immobilization of the distal limb. Care was taken to apply the bandage smoothly and evenly, and to avoid torquing the bandage (which might cause shearing of the graft away from the host site). Any repeat bandaging was performed in the same manner, with bandage changes delayed for as long as possible but no later than five to seven days apart.

Outcome

The first bandage change was performed seven days post-grafting. There was 100% take of the graft (Figure 17.F.8). Three weeks post-operatively, the grafted wound was healed, and the cat was clinically sound on the limb. At most recent follow-up two years post-operatively, the cat was reported to have normal clinical function of the operated limb. At the grafted site, there was good hair growth and favorable cosmesis (Figure 17.F.9).

Prognosis

The cat's long-term prognosis is excellent given appropriate open wound management and skin defect reconstruction has been performed. Prognosis for shearing wounds is dependent on the nature of the trauma and structures damaged. For the most part, with appropriate open wound management, most wounds will heal either by second intention or with reconstructive techniques such as free skin grafts.

Clinical Lessons

Shearing wounds are common injuries following road traffic trauma in dogs and cats. Once the patient has been stabilized appropriately, wounds should be managed as open. Gross contamination and devitalized tissue should be removed and a moist wound environment maintained to encourage healthy granulation tissue formation. Wounds can be left to heal via second intention or reconstructive techniques such as full-thickness-free skin grafts can be used to expedite wound healing and return to function.

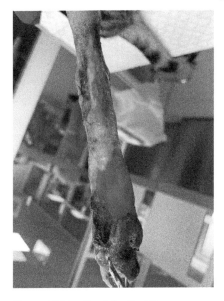

Figure 17.F.3   Day 16 – Healthy, hyperemic granulation bed on the dorsal metatarsus ready for skin grafting. *Source:* Courtesy of James D. Crowley, BVSc (Hons), MANZCVS (Small Animal Surgery).

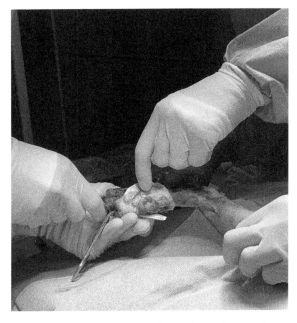

Figure 17.F.4   A sterile piece of paper is used to template the size of the dorsal metatarsal defect prior to harvest of the free skin graft. *Source:* Courtesy of James D. Crowley, BVSc (Hons), MANZCVS (Small Animal Surgery).

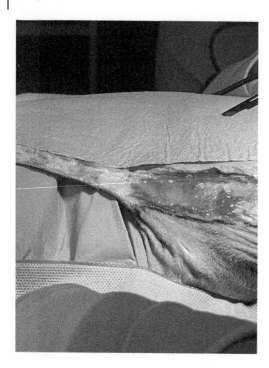

Figure 17.F.5 The free skin graft is harvested from the right lateral thorax using stay sutures to avoid excessive handling and manipulation of the graft. *Source:* Courtesy of James D. Crowley, BVSc (Hons), MANZCVS (Small Animal Surgery).

(a)

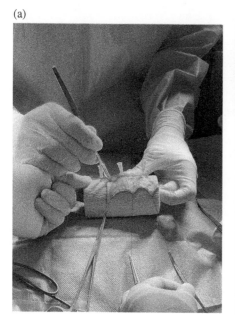

(b)

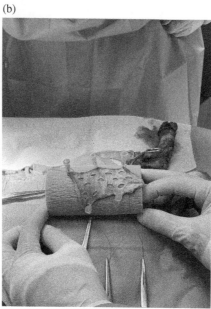

Figure 17.F.6 (a) The full-thickness skin graft is tacked to a sterile roll of bandaging material using 25 g needles and full-thickness stab incisions made in a staggered fashion to "mesh" the graft. (b) Appearance of the full thickness meshed free skin graft ready for placement into the recipient wound bed. *Source:* Courtesy of James D. Crowley, BVSc (Hons), MANZCVS (Small Animal Surgery).

Figure 17.F.7   The meshed free skin graft is placed into the recipient wound bed and the edges sutured in a simple interrupted pattern. *Source:* Courtesy of James D. Crowley, BVSc (Hons), MANZCVS (Small Animal Surgery).

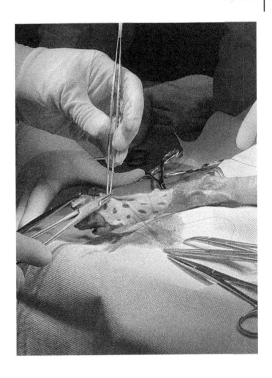

Figure 17.F.8   Appearance of the grafted wound seven days postoperative. There is nearly 100% take of the free skin graft. *Source:* Courtesy of James D. Crowley, BVSc (Hons), MANZCVS (Small Animal Surgery).

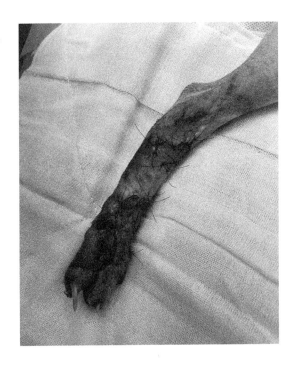

(a) (b) (c)

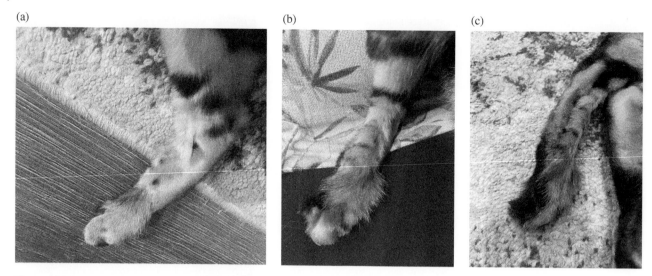

Figure 17.F.9   (a–c) Appearance of the grafted wound two years post-operative. There is excellent hair growth and cosmesis. (a) Medial aspect, (b) Dorsal aspect, (c) Lateral aspect. *Source:* Courtesy of James D. Crowley, BVSc (Hons), MANZCVS (Small Animal Surgery).

17

Specific Wounds

Subsection G: Necrotizing Fasciitis (Necrotizing Soft Tissue Infections)
Nathan Peterson

Department of Clinical Sciences, Cornell University, Ithaca, NY, USA

Presenting Signs

Necrotizing soft tissue infection (NSTI) is an uncommon but life-threatening infection, characterized by rapid onset and progression of clinical signs over the course of several hours to days that, if not recognized early and treated aggressively, can rapidly lead to death [1, 2]. This condition has many names but can best be categorized according to the deepest tissue plane affected (i.e., *necrotizing cellulitis* for infection limited to the skin and subcutis, *necrotizing fasciitis* for infection involving fascial planes, and *necrotizing myositis* when underlying muscle is affected) [3]. Presenting signs are generally vague and include recent onset malaise and fever. Significant trauma is generally absent from the history but small, seemingly innocuous accidents may be featured. Occasionally, patients have a recent history of surgery, subcutaneous fluid administration, or bite wounds. Importantly, a history of immunocompromise is absent in reports of NSTI in veterinary medicine [2].

The hallmarks of NSTI are its rapid onset and progression, and severe pain disproportionate to evident wounds. The time from initial clinical signs to the development of septic shock may be as short as a few hours [1]. The most severe pain will generally be elicited at the leading edge of the infection and may appear quite distant from identifiable wounds (Figure 17.G.1). High fever may be present but the absence of fever does not preclude NSTI due to the rapidity of progression and potential for systemic perfusion problems at presentation. Bruising or erythema of the skin may be present but often the skin overlying the infection appears normal at the time of initial evaluation. If present the leading edge should be traced with pen to allow monitoring of progression. Rapidly progressive limb swelling may also occur (Figure 17.G.2). Crepitus due to subcutaneous emphysema has high positive predictive value in humans with NSTI but is an infrequent and unreliable finding [1]. If found, the clinician's index of suspicion for NSTI should be elevated.

Laboratory findings are non-specific and usually reflective of an underlying inflammatory condition. Common findings include neutrophilia or neutropenia with left shift. Hypoglycemia, hyperlactatemia, and coagulation tests consistent with DIC may be present. Imaging may be helpful in diagnosing NSTI. Ultrasound may identify fluid pocketing along fascial planes or subcutaneous emphysema, and CT may reveal the presence of small pockets of gas accumulation [2–4]. MRI has been used to support a diagnosis of NSTI in one dog [5]. Fine needle aspiration of the affected area may yield gray to brown, non-malodorous fluid. Cytologic evaluation typically demonstrates suppurative inflammation with intracellular organisms.

Wound Characteristics

Necrotizing soft-tissue infections can occur in any location but often affect the limbs (Figures 17.G.3 and 17.G.4). The dorsal tail base and perineum may be affected in cats. Inability to locate a source of bacterial entry is relatively common so typical wound characteristics are often not identified until the time of surgery. Surgical findings associated with NSTI include identification of the previously described gray/brown (dishwater) fluid spreading along fascial planes. The fascia

Techniques in Small Animal Wound Management, First Edition. Edited by Nicole J. Buote.
© 2024 John Wiley & Sons, Inc. Published 2024 by John Wiley & Sons, Inc.
Companion website: www.wiley.com/go/buote/wounds

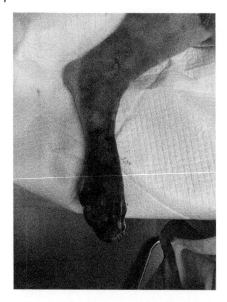

Figure 17.G.1 Photograph of a German shepherd with NSTI of the distal right pelvic limb. Note the clear demarcation between normal and necrotic tissue. This patient has no visible wound on the paw or history of known trauma. *Source:* Courtesy of Nicole Buote DVM, DACVS.

or underlying muscle may appear gray in color (Figure 17.G.3B) and muscle necrosis may be evident [3]. A common finding during surgical dissection is the ease with which the subcutaneous tissue is separated from deeper fascial structures, often referred to as a positive "finger test" [1]. Large pockets of purulent material are uncommon.

Physiologic Effects

Classic NSTI are caused by beta-hemolytic *Streptococci* sp. such as *S. canis*, and other commensal group G streptococcal organisms. Other organisms that have been identified or associated with NSTI include *S. aureus, S. psued-intermedius, P. aeruginosa, E. coli* and various *Clostridial spp., Pasturella spp., and Klebsiella spp.* Proteases produced by bacteria facilitate rapid spread of infection along tissue planes. As infection progresses, thrombosis of subcutaneous vasculature and liquefactive necrosis create an environment well suited to microbial proliferation and further promote fascial spreading [2]. Extensive necrosis of subcutaneous fat and fascia occurs secondary to direct pathogen-induced tissue injury, inflammation, edema, and thrombosis while the overlying skin is often spared [3].

The rapid growth of infective organisms can quickly overwhelm the immune response and patients may develop signs of sepsis or septic shock within hours. Sepsis is a life-threatening condition that results in organ dysfunction due to a dysregulated host immune response [6]. Multiple organ dysfunction is possible with patient's being at risk for development of acute kidney injury, disseminated intravascular coagulation, and pulmonary failure due to acute respiratory distress syndrome. Prompt recognition and treatment are necessary to prevent progression to septic shock and death. Patients presenting with evidence of hemodynamic compromise or progressing to such a state in the hospital should be aggressively resuscitated to maintain oxygen delivery to vital organs and referred for surgery as soon as possible. Stabilization of the patient might require surgery so resuscitative efforts should not significantly delay time to surgical treatment. If necessary, resuscitation can continue during surgery.

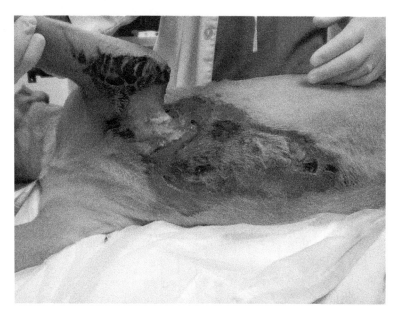

Figure 17.G.2 Photograph of a mixed breed dog with severe NSTI of the axillary and sternal regions. Skin separation is seen clearly in the left axilla and a line of demarcation with erythema and swelling adjacent. *Source:* Courtesy of Kelley Thieman DVM, MS, DACVS.

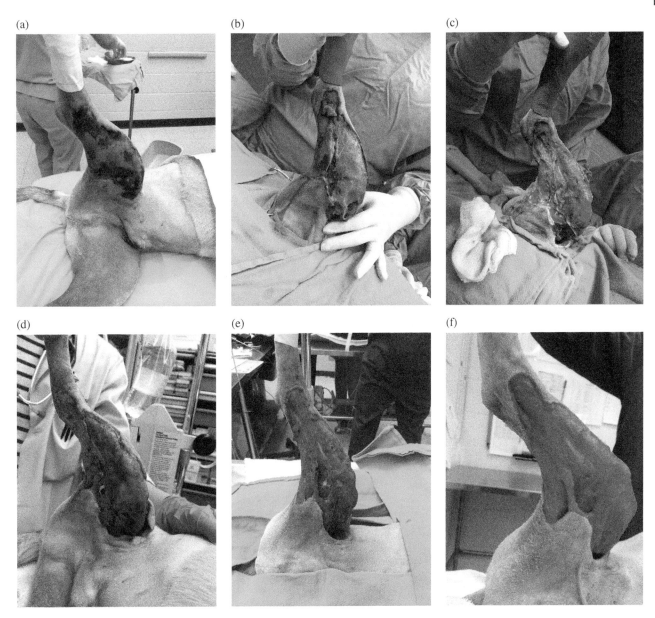

Figure 17.G.3 Photographs of a patient with diagnosed NSTI of the medial aspect of the right pelvic limb. (a) Patient at presentation. Note the line of demarcation surrounding the necrotic tissue. (b) Intraoperative (Day 0) photograph of limb with necrotic skin removed. Gray subcutaneous tissue and muscle are still present. (c) Intraoperative (Day 0) photograph after completed debridement. (d) Day 1 postoperative at bandage change. (e) Day 3 postoperative bandage change. Note continued islands of necrotic tissue. (f) Day 8 postoperative bandage change. Underlying tissue is finally healthy enough for primary closure with combination of axillary pattern flaps and second intention healing. *Source:* Courtesy of Robert Hardie DVM, DACVS, DECVS.

Shock/Sepsis

Treatment

Due to their ability to progress rapidly, NSTIs are considered to be true surgical emergencies. Clinical diagnosis alone is considered sufficient to begin treatment and surgical exploration should be recommended when clinical suspicion of NSTI is established. Early surgical debridement is the primary determinant of morbidity and mortality so diagnostic procedures, such as MRI or CT, that may delay time to surgery should be avoided.

Due to the usually extensive spread, wide surgical margins should be established and prepared pre-operatively. The initial objective of surgery is to determine the extent of infection followed by debridement of all necrotic tissue. If no necrotic tissue is identified, the wound can be closed with an active suction device in place and the patient recovered for ongoing monitoring. If necrosis is identified aggressive debridement to bleeding tissue is necessary, this may require debridement or resection of muscle and tendon. Visually determining the margins of necrosis can be challenging, especially if surgery occurs early in the course of treatment when only the fascia may be involved. Presence of persistent necrotic tissue allows infection to persist so thorough exploration of the wound is necessary. Debridement should extend beyond visible viable tissue demarcation. Most patients require surgical debridement multiple times to fully eliminate necrotic tissue so reexploration should be anticipated. If large regions of skin require resection the resulting wound should

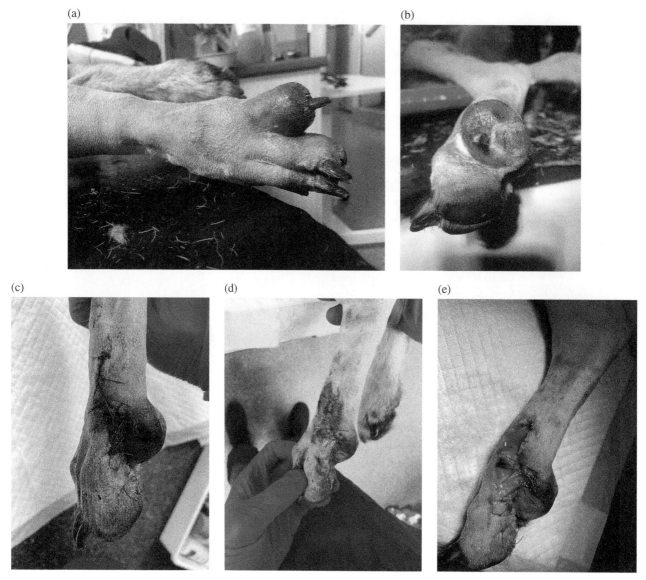

Figure 17.G.4 Photographs of a three-year-old MN German Shepherd diagnosed with NSTI of the left pelvic limb 5th digit. Initially treated via digit amputation but ultimately required a coxofemoral disarticulation amputation. (a and b) Patient's left pelvic limb 5th digit on presentation. (c) Day 1 postoperative toe amputation. (d) Patient's incision day 2 postoperative toe amputation. Note the purulent discharge already present at the incision line. (e–g) Day 5 post-toe amputation. (e) Appearance immediately following bandage removal, (f) after gentle cleaning of the wound, the wound edges were devitalized, necrotic, and peeled away from the surgical site with minimal pressure applied. (g) appearance of the wound immediately following debridement of the necrotic tissue. (h–k) Unfortunately, continued necrosis of tissue was seen at successive bandage changes (h and i) as well as a new lesion proximal to the hock (j) so the decision was made to amputate the limb (k). The patient did very well after pelvic limb amputation.
Source: Courtesy of James Crowley BVSc (Hons), MANZCVS (Small Animal Surgery).

(f)   (g)   (h)

(i)   (j)   (k)

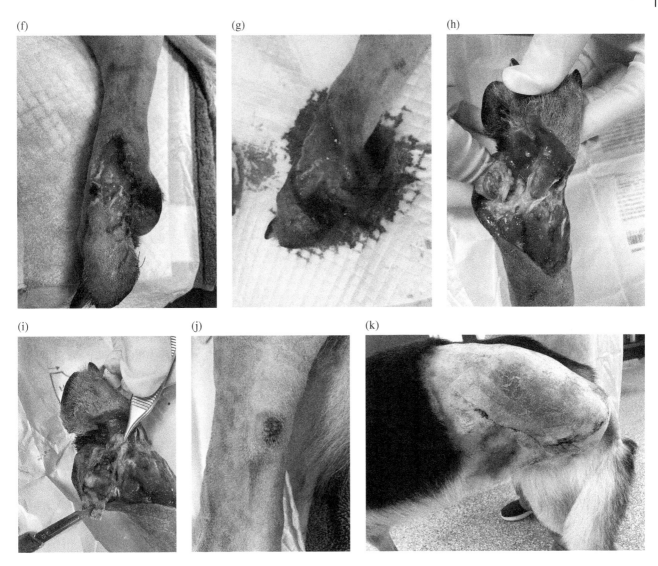

Figure 17.G.4   (Continued)

be managed open. If open management is undertaken, it can be expected that the wound will be highly exudative. Bandaged wounds should be evaluated multiple times per day to determine the necessity of additional surgical debridement.

If available, strong consideration should be given to negative-pressure wound therapy (NPWT). The application of NPWT has several advantages including: (i) increasing local blood flow and promoting angiogenesis; (ii) management of fluid accumulation and edema; (iii) reduction of bacterial load and consequent protease production; (iv) planned reoperation for evaluation and repeated debridement [7]. Reexploration is typically planned for days 2 or 3 of NPWT. If necrotic tissue is present during reexploration, debridement should proceed as before and NPWT should be reinstituted (see Chapter 10).

For NSTI-affected limbs, consideration should be given to amputation. This is particularly true for wounds that require extensive debridement since this will likely necessitate protracted bandage management. Amputation may also be considered when significant reconstruction (such as grafting) is anticipated or when owner finances preclude long hospital stays (Figure 17.G.4).

Early administration of intravenous antibiotics is recommended and efforts should be made to deliver the first dose within an hour of recognition of NSTI. Antibiotic administration should never be delayed to obtain culture results. If available, aspirates of fluid obtained at the time of diagnosis can be used for culture. The ischemic nature of the wound bed reduces antibiotic penetration and meaningful culture samples can be obtained by swabbing the wound at the time of surgery regardless of prior antibiotic administration. Initial antibiotic selection should be broad-spectrum. Ampicillin/ sulbactam, cephalosporins, or high-dose clindamycin can provide coverage for gram-positive and some gram-negative organisms. Clindamycin has the advantage of suppressing bacterial exotoxin formation and facilitation of phagocytosis of streptococcal organisms and may be the antimicrobial of choice [3]. Aminoglycosides or third-generation cephalosporins can broaden gram-negative coverage, and metronidazole can be used to further target anaerobic bacteria. Fluoroquinolone administration is not recommended for NSTI due to the potential for enhanced pathogenicity of gram-positive organisms and lack of correlation between *in vitro* susceptibility and *in vivo* effectiveness [3]. Gram staining of fluid collected at the time of diagnosis or exploration may help guide empirical antibiotic selection. As always, treatment with antimicrobial drugs should be tailored to culture and sensitivity results and de-escalation should occur as soon as susceptibility results are available.

Because of the severe pain associated with NSTI, aggressive analgesia should be provided. Constant rate infusion of an opioid such as fentanyl should be considered standard of care. Pain that is refractory to opioid administration alone may be addressed with the addition of ketamine or lidocaine as a constant rate infusion. Regional anesthesia techniques may prove useful provided they can be provided without traversing the site of infection. The use of non-steroidal anti-inflammatory drugs should be withheld initially due to the uncertainty present in the clinical course. Once hemodynamic stability has been maintained for 24 hours and future episodes of shock are not anticipated their use can be considered.

Possible Complications

The most significant complication that can be anticipated is the development of sepsis or septic shock as discussed above. Proactive monitoring is necessary to identify potentially significant harbingers early. Patients should have frequent vital sign checks and regular blood pressure monitoring and blood gas analysis should be implemented. Special attention should be paid to the possible development of acute kidney injury, particularly when aminoglycosides are being administered. Monitoring of urine output, serum creatinine, and urine sedimentation for casts is recommended.

Prolonged recumbency can predispose dogs to developing atelectasis and pneumonia as well as contribute to GI dysfunction (i.e., ileus). New fevers are cause for immediate concern and should prompt evaluation of all catheter insertion sites and consideration for thoracic radiographs or surgical reexploration.

Other possible complications include loss of limb or loss of limb function. When large limb wounds require bandage management, care should be taken to maintain the limb in a functional position.

Prognosis

For patients surviving the initial debridement and hospitalization, the ideal duration of antibiotic therapy is unknown. Typical courses in veterinary medicine average three to four weeks. The use of C-reactive protein as a biomarker for ongoing infection has been used as a guide to discontinuing antibiotic therapy for dogs with pneumonia and may hold promise for other types of infections [8, 9].

Because clinical signs can be nebulous early in the course of NSTI and the progression so rapid, the short-term prognosis may be guarded to poor, but with early recognition and aggressive surgical care, NSTI can be successfully managed. Survival statistics are limited in dogs but mortality rates likely exceed 50% and may be substantially higher [10]. Even with early and aggressive care in people, mortality rates for necrotizing fasciitis exceed 30% and may be near 100% for people with necrotizing myositis [11, 12]. True NSTI managed without surgery is generally fatal. Long-term prognosis in dogs is considered good for survival but not enough information is available to prognosticate on return to full function. People surviving NSTI have a high incidence of persistent impairment and failure to return to full work [11].

References

1 Mathews, K.A. and Singh, A. (2016). Necrotizing fasciitis. In: *Small Animal Surgical Emergencies* (ed. L.R. Aronson), 465–475. Hoboken, NJ: Wiley.

2 Rudloff, E. and Winkler, K.P. (2009). Necrotizing soft tissue infections. In: *Small Animal Critical Care Medicine* (ed. D.C. Silverstein and K. Hopper), 494–497. St. Louis, MO: Saunders.

3 Ho, V.P., Eachempati, S.R., and Baire, P.S. (2012). Surgical infections of skin and soft tissue. In: *Acute Care Surgery* (ed. L.D. Britt, A.B. Peitzman, P.S. Barie, et al.), 589–604. Philadelphia, PA: Lippincott Williams & Wilkins.

4 Mastrocco, A. and Prittie, J. (2021). Early and aggressive surgical debridement and negative pressure wound therapy to treat necrotizing fasciitis in three dogs. *Vet. Surg.* 50 (8): 1662–1669.

5 Bowlt, K.L., Pivetta, M., Kussy, F. et al. (2013). Imaging diagnosis and minimally-invasive management of necrotizing fasciitis in a dog. *Vet. Comp. Orthop. Traumatol.* 26 (4): 323–327.

6 Singer, M., Deutschman, C.S., Seymour, C.W. et al. (2016). The third international consensus definitions for sepsis and septic shock (Sepsis-3). *J. Am. Med. Assoc.* 315 (8): 801–810.

7 Buote, N.J. (2022). Updates in wounds management and dressings. *Vet. Clin. North Am. Small Anim. Pract.* 52 (2): 289–315.

8 Viitanen, S.J., Laurila, H.P., Lilja-Maula, L.I. et al. (2014). Serum C-reactive protein as a diagnostic biomarker in dogs with bacterial respiratory distress. *J. Vet. Int. Med.* 28 (1): 84–91.

9 Rodrigues, N.F., Giraud, L., Bolen, G. et al. (2022). Antimicrobial discontinuation in dogs with acute aspiration pneumonia based on clinical improvement and normalization of C-reactive protein concentration. *J. Vet. Int. Med.* 36 (3): 1082–1088.

10 Buriko, Y., Van Winkle, T.J., Drobatz, K.J. et al. (2008). Severe soft tissue infections in dogs: 47 cases (1996–2006). *J. Vet. Emerg. Crit. Care* 18 (6): 608–618.

11 Hakkarainen, T.W., Kopari, N.M., Pham, T.N. et al. (2014). Necrotizing soft tissue infections: review and current concepts in treatment, systems of care, and outcomes. *Curr. Prob. Surg.* 51 (8): 344–362.

12 Stevens, D.L. (1995). Streptococcal toxic-shock syndrome: spectrum of disease, pathogenesis, and new concepts in treatment. *Emerg. Infect. Dis.* 1 (3): 69–78.

17

Specific Wounds

Subsection H: Snakebites

Nathan Peterson

Department of Clinical Sciences, Cornell University, Ithaca, NY, USA

Presenting Signs

In North America, there are two families of venomous snakes, the Elapidae and the Viperidae. The Elapids are comprised of coral snakes that deliver a neurotoxic venom through a chewing action with their short, fixed fangs and secreting the venom into the resulting wound. Generally, the wounds resulting from Elapid bites are superficial and will not be considered further in this chapter. Vipers generally have hollow, retractable fangs through which they inject a necrogenic venom. Adult pit vipers (Crotalidae), the most clinically relevant vipers in North America, are capable of metering the dose of venom they inject into a bite victim leading to a large degree of variability in the clinical presentation of strike victims. Relevant species include water moccasins (cottonmouth), copperheads, and rattlesnakes.

The severity of a bite depends on the amount of time that has elapsed since the snake last had a meal, the motivation of the snake (defensive strike versus offensive strike), and the age of the snake. Single bites appear to be more common than multiple bites. The most common location of bite wounds is the head with up to 81% of bites occurring there [1]. Extremities account for approximately 21% of bite locations and bites to the torso are rare [1]. The delivery system that pit vipers use creates small puncture wounds similar to hypodermic needles that may easily be overlooked if no swelling or bleeding is present at the time of evaluation.

Pets presenting for possible snakebites generally have a history of known exposure to snakes or access to an environment known to be inhabited by snakes although direct observation of a strike is uncommon. Initial signs often include signs of pain and changes in behavior such as seeking or avoiding attention. Rapidly progressive swelling of the face or limbs is the most common clinical sign and may include minimal bleeding from one or two very small puncture wounds (Figure 17.H.1). Swelling and erythema around the bite wounds are generally present within 30 minutes of envenomating bites and, as a result, are usually present at the time of presentation but signs may be delayed up to 24 hours [2]. Occasionally, these early presenting signs can be mistaken for hypersensitivity reactions but a distinguishing characteristic is the pain associated with the swelling in a bite that is absent from hypersensitivity reactions (Figure 17.H.2).

Diagnosis is usually made based on history and identification of progressive swelling and bruising with characteristic puncture wounds. The presence of echinocytosis and thrombocytopenia on blood film provides supportive evidence (Figure 17.H.3). Coagulation testing may reveal prolongation of PT and aPTT. Where available viscoelastic testing with either ROTEM, TEG, or VCM has been shown to correlate with the severity of envenomation [3, 4].

Wound Characteristics

When wounds develop from envenomation, they tend to be limited to the dermis and subcutis but they may incorporate a large surface area. These wounds result from sloughing of necrotic tissue and generally develop several days following envenomation (Figure 17.H.4). Bite wounds that penetrate the myofascial compartments of the limbs may cause

Techniques in Small Animal Wound Management, First Edition. Edited by Nicole J. Buote.
© 2024 John Wiley & Sons, Inc. Published 2024 by John Wiley & Sons, Inc.
Companion website: www.wiley.com/go/buote/wounds

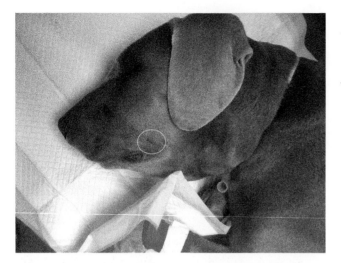

Figure 17.H.1 Photograph of a Weimeraner on presentation after a rattlesnake strike to the left muzzle. The yellow circle highlights the small external wounds created by a snake bite. Note this patient had a tracheostomy tube placed. An elbow piece is visible because cervical tissue kept occluding the tracheostomy tube. *Source:* Courtesy of Nathan Peterson, DVM, MS, DACVECC.

(a) (b)

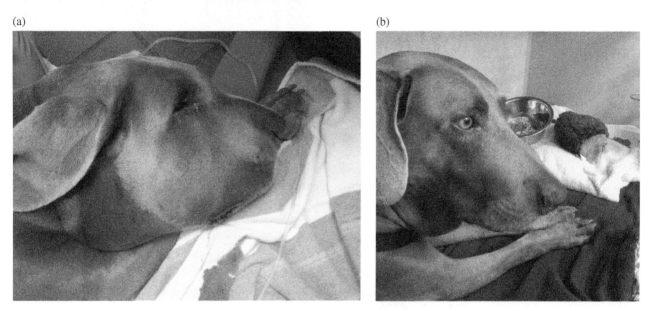

Figure 17.H.2 Photograph of the patient in Figure 17.H.1. (a) Appearance of muzzle on presentation. (b) Appearance after four days of hospitalization. *Source:* Courtesy of Nathan Peterson, DVM, MS, DACVECC.

(a) (b)

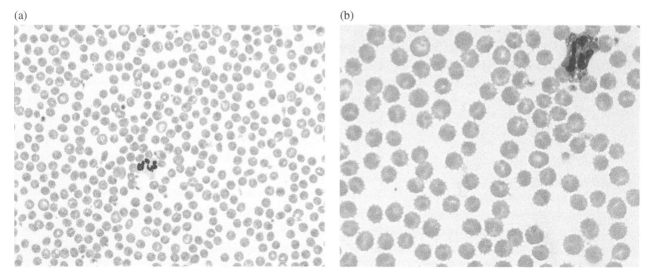

Figure 17.H.3 Photomicrographs of a blood smear of a dog after envenomation. Note the extreme echinocytosis of all red blood cells. The picture (a) is a low power (10×) view and (b) is a high power (100×) view. *Source:* Courtesy of Harold Tvedten DVM, PhD, DACVP, DECVP.

(a)

(b)

(c)

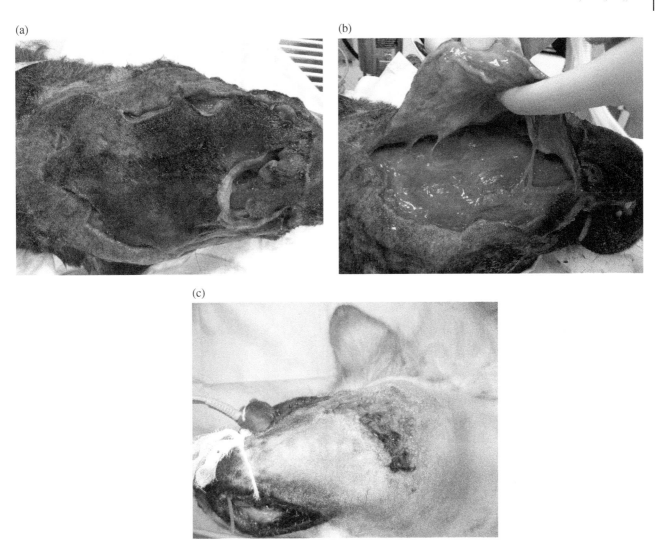

Figure 17.H.4 Photographs of dogs after snake bite wounds. (a and b) Full-thickness necrosis of skin along chin and cervical region seven days after rattlesnake bite in owner's backyard in Southern California. *Source:* Courtesy of Nicole Buote, DVM, DACVS. (c) Photograph of cervical wound from a water moccasin bite approximately five days after the initial injury. *Source:* Courtesy of Kelley Thieman, DVM, MS, DACVS.

compartment syndrome and are characterized by severe swelling and pain. Large wounds or compartment syndrome however are the exceptions. Most often, venom is delivered into the subcutaneous space and spreads along fascial planes causing hemorrhage and edema without a large wound resulting. Bruising and edema may be severe and may spread or migrate for many hours following an envenomation (Figure 17.H.5). Regions of bruising are often traced with a marker and monitored for both progression and viability.

Physiologic Effects

The composition of snake venom varies across species and geographic range so having an awareness of the species and venom characteristics in your region is beneficial. As a consequence of this diversity and the complexity of venom composition, physiologic effects will vary. Pit-viper envenomation may cause flaccid paralysis, rhabdomyolysis, coagulopathy, renal failure, cardiotoxicity, and local tissue necrosis. Hyaluronidase and collagenase present in the venom facilitate its spread and account for the potential massive tissue injury and necrosis in snake bite victims.

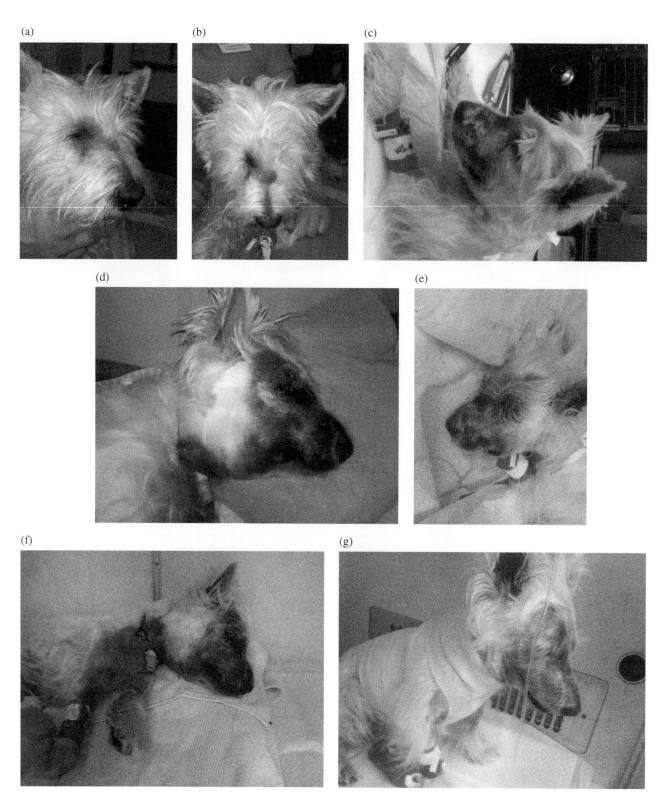

Figure 17.H.5   West Highland Terrier in the hours and days after a rattlesnake strike. (a) Right Lateral view of patient's head 90 minutes after snakebite. A small wound is visible under the right eye. (b) Dorsal view of patient 90 minutes after snakebite. (c) Left lateral view of patient four hours after snakebite and after administration of two vials of antivenom and temporary tracheostomy placement. Note the facial swelling as compared to photographs a and b. (d): Right lateral view of patient 18 hours after snakebite and after administration of six vials of antivenom. Note the progressive severe bruising with a visible line of demarcation. (e): Left lateral view of patient 28 hours after snakebite and after administration of six vials antivenom. (f) Left lateral view of patient 42 hours after snakebite. Persistent swelling and bruising are present. (g) Patient four days after snakebite. A percutaneous endoscopic gastrostomy (PEG) tube was placed but the tracheostomy tube has been removed and the patient is ready to be sent home. Note the resolution of facial swelling but continued bruising of the skin. *Source:* Courtesy of Nathan Peterson, DVM, MS, DACVECC.

The effect that pit viper envenomation has on the coagulation system can be profound and results from enzymatic activity in the procoagulant, anticoagulant, and fibrinolytic pathways. Direct activation of coagulation factors II, V, and X can lead to consumption of these factors. Inhibitors of thrombin and phospholipase A2, activators of protein C, and binding of factors IX and X promote an anticoagulant state [5]. Perhaps most importantly, fibrinolytic enzymes such as metalloproteinases and serine proteases result in defibrination of the blood. Some of these components also degrade the extracellular matrix of blood vessels and inhibit platelet binding. The end result is clinical bleeding due to consumption of fibrin that is not characterized by thrombosis or intravascular coagulation.

As noted above, some North American pit vipers, the Mojave Green Rattlesnake in particular, have a significant neurotoxic component to their venom. These neurotoxins have a predilection for peripheral nervous tissue and act as pre- or post-synaptic neuromuscular blockers by either inhibiting acetylcholine release or blocking acetylcholine receptors. Snakebites that contain a primarily neurotoxic venom usually cause an ascending flaccid paralysis with little associated tissue injury. It is uncommon to find large necrosing wounds in these circumstances.

Treatment

The treatment of snakebite begins in the field with appropriate first aid. To date, no ideal first-aid measures have been identified for managing snakebite. Incision and suction of the wound should never be recommended. The use of tourniquets for pit-viper envenomation is discouraged due to the necrogenic potential of venom. While tourniquets may limit systemic exposure to venom, they reduce the dilutional effect of spread and concentrate venom in the location of the bite allowing more time for the venom to degrade tissue. Consequently, envenomations that would otherwise not have induced necrosis might result in significant tissue loss. Cold packing has a similar effect through induction of vasoconstriction and should not be employed. However, snake envenomation often occurs in remote areas where immediate access to care is not available. When possible, owners should be instructed to immobilize the affected body region in a functional position without constricting blood flow and to seek immediate veterinary attention. A moderate number of pit-viper strikes are non-envenomating "dry bites" and may not require any further care. If a dry bite is suspected, the patient should be monitored closely for up to 24 hours for development of signs consistent with an envenomation and if they develop immediate care should be sought.

The mainstay of treatment for crotalid envenomation is the administration of antivenom products. There are currently two major types of antivenom available in the United States: polyvalent whole antibody molecule antivenom generally derived from equine serum, and polyvalent antivenom containing only the Fab portion of the antibody molecule generally derived from equine or ovine serum. Regardless of which antivenom product is selected, the mechanism of action is the same: to bind and neutralize circulating venom components. Because the effectiveness of antivenom therapy relies on the neutralization of venom by antibody binding a molar dosing regimen is utilized. This means that the volume dose of antivenom required depends on the volume of venom that was injected and not on the patient's size. Somewhat counterintuitively, smaller patients often require larger doses of antivenom. This is due to the fact that the volume of venom injected is proportionally larger in a small patient than in a larger patient. Not surprisingly, antivenom therapy is most effective when implemented early in the course of envenomation although it may be beneficial as long as free venom is present in the patient.

Antivenom therapy is expensive and may not be necessary in all cases of possible or actual pit-viper envenomation. Indications to begin antivenom therapy include: (i) rapid, progressive swelling; (ii) development of coagulopathy; (iii) severe pain; (iv) signs of systemic shock or circulatory collapse; (v) and concern that bites on the head and neck could lead to compromise of the airway. The goal when administering antivenom products should be to deliver an entire dose (usually one vial) to the patient over 30 minutes. Additional doses can be administered every 30–60 minutes as needed to control signs. Serial measurement of the affected region can be used to determine if swelling is progressive but must be distinguished from migration of edema that is already present.

Possible side effects of antivenom administration include hypersensitivity reactions including immediate type I (anaphylactic/anaphylactoid) and type III (delayed) reactions [6]. Premedication with antihistamines does not appear to be useful in mitigating these reactions. Volume overload can also result due to the colloidal properties of antivenom products so careful monitoring should be performed when administered to small patients.

Antibiotic therapy is not indicated for envenomations that do not result in the development of a wound. For those envenomations that do result in wounds, empirical treatment with a potentiated penicillin such as ampicillin/sulbactam or amoxicillin/clavulonate is generally acceptable pending culture and sensitivity results.

Debridement of wounds should occur once clear demarcation is apparent between viable and non-viable tissue. Snake envenomation can result in severe bruising with skin occasionally appearing black and still result in no wound development. If debridement of necrotic tissue is needed it can be performed as usual using either sharp debridement or bandage debridement according to patient needs (see Chapters 5, 10, 12).

Bandaging of envenomation sites in the absence of wounds is not necessary. If wounds develop, bandaging should be employed to assist with debridement and to prevent contamination of the wound with opportunistic pathogens. Unfortunately, the frequent location of wounds on the head and neck may make traditional bandaging difficult (Figure 17.H.6). Consideration should be given to using negative pressure wound therapy in patients with significant wounds of the head and neck to promote contraction of the wound and prepare a healthy granulation bed to receive reconstructive flaps or grafts if needed (see Chapters 10, 16). Occasionally, large wounds of the head, neck, or limbs require reconstructive surgery. Once a healthy recipient bed is established, reconstructive techniques such as pedicle grafts, advancement grafts, or free grafts can be employed.

Possible Complications

Infection is rare in pit-viper envenomations in which wounds do not develop. Current evidence provides little support for empirical antibiotic use [7] in such cases and, to promote good antimicrobial stewardship practices, should be withheld unless or until signs of infection are evident. If infection occurs, empirical antibiotic therapy can be instituted as above or according to hospital-specific antibiograms and should be adjusted according to the results of culture and sensitivity testing.

Occasionally, envenomations of the face or head can lead to compromise of the airways. If rapid swelling occurs and concern develops for the patency of airways, early tracheostomy is recommended. Delaying tracheostomy until overt airway compromise occurs results in a much more technically difficult procedure due to the development and migration of edema and hemorrhage in the ventral, dependent cervical region.

Envenomation of the limbs resulting in the development of large wounds may lead to partial or complete loss of function. Care should be taken to ensure limbs are immobilized in a functional position if bandaging is necessary. If large wounds develop on limbs consideration should be given to amputation if owner finances or questions about bandage compliance are a concern.

Prognosis

The short-term prognosis for pit-viper envenomation is dependent on several factors including patient characteristics, venom load injected into the patient, and delay to appropriate medical care. If patients arrive alive and without signs of systemic shock, the prognosis for recovery is generally good assuming antivenom therapy is available if needed. Patients surviving the initial envenomation and acute hospitalization are anticipated to have an excellent prognosis for long-term survival. Ultimate functional prognosis is dependent on whether or not significant necrosis occurs and the location of associated tissue loss.

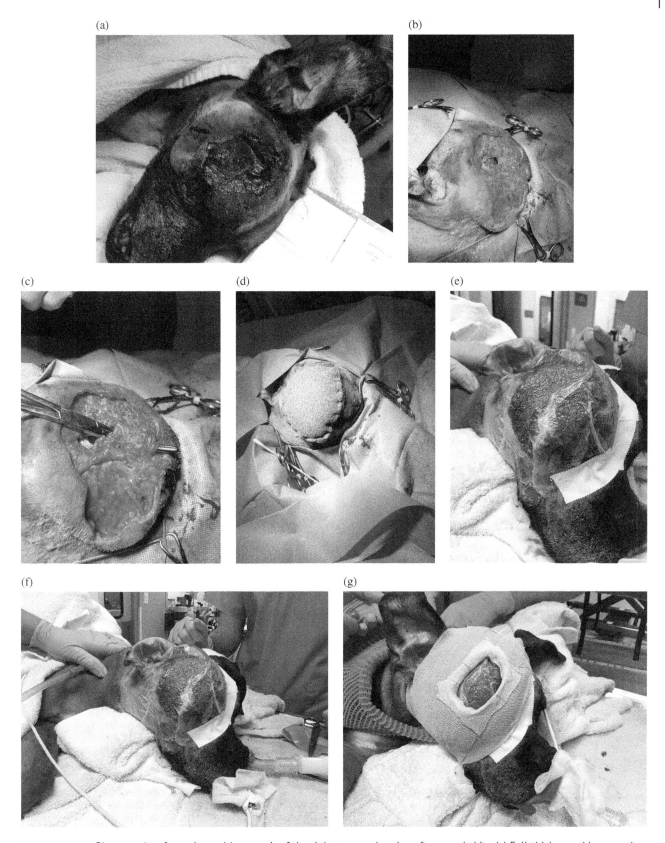

Figure 17.H.6   Photographs of a patient with necrosis of the right temporal region after a snakebite. (a) Full-thickness skin necrosis. (b and c) Debridement of necrotic tissue. (d–g) Placement of a negative pressure vacuum bandage. *Source:* Courtesy of Nicole Buote, DVM, DACVS.

References

1 Hackett, T.B., Wingfield, W.E., Mazzaferro, E.M. et al. (2002). Clinical findings associated with prairie rattlesnake bites in dogs: 100 cases (1989–1998). *J. Am. Vet. Med. Assoc.* 220 (11): 1675–1680.

2 Armentano, R.A. and Schaer, M. (2011). Overview and controversies in the medical management of pit viper envenomation in the dog. *J. Vet. Emerg. Crit. Care* 21 (5): 461–470.

3 Armentano, R.A., Bandt, C., Schaer, M. et al. (2014). Thromboelastographic evaluation of hemostatic function in dogs treated for crotalid snake envenomation. *J. Vet. Emerg. Crit. Care* 24 (2): 144–153.

4 Lieblick, B.A., Bergman, P.J., and Peterson, N.W. (2018). Thromboelastographic evaluation of dogs bitten by rattlesnakes native to southern California. *Am. J. Vet. Res.* 79 (5): 532–537.

5 Lu, Q., Clemetson, J.M., and Clemetson, K.J. (2005). Snake venoms and hemostasis. *J. Thromb. Haemost.* 3: 1791–1799.

6 McCown, J.L., Cooke, K.L., Hanel, R.M. et al. (2009). Effect of antivenin dose on outcome from crotalid envenomation: 218 dogs (1988–2006). *J. Vet. Emerg. Crit. Care* 19 (6): 603–610.

7 Kerrigan, K.R., Mertz, B.L., Nelson, S.J. et al. (1997). Antibiotic prophylaxis for pit viper envenomation: prospective, controlled trial. *World J. Surg.* 21 (4): 369–373.

17

Specific Wounds

Subsection I: Pythiosis
Kristin A. Coleman

Gulf Coast Veterinary Specialists, Houston, TX, USA

Introduction

One of the scariest and most aggressive organisms capable of causing a dermal lesion that is both minimally responsive to conservative management and behaves like a high-grade sarcoma in its invasive nature is that of a fungus: *Pythium sp.* Pythiosis is a life-threatening infectious disease of both the gastrointestinal tract and skin (cutaneous/subcutaneous) of animals caused by the aquatic filamentous eukaryotic oomycete, *Pythium insidiosum*, in the kingdom Stramenopila [1–4]. Unlike other *Pythium* species that are pathogenic to terrestrial plants, *P. insidiosum* is capable of being pathogenic to mammals, including humans, with additional species of vertebrates and invertebrates being reported each year. This *Pythium* organism is more closely related to algae than to fungi, and oospores of these pathogenic oomycetes may survive in the soil for long periods of time (possibly months to years), which allows the pathogen to persist in the environment, such as through a mild winter. During certain favorable conditions, including an ideal temperature range of 90–98 °F (32–36 °C), the oospore germinates, forming sporangia from which zoospores are released and provide an inoculum for infection of susceptible host tissues [3–6]. The zoospores then encyst in susceptible host tissue, such as a defect in the skin, and form a thick cell wall to produce a germ tube that penetrates the tissue via "penetration pegs" and forms hyphal structures. Sporangia may then form directly from mycelia in infected tissue, and thus, the repeated cycle of reinfection of the tissue propagates to create a fungal lesion in the cutaneous and/or subcutaneous tissue [3, 4, 6, 7].

The first reported lesions occurred in humans in 1884 [8], and when it was again reported in 1974 in horses, the organism causing the lesion was identified as *Pythium* sp. Other names throughout history for pythiosis, which are all derived from the common mode of infecting animals in an aqueous environment via their open wounds or cutaneous defects, include: phycomycosis, bursattee, espundia, horse leeches, granular dermatitis, summer sore, and swamp cancer [9]. In a recent study investigating the global distribution and clinical features of pythiosis [9], there were 4203 cases of pythiosis in humans, dogs, cattle, horses, cats, sheep, other vertebrate species, and several invertebrate species, such as shrimp. These were reported from tropical, subtropical, and temperate countries around the world with 79.2% of animal cases being reported in the U.S.A. and Brazil with optimal growth temperature of *P. insidiosum* being between 28 and 37 °C. The most common form in animals is the cutaneous/subcutaneous manifestation on the face, limb, trunk, or abdomen, which accounts for 89.8% of all affected animals [9], and these animals often have a history of recurrent exposure to warm, freshwater habitats [2, 10].

Presenting Signs

Pythiosis commonly presents as an ulcerated or draining granulomatous lesion, and it is initiated by the individual coming into contact with the zoospores of the fungus, which is mostly by exposure to freshwater containing the zoospores that are attracted to hair, broken skin, or open wounds [2, 4]. These affected animals with cutaneous pythiosis often have

Techniques in Small Animal Wound Management, First Edition. Edited by Nicole J. Buote.
© 2024 John Wiley & Sons, Inc. Published 2024 by John Wiley & Sons, Inc.
Companion website: www.wiley.com/go/buote/wounds

persistently growing cutaneous lesions, non-healing wounds, and/or chronic draining tracts [11–13]. Locations on the body most commonly affected include the face, limbs, ventral aspect of the thorax, perineum, tailhead, and abdomen [9, 11, 12]. Other than the most commonly reported cutaneous/subcutaneous and gastrointestinal forms, the remaining clinical manifestations are classified into ocular, vascular, pulmonary, prostatic, and disseminated pythiosis [9].

Occurrence has been documented in several species, including humans, dogs, cats, sheep, horses, and cattle, and while water is usually involved as part of the history of infection due to the fungal life cycle, the overall geographical extent is unknown. Even with a single cutaneous lesion, this is considered a systemic fungal infection, and it is not uncommon to see intermittent lethargy and decreased appetite with the cutaneous/subcutaneous form. It may appear as a quickly growing mass despite topical or oral treatments [14].

According to one study [11], most dogs who were presented with cutaneous/subcutaneous pythiosis were young (median age of 22 months) and represented breeds were over 20 kg. Lesions were chronic, ulcerated, and nodular with multiple draining tracts on the limbs, thoracic wall, or perineal regions. There was occasionally the history of swimming. Differential diagnoses for these lesions include subcutaneous mycosis, lymphoma, and parasitic and bacterial infections.

Diagnosis

Diagnosis of a *P. insidiosum* lesion usually begins with bloodwork and cytology of the mass, and once a presumptive diagnosis of pythiosis is confirmed, there are several studies investigating confirmatory tests and stains to be performed on an incisional biopsy of the tissue. Non-specific but common hematologic and biochemical findings include anemia, eosinophilia, hypoalbuminemia, and hyperglobulinemia [3], and if cytology is performed, about 50% will reveal hyphae from the lesion.

Incisional biopsy is the next step and can reveal severe necrotizing and fibrosing granulomatous and eosinophilic dermatitis and cellulitis and/or pyogranulomatous panniculitis [14]. Histopathological evaluation of the tissue using the Gomori Methenamine Silver (GMS) stain was the most useful for providing presumptive evidence of cutaneous pythiosis.

Pythiosis may be diagnosed via culture identification and zoospore induction, histological examination with immunostaining (neutral-buffered 10% buffered formalin for H&E) [15], serological tests (i.e., immunodiffusion [ID], Western blot [WB], enzyme-linked immunosorbent assay [ELISA], hemagglutination [HA], and immunochromatography [ICT]), molecular assays (i.e., PCR and sequence homology analysis), and proteomic approaches [9, 10, 16]. Other dermatopathologic testing may use GMS, periodic acid-Schiff, and Brown-Brenn stains on the tissue samples. Microscopically, the characteristics of *P. insidiosum* include broad hyphae (4–7 μm in diameter), perpendicular branching, coenocyte in young hyphae, sparse septation in an aged organism, and rounded hyphal tips [9]. The most practical diagnosis is by culture on antibiotic-containing selective media [17], Campy blood agar or vegetable extract agar amended with streptomycin and ampicillin [10] with resultant hyphal growth and subsequent identification of the *Pythium insidiosum* morphology in addition to incisional biopsy with GMS staining is one of the most reliable methods to diagnose pythiosis. It is very important to accurately diagnose *P. insidiosum* since it is addressed differently than *Lagenidium* but appears grossly similar.

Diagnostic imaging, especially CT scan, should be considered to determine the extent of disease of the cutaneous lesion prior to aggressive surgical resection and to aid in surgical planning. Lymphadenomegaly is occasionally noted on CT scan, so fine needle aspiration and cytologic interpretation should be done with GMS-stained slides to rule out disseminated pythiosis before surgery [14]. CT scan in particular is able to identify soft tissue changes that are not possible to detect on palpation, so the recommended 5-cm surgical margins may be measured from the CT-identified ill-defined area of contrast-enhancing diseased tissue, which may extend several centimeters beyond the palpable edge of the fungal mass.

Wound Characteristics

Cutaneous/subcutaneous pythiosis may appear as ulcerative pyogranulomatous lesions, cellulitis, and/or subcutaneous lumps or nodules anywhere on the body with or without draining tracts (Figures 17.I.1 and 17.I.2). Prior to considering surgical excision, a CT scan is recommended due to the ill-defined peripheral and deep margins with the need for wide surgical excision as treatment. Regrowth of the lesion is relatively rapid with marginal or anything less than wide excision.

Physiologic Effects

In a recent study, looking at animals and humans infected with pythiosis [9], there is a 33.5% mortality rate considering all clinical manifestations in animals. With regards to the cutaneous/subcutaneous form, there was a 71.0% mortality rate in dogs and a 62.5% mortality rate in cats. Affected animals often have a history of coming into contact with fresh water, notably swampy areas that may harbor *P. insidiosum*, such as rice fields, rivers, and water reservoirs [9]. Once the motile zoospore, which is the infective flagellate unit of the oomycete, or hyphae attach and penetrate any exposed wound or damaged skin of the animal host after direct contact with the contaminated water, pythiosis ensues with the clinical form dictated by the site of entry. Fortunately, pythiosis is not zoonotic and has never been reported to transmit from animal to animal or from animal to human.

Affected tissues contain several foci of necrosis surrounded and infiltrated by neutrophils, eosinophils, and macrophages, and vasculitis is occasionally present. The *P. insidiosum* organisms are usually found within areas of necrosis or at the center of the lesion [7]. The areas of inflammation are often located in the deep dermis and subcutaneous layers. This results in cutaneous pythiosis, which typically causes severe nodular to diffuse ulcerative dermatitis and panniculitis.

![Figure 17.I.1 Dorsal lumbar cutaneous/subcutaneous pythiosis lesion on a dog.](placeholder)

Figure 17.I.1 Dorsal lumbar cutaneous/subcutaneous pythiosis lesion on a dog. *Source:* Courtesy of Kristin Coleman, DVM, MS, DACVS.

Treatment

The etiologic agent of pythiosis has limited sensitivity to conventional antimicrobial agents, so surgical intervention with excision of the infected tissue, whether cutaneous or intestinal, is the current primary treatment for pythiosis and may even provide the ability to cure. Excision with 5-cm skin margins and two fascial planes has been described with long-term (36-month) resolution of the initial lesion [14]; however, guidelines for aggressiveness of surgical excision are ambiguous with one source simply recommending wide surgical excision if addressing a truncal lesion and amputation if addressing a lesion on an extremity [13]. The concept for this wide surgical excision is derived from the surgical oncologic recommendation regarding wide surgical excision of vaccine-associated sarcomas [14, 18]. If these margins are not feasible due to the size of the lesion or the anatomic location on the patient's body, such as the large, ulcerated lesion in Figure 17.I.3 on the right shoulder, brachium, and cranial thorax, palliative care or euthanasia are the only remaining options.

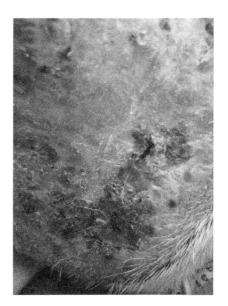

Figure 17.I.2 Cutaneous/subcutaneous pythiosis lesion on 6-year-old mixed breed dog. *Source:* Courtesy of Kristin Coleman, DVM, MS, DACVS.

The author of this chapter had similar success of over three years local control of a dorsal lumbar cutaneous pythiosis lesion (Figure 17.I.4–17.I.12) utilizing the wide surgical excision with 5-cm lateral and two fascial planes deep, a right caudal superficial epigastric axial pattern skin flap with a dorsal single pedicle advancement flap to cover the defect, and five months of oral anti-fungal therapy using terbinafine and itraconazole postoperatively. Prior to a wide surgical excision of this magnitude, there are three criteria that must be met: (i) the area of the lesion is amenable to wide surgical excision of 5-cm lateral margins and two fascial planes deep, (ii) there is no evidence of regional lymph node pythiosis infection, and (iii) there is no evidence of distant spread on the body of the pythiosis.

While surgical excision guidelines for cutaneous pythiosis are lacking, the generally accepted recommendation is to amputate if the lesion is on a limb or tail and to widely excise if the lesion is on the truncal region. The dimension

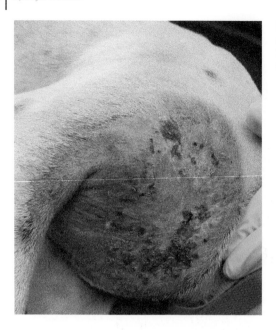

Figure 17.I.3 Large ulcerative crusting invasive cutaneous/subcutaneous *P. insidiosum* lesion of the right shoulder, brachium, cranial elbow, and cranial thoracic areas of this 6-year-old mixed breed dog. *Source:* Courtesy of Kristin Coleman, DVM, MS, DACVS.

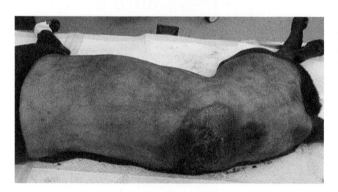

Figure 17.I.4 Anesthetized canine patient being prepared for wide surgical excision of the dorsal lumbar cutaneous/subcutaneous pythiosis lesion. *Source:* Courtesy of Kristin Coleman, DVM, MS, DACVS.

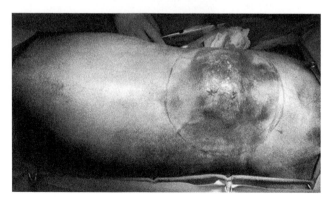

Figure 17.I.5 Surgical marker is used to adequately outline the wide surgical excision of 5-cm lateral skin margins. In the image, the patient's head is to the left, and the dorsal lumbar *P. insidiosum* lesion is going to be excised in this staged procedure. *Source:* Courtesy of Kristin Coleman, DVM, MS, DACVS.

guidelines set forth by Thieman et al. in their 2011 case report, which chose margins suggested for resection of high-grade soft tissue sarcomas in animals, were gleaned from the STS guidelines [14, 18]. With such a large portion of tissue being resected from somewhere on the trunk and attaining two fascial planes of tissue below that of the lesion, an axial pattern flap is strongly encouraged to transpose into the defect. If a single-session surgery is elected, an axial pattern flap does not require a granulation bed and may be placed on most organic substrates.

Figure 17.1.6 If the lesion to be resected is on the truncal region, an axial pattern flap, such as a caudal superficial epigastric flap, is often utilized to cover the defect created by the fungal lesion excision. In this image, the patient's head is to the right, and a right CSE flap is being planned. *Source:* Courtesy of Kristin Coleman, DVM, MS, DACVS.

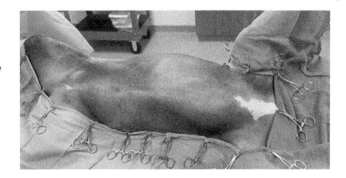

Figure 17.1.7 The patient's head is on the right in this image, and in this staged procedure, the CSE flap is elevated then sutured into the bridging incision. *Source:* Courtesy of Kristin Coleman, DVM, MS, DACVS.

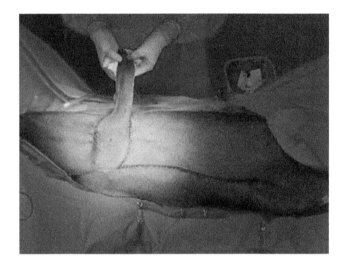

Figure 17.1.8 The patient's head is on the right in this image, and after elevating the right CSE flap and isolating the flap in sterile moistened laparotomy sponges in the foreground of the image, the dorsal lumbar fungal lesion is then excised. *Source:* Courtesy of Kristin Coleman, DVM, MS, DACVS.

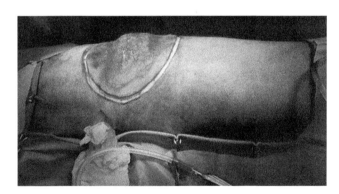

Figure 17.1.9 The patient's head is on the right in this image, and after excising the fungal lesion and changing gloves and surgical instruments, the flap is then sutured into the defect. *Source:* Courtesy of Kristin Coleman, DVM, MS, DACVS.

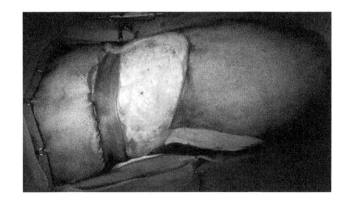

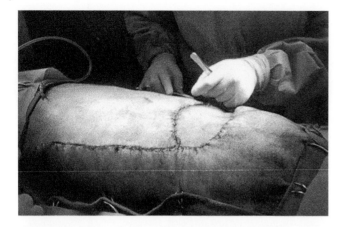

Figure 17.I.10 The patient's head is on the left in this image, and after apposing the cutaneous trunci muscle of the single pedicle advancement flap and the right CSE flap to cover the large dorsal lumbar defect with 2-0 medium-lasting synthetic monofilament absorbable suture, subcutaneous and skin layers were closed routinely. *Source:* Courtesy of Kristin Coleman, DVM, MS, DACVS.

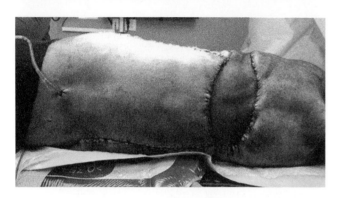

Figure 17.I.11 A closed suction drain was placed and kept indwelling for five days postoperatively to reduce the risk of seroma formation due to the extreme amount of dead space created with the two skin flaps. *Source:* Courtesy of Kristin Coleman, DVM, MS, DACVS.

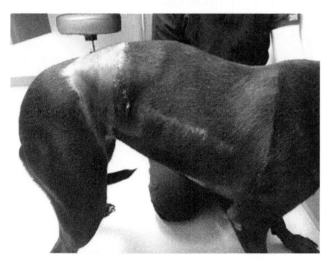

Figure 17.I.12 The patient was presented for suture removal three weeks following surgery. At this time, all incisions were deemed healed. *Source:* Courtesy of Kristin Coleman, DVM, MS, DACVS.

At the time of single-session surgery, it is recommended to include both the lesion and the donor site for the skin flap, as well as all surrounding tissue, to adequately drape all areas in the operating room (Figure 17.I.6). Between wide surgical excision of the fungal lesion and creation and closure of the skin flap, be sure to change gloves and instruments to reduce the risk of reinfection. To adequately assess completeness of excision, ink all cut edges of the excised tissue, which should be submitted *en bloc*. If dirty margins remain, scar revision should be performed, so denoting which edges of the *en bloc* tissue are cranial, proximal, etc. is important and may be done by placing sutures of varying suture patterns or colors (e.g., cruciate mattress in the cranial edge, simple interrupted in the caudal edge) to help the pathologist distinguish anatomic location of the mass.

There have been efforts made in using immunotherapy with *P. insidiosum* antigens [19], but the efficacy is currently lacking for this treatment modality [9]. Due to the systemic nature of this fungal infection, medical treatment in the form of itraconazole (9 mg/kg [4 mg/lb] PO q 24 hours) and terbinafine (11 mg/kg [5 mg/lb] PO q 24 hours) administration for three months is also commonly initiated in combination with surgical excision of the lesion, especially if serology confirms active pythiosis [14].

Medical treatment alone is rarely successful with <20% of animal patients responding to the anti-fungal combination of itraconazole and terbinafine when not administered with surgical excision of the lesion [13, 14]. Immunotherapy or anti-fungal therapy using amphotericin B, liposomal nystatin, and ketoconazole were also unsuccessful when not combined with wide surgical excision of the lesion. The theory of why pythiosis does not respond to anti-fungal therapy is that these medications target ergosterol, which is generally absent in the oomycete cytoplasmic membrane of *Pythium sp.* Instead of chitin in their cell walls like other fungi, *P. insidiosum* has B-glucans and cellulose [20]. Due to this cellular variation and the resultant poor response to anti-fungal therapy alone, surgery is the treatment of choice for pythiosis when the lesions are in a potentially resectable anatomic location.

Possible Complications

Local recurrence is the most concerning of the potential postoperative complications, which is why such aggressive surgical excision should be performed with lesion removal.

Prognosis

The general prognosis for pythiosis is poor, primarily due to the delayed treatment when this deadly fungal lesion is misdiagnosed as another fungal infection with similar clinical manifestations. In dogs with gastrointestinal lesions, there is a reported 86.4% mortality rate, and there is a 100% mortality rate in those with disseminated infection. Although it is difficult to prevent disease in endemic tropical areas, avoiding stagnant water is recommended, especially if wounds are present on the tissue being exposed to the water [8].

References

1 Foil, C., Short, B., Fadok, V. et al. (1984). A report of subcutaneous pythiosis in five dogs and a review of the etiologic agent Pythium spp. *J. Am Anim. Hosp. Assoc.* 20: 959–966.

2 White, S.D., Ghoddusi, M., Grooters, A.M. et al. (2008). Cutaneous pythiosis in a nontravelled California horse. *Vet. Dermatol.* 19: 391–394.

3 Berryessa, N.A., Marks, S.L., Pesavento, P.A. et al. (2008). Gastrointestinal pythiosis in 10 dogs from California. *J. Vet. Intern. Med.* 22: 1065–1069.

4 Mendoza, L., Hernandez, F., and Ajello, L. (1993). Life cycle of the human and animal oomycete pathogen *Pythium insidiosum. J. Clin. Microbiol.* 31: 2967–2973.

5 Martins, T., Kommers, G., Trost, M. et al. (2012). A comparative study of the histopathology and immunohistochemistry of pythiosis in horses, dogs and cattle. *J. Comp. Pathol.* 146: 122–131.

6 Oldenhoff, W., Grooters, A., Pinkerton, M.E. et al. (2014). Cutaneous pythiosis in two dogs from Wisconsin, USA. *Vet. Dermatol.* 25: 52–e21.

7 Miller, R.I. (1983). Investigations into the biology of three phycomycotic agents pathogenic for horses in Australia. *Mycopathologia* 81: 23–28.

8 Gaastra, W., Lipman, L.J., De Cock, A.W. et al. (2010). *Pythium insidiosum*: an overview. *Vet. Microbiol.* 146: 1–16.

9 Yolanda, H. and Krajaejun, T. (2022). Global distribution and clinical features of pythiosis in humans and animals. *J. Fungi (Basel)* 8 (2): 182. https://doi.org/10.3390/jof8020182. PMID: 35205934; PMCID: PMC8879638.

10 Grooters, A.M. and Foil, C.S. (2012). Miscellaneous fungal infections. In: *Infectious Diseases of the Dog and Cat*, 4e (ed. C.E. Greene), 677–680. St Louis, MO: Elsevier.

11 Dykstra, M.J., Sharp, N.J.H., Olivry, T. et al. (1999). A description of cutaneous-subcutaneous pythiosis in fifteen dogs. *Med. Mycol.* 37: 427–433.

12 Neto, R.T., De MG Bosco, S., Amorim, R.L. et al. (2010). Cutaneous pythiosis in a dog from Brazil. *Vet. Dermatol.* 21: 202–204.

13 Grooters, A.M. (2003). Pythiosis, lagenidiosis, and zygomycosis in small animals. *Vet. Clin. North Am. Small Anim. Pract.* 33: 695–720.

14 Thieman, K.M., Kirkby, K.A., Flynn-Lurie, A. et al. (2011). Diagnosis and treatment of truncal cutaneous pythiosis in a dog. *J. Am. Vet. Med. Assoc.* 239: 1232–1235.

15 Thomas, R.C. and Lewis, D.T. (1998). Pythiosis in dogs and cats. *Compend. Cont. Educ. Pract. Vet.* 20: 63–74.

16 Grooters, A.M. and Gee, M.K. (2002). Development of a nested polymerase chain reaction assay for the detection and identification of *Pythium insidiosum*. *J. Vet. Intern. Med.* 16: 147–152.

17 Grooters, A.M., Whittington, A., Lopez, M.K. et al. (2002). Evaluation of microbial culture techniques for the isolation of *Pythium insidiosum* from equine tissues. *J. Vet. Diagn. Invest.* 14: 288–294.

18 Vaccine-Associated Feline Sarcoma Task Force (2005). The current understanding and management of vaccine-associated sarcomas in cats. *J. Am. Vet. Med. Assoc.* 226: 1821–1842.

19 Wanachiwanawin, W., Mendoza, L., Visuthisakchai, S. et al. (2004). Efficacy of immunotherapy using antigens of *Pythium insidiosum* in the treatment of vascular pythiosis in humans. *Vaccine* 22: 3613–3621.

20 Schurko, A., Mendoza, L., de Cock, A.W. et al. (2003). Evidence for geographic clusters: molecular genetic differences among strains of *Pythium insidiosum* from Asia, Australia and the Americas are explored. *Mycologia* 95: 200–208.

17

Specific Wounds

Subsection J: Eyelid Wounds
Brian Marchione

Ocuvet Inc., Los Angeles, CA, USA

Introduction

The most common types of eyelid wounds are traumatic, infectious, inflammatory, and neoplastic in origin. Acting as a physical barrier to the outside world and a layer of protection for the globe, the eyelids are susceptible to **traumatic wounds** such as lacerations from an animal bite, claw, or sharp object in the environment. Additionally, wounds to the periocular skin can occur secondary to a number of **infectious agents** and **inflammatory conditions** arising from the skin and the meibomian glands within the eyelid. **Neoplasia** may arise from the meibomian glands or nearby skin and conjunctiva. **Surgical wounds** may occur as a result of resection of eyelid or periocular masses. **Cicatricial wounds** can occur secondary to severe wounds that heal with significant scar tissue formation or incorrect apposition of the eyelid margin during attempted eyelid mass removal or laceration repair.

Treatment of eyelid wounds is dependent on the nature of the wound and wound severity. Minor wounds to the eyelid will often heal with appropriate medical management and without surgical intervention because the eyelids are highly vascularized. When trauma, neoplasia, or severe chronic wounds disrupt the eyelid margin and the margin's position relative to the ocular surface; however, surgical intervention may be required to reestablish normal eyelid position and function.

Noteworthy anatomical points of the eyelids:

- Four Regions: The eyelids are divided into 4 regions: (i) the upper (dorsal) eyelid; (ii) the lower (ventral) eyelid; (iii) a relatively immobile medial canthus; (iv) and a relatively more mobile lateral canthus (Figure 17.J.1).
- Upper Eyelid Mobility: The upper eyelid is much more mobile compared to the lower eyelid, as it is responsible for blinking. If surgery is performed, care should be taken to ensure the eyelid maintains this function.
- Lacrimal Puncta and Canaliculi: The upper and lower lacrimal puncta reside in the medial portions of the palpebral conjunctiva, which are approximately 5 mm lateral to the medial canthus. Care should be taken to avoid surgical trauma to the punctum and/or the lacrimal canaliculi which extend medially deep to the punctum (Figure 17.J.1).
- Meibomian Glands: The meibomian glands are located within the eyelid, with their openings located on the surface of the eyelid margin. These gland openings along the eyelid margin are referred to as the "gray line." The "gray line" typically provides an easy-to-identify landmark for placing sutures within the eyelid margin so that they do not rub on the corneal surface (Figure 17.J.2).
- Highly Vascularized: The eyelids are highly vascularized and therefore, minimal freshening of edges is needed prior to a laceration repair.

Techniques in Small Animal Wound Management, First Edition. Edited by Nicole J. Buote.
© 2024 John Wiley & Sons, Inc. Published 2024 by John Wiley & Sons, Inc.
Companion website: www.wiley.com/go/buote/wounds

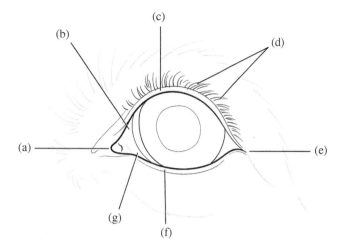

Figure 17.J.1   Noteworthy anatomical landmarks. a – medial canthus, b – Dorsal (upper) lacrimal punctum, c – Dorsal (upper) eyelid, d – Cilia (eyelashes), e – Lateral canthus, f – Ventral (lower) eyelid, g – Ventral (lower) lacrimal punctum.

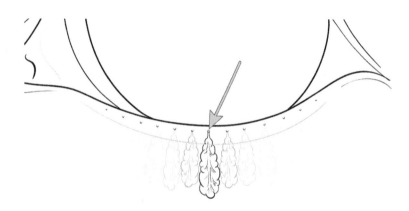

Figure 17.J.2   Note the meibomian glands within the eyelid and their openings along the eyelid margin (arrow). These openings represent the "gray line" and provide a useful surgical landmark.

Presenting Signs

Trauma

Traumatic wounds to the eyelid and periocular skin typically present with an acute injury to the eyelid margin or periocular skin. Any ocular discharge or hemorrhage should be gently cleansed away with purified water eye wash or a balanced saline solution to allow for visualization of the wound. The wound may involve the eyelid margin, the periocular skin, or both. The wound may be full or partial thickness and, when involving the eyelid margin, may run perpendicular or diagonal relative to the margin (Figure 17.J.3).

When assessing an eyelid wound, the ocular surface should also be closely evaluated for trauma to the globe itself. Trauma to the globe can range from a simple, superficial corneal ulcer or conjunctival laceration that will heal without surgical intervention, to a full-thickness corneal or scleral laceration (Figure 17.J.4). Corneal or scleral lacerations should be evaluated by an ophthalmologist to determine if surgical intervention is needed. If the traumatic injury is not acute, the wound may already be healing by second intention, in which case poor apposition of the eyelid margin, secondary trichiasis, or large defects in the eyelid may be present.

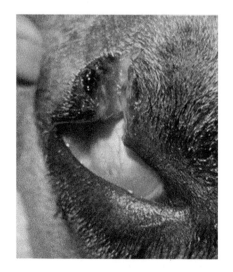

Figure 17.J.3   Full-thickness laceration to the upper eyelid running perpendicular to the eyelid margin. *Source:* Courtesy of Brian Marchione DVM, DACVO.

Figure 17.J.4 Full-thickness laceration to the lateral cornea. Note the fibrin plug sealing the laceration site and extending onto the lateral canthus. *Source:* Courtesy of Brian Marchione DVM, DACVO.

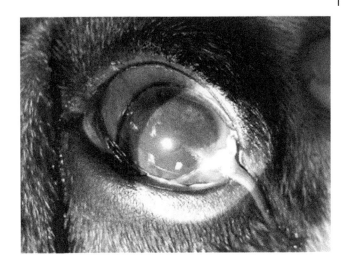

Figure 17.J.5 Medial canthal ulcerative blepharitis. *Source:* Courtesy of Brian Marchione DVM, DACVO.

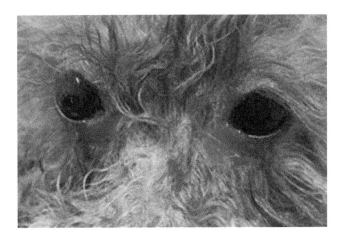

Inflammation

Inflammation of the eyelids (blepharitis) is common in dogs. The presenting signs can vary depending on the underlying cause, including: parasites, bacteria, and immune-mediated diseases such as pemphigus and medial canthal ulcerative blepharitis [1]. Lesions can be focal or diffuse and may affect one or both eyes. Parasitic blepharitis, from agents such as demodex, present with periocular alopecia, hyperemia, and pruritus. Pruritic lesions will result in the patient rubbing vigorously at the eyelids and periocular skin, making it difficult to differentiate the primary lesions from lesions caused by self-trauma. Bacterial blepharitis often presents as swelling of the lids, either generalized or in nodules or may cause ulcerations along the eyelid margin and periocular skin. If these lesions become chronic, alopecia and fibrosis of the skin may occur. If severe enough, the fibrosis may result in contraction of the skin leading to secondary ectropion or entropion and incomplete eyelid closure. Diseases of the pemphigus complex and medial canthal ulcerative blepharitis present with ulcerative wounds along the eyelids (Figure 17.J.5).

Neoplasia

In the case of eyelid neoplasms, most are benign and will present with a history of a progressive lesion that may or may not be ulcerative and/or pigmented. If the mass is rubbing on the ocular surface, there may also be ocular irritation and blepharospasm. Eyelid masses such as meibomian gland adenomas and papillomas are often friable and will break apart causing hemorrhage from the site. The hemorrhage noted by the owner may be the reason for presentation. If the masses are large

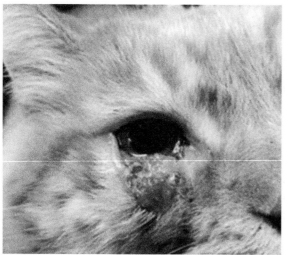

Figure 17.J.6 Squamous cell carcinoma infiltrating the lower eyelid and periocular skin. *Source:* Courtesy of Brian Marchione DVM, DACVO.

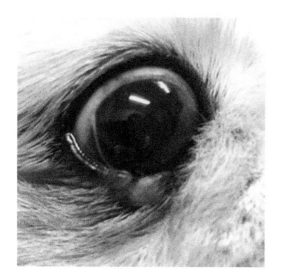

Figure 17.J.7 Previous eyelid laceration allowed to heal by secondary intention. Note the gap in the lower eyelid margin. *Source:* Courtesy of Brian Marchione DVM, DACVO.

enough, they may also prevent complete eyelid closure. Squamous cell carcinoma, another common eyelid neoplasia, will appear ulcerative and infiltrative with a more rapid onset and progression (Figure 17.J.6).

Physiologic Effects

Opening and closing of the eyelid effectively spread the precorneal tear film across the ocular surface. Tears provide oxygen, antimicrobial defense, nutrients, and lubrication to the ocular surface. Therefore, complete eyelid closure with a smooth and intact eyelid margin is imperative for ocular health and comfort. If eyelid closure is not complete, or if periocular hairs are contacting the corneal surface, corneal lesions such as vascularization, fibrosis, pigmentation, and ulceration will often occur.

Treatment

Infectious and inflammatory causes of blepharitis will often require a definitive diagnosis via skin scraping, cutaneous cytology, culture, or biopsy to determine appropriate treatment for the underlying cause. Parasitic and bacterial blepharitis will respond to antimicrobial treatment targeting the causal agent, whereas most cases of immune-mediated blepharitis will resolve with topical ophthalmic antibiotic and corticosteroid treatment. Severe cases of immune-mediated blepharitis, however, will require systemic corticosteroid treatment for resolution [2]. If the periocular skin heals without affecting the mobility or the position of the eyelids, surgery is not required. If, however, contraction of the skin results in entropion, ectropion, trichiasis, or exposure of the ocular surface, surgical correction will be necessary.

Eyelid tumors and wounds, such as eyelid lacerations that disrupt the eyelid margin, will require surgical intervention to appose the eyelid margin and restore normal eyelid function. Similarly, wounds that leave a defect in the eyelid margin, which are left to heal by second intention, are unlikely to appose normally during healing and will require corrective surgery. Abnormal apposition will lead to trichiasis or entropion with secondary ocular irritation and corneal ulceration (Figure 17.J.7).

Surgical Preparation of the Periocular Skin, Eyelids, and Ocular Surface

The periocular region and ocular surface should be appropriately prepared prior to surgery of the eyelids. The periocular hair in the surgical field should be removed with clippers; however, care should be taken not to traumatize the skin or further damage the eyelid margin. A petrolatum-based ointment may be placed on the ocular surface to collect any hair removed during shaving. The ointment and any gathered hair may be rinsed away using 0.9% saline and a cotton-tipped applicator. Then, the ocular surface and periocular skin should be cleansed with a diluted (1 : 50) povidone-iodine aqueous solution followed by rinsing with 0.9% saline

Cicatricial Ectropion and Entropion

If contraction of a wound results in ectropion and overexposure of the ocular surface (Figure 17.J.8), a V to Y Plasty should be considered to release tension from the eyelid, and to allow for better mobility of the lid and a return to normal position. (Figure 17.J.9) If entropion develops as a result of wound contraction (Figure 17.J.10), a Y to V Plasty may be performed to roll the eyelid outward and return it to normal position (Figure 17.J.11) [3].

Eyelid Laceration

Necrosis of the eyelid tissue is unlikely because the eyelids are highly vascularized, so minimal freshening of the wound edges is needed in preparation for surgery. When surgically correcting an eyelid margin wound, the most important and tedious part of the surgery is correct apposition of the eyelid margin, as a poorly apposed lid margin will result in periocular hairs rubbing on the ocular surface. In cases where the laceration is full thickness, the subcutaneous tissues should be closed first with 4-0 to 6-0 absorbable suture using a simple continuous pattern, followed by apposition of the eyelid margin with 4-0 to 6-0 nonabsorbable suture. Apposition of the eyelid margin is most consistently performed using a figure of 8 suture pattern (Figure 17.J.12). This procedure also allows for the margin to be sutured and the suture tags

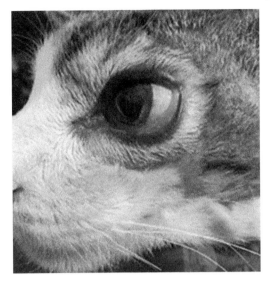

Figure 17.J.8 Cicatricial ectropion secondary to a previous facial wound. The tension created by the healed wound resulted in the lower eyelid being pulled ventrally and outward with exposure to the palpebral conjunctiva. *Source:* Courtesy of Brian Marchione DVM, DACVO.

to remain away from the corneal surface. Once the eyelid margin is apposed, the remaining laceration may be closed in the same manner that a normal skin laceration would be closed using a simple continuous or interrupted, nonabsorbable suture. Care should be taken to make sure suture tags are either cut close, directed away from the ocular surface, or incorporated into other knots so that they do not rub on the ocular surface (17.J.13) [4]. A periocular laceration to the skin that does not affect the eyelid margin may be closed as a normal skin laceration, but care should be taken to make sure that tension is not placed on the eyelids thereby preventing complete eyelid closure.

Figure 17.J.9 V to Y Plasty can be performed to correct an eyelid that is rolling outward secondary to scarring. The top of the V incision should be performed 1–2 mm from the lid margin and extend into the scarred area (a). A V-shaped skin flap is then created by separating the underlying and adjacent tissues and excising any scar tissue within the subcutaneous layer with tenotomy scissors. This will allow for a more movable skin flap and resolution of the ectropion (b). The wound is apposed in a Y-shaped closure with 4-0 to 6-0 simple interrupted nonabsorbable sutures (c and d).

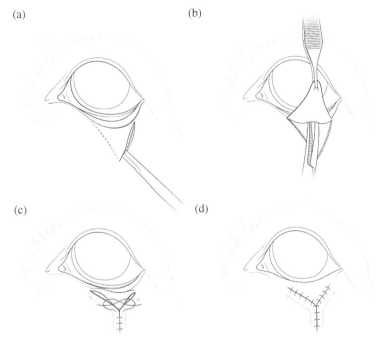

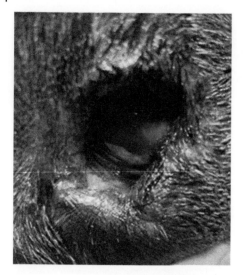

Figure 17.J.10 Cicatricial entropion secondary to previous injury to the eyelid margin. *Source:* Courtesy of K. Michael Chang DVM, DACVO.

Eyelid Neoplasia

Neoplasia affecting the eyelid margin, such as large meibomian gland adenomas, will need to be completely excised and the resulting surgical wound repaired in a way that can restore normal eyelid function. This will require appropriate apposition of the lid margin while minimizing tension on the remaining eyelid. If removal of an eyelid mass results in a surgical defect that is less than 1/3 of the eyelid margin and full-thickness excision is needed, a 4-sided resection is usually sufficient to correct it (Figures 17.J.14 and 17.J.15). Any surgical wound larger than 1/3 of the length of the margin will require a sliding skin flap or other grafting procedure to allow for a smooth, hairless eyelid margin that is not under tension (Figure 17.J.16) [5].

Possible Complications

Lagophthalmos

Incomplete closure of the eyelids (i.e., lagophthalmos) brought about by scarring or by an eyelid mass preventing closure will cause exposure of the corneal surface resulting in corneal inflammation in the form of vascularization, fibrosis, and pigmentation. This opacification of the cornea may become significant enough to impair vision.

Poor Eyelid Apposition

Wounds to the eyelid margin that are left to heal by second intention may result in trichiasis with secondary irritation to the ocular surface and corneal ulceration. If this occurs, surgical correction may be accomplished by performing a four-sided resection (as discussed above) of the affected area and reapposing the eyelid margin.

(a) (b)

(c) (d)

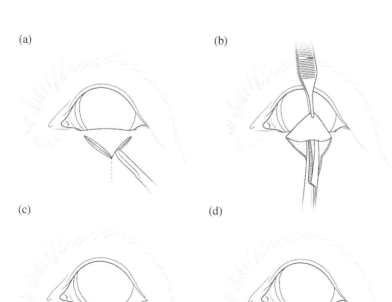

Figure 17.J.11 Y to V Plasty can be performed to correct cicatricial entropion caused by a healing and secondary scarring from a chronic periocular skin wound. The top of the Y incision should be performed 1–2 mm from the lid margin. The incision should extend away from the eyelid margin long enough to provide correction of the entropion (a). Once the Y shape incision is made, the flap should be separated from the underlying tissues carefully with blunt dissection using tenotomy scissors (b). The tip of the flap is apposed to the bottom and sides with 4-0 to 6-0 simple interrupted sutures in a V-shaped pattern (c and d).

Figure 17.J.12   The figure of 8 suture pattern allows for exact apposition of the eye eyelid margin. The needle is passed through the skin approximately 2–3 mm from the cut edge and exits the cut surface (1). The needle is then passed through the opposite cut surface and out through the eyelid margin approximately 2–3 mm from the cut edge using the meibomian gland openings as a landmark (2). The suture then crosses over the cut lid margin and the needle enters into the opposite eyelid margin (3). The needle is then passed through the opposite cut surface and out of the skin (4).

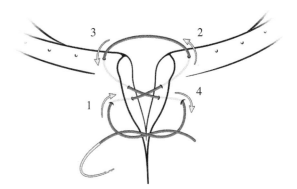

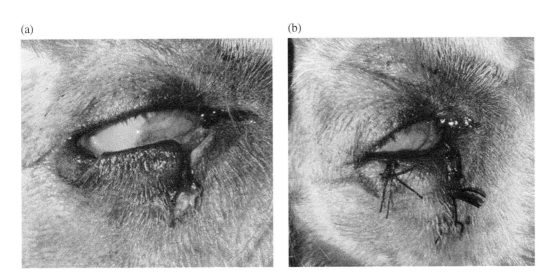

Figure 17.J.13   (a) Two full-thickness eyelid lacerations affecting the medial portion and lateral portion of the lower eyelid. *Source:* Brian Marchione (Chapter Contributor). (b) Immediate postoperative appearance. Note that suture tags are incorporated into distal knots to prevent rubbing on the corneal surface. *Source:* Courtesy of Brian Marchione DVM, DACVO.

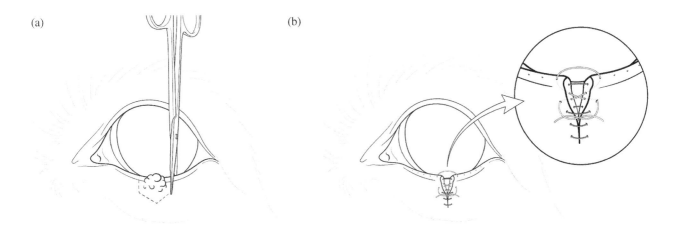

Figure 17.J.14   A four-sided resection may be used to excise eyelid masses involving the eyelid margin. Tenotomy scissors or scalpel blades are used to remove the tumor and surrounding eyelid resulting in a four-sided defect in the eyelid (a). The resulting wounded is apposed in two layers. Subcutaneous tissues are closed with 4-0 to 6-0 absorbable suture in a simple interrupted or continuous pattern. The eyelid margin is then apposed with a figure of 8 suture pattern using non-absorbable, 4-0 or 6-0 suture. The skin distal to the eyelid margin is closed in a simple interrupted or continuous pattern using a non-absorbable 4-0 to 6-0 suture (b).

(a)

(b)

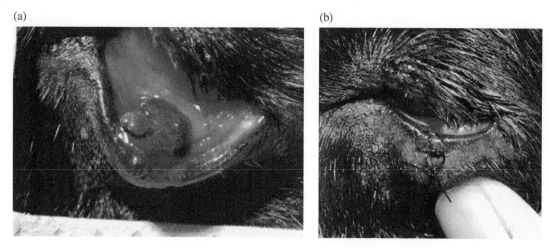

Figure 17J.15   (a) Meibomian gland adenoma affecting the central portion of the lower eyelid. The mass is effacing the eyelid margin. *Source:* Brian Marchione (Chapter Contributor). (b) Postoperative appearance after the mass was removed via a four-sided excision. The eyelid margin apposed using a figure of 8 suture pattern. *Source:* Courtesy of Brian Marchione DVM, DACVO.

(a)

(b)

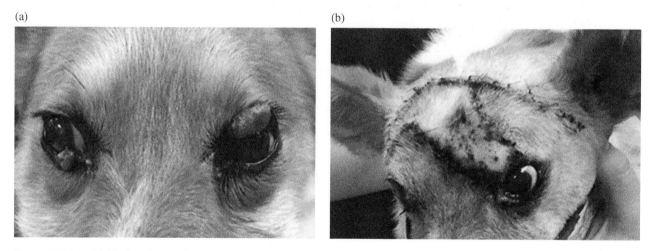

Figure 17J.16   (a) Histiocytic neoplasia affecting ½ of the left upper eyelid. Due to the amount of eyelid involvement, a caudal auricular skin flap was placed to fill the defect left by excision of the tumor. *Source:* Brian Marchione (Chapter Contributor). (b) Two-week postoperative appearance. *Source:* Courtesy of Brian Marchione DVM, DACVO.

Entropion/Ectropion

Potential surgical complications that may arise when correcting entropion or ectropion may be **under or overcorrection of the eyelid**. When performing these corrective procedures, care should be taken to approximate the amount of tissue that should be removed to correct entropion and how much tissue to release when correcting ectropion.

Wound Dehiscence

Complications arising from an eyelid laceration repair or eyelid mass removal may include **wound dehiscence** if the patient is not in a cone collar and is allowed to rub at the surgical site.

Corneal Ulceration

If the sutures along the eyelid margin rub against the corneal surface, discomfort and/or corneal ulceration may occur. Any associated self-trauma may also increase the risk for wound dehiscence. This can be prevented by making sure that any sutures along the lid margin do not sit posterior to the meibomian gland openings (i.e., the gray line), and through appropriate management of suture tags.

Prognosis

Wounds to the periocular skin and eyelid margin tend to carry a good prognosis when impairment to the normal function of the eyelid is corrected and normal apposition is restored. The likelihood of a good prognosis will depend on the severity of the lesion to the eyelids, the periocular skin, and the expertise of the surgeon. Eyelid neoplasms are typically benign and, therefore, complete removal is typically curative. Malignant eyelid neoplasms, such as squamous cell carcinoma, can still carry a favorable prognosis if early intervention and complete excision are achieved, and if appropriate adjunctive treatment is performed.

References

1 Stades, F.C. and Van der Woerdt, A. (2021). Diseases and surgery of the canine eyelid. In: *Veterinary Ophthalmology*, 6e (ed. K.N. Gelatt, G. Ben-Shlomo, B.C. Gilger, et al.), 923–987. Hoboken: Wiley Blackwell.

2 Maggs, D.J. (2013). Eyelids. In: *Slatter's Fundamentals of Veterinary Ophthalmology*, 5e (ed. D.J. Maggs, P.E. Miller, and R. Ofri), 110–139. Elsevier Inc.

3 Hamilton, H.L., McLaughlin, S.A., Whitley, R.D. et al. (1998). Surgical reconstruction of severe cicatricial ectropion in a puppy. *J. Am. Anim. Hosp. Assoc.* 34: 212–218.

4 Gelatt, K.N., Gellatt, J.P., and Plummer, C.E. (2022). Surgery of the eyelids. In: *Veterinary Ophthalmic Surgery*, 2e, 102–147. Elsevier ltd.

5 Van der Woerdt, A. (2004). Adnexal surgery in dogs and cats. *Vet. Ophthalmol.* 7: 284–290.

17

Specific Wounds

Subsection K: Lip Wounds

off

Nicole J. Buote

Department of Clinical Sciences, Cornell University, Ithaca, NY, USA

Introduction

Lip wounds happen to multiple traumatic causes in veterinary patients. Most commonly we see them after animal-on-animal attacks (Figures 17.K.1 and 17.K.2) or association with severe facial trauma from falls from heights (windows, trees) but other injuries (Figure 17.K.3), envenomations and severe infections (Figure 17.K.4) can also lead to lip wounds. Reconstructions for neoplasia are more common than trauma but the same techniques apply (see Chapter 16) and multiple references are available discussing a wide variety of options [1, 2]. Injuries to the face are particularly challenging because owners tend to be as interested in cosmesis as they are in function restoration. Dogs usually have more elastic skin and larger lips (especially maxillary) compared to cats [2] therefore advancement flaps can be easily used for lip reconstruction in this species. In cases where adjacent skin is not readily available (cats, certain dogs), axillary pattern flaps may need to be employed. Keep in mind that any rotational flaps in long-haired patients may lead to hair growth in a different direction or color, and these changes, while completely cosmetic, should be discussed with owners prior to surgery.

Anatomic Considerations

Lips wounds are usually easy to diagnose due to the relatively short fur on most animal's face and the noticeable bleeding that accompanies them. The appearance of lips varies widely among dog breeds with some patients having very large loose lips and others having smaller tight lips. These differences affect the size of the vestibule which is the space lateral to the teeth and gingiva and medial to the lip. Lips have an outer skin and an inner mucosal surface. It is very important when reconstructing lips to ensure both surfaces are appropriately repaired although some techniques do rotate haired skin into the oral cavity [3]. Muscles of the lip and nose include orbicularis oris, zygomaticus, superior and inferior incisivus, levator labii superioris, caninus, buccinator, mentalis, and levator nasolabialis [4]. The orbicularis oris is the largest superficial muscle and spans both the maxillary and mandibular lip. This muscle closes the lips and is involved in moving the nose (sniffing). The buccinator is one of the deep muscles of the lip, comprised two different parts (molar and buccal), and is important for returning food from the cheek to the masticatory surface of the teeth [4].

The lips have a rich blood supply based on the facial artery which divides into a superior labial artery, inferior labial artery, and the angularis oris artery (important for the axial pattern flap named after it, see Chapter 16). The infraorbital and mental arteries also contribute blood supply to the maxillary and mandibular lips respectively. The advantage of this abundance in collateral blood supply is a high likelihood of success in lip reconstructions. The disadvantage is that lip wounds bleed robustly therefore surgeons should have access to hemostatic agent/equipment when performing surgery in this region. The parotid and zygomatic salivary gland ducts open in the maxillary lip opposite the 4th upper premolar and 1st molar respectively and can be damaged with trauma to the maxillary lip. The mandibular and monostomatic sublingual salivary gland duct opens ventral to the body of the tongue and is not usually injured with lip wounds.

Techniques in Small Animal Wound Management, First Edition. Edited by Nicole J. Buote.
© 2024 John Wiley & Sons, Inc. Published 2024 by John Wiley & Sons, Inc.
Companion website: www.wiley.com/go/buote/wounds

(a)
(b)
(c)

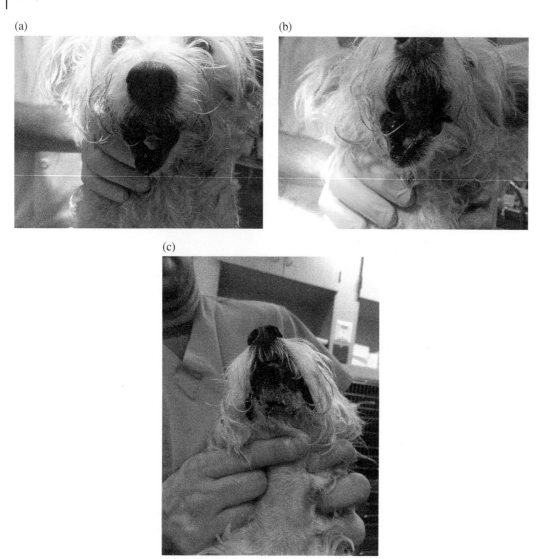

Figure 17.K.1   Photographs of adult West Highland terrier after a big-dog-little-dog attack. The rostral mandibular lip has been avulsed off the mandible and torn. (a) The lip is ventrally deviated and the gloved hand of the assistant can be seen through the hole that was created. (b) The periosteum of the mandible below the incisors is visible. (c) Repair of the chin wound was performed primarily. The lip was reattached by drilling holes in the mandible. *Source:* Courtesy of Nicole Buote, DVM, DACVS.

Wound Characteristics

Lip wounds can be characterized by location and type (Table 17.K.1). Regardless of the type of wound, closures must also take into account the function of the mouth and jaw in order to ensure comfortable postoperative mastication. Traumatic lateral lip wounds usually present with jagged edges requiring some degree of debridement before repair. Due to the excellent blood supply to the lip, these wounds can be repaired primarily after the typical "Golden Period" of six hours but every effort to reconstruct them in a timely fashion should still be made. Avulsion injuries of the rostral lip attachments are commonly seen in animals after being struck by vehicles or falling from an elevated height.

Surgical Treatments

Surgical repair of lip wounds is usually performed in two layers. *Always* suture the lip edge first with a simple interrupted suture to ensure appropriate apposition and cosmesis. Suture the mucosa first with 3-0 to 5-0 monofilament (Monocryl®)

(b)

(a)

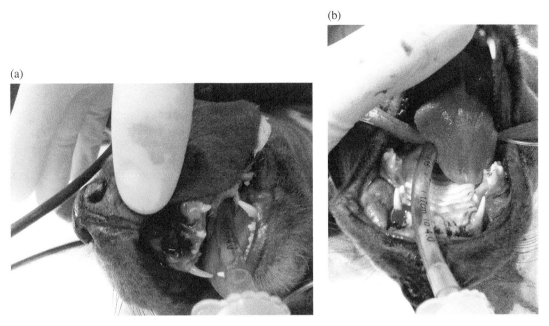

Figure 17.K.2   Photographs of a canine patient after a dog attack. (a) The rostral maxillary lip has been avulsed from the underlying incisive bone, (b) the lip has been reattached with suture passing through the hard palate. *Source:* Courtesy of Katie Barry, DVM, DACVS.

(a)   (b)

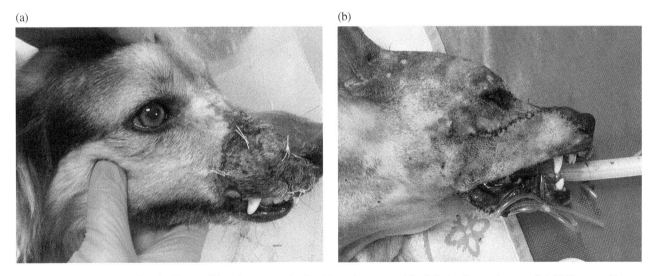

Figure 17.K.3   Photographs of a 7-year-old male neutered, mixed breed, presented for failed primary closure of right lip wound/ laceration from fence. (a) Visible necrosis of the rostral right maxillary lip. (b) Labial advancement flap. *Source:* Courtesy of Andy Law, BVetMed, DACVS-SA.

or braided sutured (Vicryl®) in an interrupted or continuous pattern. While braided sutures do trap bacteria more readily than monofilament sutures, newer antibiotic-impregnated braided sutures (Vicryl Plus Antibacterial) have been created and due to the robust blood supply lip wounds rarely become infected. Braided sutures are soft and therefore do not bother the patients as much which means they may not paw or rub at the incision line. Suturing the mucosa is usually performed from the lateral (outside) aspect of the lip with the knot being placed in the submucosal layer. The skin is then apposed routinely – it is not usually necessary to place sutures in the subcutaneous or muscle layer unless excessive tension is appreciated. Fight the urge to place more sutures than necessary as this may damage the blood supply to the tissue.

(a)

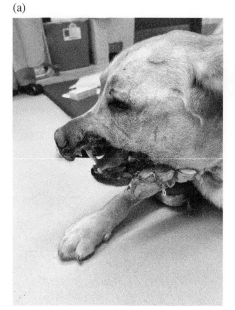

(b)

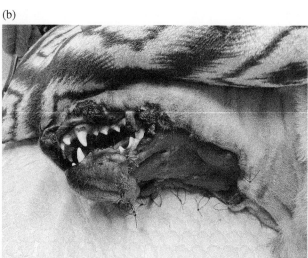

Figure 17.K.4 Photographs of a two-year-old Labrador retriever presenting after a bite of unknown origin created a severe facial abscess. (a) Lateral view illustrating full-thickness necrosis of the rostral portion of the left maxillary lip. (b) This patient also had significant skin loss to the left lateral mandibular lip and chin. *Source:* Courtesy of Nicole Buote, DVM, DACVS.

Table 17.K.1   Lip wound characteristics and recommended treatments.

Location	Treatment
Lateral lip-maxillary	*Minor*: primary repair after debridement, wedge resection *Medium-Large wounds*: advancement flap, buccal transposition flap, +/− Angularis oris flap (depending on location of wound)
Lateral lip-mandibular	*Minor*: primary repair after debridement, wedge resection *Medium-Large wounds*: advancement flap, Angularis oris flap
Rostral lip	Primary repair, advancement flap
Type	
Avulsion	Primary repair Suture loop around incisors Suture placed through K-wire holes Postoperative antibiotics usually not necessary
Lacerations	Minimal debridement Primary repair or reconstructions (see above) as soon as possible Postoperative antibiotics usually not necessary
Envenomation	If a necrotic wound is created, serial debridements must be performed until the wound bed is healthy Reconstructive techniques required (see above) Antibiotics required
Bite wounds	If a necrotic wound is created, serial debridements must be performed until the wound bed is healthy +/− Primary repair if adequately cleaned and lavaged Reconstructive techniques required (see above) Antibiotics required

Avulsion Injuries

Avulsion wounds can be primarily closed if sufficient gingiva is preserved but most times this is not the case (Figures 17.K.1 and 17.K.2). In those cases, sutures from the lip may be placed around the incisors if possible or through holes drilled into the mandible/maxilla using a K-wire. The author prefers monofilament absorbable suture (4-0 to 5-0) for this repair, and it should be undertaken as soon as possible to avoid excessive tissue damage from drying out or decreased blood supply.

Primary Repair

Primary repair is the easiest technique when possible. If the wound has occurred recently and minimal debridement is required, lip edges can be reapposed primarily in a two-layer closure. If a wound creates a defect (square, rectangular), closure can be performed to create a "Y" incision (see Chapter 16).

Wedge Resection Techniques

A triangular wedge resection can be employed in some cases if lip wounds create devitalized tissue that must be removed [1, 2]. A wedge technique centers the apex of the triangle pointing dorsally or ventrally depending on the location of the wound with the arms of the triangle to either side of the wound edges. Be sure to remove as little additional tissue as possible and start the reconstruction at the lip margin to ensure appropriate apposition.

Full-Thickness Advancement Flaps Full-Thickness

Advancement flaps are one of the most useful and versatile closure techniques for the lips in dogs and cats. These flaps utilize a full-thickness incision and dissection of a longitudinal flap which is advanced into the wound [1, 2]. If a square or rectangular piece of lip is removed traumatically or needs to be removed due to trauma, these flaps can be slid into place from the adjacent lip (Figures 17.K.3 and 17.K.5). If a large defect is created, these flaps may need to include the commissure, requiring two full-thickness incisions. Important considerations for these flaps include (i) Always leave a strip of lip gingiva to suture to if possible as the gingiva does not hold suture well, (ii) Tension along the flap must be alleviated carefully to avoid disrupting the blood supply, and (iii) Depending on the length of the flap, the lip commissure may be moved rostrally – you must check that this does not affect opening/closing of the mouth. Closure is in two layers as described for wedge resections.

Buccal Transposition (Rotation) Flap

Recently, a study investigated the use of a buccal transposition flap for closure of maxillary wounds created for oncologic treatments [5]. This technique was initially described by Pavletic for mid-large maxillary reconstructions, but the commissure was not incised but instead advanced rostrally at that time [1]. This technique can also be used for mandibular wounds. The recent method involves incising the commissure, rotating the maxillary flap rostrally and dorsally, apposing buccal mucosa to maxillary mucosa, and reconstructing the commissure by suturing rotated buccal tissue to the mandibular lip [5]. Proposed advantages to this technique include decreased tension and more anatomic range of motion to mouth. The clinical study on five dogs reported 100% flap survival and cosmetic and functional outcomes were considered satisfactory in all dogs. Complications described included two oronasal fistulas and one partial dehiscence [5]. This flap appears to be supplied by branches of the angularis oris and superior labial artery.

Axial Pattern Flaps

The angularis oris flap (discussed in Chapter 16) is the most robust axial pattern flap of the lateral face/cheek region (Figure 17.K.6). A small case series on it's use in dogs included indications such as tumor resection (six dogs), trauma (two dogs), and a chronic, nonhealing wounding (one dog) [6]. Anatomic regions covered by this flap include chin,

(a)

(b)

(c)

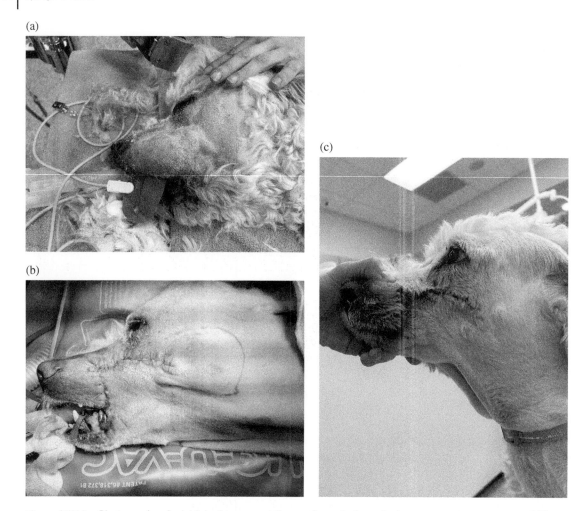

Figure 17.K.5 Photographs of a labial advancement flap performed after soft tissue sarcoma tumor removal. The same technique can be performed for traumatic wounds. (a) Preoperative, (b) Postoperative, (c) Appearance at two-week recheck. *Source:* Courtesy of Daniel Linden, DVM, MS, DACVS.

nasomaxillary area rostral to the eyes, and region ventral to orbit/ear. In the study by Loskinki, all flaps healed with acceptable functional and cosmetic outcomes but minor complications including flap edema (eight dogs), partial incisional dehiscence (three dogs), distal tip necrosis (two dogs), and oroantral (epithelialized pathological communication between oral cavity and maxillary sinus) fistula recurrence (one dog) [6]. For large lateral reconstructions of the maxillary and mandibular lip and chin, this is the author's preferred technique.

The author has also used the caudal auricular flap for mandibular lip reconstructions (Figure 17.K.7). This technique can mobilize a moderately sized flap but distal venous congestion is common and treatments such as medicinal leeching may be required. A multicentered study reported partial flap necrosis in 63% (10/16) of dogs and 42% (5/12) of cats with revision surgeries being performed in 50% of dogs and 25% of cats [7].

Lip-to-Lid and Lip-to-Nose Transposition Flaps

Composite mucocutaneous subdermal plexus flaps have been successfully used to close facial wound defects, oncologic resections as well as congenital defects (eyelid agenesis) in veterinary patients (Figure 17.K.8) [8–13]. These flaps consist of lip mucosa, a subcutaneous musculofascial layer and skin making them ideal for closures of adjacent lip, nasal cavity, oral cavity (hard or soft palate), and eyelid. These flaps are supplied by the superior and inferior labial arteries and veins. A study by Doyle et al. illustrated the rich arterial blood supply including extensive choke anastomoses to the infraorbital

(a)

(b)

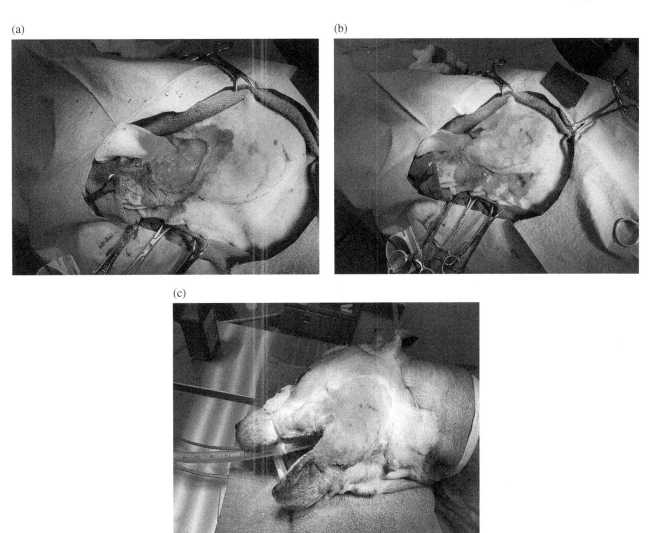

(c)

Figure 17.K.6 Photographs of an adult Boxer after resection of a grade two mast cell tumor on the mandibular lip. (a) Post resection with wide margins, (b) creation of the flap based on the angularis oris artery, (c) Sutured flap. *Source:* Courtesy of Rodrigo Rosa, MV, CVPP, MANZCVS (SA Surgery), DABVP (canine/feline).

and mental arteries supporting the numerous transposition flaps that can be created in this region [13]. When reconstructing the eyelid, special attention must be paid to the mucosa to conjunctival apposition in order to decrease the chance of contracture and corneal damage [11]. Lip-to-nose flaps can be particularly helpful when faced with nasal trauma as the lip mucosa can replace the nasal mucosa which is preferred to free mucosal grafts or xenografts (porcine small intestinal submucosa) [9, 10].

Postoperative Care

Patients recovering from facial surgery must be sent home with an E-collar to prevent the patient from scratching or pawing at their face. Alternative to E-collars (inflatable collars, neck braces) can be considered on a patient-by-patient basis but in the author's experience most patients can get paws around them therefore they should be avoided. Feeding patients soft food may not be necessary for lip reconstructions (as compared to oral surgery) but the author does recommend this for the first week to decrease any discomfort the patient may have. The need for postoperative antibiotics is based on the type of wound (bite wound versus laceration) and patient factors (comorbidities).

(a) (b) (c)

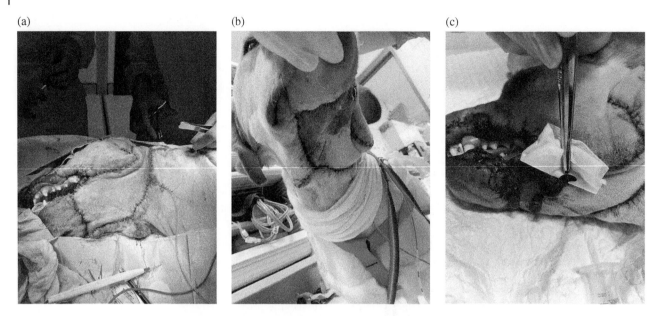

Figure 17.K.7 Photographs of patient seen in Figure 17.K.3 after a caudal auricular flap was used to close the mandibular lip and chin wound. (a) Immediate postoperatively, (b) Day 1 postoperatively- note the discoloration (venous congestion) of the distal tip of the flap, (c) medicinal leeching therapy was used to address the venous congestion. *Source:* Courtesy of Nicole Buote, DVM, DACVS.

(a)

(b)

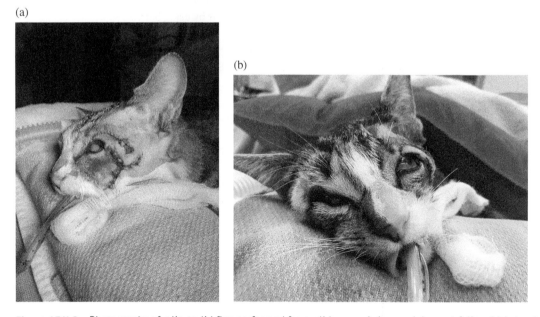

Figure 17.K.8 Photographs of a lip-to-lid flap performed for eyelid agenesis in an adolescent feline. (a) Lateral view, (b) Rostral view. *Source:* Courtesy of Nicole Buote, DVM, DACVS.

Complications

Complications associated with lip wounds include dehiscence, ongoing necrosis, infection, and hemorrhage. Dehiscence can be associated with excessive tension, inappropriate tissue handling, or patient-related factors such as licking, scratching, or rubbing the incision line (Figure 17.K.9). Ongoing necrosis and infection are always possible in traumatic wounds but the robust blood supply to the lips make these complications less common in the author's experience. A complication specific to lip wounds includes hindrance of mastication due to flap advancement. While not detrimental to survival in most cases, decreasing the patient's ability to open their mouth may also prevent playing with certain toys and or jobs (working police dogs).

Prognosis

No specific studies have been performed on the prognosis of lip reconstructions after trauma in veterinary patients. In the author's experience, the prognosis for most lip wounds is excellent if timely repair is performed. Multiple reconstructive options exist, and the tissue heals readily due to its excellent blood supply if appropriate surgical principles are followed.

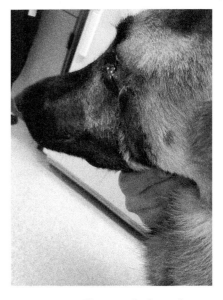

Figure 17.K.9 Photograph of a canine patient with evidence of dehiscence of his lip-to-lid flap from the conjunctiva. *Source:* Courtesy of Nicole Buote, DVM, DACVS.

References

1 Pavletic, M.M. (1990). Reconstructive surgery of the lips and cheek. *Vet. Clin. North Am. Small Anim. Pract.* 20 (1): 201–226.
2 Degner, D.A. (2007). Facial reconstructive surgery. *Clin. Tech. Small Anim. Pract.* 22 (2): 82–88.
3 Nakahara, N., Mitchell, K., Straw, R., and Kung, M. (2020). Hard palate defect repair by using haired angularis oris axial pattern flaps in dogs. *Vet. Surg.* 49 (6): 1195–1202.
4 Hermanson, J.W., de Lahunta, A., and Evans, H.E. (2020). Muscles of the head. In: *Miller and Evans' Anatomy of the Dog*, 5e (ed. J.W. Hermanson, A. de Lahunta, and H.E. Evans), 214–236. St. Louis, MO, USA: Elsevier.
5 Hildebrandt, I.M., Skinner, O.T., Souza, C.H.M. et al. (2023). Buccal transposition flap for closure of maxillary lip defects in 5 dogs. *Vet. Surg.* 52 (2): 276–283.
6 Losinski, S.L., Stanley, B.J., Schallberger, S.P. et al. (2015). Versatility of the angularis oris axial pattern flap for facial reconstruction. *Vet. Surg.* 44 (8): 930–938.
7 Proot, J.L.J., Jeffery, N., Culp, W.T.N. et al. (2019). Is the caudal auricular axial pattern flap robust? A multi-centre cohort study of 16 dogs and 12 cats (2005 to 2016). *J. Small Anim. Pract.* 60 (2): 102–106.
8 Pavletic, M.M. (2021). Full-thickness labial flaps to reconstruct facial defects in four dogs. *Vet. Surg.* 50 (6): 1338–1349.
9 Massari, F., Chiti, L.E., Lisi, M.L.P. et al. (2020). Lip-to-nose flap for reconstruction of the nasal planum after curative intent excision of squamous cell carcinoma in cats: description of technique and outcome in seven cases. *Vet. Surg.* 49 (2): 339–346.
10 Chiti, L.E., Montinaro, V., Lisi, M.L.P. et al. (2018). Lip-to-nose flap for nasal plane reconstruction in dogs: a cadaveric and in vivo feasibility study. *Vet. Surg.* 47 (8): 1101–1105.
11 Whittaker, C.J., Wilkie, D.A., Simpson, D.J. et al. (2010). Lip commissure to eyelid transposition for repair of feline eyelid agenesis. *Vet. Ophthalmol.* 13 (3): 173–178.
12 Hunt, G.B. (2006). Use of the lip-to-lid flap for replacement of the lower eyelid in five cats. *Vet. Surg.* 35 (3): 284–286.
13 Doyle, C.P. and Degner, D.A. (2019). Evaluation of the superior labial musculomucosal flap in dogs: an angiographic study and case report. *Vet. Comp. Orthop. Traumatol.* 32 (2): 133–138.

17

Specific Wounds

Subsection L: Pinna Wounds

Nicole J. Buote

Department of Clinical Sciences, Cornell University, Ithaca, NY, USA

Anatomic Considerations

The external ear varies widely between breeds in the canine species but is consistent among cats with the exception of Scottish folds. The purpose of the pinna from an evolutionary standpoint was to direct sound to the external acoustic meatus although in some breeds this is clearly not the case (Cocker spaniel, basset hound, etc.). Each ear can be independently manipulated by multiple muscles of varying sizes which allows the pinna to be utilized as an expressive appendage much like the tail. The pinna is also called the auricle [1] and can be categorized as pendulous or upright. There is a convex (outer) and concave (inner) surface to the pinna. The auricular cartilage is perforated by multiple foramina to allow blood vessels and nerves to traverse from the concave surface to the convex surface, explaining why injuries to the pinna are known to cause troublesome hemorrhage (aural hematomas). The scapha is the large flat inner surface of the pinna separated from the external acoustic meatus by the anthelix, a transverse fold of cartilage. The free margins of the pinna are the helix (medial and lateral), with a small pocket of skin found on the lateral surface near the base of the ear named the cutaneous marginal pouch (or Henry's pocket). The tragus and antitragus create the rostral border of the external ear canal. The blood supply to the pinna is provided by the caudal auricular artery a branch of the external carotid artery [1].

Wound Characteristics

Pinna wounds are most commonly bite or scratch wounds creating laceration-type injuries [2–4]. As noted above, there are also wounds created by crushing and circumferential injuries when pinna are tied up to try and create an upright appearance (Figure 17.L.1). Wounds may be full-thickness (through inner and outer skin and auricular cartilage) or partial thickness (only including one skin surface +/− underlying cartilage). Specific considerations for the repair of these wounds include protection of the blood supply to the pinna and attention to the auricular cartilage. The arborizing blood supply along the convex surface of the pinna means that any damage to the larger first-order vessels at the base of the ear can have disastrous complications for the skin and cartilage toward the apex. This is why simple interrupted sutures placed for aural hematomas are always positioned parallel to the long axis of the pinna to decrease the chance of ligating secondary or tertiary vessels. The presence of the auricular cartilage between the inner and outer skin means that skin cannot be easily rotated or advanced. Dissecting skin off the underlying cartilage can be performed closer to the base of the pinna but the skin is thin and tightly adhered at the apex.

Techniques in Small Animal Wound Management, First Edition. Edited by Nicole J. Buote.
© 2024 John Wiley & Sons, Inc. Published 2024 by John Wiley & Sons, Inc.
Companion website: www.wiley.com/go/buote/wounds

(a)   (b)   (c)

(d)   (e)   (f)

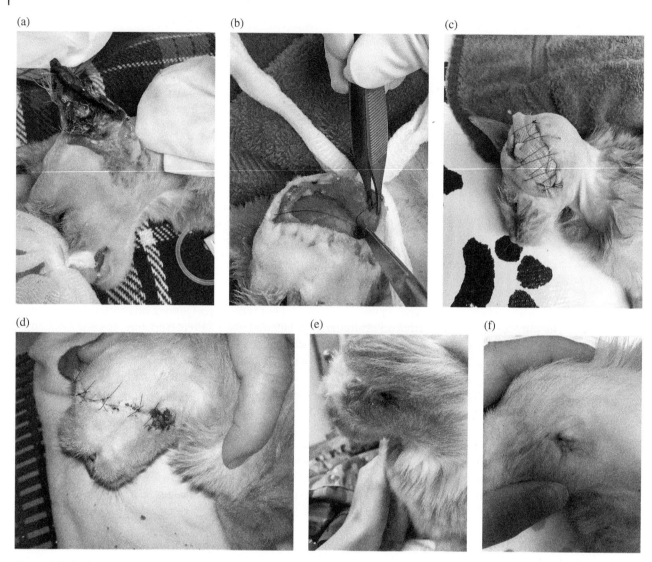

Figure 17.L.1   Photographs of a feline patient after sustaining wounds from being caught in an engine compartment when it was turned on. Note the left pinna was avulsed from the blood supply leading to complete necrosis of the pinna, the vertical ear canal was also avulsed. (a) Preoperative photograph on admission, note the entire pinna is black and necrotic. (b) Photograph of the wound after pinnectomy and multiple wet-to-dry bandages had been placed to clean and debride the wound. (c) Wet-to-dry bandage placement in wound. (d) In this patient, athe remaining horizontal ear canal was sutured to skin once the tissue was healthy. This photograph shows the ear canal stoma at ~1 week postop. Note there is moderate discharge at the ear canal incision line. (e and f) Photographs of ear canal fully healed at suture removal. *Source:* Courtesy of Katie Barry, DVM, DACVS.

Surgical Treatments

Just as with all traumatic wounds, wounds to the pinna must be appropriately cleaned and assessed for nonviable tissue. If presented soon after injury, primary repair may be possible and is recommended over healing by second intention. When the pinna heals by second intention contracture distorts, the tissues of the ear leading to curling [1]. Depending on location of the injury, lacerations to the pinna may disrupt blood supply to the distal portion (apex) so specific attention should be paid to the viability of tissue before primary repair is performed. Suture placement should be performed parallel to the long axis of the ear to reduce the chance of ligation of downstream branches.

Primary Repair

Surgical repair of pinna wounds can be performed in one layer incorporating both concave and convex skin toward the apex in patients where the pinna is thin. If both skin surfaces are torn in a thicker region of the pinna, they may be repaired individually [4]. Primary repair of the cartilage can be included in one of the skin layers in order to maintain rigidity in the ear. When performing primary repair of a pinna laceration, suture the edge (helix) first with a simple interrupted suture to ensure appropriate apposition and cosmesis. The author prefers 3-0 to 4-0 monofilament (Monocryl®) simple interrupted sutures because they will dissolve eliminating the need for sedation for suture removal. Vertical mattress sutures can also be utilized on one surface, but care must be taken not to impinge on the blood supply depending on orientation of the laceration [5]. If a long segment of the helix is sutured (such as in a partial pinnectomy), a continuous pattern can be used.

Pinnectomy

Partial or complete pinnectomy can be performed when damage to the pinna is extensive (Figures 17.L.1–17.L.4). Pinnectomy can be performed with sharp dissection (Mayo or cartilage scissors), monopolar electrosurgery or CO_2 laser. The author prefers CO_2 laser transection as it cuts and reduces hemorrhage without creating excessive char which can sometimes be seen with monopolar electrosurgery. Once the affected tissue is resected, the skin on the convex surface is generally pulled over the auricular cartilage and sutured to the concave skin in a simple continuous pattern with 3-0 to 4-0 monofilament absorbable or delayed absorbable suture. There is no need to incorporate the cartilage in this closure.

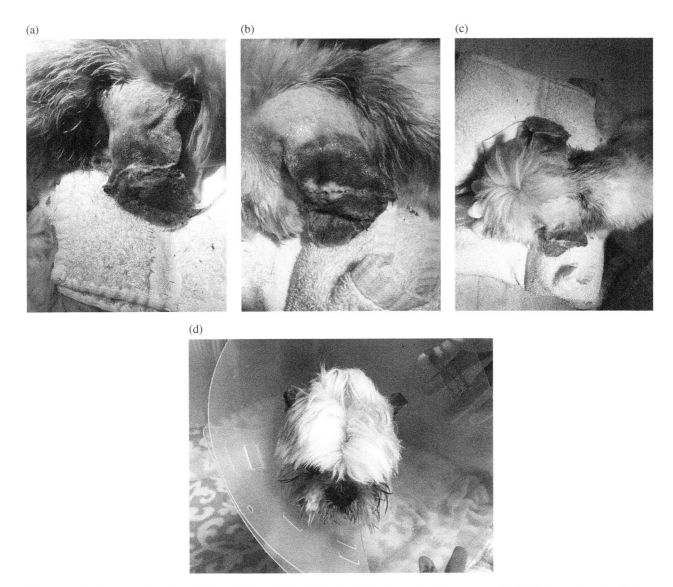

(a) (b) (c)

(d)

Figure 17.L.2 Photographs of a patient sustaining bilateral injuries to the pinna after the owner applied hair ties to the pinna to try to "train" the ears to stand in an upright fashion. (a) Preoperative photograph of right pinna; (b) Preoperative photograph of left pinna; (c) Preoperative photograph of dorsal view; (d) Postoperative photograph. *Source:* Courtesy of Nicole Buote, DVM, DACVS.

(a) (b) (c)

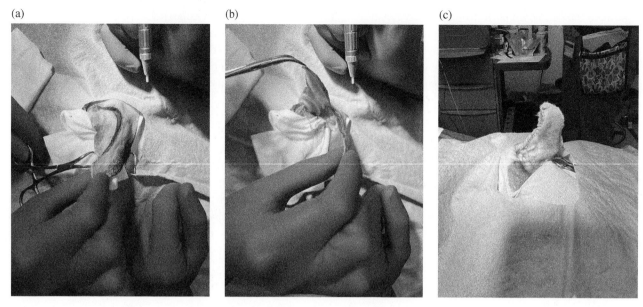

Figure 17.L.3 Intraoperative photographs of a feline partial pinnectomy. While this procedure was performed for squamous cell carcinoma of the pinna helix, the procedure is the same for trauma. (a) A CO_2 laser has been used to start the incision along the convex (outer) surface of the pinna. Note the minimal bleeding. (b) This incision has been continued to full thickness through the auricular cartilage and concave (inner) skin surface. (c) Postoperative photograph of partial pinnectomy. *Source:* Courtesy of Nicole Buote, DVM, DACVS.

Reconstructions

Reconstructive surgery for a degloving wound to the pinna has been reported [1] with the caudal auricular flap (Figure 17.L.5). This flap was successful in this case allowing for continued movement of the pinna and acceptable cosmesis but dedicated postoperative care was required. Cartilage loss due to the injury and contraction still led to caudal folding of the apex of the reconstructed pinna. Vascular compromise was not appreciated during healing, but cellulitis was a persistent symptom for three months and may have contributed to head shaking a mild otitis externa. Local rotation (Figure 17.L.6) or advancement flaps can also be considered if injuries are closer to the base of the ear, or the ears are short in length, but all flaps carry the risk of complications and owners must be prepared [6]. Even with perfect apposition, contraction anecdotally occurs during healing in this location leading to unpredictable cosmesis.

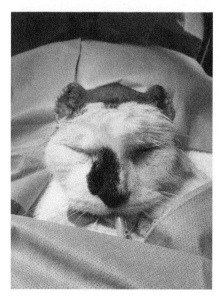

Figure 17.L.4 Postoperative photograph of a feline patient with bilateral near-total pinnectomies. *Source:* Courtesy of Nicole Buote, DVM, DACVS.

Postoperative Care

Depending on the type of wound management, postoperative care may include bandaging or an Elizabethan collar. The decision to bandage an ear is usually made to decrease the effects of postoperative head shaking and to help with compression. If a flap is performed, a bandage will cover the site and make it more difficult to assess flap viability so the author does not recommend them with those cases. Bandages are also not usually needed for partial or complete pinnectomies in upright ears but may be considered in breeds with pendulous ears (bloodhounds, bassets, etc.). If the ear is not covered in a bandage an E-collar should always be placed to protect the repair from scratching or rubbing. Pain medications and antibiotics are provided as appropriate.

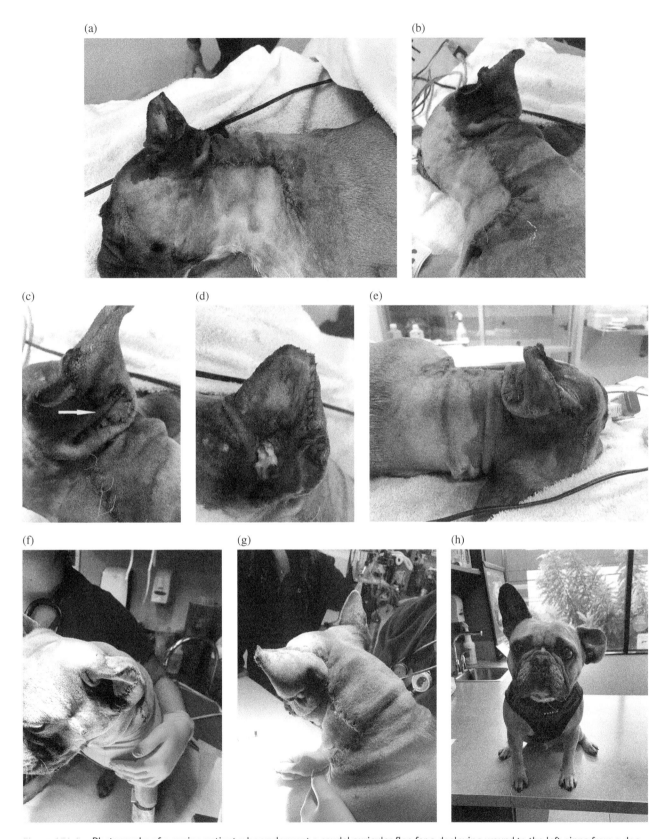

Figure 17.L.5   Photographs of a canine patient who underwent a caudal auricular flap for a degloving wound to the left pinna from a dog attack (kata). (a–e) Immediate postoperative photographs, (a) Lateral view of caudal auricular flap donor site and reconstructed pinna, (b) Caudal view, (c) Close-up view of ear base where flap is rotated onto to pinna surface (yellow arrow), (d) Close-up of the frontal view of the reconstructed pinna (inner surface) – note the flap has been pulled over the edge of the pinna for closure and the closure starts at the cutaneous marginal pouch and finishes at the apex, (e) Dorsal view of the completed reconstructed pinna. (f and g) Day 1 postoperative photographs illustrating swelling of the flap near the base (f: frontal view, g: caudal view). (h) Frontal view photograph 28 days postoperatively – note the low ear carriage and caudal orientation of the apex of the pinna, this is due to a lack of cartilage from the initial trauma and contraction. (i and j) Photographs the patient at final recheck (~6 months postoperatively) – note the ear carriage is improved but the caudal tipping to the apex remains. (i: Photograph of author with patient in frontal view, j: Lateral close-up view).
Source: Courtesy of Nicole Buote, DVM, DACVS.

(i)   (j)

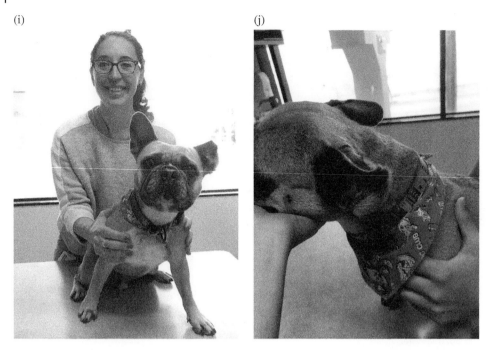

Figure 17.L.5   (Continued)

(a)   (b)

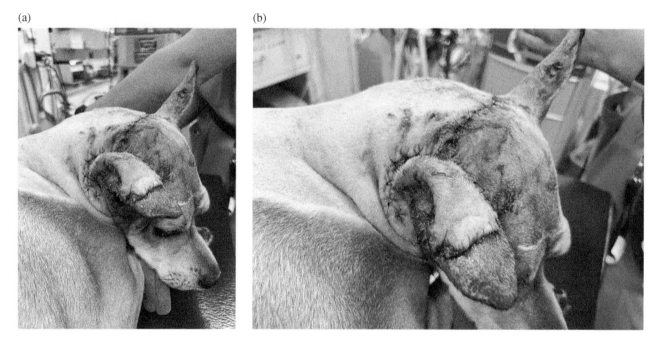

Figure 17.L.6   Photographs of a canine patient postoperatively. (a) He sustained bite wounds to his head and required primary closure over the dorsum of the cranium as well as a small rotational flap based on the caudal auricular artery to cover a wound on his right pinna. (b) Close-up of the rotational flap. *Source:* Courtesy of Nicole Buote, DVM, DACVS.

Complications

The major complications seen with repair of pinna wounds include hemorrhage and dehiscence. Both complications usually occur due to head shaking or self-trauma. E-collars can disrupt normal air flow around the ear canal leading to overgrowth of yeast or bacteria and surgical inflammation can lead to swelling of the tissues predisposing patients to otitis externa. Owners should be encouraged to contact the veterinarian if they see increased head shaking or appreciate any bleeding or foul odor from the ear as an infection may need to be treated.

Prognosis

Wounds to the pinna have an excellent prognosis. Primary repair and pinnectomy are simple procedures with a low rate of complications. Dedicated owners may opt for reconstructive surgeries and satisfactory outcomes can be achieved although a longer recovery should be expected.

References

1 Hermanson, J.W., de Lahunta, A., and Evans, H.E. (2020). The ear. In: *Miller and Evans' Anatomy of the Dog*, 5e (ed. J.W. Hermanson, A. de Lahunta, and H.E. Evans), 839 857. St. Louis, MO, USA: Elsevier.

2 Lanz, O.I. and Wood, B.C. (2004). Surgery of the ear and pinna. *Vet. Clin. North Am. Small Anim. Pract.* 34: 567–599.

3 Fossum, T.W. (2018). Surgery of the ear. In: *Small Animal Surgery*, 5e (ed. T.W. Fossum), 302–330. Philadelphia, PA, USA: Elsevier.

4 Bacon, N.J. (2018). Pinna and external ear canal. In: *Veterinary Surgery: Small Animal*, 2e (ed. S.A. Johnston and K.M. Tobias), 2309–2340. St. Louis, MO, USA: Elsevier.

5 Horne, R.D. and Henderson, R.A. (2003). Pinna. In: *Textbook of Small Animal Surgery*, 3e (ed. D. Slatter), 1737–1745. Philadelphia, PA, USA: WB Saunders.

6 Field, E.J., Kelly, G., Pleuvry, D. et al. (2015). Indications, outcome and complications with axial pattern skin flaps in dogs and cats: 73 cases. *J. Small Anim. Pract.* 56: 698–706.

17

Specific Wounds

Subsection M: Circumferential Wounds – A Case Study

Nicole J. Buote

Department of Clinical Sciences, Cornell University, Ithaca, NY, USA

Introduction

Circumferential wounds can be produced by many causes including rope/chain/rubber band injuries (malicious and accidental) as well as bandage-related, trauma injuries, and surgical incisions. Any injury that creates a 360° disruption in arterial or venous blood flow and tissue damage can be categorized as a circumferential wound. The most common region for these wounds in the author's experience is the limbs [1, 2] and the most common presenting physical exam sign is swelling of the distal tissues. These animals may present after surgical procedures or bandage placement as well so clinicians must be ever vigilant as treatment should be instituted promptly.

Venous congestion occurs when an imbalance between arterial inflow and venous outflow results in stasis of blood. Reduction in venous outflow occurs with constrictive wounds because of the thin walls of the low-capacitance veins are easily collapsed. The physical manifestations of venous congestion include a bluish/purple color to the skin, edema, brisk capillary return, and warmth in the tissue. When venous blood flow is slowed, arterial blood cannot perfuse tissue leading to hypoxia, acidosis, arterial thrombi formation, and tissue necrosis. Medicinal leeching (see Chapter 11A) can be used for circumferential wounds when venous congestion is present as can other types of bloodletting such as chemical leeching (heparin injection) or pricking the tissue and allowing it to bleed freely. Releasing restrictive tissue or implants is *the* most important primary treatment for these wounds. In some cases, the material (leashes, wires, etc.) may be deeply embedded and advanced diagnostics may be needed to appreciate their presence.

Case 1

Presenting Signs

A 4-year-old male castrated Yorkshire terrier was presented after a neighbor's dog attacked him while on a walk. On initial physical exam, he was diagnosed with tarsometarsal fracture luxation as well as various bite wounds (Figure 17.M.1). The patient had no comorbidities and was not on any chronic medications. The patient was stabilized, wounds cleaned, and the limb splinted overnight. Antibiotics (Clavamox 13.75 mg/kg PO BID) and pain medication (Methadone 0.2 mg/kg IV TID) were provided overnight.

Surgery and Postoperative Management

The following day the patient underwent a partial tarsal arthrodesis with a lateral bone plate and medial Kirshner wire (Figure 17.M.2). A modified Robert Jones bandage was placed on the limb postoperatively. Two days postoperatively increased limb swelling and bruising were identified, and the paw was cold to the touch (Figure 17.M.3). The swelling was

(a)

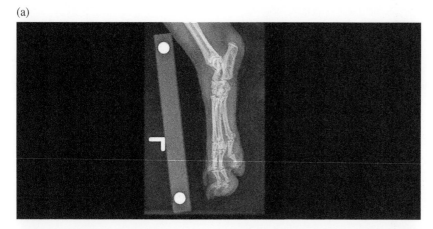

Figure 17.M.1 Orthogonal view radiographs of tarsometatarsal fracture luxation patient 1 sustained (a-lateral, b-craniocaudal). *Source:* Courtesy of Nicole Buote, DVM, DACVS.

(b)

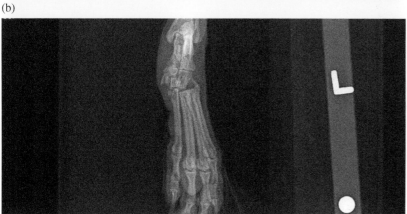

managed with the release of a few medial skin sutures, massage, and rewrapping of the limb with a looser bandage in the morning. In the afternoon, a decision was made to release additional skin sutures on the lateral aspect and remove the bandage entirely. The following morning his limb swelling was static to worsened (Figure 17.M.4) and soaking in Epsom salts and continued massage did not improve the appearance, so the decision was made to initiate medicinal leech therapy (MLT, see Chapter 11A for more information).

The limb was gently cleaned with sterile saline and multiple leeches were placed on the limb to decrease venous congestion (Video 17.M.1 ⊜). After MLT, the limb was rebandaged in a loose soft padded bandage to capture any residual bleeding. The patient was started on a fluoroquinolone to protect against leech flora. The patient underwent MLT twice daily for two days and the swelling markedly decreased (Figures 17.M.5 and 17.M.6). At that point, a honey-impregnated dressing was applied over the open surgical incisions, and a soft padded bandage applied. The patient was discharged with instructions to watch for any change in limb use or increased swelling of the toes.

Follow-Up

The patient returned for multiple visits over the following two months. Presumed incisional infections (treated empirically with broad-spectrum antibiotics) and discomfort (treated with oral gabapentin) were treated and eventual implant explant performed three months after initial presentation. Limb swelling/venous congestion did not reoccur post-MLT.

Outcome

Patient is weight-bearing on the limb and no skin or digit loss occurred due to venous congestion.

Figure 17.M.2 Orthogonal view radiographs of patient 1's postoperative tarsometarsal fracture luxation repair (a-lateral, b-craniocaudal lateral). *Source:* Courtesy of Nicole Buote, DVM, DACVS.

(a)

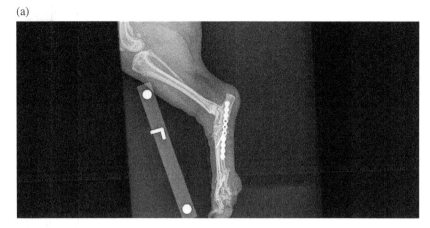

(b)

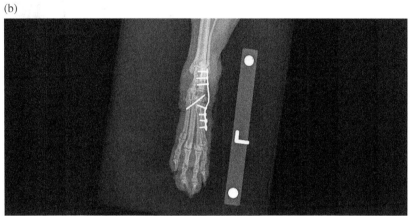

Figure 17.M.3 (a) (lateral) and (b) (craniocaudal) photographs of patient 1's limb two days postoperatively. Note the severe swelling with the nails pointing to the sides and the deep bruising of the skin. *Source:* Courtesy of Nicole Buote, DVM, DACVS.

(a)

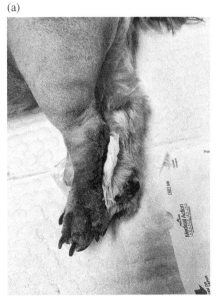

(b)

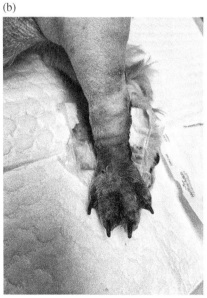

(a)

(b)

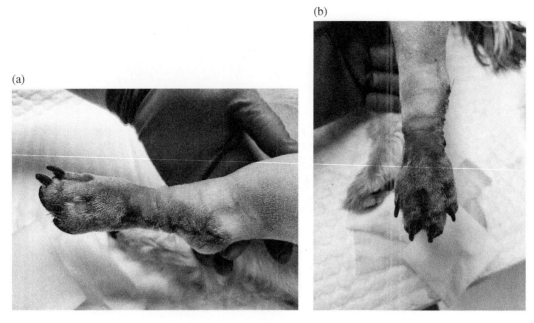

Figure 17.M.4   (a) (lateral) and (b) (craniocaudal) photographs of patient 1's limb three days postoperatively in the morning before medicinal leech therapy (MLT) was instituted. The paw remains swollen and bruised in the face of Epsom salt soaks and the release of skin sutures bilaterally. *Source:* Courtesy of Nicole Buote, DVM, DACVS.

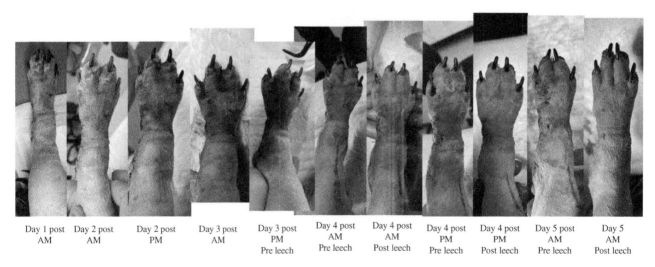

| Day 1 post AM | Day 2 post AM | Day 2 post PM | Day 3 post AM | Day 3 post PM Pre leech | Day 4 post AM Pre leech | Day 4 post AM Post leech | Day 4 post PM Pre leech | Day 4 post PM Post leech | Day 5 post AM Pre leech | Day 5 AM Post leech |

Figure 17.M.5   Image of multiple craniocaudal photographs of patient 1's paw taken from day 1 through day 5 postoperatively. Decreased swelling and bruising is noted after MLT was instituted twice daily. *Source:* Courtesy of Nicole Buote, DVM, DACVS.

Prognosis

The long-term prognosis for this patient is fair-good from a limb use perspective. Due to the initial injury, (tarsometatarsal fracture luxation) the patient will be at risk for ongoing osteoarthritis even with a stable arthrodesis. Vascular compromise was effectively treated, and once implants are removed, no ongoing source for biofilm or chronic infection should persist.

Figure 17.M.6   (a) (lateral) and (b) (craniocaudal) photographs of patient 1's paw on day 5 postoperative after two days of MLT (this was the last day of MLT). *Source:* Courtesy of Nicole Buote, DVM, DACVS.

(a)

(b)

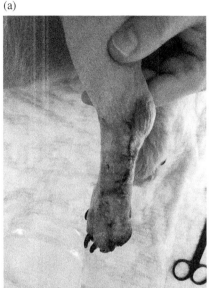
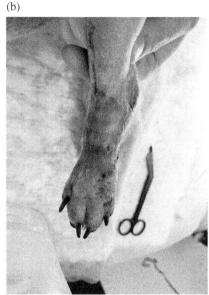

Other Examples of Circumferential Injuries (see Chapter 11A)

Not all examples of circumferential wounds occur on the limb. Unfortunately, injuries to the face (muzzle and ears), neck, and abdomen can occur due to malicious or accidental causes as well as iatrogenic surgical procedures [3, 4]. No matter the cause, constrictive wounds must deal with the venous congestion that accompanies them if the distal tissues are to heal.

Case 2

This 8-month-old male intact Maltese cross was presented for purulent discharge from his face. The owner's child had placed a rubber band around the muzzle which had gone unnoticed until the infection was obvious. Figures 17.M.7a (dorsal view) and 17.M.7b (lateral view) are photographs of the patient on presentation after sedation. Purulent material is obvious in a circumferential pattern, but the extent of the wound is not evident. Figure 17.M.7c is a photograph after the patient was anesthetized. No damage to the underlying maxillary gingiva was present as seen when the lip was retracted dorsally by the tongue depressor. Figure 17.M.7d is a photograph of the right lateral muzzle after clipping and cleaning have been performed. Now the full extent of the injuries is visible. This wound was present long enough to allow for full-thickness laceration through the maxillary skin and underlying muscle to the level of the bone and for granulation tissue to begin to form. The injury to the mandibular lips was less severe and primary closure was not necessary. Figure 17.M.7e is a photograph of the closure procedure for the maxillary injury. The nose and distal skin were monitored closely for venous congestion and edema. Warm packing of the muzzle was performed four times daily for the first two days and the patient healed uneventfully.

Case 3

This adult male intact mixed breed dog was presented after a rescue organization adopted him from a shelter. On the initial exam, the patient had a hunched posture and a short-strided pelvic limb gait. A deep scar was present 360° around the caudal abdomen from what had been reported to be a chain left on the dog for weeks on end. Figure 17.M.8a,b photographs of this patient after surgery was performed to loosen the cicatrix and re-appose the tissue. (a) Global view of the circumferential repair. The wound was directly cranial to the prepuce and special care was taken during reconstruction not to affect this region. (b) Close-up view of the primary repair. The injury had transected more deeply dorsally lacerating the skin,

(a) (b) (c)

(d) (e)

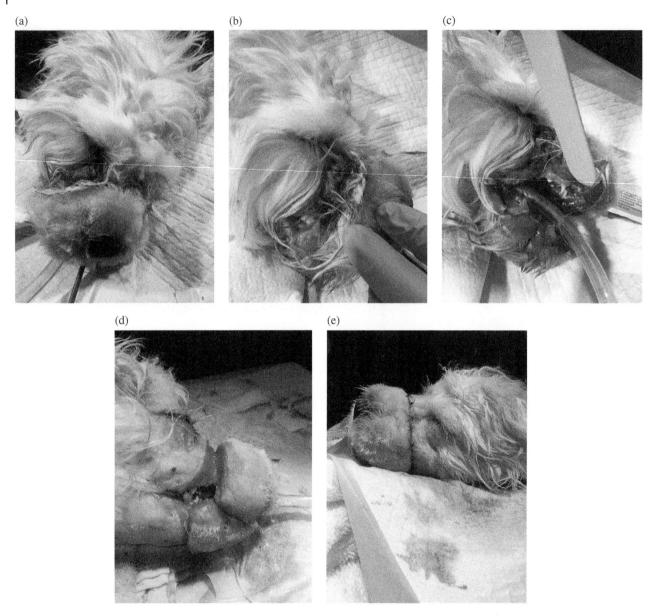

Figure 17.M.7 (a–e) Photographs of patient with muzzle injuries due to a rubber band being left in place maliciously. (a): dorsal view pre-clip; (b): right lateral view pre-clip; (c): right lateral view with maxillary lip retracted dorsally to assess the maxillary gingiva; (d): Right lateral view post-clip and clean; (e): Left lateral view post-repair. *Source:* Courtesy of Nicole Buote, DVM, DACVS.

subcutaneous tissue and fascia of the dorsal epaxial muscles. Resection of adjacent skin was minimal due to the decreased elasticity of the patient's skin and size of the wound. This patient went on to heal uneventfully with no functional limb abnormalities, but full extension of the pelvic limbs was still decreased.

Clinical Lessons

While the author has seen constrictive wounds from inappropriate bandages and leashes/rubber bands, etc., I chose the primary case above because iatrogenic constriction due to surgical procedures may be unanticipated and therefore undetected. The distal limbs are at exceptional risk of this injury due to the unforgiving skin with little ability to stretch with swelling. The use of MLT in these cases is probably underperformed and clinicians should have multiple therapies available when treating these wounds.

(a)

(b)

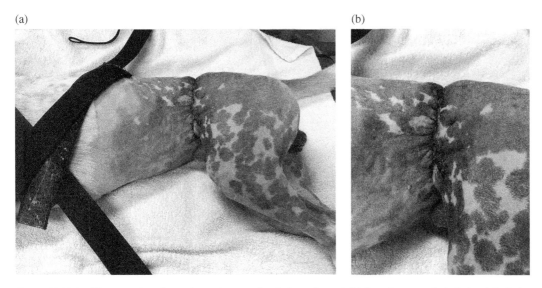

Figure 17.M.8   Photographs of a patient who sustained circumferential injury due to a chain being left tied around his waist for many weeks. (a): global view shows location of wound in referenced to prepuce and caudal abdomen. (b): close-up view of surgical repair. *Source:* Courtesy of Nicole Buote, DVM, DACVS.

References

1 Buote, N.J. (2014). The use of medical leeches for venous congestion. A review and case report. *Vet. Comp. Orthop. Traumatol.* 27 (3): 173–178.

2 Brisson, B.A. and Théoret, M.C. (2008). Osteolysis of the radius and ulna induced by a circumferential foreign body in a cat. *J. Am. Vet. Med. Assoc.* 233 (7): 1117–1120.

3 Stelmach, D., Sharma, A., Rosselli, D., and Schmiedt, C. (2014). Circumferential cervical rubber band foreign body diagnosis in a dog using computed tomography. *Can. Vet. J.* 55 (10): 961–964.

4 Westermeyer, H.D., Tobias, K.M., and Reel, D.R. (2009). Head and neck swelling due to a circumferential cicatricial scar in a dog. *J. Am. Anim. Hosp. Assoc.* 45 (1): 48–51.

17

Specific Wounds

Subsection N: Preputial Reconstruction – Hypospadia Case Study

Galina Hayes

Department of Clinical Sciences, Cornell University, Ithaca, NY, USA

Presenting Signs

An 18-month-old intact male Labrador retriever was presented with a history of chronic trauma and intermittent injury to the penile tip secondary to congenital hypospadia. Routine castration had been performed at six months of age. There was no history of urinary tract infections, and the dog was reported to pass a normal urine stream without difficulty.

Examination and Wound Characteristics

Physical exam was unremarkable apart from the penis/preputial area. Urinary function and urethral anatomy were relatively normal, although the urethral orifice was located on the ventral aspect of the penis, close to the penile tip. The penis was short and angled ventrocaudaly. An area of mucosal tissue was present cranial to the penis, containing the longitudinal folds typical of the preputial mucosa (Figure 17.N.1a,b). The scrotum was absent, but at least one testicle could be palpated caudal to the base of the penis.

Diagnostics

CBC, serum chemistry profile, and urinalysis were unremarkable. Focal urinary ultrasound revealed no additional anatomic abnormalities of the urinary tract. Both testes could be identified on ultrasound in the inguinal area, external to the abdominal cavity.

Surgical Procedure

The patient was positioned in dorsal recumbency and clipped and prepared for aseptic surgery. A urethral catheter was placed. The island of preputial mucosa was incised and raised circumferentially, maintaining dorsal midline attachments (Figure 17.N.2). Stay sutures were placed. The testes were then identified in the external inguinal canals, and a routine closed castration was performed (Figure 17.N.3). The paired retractor penis muscles were identified and found to be shortened and contracted, creating the caudal and ventral deviation of the penis. These were transected, allowing the penis to be returned to a more normal position (Figure 17.N.4). The preputial mucosa was closed in two layers into an inverted tube around the penis, starting at the penile base (Video 17.N.1 ☺) (Figure 17.N.5). The abdominal skin was then closed in two

Techniques in Small Animal Wound Management, First Edition. Edited by Nicole J. Buote.
© 2024 John Wiley & Sons, Inc. Published 2024 by John Wiley & Sons, Inc.
Companion website: www.wiley.com/go/buote/wounds

(a)

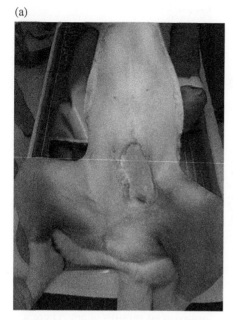

(b)

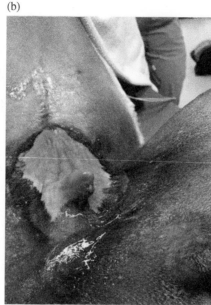

Figure 17.N.1   (a and b) Ventral abdomen showing the abnormal penis and preputial mucosa. *Source:* Courtesy of Galina Hayes, BVSc, DVSc, PhD, DACVECC, DACVS.

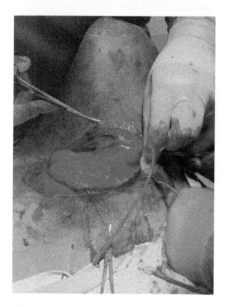

Figure 17.N.2   Island of preputial mucosa circumferentially incised while maintaining dorsal attachments. *Source:* Courtesy of Galina Hayes, BVSc, DVSc, PhD, DACVECC, DACVS.

layers cranially on the midline and then apposed circumferentially around the new preputial orifice (Figure 17.N.6) leaving a defect at the base of the penis. A flank fold flap was then marked and raised from the cranial aspect of the left thigh (Figure 17.N.7a,b). Stay sutures were placed in the tip of the flap and the soft tissues at the base were progressively released until the desired coverage was achieved (Figure 17.N.8a,b). The flap was then sutured in place in the new position in a two-layer appositional closure at the margin and with several simple interrupted sutures placed on the deep surface of the flap while avoiding the urethra (Figure 17.N.9a,b). Routine postoperative analgesic coverage was provided using opioids and an NSAID and an indwelling urinary catheter was maintained for the first 12 hours postoperatively. Following removal, the dog was able to urinate without difficulty and was discharged on the first postoperative day with a 5-day course of carprofen (2 mg/kg bid).

Outcome

The incisions had healed well by suture removal 14 days later (Figure 17.N.10).

Prognosis

This dog's long-term prognosis is excellent given that appropriate coverage of the delicate penile mucosa has been achieved.

Clinical Lessons

Hypospadia can have a range of clinical presentations, and the reconstruction approach, if one is needed, should be tailored to the clinical concerns of each patient. Excellent results can be achieved with careful planning.

Figure 17.N.3   Right testicle being exteriorized from the inguinal canal – the cremaster muscle is about to be incised. *Source:* Courtesy of Galina Hayes, BVSc, DVSc, PhD, DACVECC, DACVS.

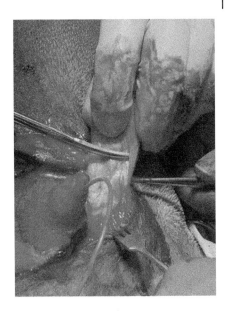

Figure 17.N.4   The penis is now in a more normal orientation, and the preputial mucosa is starting to be closed into an inverted tube starting around the penile base. *Source:* Courtesy of Galina Hayes, BVSc, DVSc, PhD, DACVECC, DACVS.

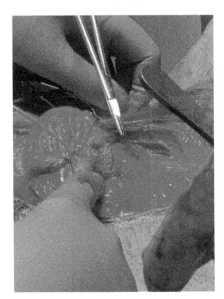

Figure 17.N.5   Completed closure of the preputial mucosa to achieve penile coverage. *Source:* Courtesy of Galina Hayes, BVSc, DVSc, PhD, DACVECC, DACVS.

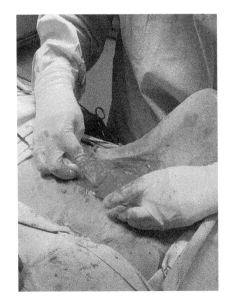

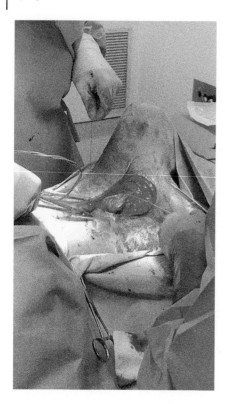

Figure 17.N.6   The skin of the abdominal wall was then closed in two layers cranial to the prepuce prior to apposition circumferentially around the new preputial orifice. *Source:* Courtesy of Galina Hayes, BVSc, DVSc, PhD, DACVECC, DACVS.

(a)

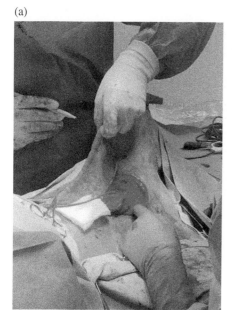

(b)

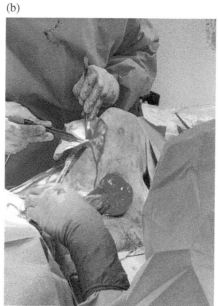

Figure 17.N.7   (a and b) Following partial closure of the cranial aspect of the prepuce, a flank fold flap was raised from the cranial aspect of the left thigh and boundaries marked. This was used to close the caudal wound. *Source:* Courtesy of Galina Hayes, BVSc, DVSc, PhD, DACVECC, DACVS.

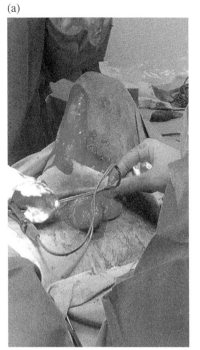

Figure 17.N.8   (a and b) The flank
fold flap was progressively mobilized
from the base until the desired
coverage around the caudal aspect of
the reconstructed prepuce was
achieved. The donor site was then
closed routinely in two layers. *Source:*
Courtesy of Galina Hayes, BVSc, DVSc,
PhD, DACVECC, DACVS.

(a)

(b)

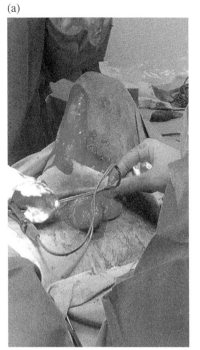
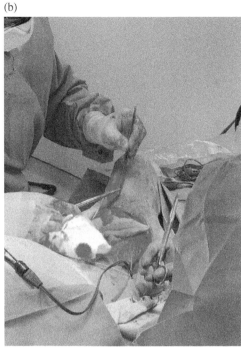

Figure 17.N.9   (a and b) Placement
of the flap and closure in the new
position. *Source:* Courtesy of Galina
Hayes, BVSc, DVSc, PhD,
DACVECC, DACVS.

(a)

(b)

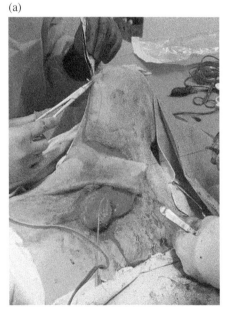
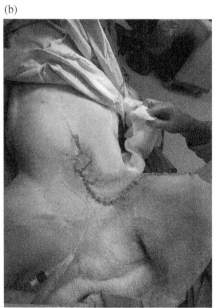

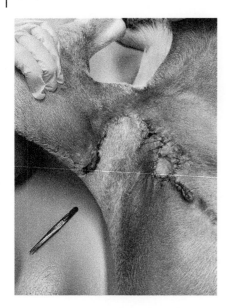

Figure 17.N.10 Clinical appearance at suture removal 14 days postoperatively.
Source: Courtesy of Galina Hayes, BVSc, DVSc, PhD, DACVECC, DACVS.

Index

Note: *Italic* page numbers refer to *figures* and **Bold** page numbers refer to **tables**.

Techniques in Small Animal Wound Management, First Edition. Edited by Nicole J. Buote.
© 2024 John Wiley & Sons, Inc. Published 2024 by John Wiley & Sons, Inc.
Companion website: www.wiley.com/go/buote/wounds